THE KNEE

Form, Function, Pathology, and Treatment

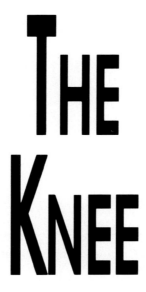

THE KNEE

Form, Function, Pathology, and Treatment

edited by

Robert L. Larson, M.D.
Clinical Professor of Surgery
Division of Orthopedics and Rehabilitation
School of Medicine
Oregon Health Sciences University
Portland, Oregon
Private Practice
Orthopedic and Fracture Clinic
Eugene, Oregon

William A. Grana, M.D.
Clinical Professor
Department of Orthopedic Surgery
and Rehabilitation
University of Oklahoma College of Medicine
Medical Director
Oklahoma Center for Athletes
Oklahoma City, Oklahoma

W. B. SAUNDERS COMPANY
Harcourt Brace Jovanovich, Inc.
Philadelphia   London   Toronto   Montreal   Sydney   Tokyo

W. B. SAUNDERS COMPANY
Harcourt Brace Jovanovich, Inc.

The Curtis Center
Independence Square West
Philadelphia, Pennsylvania 19106

Library of Congress Cataloging-in-Publication Data

The knee: form, function, pathology, and treatment / [edited by] Robert L. Larson, William A. Grana.

p. cm.

ISBN 0–7216–3495–8

1. Knee—Wounds and injuries.   2. Knee—Wounds and injuries—Surgery.   3. Knee—Diseases.   4. Knee—Surgery.   I. Larson, Robert L.   II. Grana, William A. [DNLM: 1. Joint Diseases—therapy.   2. Knee—physiology.   3. Knee Injuries—therapy. WE 870 K6748]

RD561.K575 1993   617.5'82—dc20   92–7915

The Knee: Form, Function, Pathology, and Treatment   ISBN 0–7216–3495–8

Printed in the United States of America.

Last digit is the print number: 9   8   7   6   5   4   3   2   1

Contributors

GREGORY W. BRICK, FACS
Clinical Instructor, Harvard Medical School; Orthopedic Surgeon, Brigham and Women's Hospital, West Roxbury Veterans Administration Hospital, Boston, Massachusetts
Arthritis and Arthroplasty

ROBERT S. BURGER, M.D.
Assistant Clinical Professor, Orthopaedic Surgery, University of California, Davis Medical Center; Attending Orthopaedic Surgeon, Kaiser Permanente Medical Center, Sacramento, California
Acute Dislocations
Acute Ligamentous Injury
Chronic Anterior, Anterolateral, and Anteromedial Instability

W. DILWORTH CANNON, JR., M.D.
Professor of Clinical Orthopaedic Surgery and Director of Sports Medicine, University of California, San Francisco
Problems of the Menisci and Their Treatment

JOHN C. GARRETT, M.D.
Assistant Clinical Professor, Emory University School of Medicine, Atlanta, Georgia
Osteochondral Allografts for Reconstruction of Articular Defects
Osteochondritis Dissecans

WILLIAM A. GRANA, M.D.
Clinical Professor, Department of Orthopedic Surgery and Rehabilitation, University of Oklahoma College of Medicine; Medical Direc-
tor, Oklahoma Center for Athletes, Oklahoma City, Oklahoma
Functional and Surgical Anatomy
Physiologic and Biomechanical Considerations
Diagnostic Evaluation
Extra-Articular and Overuse Problems
Rehabilitation
Patellofemoral Pain Problems
Chronic Posterior and Posterolateral Laxity
Allograft and Synthetic Reconstruction of the Ligaments of the Knee

JONATHAN GREENLEAF, M.D.
Staff Orthopedist, Cook Clinic, Tualatin; Attending Surgeon, The Shriner's Hospital for Crippled Children, Portland, Oregon
Complications in Arthroscopic and Ligamentous Knee Surgery

ROBERT L. LARSON, M.D.
Clinical Professor of Surgery, Division of Orthopedics and Rehabilitation, School of Medicine, Oregon Health Sciences University, Portland, Oregon
Introduction and Historical Perspective
Functional and Surgical Anatomy
Clinical Evaluation
Evaluation and Decision Making for Ligamentous Injury
Acute Dislocations
Acute Ligamentous Injury
Chronic Anterior, Anterolateral, and Anteromedial Instability
Complications in Arthroscopic and Ligamentous Knee Surgery

JOHN F. MEYERS, M.D.
Clinical Associate Professor in Orthopaedic Surgery, Medical College

of Virginia; Director, Orthopaedic Research of Virginia, Richmond, Virginia
Arthroscopy

H. DAVID MOEHRING, M.D.
Assistant Professor of Clinical Orthopaedic Surgery, University of California at Davis; Staff, University of California at Davis Medical Center, Sutter General Hospital, Mercy General Hospital, Sacramento; Mercy Hospital, Folsom, California
Regional Fractures of the Knee

DEMPSEY S. SPRINGFIELD, M.D.
Associate Professor of Orthopaedics, Harvard Medical School, Cambridge; Visiting Orthopaedic Surgeon, Massachusetts General Hospital, Boston, Massachusetts
Tumors and Their Treatment

J. ANDY SULLIVAN, M.D.
Professor, Vice-Chair, Chief of Pediatric Orthopedics, Department of Orthopedic Surgery and Rehabilitation, University of Oklahoma, College of Medicine; Chief, Pedi-

atric Orthopedics, Children's Hospital of Oklahoma, Oklahoma City, Oklahoma
Congenital and Developmental Problems of the Knee
Infectious and Inflammatory Processes of the Knee

THOMAS S. THORNHILL, M.D.
Associate Clinical Professor of Orthopedics, Harvard Medical School; Staff, Brigham and Women's Hospital, New England Baptist Hospital, Boston, Massachusetts
Arthritis and Arthroplasty

WILLIAM W. TOMFORD, M.D.
Associate Professor of Orthopaedics, Harvard Medical School, Cambridge; Associate Orthopaedic Surgeon, Massachusetts General Hospital, Boston, Massachusetts
Tumors and Their Treatment

PAUL J. TSAHAKIS, M.D.
Chief, Arthritis Research, Carolinas Medical Center, Miller Orthopaedic Clinic, Charlotte, North Carolina
Arthritis and Arthroplasty

Preface

The knee has been a challenge to the practicing physician over the years. The complexity of its motion, the occasional controversy and confusion over diagnosis and treatment, the necessity for functional stability in athletic endeavors, and the importance of this joint for everyday activities are evidence of the need for continual update in knowledge that focuses on this joint. The enormity of the task of treating knee problems has produced a compartmentalization of information into specialized texts, each dealing with a different aspect of knee pathology. The purpose of this text is to provide a consolidation of information about the knee that will aid physicians whether their interests are general orthopaedics, sports medicine, pediatric orthopaedics, or joint replacement.

We have attempted to provide information on all aspects of the anatomy and physiology—the form—of the knee; to elicit an understanding of the biomechanics and function of the knee in everyday activity, as well as in strenuous work and athletic activities; to present the pathologic conditions that beset the knee (developmental and congenital, tumorous, infectious and inflammatory, and traumatic, especially that frequent initiator of knee dysfunction, sports trauma); and to render a treatment protocol for these problems with modern concepts that integrate all of these factors.

We have been privileged and honored by the contributions of several authors who have been called upon to provide their expertise in special aspects of knee pathology. The individual chapters that present the knowledge accumulated by these authorities on their selected topics provide the reader with the most up-to-date methods of diagnosis and treatment for the many pathologic conditions of the knee. We are extremely appreciative and grateful for the dedication and detail that these contributors have brought to their task.

We recognize that no treatise can be everything to everyone. Readers who desire more detailed information about particular topics will find extensive references for each chapter.

The knee has afforded us the major portion of our livelihood over the years of orthopaedic practice. It is, therefore, with a certain sense of indebtedness that this text is produced. The quotation, from whom we know not, "authors never finish a book, they merely abandon it" reflects the frustration encountered in supplying the most recent and modern technology available. It is our modest hope that we have produced a reference that is useful and practical for readers whose chief or partial livelihood may also depend on the treatment of problems of the knee.

Robert L. Larson, M.D.
William A. Grana, M.D.

Contents

CHAPTER 14

CHAPTER 15

CHAPTER 16

CHAPTER 17

PART IV
Orthopaedic Sports Traumatology: Laxity of the Knee..... 489

THE KNEE

Form, Function, Pathology, and Treatment

PART I

Basic

Considerations

■

CHAPTER 1

Introduction and Historical Perspective

ROBERT L. LARSON, M.D.

∎

Attention given to injuries of the knee has provoked considerable interest, not only because of the publicity that top athletes receive after such injuries, but also because of the personal involvement by the growing number of recreational athletes as well as patients who have experienced wear changes in the knees that require operative intervention such as total knee replacements. The understanding of the biomechanics of the knee has been considerably refined, the anatomic structure has become better appreciated, and both the ability to diagnose problems of the knee joint and the treatment of these conditions have improved dramatically. Noninvasive procedures such as computerized axial tomography (CAT scan), magnetic resonance imaging (MRI), radioactive bone scans, and ultrasonography of the soft tissues have provided physicians with the ability to evaluate the bone and the soft tissue around the knee with a thoroughness not possible in the past. Arthroscopic evaluation of the knee, arthroscopic surgery of the knee, total knee replacement, whole allograft replacement surgery, and newer techniques of knee ligament surgery attest to the modernization in the treatment of knee maladies.

Complexities of knee joint function allow balance at rest and during walking, running, jumping, and kicking. The knee is a vital part of the lower extremity linkage mechanism that provides a propulsion and re-straining mechanism and a stable pedestal for power of body movements, and yet it allows for adaptation to sudden changes in movement forces or rapid changes in direction, acceleration, or deceleration.[10] The exposed position of the knee and the lack of any efficient protective device that allows all of the functions just listed to occur effectively are conducive to frequent injuries to this joint in athletic participation; in some sports, it is knee injuries that most frequently result in a loss of ability to participate.

The knee joint is also exposed to the constant impact load of daily activity. Constitutional factors not yet understood cause wear changes in the articular cartilage that lead to pain, disability, and malfunction. Although such degenerative changes may be produced or enhanced by trauma, there is no way to equate the trauma and the resultant degener-ative change that develops. Malalignment from either congenital or de-velopmental causes may lead to abnormality of function or increased wear of the joint surfaces. The extensor mechanism, including patellofemoral articulation, is particularly vulnerable to such malalignment abnormalities, which may produce pain with use or a functional disability.

This joint, like others, is vulnerable to fracture, systemic conditions, infections, tumors, and other conditions that sometimes defy specific categorization.

HISTORICAL REVIEW

Hippocrates provided medical practitioners with an awareness of muscle and joint function: "that which is used develops, and that which is not wastes away." Galen[8] first described the anatomy of the knee, and his description included the anterior cruciate ligament (ACL). He recognized the importance of ligaments as supporting structures that help stabilize the joint and restrict abnormal motion. The dynamics of knee motion were introduced by the Weber brothers of Gottingen and Leipzig in a treatise published in 1836.[3] They described the mechanics of joint motion and helped clarify the functions of important intra-articular and periartic-ular components.

Meyer of Zurich in 1873 recognized and described the "screw move-ment" of the knee joint. This important concept introduced the notion of the rotation aspect produced by the inequality of the femoral condyles that convert the knee joint from a muscular ligament-supported mecha-nism to a weight-bearing skeletal structure. As indicated by Bick,[3] "These anatomic studies established the function of the several components of the joints—the cruciate ligaments, the intra-articular fibrocartilage, and the lateral ligaments." In 1941, Brantigan and Voshell[5] provided an extensive review of the literature and a study of the knee joint in 100 cadaver specimens and concluded, "A comprehensive review of the literature reveals no unanimity of the opinion concerning the function of the knee-joint ligaments, and often equivocal statements are made. A study of the literatures leaves one bewildered."

Early treatment of knee disorders was focused on septic conditions such as tuberculosis. A quotation by Crowther in 1797 suggests the frustration experienced in the handling of such problems: "Patients afflicted with white-swelling are often encouraged by practitioners to hope that the complaint may terminate in ankylosis; but this, unfortunately, is a very infrequent occurrence, and cannot reasonably be expected; whilst the disease is suffered to proceed."[3]

The first surgical correction of a knee dysfunction was probably performed by Paré, who in 1558 first reported the removal of a loose body within the joint. Although Hippocrates had recognized mechanical de-rangements of the knee, it was not until 1784 that the term "internal derangement of the knee joint" was used by William Hey of Leeds to categorize this group of problems that interfere with knee motion. Surgery was not a popular method of treatment because of the high frequency of postoperative infections and because the search for the loose body fre-quently took more time than was available before the advent of anesthesia. Even Hey advocated conservative treatment by prolonged immobilization.[3]

The first surgical removal of a displaced medial meniscus was per-formed by Brodhurst in 1866. Arthrotomy was popularized by Annandale, the successor to Lister at the University of Edinburgh. In 1879, he published on removal of "loose cartilages" in the knee joint with antiseptic precautions. Allingham described several modifications in the technique of arthrotomy and in 1889 reported a method of suturing the loose meniscus in place rather than excising it.[3]

Until Annandale's introduction of antiseptic precautions in knee joint surgery, attempts at surgical treatment of knee joint problems had been confined to the drainage of septic joints. *Pathology and Surgery of Diseases of the Joint* by Brodie, published in 1819, was the standard monograph on the subject during the first half of the 19th century. New techniques were gradually introduced. One of the first was synovectomy for the treatment of nontubercular chronic arthritis. Goldthwait first introduced this opera-tion in the United States in 1900, although it had been used in Europe by Volkman earlier for tuberculosis of the joint. It was recognized that this treatment was not adequate for tubercular infection of the knee joint. Partial synovectomy, however, became a frequent part of knee operations.[3]

Arthrodesis of the knee joint was introduced by Albert of Vienna in 1878 as a means to eliminate the use of braces in the presence of instability of the lower extremities, especially the knee. Other indications for its use became evident, and in 1911 Hibbs fused a knee joint destroyed by tuberculosis.[3]

Arthroplasty of the knee joint was first used in an attempt to prevent fusion of a resected joint and later to restore motion of a fused joint. Verneuil in 1860 first introduced the concept of interposing soft tissue between resected bone ends to prevent fusion. Ollier published a report on the interposition of soft tissues in the noninfected joint in 1885. The technique was introduced in the United States by Murphy of Chicago in 1902, who used a pedicle flap of para-articular fat and fascia in the knee. During this period, many surgeons used foreign materials because of the resorption of autogenous tissue.[3]

A new era of knee joint surgery began in 1925, when Smith-Petersen used prefabricated molds as interposition material for arthroplasty. Other surgeons used materials such as glass (Pyrex), viscaloid, Bakelite, and Vitallium after its introduction by Venable and Stuck. Campbell reported in 1940 on the use of Vitallium plates made to conform to the condyles of the femur for arthroplasty of the knee.[3] The validity of total joint replacement was thus inaugurated.

Other techniques to surgically treat knee problems were introduced in the late 1800s and early 1900s. In 1850, Heller treated recurrent dislocation of the patella by scarifying the medial capsule in order to produce contracture of the tissues, which would induce stabilization. In 1899, Hoffa described reefing of the soft tissues parallel to the patellar tendon, and in 1904, Goldthwait, using a split patellar tendon, brought the outer half beneath the medial half to provide such stabilization. In 1916, Jones described a more aggressive treatment of elevating and wedging forward the lateral femoral condyle, and Albee added a bone graft to this procedure in order to maintain the position as a means of preventing recurrent patellar dislocation.[3]

The recognition and treatment of an ACL injury was first reported by Stark in 1850.[17] Cast immobilization was used. Battle[2] and Robson[14] reported on surgical repair of the ACL performed 2 and 8 years earlier. In 1906, Hogarth and Pringle reported on the reattachment of the anterior tibial spine after its avulsion with the ACL.[3] In 1913, Goetjes wrote a detailed paper on the mechanism of rupture of the ACL, as determined from cadaver studies.[15] He advocated surgical repair for fresh injuries, replacement of avulsed tibial spine injuries, and conservative treatment for the neglected case. He also introduced examination under anesthesia for difficult diagnostic problems.

The concept of reconstruction of the ACL was introduced by Hey Groves (Fig. 1–1) in 1917.[9] He used a band of the iliotibial tract detached from its tibial insertion and directed through drill holes in the femur and the tibia that matched the attachment sites of the normal ACL.

Collateral ligament injuries were generally treated by cast immobilization. The significance of associated collateral and cruciate injuries was not appreciated. Alwyn Smith,[1] a contemporary of Hey Groves, modified the operation of Hey Groves by bringing the end of the graft, after its passage through the tibial drill hole, up toward the medial femoral condyle in order to reinforce the medial collateral ligament in old injuries. He also advanced the sartorius insertion. In 1936, Campbell[6] recognized the frequent association of a torn medial meniscus, a torn medial collateral

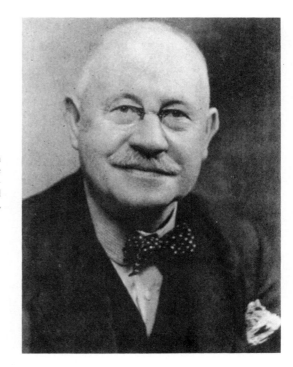

FIGURE 1–1. Ernest W. Hey Groves, M.D., English physician who first described the intra-articular reconstruction of the anterior cruciate ligament in 1917. (Reproduced with permission from the Editor of the *British Journal of Surgery* and by permission of the publishers, Butterworth-Heinemann Ltd, London, England.)

ligament, and a torn ACL. At this time, he also introduced a reconstruction of the ACL in which a strip of patellar tendon was directed through tibial and femoral drill holes.

The first extra-articular approach to resolve an ACL deficiency was described by Bosworth and Bosworth[4] in 1936. They used free fascial lata grafts woven in cruciate manner on the medial or lateral side of the knee.

In 1938, Ivar Palmer (Fig. 1–2) wrote a comprehensive treatise entitled *On the Injuries to the Ligaments of the Knee Joint.*[13] The anatomy, biomechanics, and pathology and treatment of knee ligament injuries, as well as the current state of the art in evaluation and treatment, were reviewed, and newer concepts of the biomechanics after injury and methods of surgical treatment were provided. This work was monumental in contributing a modern philosophy to the topic of ligamentous injury to the knee.

In the United States in 1950, the published results of O'Donoghue (Fig. 1–3) provided the stimulus to reevaluate the treatment of knee ligament injuries.[11] By documenting good results and advocating repair of torn ligament tissue by using the example of the triad of meniscal injury, torn medial collateral ligament, and torn ACL, he disproved the then-held concept that such injuries tend to be devastating and therefore should be treated by conservative measures.

The historical perspective of the treatment of knee problems would not be complete without mention of two other developments that have had significant impact. The first was the introduction of chemotherapeutic agents to treat infection. Since 1908, sulfonamide derivatives had been the subject of experimentation and trial, but the introduction of the use of sulfonamide as an effective chemotherapeutic agent by Domagk in 1935 initiated the "greatest contribution to orthopedic surgery as to the entire field of surgery in this generation and overshadowing by far all other

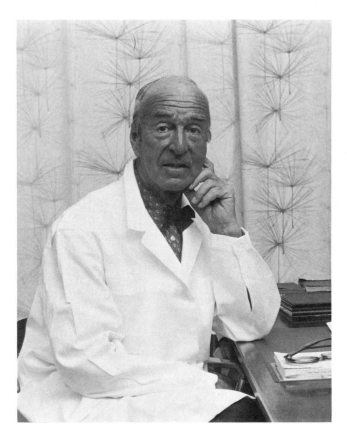

FIGURE 1–2. Ivar Palmer, M.D., Swedish surgeon whose 1938 thesis *On the Injuries to the Ligaments of the Knee Joint* contributed to the modern concepts on the functional anatomy, biomechanics, and pathology and treatment of knee ligament problems. (From Eriksson E: Ivar Palmer: A great name in the history of cruciate ligament surgery. Clin Orthop 172:3, 1983.)

considerations."[3] Antibiotics not only took away infections of the joints as one of the major preoccupations of the orthopaedic surgeon but also provided more safety in surgery and an acceptable treatment method should postoperative infection occur.

The second development that has allowed considerable improvement in the ability to treat orthopaedic conditions is the progress in diagnosis of conditions affecting the knee joint. The evolution of this progress began with the improvement of radiologic diagnosis, especially arthrography. In the early 1900s, Rauenbusch injected the knee joint with oxygen in order to see defects and lesions of the menisci and cartilage. Werndorff and Robinson repeated the use of the gas arthrogram of the knee in 1905. Further attempts at this procedure were made, but the results continued to be inadequate, and one fatal air embolism resulted from its use.[3] Double-contrast arthrography was described in 1930 by Bricher and Oberholzer. It was not until the introduction of water-soluble media and better technical developments in radiology in the late 1950s that arthrographic outcomes became more predictable and the technique became popular.[16]

In 1918, Takagi in Japan attempted to actually visualize the interior of the knee joint with the use of a cystoscope.[18] A practical arthroscope, developed in 1931, enabled Watanabe in 1955 to perform the first successful arthroscopic surgery: the removal of a benign tumor of the knee. Researchers in Europe and the United States were also investigating these

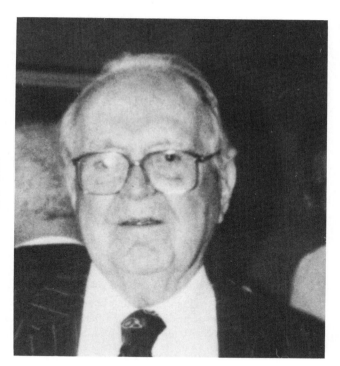

FIGURE 1–3. Don H. O'Donoghue, M.D., orthopaedist from Oklahoma City who advocated and in 1950 reported on the surgical treatment of acute knee ligament injuries in athletes. His reports provided the impetus for research and treatment for ligament disruption, particularly in athletes.

techniques. In Europe, Bircher reported in 1922 on the use of the Jacobaeus laparoscope introduced into the articular cavities of 32 patients before operation on a diseased joint and confirmed the diagnoses in all. In the United States, Kreuscher in 1925 and Burman, Mayer, and Finkelstein in 1931 reported on the direct visualization of joints by the use of the arthroscope.[16] Fiberoptics enabled the development of smaller and self-focusing arthroscopes, which were introduced in 1970. The explosion in the development of arthroscopic equipment and in improvements in techniques and surgical procedures has made arthroscopy the orthopaedic procedure most commonly performed.

Modern concepts relating to the biomechanics, biochemistry, and physiology of articular cartilage are being developed. It has become evident that biochemical and enzymatic changes occur in the knee joint as responses to disease, trauma, and wear. The ability of the proteoglycans to absorb water, which is a natural process of articular metabolism, is interfered with by any insult to the articular cartilage. An increase in neutral proteinases, such as collagenase, occurs in osteoarthritis, in rheumatoid arthritis,[7] and as a response to artificial ligament wear particles produced in the joint when these devices are used.[12] Studies in these areas represent yet another facet of investigation to help in understanding the pathophysiologic processes of the knee joint.

PHILOSOPHY OF THE TREATMENT OF KNEE PROBLEMS

The ability to better diagnose knee problems and the improvement in many treatment modalities have led to a consensus of the appropriate management of many knee disorders. Arthrodesis of the knee for degenerative or rheumatoid joint disease is rarely used because of the success of total joint replacement. The nonoperative management of isolated medial collateral ligament tears has proved to be as effective as surgical repair. This conclusion is possible because of the arthroscopic diagnosis of the extent of injury. ACL reconstruction techniques have provided an improvement in joint function in patients with a functional disability. The early rehabilitation in nearly all knee surgeries has provided a lessening of morbidity rates and an early return to the activities of daily living.

There still remain areas in which reliable and reproducible results have not occurred. Problems of the patellofemoral joint remain enigmas without a readily identifiable solution. Intra-articular ligament surgery, although providing functional improvement, has yet to produce reconstruction so that the ligament is as strong or biomechanically adept as it was originally. There is, therefore, a continuing quest for final solutions to the many problems that beset the knee.

The surgeon who performs knee surgery is challenged by the congenital, traumatic, degenerative, infectious, metabolic, and tumorous conditions that occur in the knee. A constant update of information and a rethinking of indications and treatment are appropriate.

REFERENCES

1. Alwyn Smith S: The diagnosis and treatment of injuries to the crucial ligaments. Brit J Surg 6:176–189, 1917.
2. Battle WH: A case after open section of the knee joint for irreducible traumatic dislocation. Clin Soc London Trans 33:232, 1900.
3. Bick EM: Source Book of Orthopaedics. Baltimore: Williams and Wilkins, 1948.
4. Bosworth DM, Bosworth BM: Use of fascia lata to stabilize the knee in cases of ruptured crucial ligaments. J Bone Joint Surg 18A:178–179, 1936.
5. Brantigan OC, Voshell AF: The mechanics of the ligaments and menisci of the knee joint. J Bone Joint Surg 23:44–66, 1941.
6. Campbell WC: Repair of ligaments of the knee. Surg Gynecol Obstet 62:964–968, 1936.
7. Evans CH, Mears DC, Cosgrove JL: Release of neutral proteinases from mononuclear phagocytes and synovial cells in response to cartilagenase wear particles in vitro. Biochem Biophys Acta 677:287–294, 1981.
8. Galen C: On the Usefulness of the Parts of the Body (May MT, trans). Ithaca, NY: Cornell University Press, 1968.
9. Hey Groves EW: Operation for the repair of the crucial ligaments. Lancet 11:674, 1917. (Reprinted in Clin Orthop 147:4–6, 1980.)
10. Nicholas JA: Glossary of sports maneuvers in which the knee is immediately involved. Presented at The Injured Knee in Sports: Special Reference to the Surgical Knee. Eugene, OR: American Academy of Orthopaedic Surgeons Postgraduate Course, July 1973.
11. O'Donoghue DH: Surgical treatment of fresh injuries to the major ligaments of the knee. J Bone Joint Surg 32A:721–738, 1950.
12. Olson EJ, Kang JD, Fu FH, et al: The biochemical and histological effects of artificial ligament wear particles: in vitro and in vivo studies. Am J Sports Med 16:558–570, 1988.
13. Palmer I: On the injuries to the ligaments of the knee joint—a clinical study. Acta Chir Scand 81 (Suppl 53):2–282, 1938.
14. Robson MAW: Ruptured crucial ligaments and their repair by operations. Ann Surg 37:716, 1903.
15. Snook GA: A short history of the anterior cruciate ligament and the treatment of tears. Clin Orthop 172:11–13, 1983.
16. Snook GA: The ACL: a historical review. In Feagin JA (ed): The Crucial Ligaments, pp. 157–160. New York: Churchill-Livingstone, 1988.
17. Stark J: Two cases of rupture of the crucial ligament of the knee-joint. Edinb Med Surg 74:267, 1850.
18. Watanabe M, Takeda S, Ikeuchi H: Atlas of Arthroscopy. New York: Springer-Verlag, 1969.

CHAPTER 2

Functional and Surgical Anatomy

WILLIAM A. GRANA, M.D.

ROBERT L. LARSON, M.D.

■

In order to repair an acute injury of the knee or to devise reconstructive procedures to improve knee stability, a surgeon must understand the basic supporting structures, the surrounding musculature, and the three-dimensional motion of the knee.

To describe the knee in a static anatomic sense is analogous to describing a tornado as an atmospheric change in air pressure. The knee is composed not of ligaments, bone, and muscle alone but of a series of dynamic guy wires, cams, and articulating processes; thus it is an integrated mechanism that produces multiplane motion that is stable with function (Fig. 2–1). Therefore, the knee enables motion of different complexity for the different physical demands of such activities as walking, running, jumping, and kicking, and yet it is stable in all these activities (Fig. 2–2).

Functional stability of the knee is provided by both passive and active stabilizers. The passive stabilizers include the ligaments around the knee, the osseous structures, and the menisci. The active stabilizers are the muscles that surround the knee.

Palmer[59] described the knee as a physiologic joint in which all components work toward the integrity of the whole. He also described the ligamentomuscular reflex, which causes the muscles to reflexively

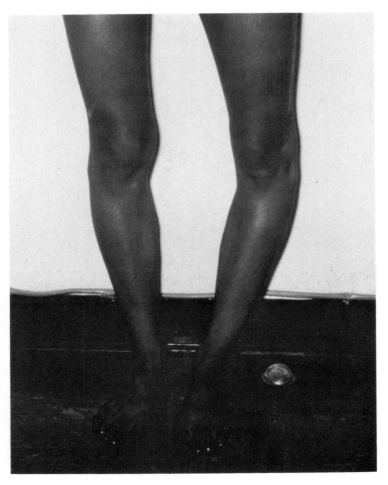

FIGURE 2–1. The muscles, ligaments, and menisci (stability structures) provide an integrated mechanism to produce multiplane motion. When injured, complex deformity occurs, such as the posterolateral laxity and varus deformity depicted here.

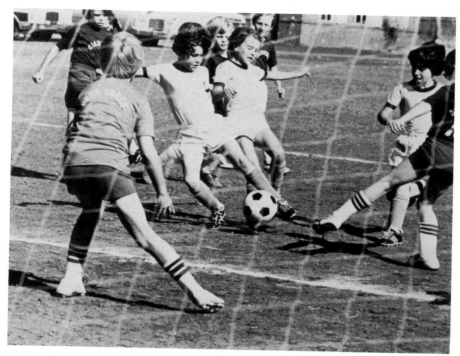

FIGURE 2–2. Sports such as soccer place heavy demands on the knee, hence the need for more complex integration of the anatomic restraints to motion.

tighten as ligamentous tension is produced around the knee. The first line of defense, therefore, is the muscle strength, which helps compress the joint by the increased tone of muscles. Should the muscles fail, the ligaments then act as passive stabilizers to restrict motion beyond the normal limits. However, this muscle reflex is often too slow in response to protect the ligaments against stress when large forces are suddenly applied to the knee, as in an injury.[40] Ligaments that have been stretched or torn enable abnormal motion of the knee and may produce functional deficits that cause disability for the patient in certain activities. When functional use of the knee is limited, the surgeon must consider surgical measures designed to improve stability and to restore knee function.

Although each ligament contributes to the stabilizing function of the other ligaments, individual ligaments have a primary stabilizing role in guiding and restraining certain motions of the knee. The basic supporting structures of the medial side of the knee are the medial retinaculum, the medial collateral ligament (superficial tibiocollateral ligament), the medial capsular ligament, the pes anserinus, and the semimembranosus muscle complex. The posterior aspect derives support from the posterior capsule, ramifications of the semimembranosus muscle (the oblique popliteal ligament), the arcuate ligament, the popliteus muscle, and the ligaments of Wrisberg and Humphry.

On the lateral side of the knee, the important stabilizing structures are the iliotibial tract, the lateral collateral ligament (fibular collateral ligament), the short collateral ligament, the biceps tendon, the popliteus tendon, and the retinacular extension of the vastus lateralis. The anterior and posterior cruciate ligaments prevent abnormal anterior (forward) and posterior (backward) displacement of the tibia on the femur, hyperextension, and excessive rotation.

Internal structures of the knee—the menisci and the cruciate ligaments—contribute to stabilize and help guide the knee through its normal arc of motion. The anterior cruciate ligament (ACL) is like a hub of a wheel, enhancing stabilization both medially and laterally as well as rotationally. Attempts to repair, augment, and replace this vital structure are among the more commonplace procedures in reconstructive knee surgery.[1, 14, 15, 19, 20, 27, 41, 55, 58, 59, 60]

OSSEOUS STRUCTURES

The knee is conveniently classified as three separate joints provided by the osseous structures: the patella, the femoral condyles, and the tibial plateaus. The knee is not a simple hinge; rather, it involves a rotatory component as well as flexion and extension. The femoral condyles glide, rock, and rotate on the tibial plateau as motion occurs.

FEMORAL CONDYLES. The distal end of the femur, which comprises the femoral condyles, is covered with articular cartilage, which is divided into the portion beneath the patella and its articulation and the portion above the tibial plateaus and their articulations by two superficial grooves that run obliquely across the anterior part of the articular surface of each femoral condyle. These grooves, the sulci terminales, may be seen on lateral radiographic views of the knee as shallow indentations in the convex contour of the condyle. As a rule, the sulcus terminalis of the lateral femoral condyle is more distinct than that of the medial femoral condyle and is an identifying landmark of the lateral femoral condyle (Fig. 2–3). The articular surface toward the patella—the patellofemoral groove (trochlea or facies patellaris or sulcus)—spreads over the anterior part of the distal femur, and the bulk of this surface is situated on the lateral condyle, which reaches to a higher level than does the medial condyle. The portion of the femoral condyles that articulates with the tibia (facies tibialis) is divided by the intercondylar fossa into the medial and lateral femoral condyles.

The femoral condyles are eccentrically curved, the anterior portion being part of an oval and the posterior portion part of a sphere. As the knee flexes, the spherical condylar portions articulate with the tibia, which is deepened by the medial and lateral menisci and in essence becomes a modified ball-and-socket joint with limited rotatory motion.

Anteriorly, the condyles are somewhat flattened, the lateral slightly more so than the medial, and this flattening provides a larger surface area for contact and weight transmission. The articular surface of the lateral condyle is longer and wider than that of the medial condyle. The long axis of the lateral condyle is oriented essentially along the sagittal plane, whereas that of the medial condyle is usually at about a 22° angle to the sagittal plane.[45] This asymmetry of construction is essential for the mechanics of knee motion, which is discussed in the "Mechanics of Knee Motion" section (Fig. 2–4). The asymmetry of the knee joint both in design and in motion was studied by Dye and found to exist in the prehistoric tetrapods, which were common ancestors of modern-day reptiles, birds, and mammals.[13] The persistence of such asymmetry

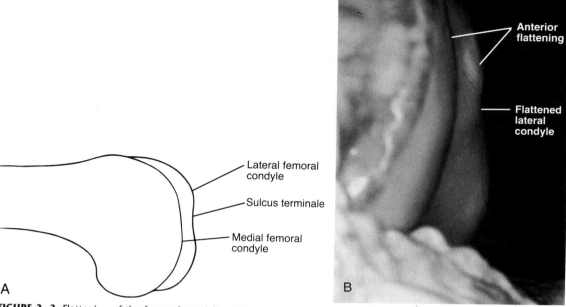

A

B

Lateral femoral condyle

Sulcus terminale

Medial femoral condyle

Anterior flattening

Flattened lateral condyle

FIGURE 2–3. Flattening of the femoral condyle, more prominent on the lateral side and in the anterior portion of each condyle for weight bearing.

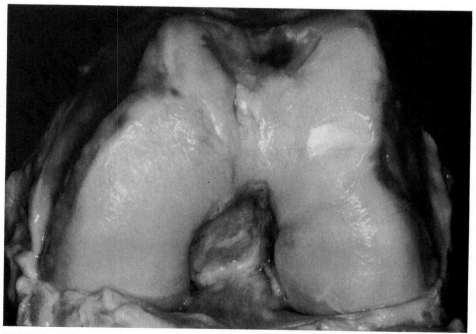

FIGURE 2–4. The asymmetry of the femoral condyle is an essential part of the mechanics of knee motion. Lateral condyle *(right)* is larger than the medial *(left)*.

through an evolutionary period of 320 million years indicates that the knee is a profoundly adaptive biomechanical system that has undergone little modification despite major modifications of functional demand.

TIBIAL PLATEAU. McLeod and associates[53] examined tibial plateau topography to study its contribution toward knee stability. The medial tibial plateau shows no significant concavity when viewed in the coronal plane, whereas the lateral tibial plateau shows a slight concavity. In the sagittal plane, the lateral tibial plateau appears convex, whereas the medial condyle is concave. Neither side of the tibial plateau, according to these topographic studies, provides much assistance in stabilizing the knee.

Other studies, however, have shown that the convexity may help protect the ligaments and the capsule. As the knee is flexed, the lateral femoral condyle is displaced slightly more anteriorly to ride upward on the convexity of the lateral tibial condyle. This upward motion absorbs energy and reduces the requirement of the ligamentous capsule to stabilize the knee. The intercondylar eminence of the tibia aids in this stabilization. The eminence is roughly conical in shape, when viewed from the front, which helps control the amount of rotation possible within the joint. As rotation of the knee occurs, the femur necessarily rides upward on the intercondylar eminence if the supporting structures of the capsule and ligament are intact. With this elevation of the femur, energy is absorbed so as to minimize the load on the capsule and ligaments as rotation occurs (Fig. 2–5).[40]

McLeod and associates[53] suggested that the lateral femoral condyle slides slightly laterally, pulling the medial femoral condyle against the medial tibial spine in order to help maintain stability.

THE PATELLA AND THE PATELLOFEMORAL GROOVE. The patella is a triangular sesamoid bone situated in the extensor mechanism between the quadriceps tendon and the patellar tendon. The proximal wider portion is the base of the patella, and the narrower distal pole is the apex. The articular surface is divided by a vertical ridge, which creates a small

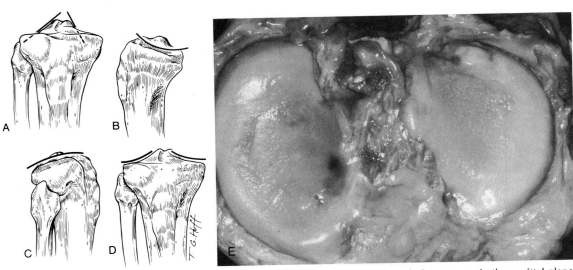

FIGURE 2–5. *(A)* Slope of the intercondylar eminence. *(B)* Concavity of mediolateral plateau seen in the sagittal plane. *(C)* Convexity of lateral tibial plateau in the sagittal plane. *(D)* Coronal view shows slight concavity both medially and laterally. *(E)* Seen from above, the two surfaces provide little stable contact without the menisci and ligaments.

medial and a large lateral articular facet. In addition to the medial and lateral facets, Goodfellow and colleagues[22] described the odd facet on the medial border of the patella, separated from the medial facet by a small ridge (Fig. 2–6). Through movement of the knee from 0° to 90° flexion, a band of contact occurs between the patella and the patellofemoral groove of the femur, from the inferior to the superior pole. During flexion of between 90° and 135°, the patella rotates in the ridge between the medial and odd facets and engages the femoral condyle. At 135° of flexion, the patella slides off the true patellar facets of the femur, and the odd facet makes contact with the femoral condyles and the facies tibialis of the femur. At this degree of flexion, the patella has slipped into the intercondylar notch and rotates about a vertical axis as it shifts laterally. The odd facet engages the medial femoral condyle. The odd facet is thus the only part of the patella that never makes contact with the true patellar facets of the femur and is the only part of the patella that makes contact with the true tibial articular surfaces of the medial femoral condyle of the femur.

During flexion and extension, the patella moves 7 to 8 cm in relation to the femoral condyles. As flexion occurs, contact pressure is shifted from the lateral facet to the medial facet (Fig. 2–7).

The shapes of the patella and of the patellofemoral groove are important components of the extensor mechanism stability. The patellofemoral groove is concave medially to laterally and convex proximally to distally. The lateral aspect of the patellofemoral groove projects higher anteriorly than does the medial aspect, producing a somewhat asymmetric sulcus. The asymmetry of the groove from the proximal portion is well adapted to the triangular shape of the articular surface of the patella. The groove, however, loses its asymmetric shape distally, becoming deeper

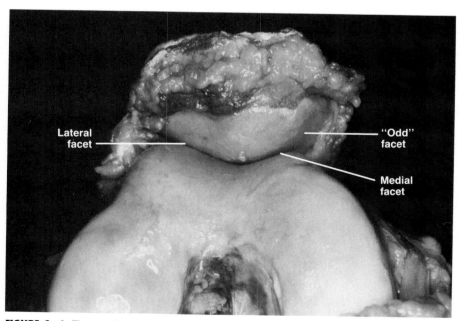

FIGURE 2–6. The smaller medial and larger lateral facets of the patella provide articulation with the trochlear groove of the femur. The odd facet is on the medial side, separated by a ridge from the medial facet.

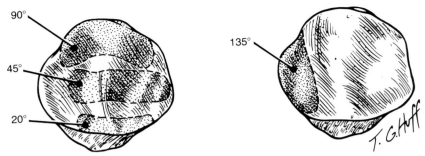

FIGURE 2–7. Femoral contact areas on the patella at 20°, 45°, 90°, and 135° of knee flexion.

and wider. The protection provided by the high lateral femoral condyle in the proximal portion of the groove against lateral displacement is replaced by the deepening of the groove distally until the sulcus terminalis is approached at the boundary between the articular surface of the patella and the articular surface of the tibia on the femoral condyles.

Wiberg[80] first described three patellar configurations. This description was later expanded by F. Baumgartl (Das Knieglenk, Berlin, Springer-Verlag, 1944) to include six basic types. Type I consists of equal-sized facets that are slightly concave. Type II consists of a smaller medial facet, but both the facets are concave. Type III consists of a smaller medial facet, but it is convex; the lateral facet in both types is concave. Type II/III consists of a flat medial facet, and type IV consists of a very small medial facet; the lateral facet in both types is concave. Type V (Jägerhut) consists of no medial facet and no central ridge and is often associated with patellar instability (Fig. 2–8).

The patellar shape and the patellofemoral groove and the congruence of these two structures are best evaluated with tangential roentgenograms of the patellofemoral joint.[29, 49, 54] Several methods, such as those of Hughston,[29] Merchant and collaborators,[54] and Laurin and colleagues,[49] have been used to assess the configuration of the patella and the groove and the congruency of the patella in the groove at the various positions of knee flexion.

THE QUADRICEPS MECHANISM. The rectus femoris, the vastus medialis, the vastus lateralis, and the vastus intermedius are the muscles that make up the quadriceps mechanism. They form a trilaminar quadriceps tendon that is attached to the proximal pole of the patella. The tendon of the rectus femoris is the anterior lamina, which inserts at the anterior edge of the proximal pole. The tendon of the vastus intermedius is the deepest lamina and inserts into the posterior edge of the proximal pole. The middle lamina is formed by the concurrent edges of the vastus lateralis and the vastus medialis. The convergent edges of these two muscles insert onto the medial and lateral margins of the patella. Some superficial fibers pass over the anterior surface of the patella in a distal direction and blend with the patellar tendon, which originates from the distal pole of the patella and inserts distally into the tibial tubercle.

The tendinous fibers originate from the vastus medialis and the vastus lateralis, pass in a distal direction along the margins of the patella, and insert into the tibia medially and laterally to the tuberosity. Beneath these

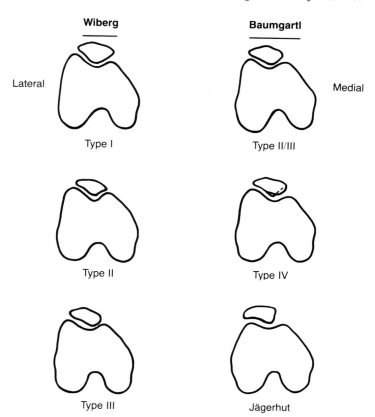

FIGURE 2–8. Patellar configurations as described by Wiberg and Baumgartl. Except for types I and II, unequal stresses are applied to the patellar articular surfaces. (Redrawn from Larson RL, Jones DC: II. Dislocations and ligamentous injuries of the knee. *In* Rockwood CA, Green DP [eds]: Fractures, 2nd ed, vol II, p. 1481. Philadelphia: JB Lippincott, 1984.)

longitudinally oriented fibers is a layer of transverse tendinous fibers originating from the medial and lateral epicondyles; these transverse fibers attach to the medial and lateral margins of the patella. The longitudinal and transverse fibers make up the medial and lateral retinaculum. Kaplan[43] called the transverse fibers, which play an important role in the stabilization of the patella in the groove, the patellofemoral ligaments. These ligaments help guide the patella through the groove and limit the mobility of the patella sideways. In traumatic patellar dislocation, the patellofemoral ligaments are torn or stretched. The lateral patellofemoral ligaments may be congenitally shortened or may develop contracture, producing either enhancement of patellar subluxation or increased patellar compression as the patella moves through the patellofemoral sulcus.

The vastus medialis is divided into the longitudinally oriented fibers (vastus medialis longus) and the more obliquely oriented fibers (vastus medialis obliquus). The vastus medialis obliquus is the major stabilizer of the patella, maintaining its centralization in the sulcus as the patella moves through the groove with knee flexion.[34]

The distal extension of the quadriceps mechanism from the patella is the patellar tendon. It is approximately 5 to 6 cm long and 5 to 6 mm thick, and its width varies from 3 cm at the upper end to 2 cm at the lower end. The patella is reinforced by fibers from the vastus medialis and vastus lateralis muscles, as mentioned earlier. The patellar tendon is vascularized by the anastomotic circle of arteries around the patella, distributed over a fine vasiferous membrane that surrounds the ligament. These arteries run vertically, giving off intraligamentary branches that pass through the ligament from front to back. Some blood supply is also derived from the fat pad lying at the proximal end of the patellar tendon on its undersurface. Arterial supply to the middle third of the tendon is reduced in adults in comparison with that supply in children.[26]

Strengthening of the quadriceps muscle has long been known to be a deterrent to possible ligament injury in active knee use. The quadriceps muscle is more than a motor for extension of the knee. In the sagittal plane, the quadriceps muscle acts through the contact pressure of the patella against the patellofemoral groove, preventing flexion of the knee that is caused by the action of body weight. As the quadriceps muscle contracts, it also acts as a force at the level of the tibial tuberosity, producing a compression between the articular surfaces of the femur and of the tibia and thus enhancing joint stability. Because of its orientation, anterior to the transverse axis of rotation of the distal femur as it attaches to the tibial tubercle, the quadriceps muscle acts in concert with the posterior cruciate ligament (PCL) in preventing posterior subluxation of the tibia on the femur. Through the patellomeniscal bands running from the anterior horns of the menisci to the patella, the quadriceps muscle helps to pull the menisci forward as the knee is extended.[44]

The role of the quadriceps muscle in dynamically protecting the medial collateral ligament from abduction stress was demonstrated in cadaver experiments by White and Raphael.[79] Using strain-gauge transducers attached to the anterior fibers of the medial collateral ligament, they noted a decrease in strain as load was applied to the quadriceps mechanism, regardless of the degree of flexion at the time of loading. Abduction stresses to the knee created increased strain to the medial ligaments; however, this strain was reduced by simultaneously loading the quadriceps mechanism.

Johnson and Pope[40] contrasted the antagonistic effect of the quadriceps muscle with the stabilizing effect of the ACL. The ACL must constantly resist the anterior vector of force being placed on the proximal tibia by the patellar tendon attachment to the tibial tubercle. After analysis of forces produced, Johnson and Pope pointed out that if 140 pounds of force (which is necessary to lift a nonweighted adult leg) is applied to the quadriceps mechanism, the ACL must resist as much as 27 pounds in order to prevent anterior subluxation of the tibia on the femur. This is even more graphically illustrated in the example of climbing stairs. According to these studies, 422 pounds of force is generated by the quadriceps muscle in climbing stairs, and the ACL resists up to 85 pounds of force to prevent anterior displacement of the tibia.

MECHANICS OF KNEE MOTION

If the shaft of the femur is held vertically, the medial femoral condyle projects farther distally than does the lateral femoral condyle. Physiologic valgus of the knee, from approximately 6° to 8°, enables these two condylar surfaces to be on the same plane in the normal upright posture. The mechanical axis of the femur passes through the center of the knee and the center of the hip joint in a vertical direction. The anatomic axis of the femur passes through the center of the knee joint along the femoral shaft and is inclined laterally, producing an angle of 6° between the mechanical axis and the anatomic axis.

The eccentrically shaped femoral condyles and the disparity between the lengths of the articular surface of the femoral and tibial condyles provide a rotating cam action, the extremes of which are controlled by the cruciate ligaments. Two types of motion occur during flexion-extension of the knee. The first is a rocking motion. Different points on the tibia contact different points on the femur, each of which is equidistant from the beginning point. The second type of motion is the gliding motion in which a constant point on the tibia comes in contact with ever-changing points on the femur.[72]

In the first 20° to 30° of knee flexion, a rocking or rolling action[64] between the femur and the tibia occurs; the excursion of the lateral side is more extensive than that of the medial side. At more than 30° of flexion, the sliding action occurs, during which the tibial condyles are kept centered beneath the femoral condyles by the tethering effect of the cruciate ligaments. Loss of this continuity allows the tibia to shift too far anteriorly (in the case of ACL loss) or too far posteriorly (in the case of PCL loss). Other secondary restraints help control this laxity, and if they are also inadequate, higher degrees of instability and more complex instabilities occur.

The four-bar linkage has been described as the mechanical manifestation of the attachment to the cruciate ligaments on the femur. Because both ligaments have attachment sites on both the tibia and the femur, each contributes to the rolling and rocking action and the tethering effect as flexion-extension of the knee occurs. The attachment sites of the cruciate ligaments on the femur lie on a line that forms a 40° angle with the long axis of the femur. With the tibial attachments acting as a coupler between the two femoral attachments of the cruciate ligaments as knee motion occurs, the tibia is confined to the arc of the normal contour of the femoral condyles (Fig. 2–9).[55] Some authors have challenged the crossed four-bar linkage explanation as too simplistic because of the rotational aspects of the knee motion. This concept does, however, emphasize the contributions that the cruciate ligaments make to one another in their stabilizing action.

The vertical rotational axis of the knee passes through the medial tubercle of the intercondylar eminence near the femoral attachment of the PCL.[68] Total rotation of the knee has been found to be approximately 36°; internal rotation is 15°, and external rotation is 21°.[63] The lateral condyle of the femur on the tibia has more latitude of rotation than does the medial condyle. This latitude has been calculated by Dye[13] to be a 24-mm excursion on the lateral side and an approximately 10-mm excursion on the medial side. This asymmetry of rotational motion is an ancient feature seen in all of the mammals examined by Dye in his comparative study of the knee. Maximal rotation occurs in the normal knee at approximately 45° to 60° of flexion as the more spherical portions of the condyles articulate with the tibia.[62] In complete extension, the knee has little or no rotation.[24]

ATMOSPHERIC PRESSURE

Another stabilizing factor in the knee is atmospheric pressure, as demonstrated by Semlak and Ferguson.[67] They showed that in the normal knee, no widening of the normal joint space was produced by a valgus

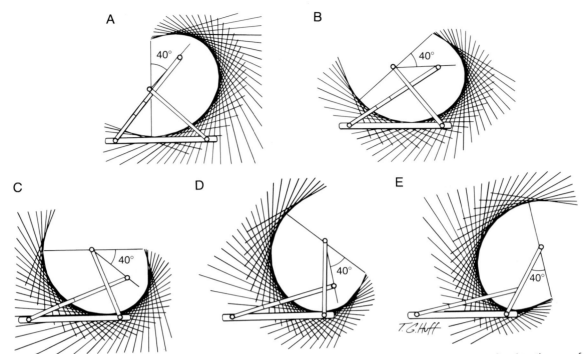

FIGURE 2–9. The crossed four-bar linkage is a mechanical concept that explains how the tibia is confined to the arc of the normal contour of the femoral condyle by the configuration of the cruciate ligaments. Tibia is represented as the fixed horizontal bar. (Redrawn from Müller W: The Knee: Form, Function, and Ligament Reconstruction, p. 11. Berlin: Springer-Verlag, 1982.)

load until more than 4.5 kg was applied to the tibia. If the load exceeded 4.5 kg, the effect of atmospheric pressure was overcome as vaporization occurred. When an effusion and torn medial structures were present, the knee distracted with no vaporization occurring. Semlak and Ferguson concluded that varus and valgus stresses do not produce joint opening until the effect of atmospheric pressure is exceeded. Atmospheric pressure thus provides a protective function; however, this protective function is lost when effusion or communication of the joint with the atmosphere has developed. In the presence of mild laxity of the collateral ligaments without effusion, the atmospheric pressure phenomenon may thus provide some protection.

STABILIZING STRUCTURES OF THE KNEE

Muscles and ligaments around the knee that act as active and passive stabilizers work as an integrated mechanism. They stabilize the knee against excesses of translation and rotary movements. Three types of translations occur: anterior-posterior displacement, medial-lateral displacement, and distraction-compression displacement. There are three types of rotations: valgus-varus rotation, axial-tibial rotation, and flexion-extension rotation. Normal motion is a combination of rotation and slight translation that provides a helicoid of knee action. Pathologic laxity of the supporting structures can lead to a combination of increased translation and rotation that may interfere with the normal function of the knee.[23]

The supporting structures of the medial, posterior, and lateral aspects of the knee constitute three layers of support: the capsular layer, the ligamentous layer, and the muscular layer,[78] usually in that order from innermost to outermost.

Medial Aspect

The capsule forms a sleeve around the knee that is interrupted anteriorly by the extensor mechanism. It is divided above and below the joint line into the meniscofemoral and meniscotibial portions. The capsule on the medial side of the knee can be divided into anterior, middle, and posterior thirds. The anterior third is reinforced by expansions of the vastus medialis and thus is actively controlled by contractions of that muscle. This portion extends from the medial border of the patella and patellar tendon posteriorly to the medial edge of the medial collateral ligament (superficial tibiocollateral ligament). The middle capsular ligament is the portion of the capsule that lies beneath the medial collateral ligament. It is primarily a thickening of the capsular ligament reinforced by the overlying medial collateral ligament.

The third portion of the capsular ligament is the posterior capsular ligament. Hughston and Eilers[33] coined the term "posterior oblique ligament of the knee" for this portion (Fig. 2–10). It is the area of the capsule that lies between the medial collateral ligament anteriorly and the posterior capsule posteriorly, and it protects the knee against rotary instability. It is a confluence of several groups of fibers. The posterior edge of the medial collateral ligament has fibers that sweep from above downward in an oblique direction and fibers that sweep from below upward and are intimately bound to the posterior third of the capsular ligament. The deeper vertical fibers of the posteromedial capsule cover the anteromedial limb of the semimembranosus muscle as it runs along the superior edge of the tibial condyle. The posterior portion of the posteromedial capsule is reinforced by the semimembranosus muscle attachments to the medial meniscus. This area of confluence of the medial capsular ligament, the fibers from the medial collateral ligament, and attachments of the semimembranosus muscle form the posterior oblique ligament (Fig. 2–11). (In the French literature, this structure is termed the posterior medial aspect of Trillat.)

The posterior third of the posterior capsular ligament forms a sling around the posterior aspect of the medial femoral condyle as it blends with the posterior capsule. This sling is quite tense in full extension, but as flexion occurs, it becomes relaxed. The attachment of the semimembranosus muscle in this area, however, dynamically helps tighten the sling with flexion. The medial capsular layer is intimately attached to the medial meniscus, and disruptions of this attachment can enhance the meniscus mobility and produce problems with meniscal catching in the joint or increased meniscal wear.

The ligamentous layer of the medial side of the knee is composed of the medial collateral ligament. This is a broad, fibrous band, approximately 10 to 12 cm long, attaching superiorly to the medial epicondyle of the femur and distally about a hand's breadth below the joint line into the medial aspect of the tibia. The anterior border, which consists of dense

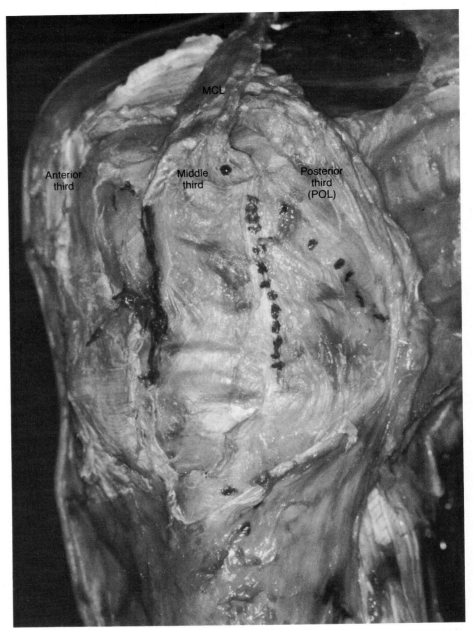

FIGURE 2–10. The medial capsular ligament (MCL) is divided into thirds. With the MCL reflected superiorly, the capsular ligament is apparent.

vertical collagen fibers, is quite distinct. The width of the dense fibers is about 1 cm at its femoral attachment and increases to approximately 2 cm at the level of the joint cavity. This portion of the ligament is covered superficially by the fascia extending distally from the vastus medialis (medial retinaculum), which attaches to the superior edge of the fascia of the pes anserinus. The distal attachment of the collateral ligament is directly beneath the anterior and medial portions of the pes anserinus group of tendons, which attach just anteriorly on the tibia (Fig. 2–12).

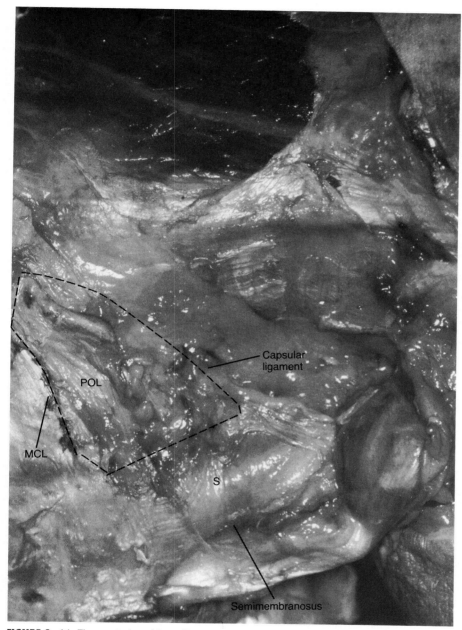

FIGURE 2–11. The posterior oblique ligament (POL) is the confluence of the MCL, the medial capsular ligament, and the semimembranosus. (Anterior is to the left.)

The medial collateral ligament and the medial capsular ligament are separated by a bursa that enables the medial collateral ligament to glide forward in extension and backward with flexion. Should adhesions develop between the superficial and deep structures, knee motion may be restricted. The proximal insertion of the medial collateral ligament forms an oval, approximately 2 cm wide, whose long axis is in a vertical direction when the knee is extended. With flexion, the femoral attachment becomes more horizontal, and the anterior fibers tighten as the posterior fibers

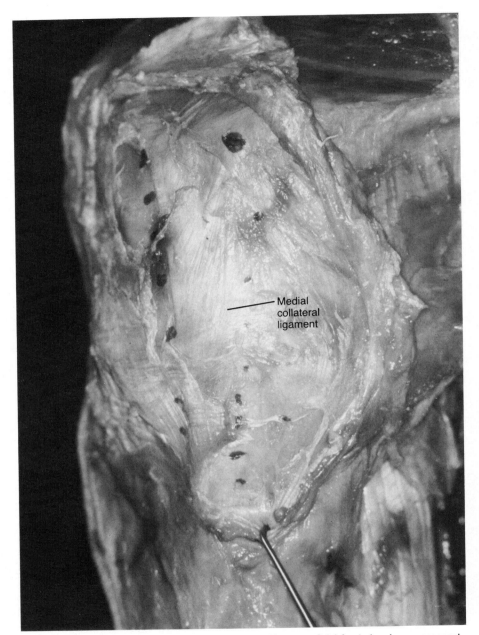

Medial
collateral
ligament

FIGURE 2–12. Outlined by the marker is the MCL. The superficial fascia has been removed.

relax. Wang and associates[76] showed that the medial collateral ligament is more taut in extension and shortens by 15 to 20 per cent on flexion of the knee from 0° to 120°. A slight laxity noted on valgus testing of the knee at 30° flexion is thus caused by the slight physiologic laxity that occurs.

The medial collateral ligament and the deep capsular ligament stabilize the knee not only against excessive abduction of the tibia on the femur but also against excessive external rotational movement of the tibia. These medial structures are in a better position biomechanically to resist the rotational forces and the valgus forces than are the centrally located cruciate ligaments.[24, 45, 77]

Structures of the posteromedial corner of the knee have been termed the semimembranosus complex. It consists of the posterior oblique ligament, the semimembranosus muscle, and the medial meniscus. The synergistic action of the semimembranosus complex and the ACL has been emphasized by Müller[55] (see Fig. 20–2). When the tibia is displaced anteriorly, the ACL comes under tension to restrain it. At the same time, the femoral condyle moves posteriorly and must push the posterior horn of the medial meniscus backwards or ride up on it. Because the meniscus is firmly attached to the posterior oblique ligament, its backward displacement is checked by these fibers together with the meniscofemoral portion of the posterior oblique ligament. This system functions as an intact unit. A lesion of this unit leads to the first stages of anteromedial rotatory instability. As has been emphasized both by Hughston and Eilers[33] and by Müller,[55] accurate repair of this area in an isometric fashion with the preservation of the medial meniscus provides considerable improvement of the anteroposterior stability to the medial joint. If in addition to damage to the posteromedial structures the ACL is torn, considerable anterior displacement can occur. Because the lateral tibial condyle has more mobility, a pivot shift may develop, causing a functional disability.

The muscular layer is composed of the pes anserinus group of muscles—the sartorius, the gracilis, and the semitendinosus—that cover the tibial attachment of the medial collateral ligament. The other component of the muscular layer covering the posteromedial aspect of the knee is the semimembranosus muscle, which is a very important dynamic stabilizing element of this aspect. The vastus medialis obliquus muscle fascia extends distally as the medial retinaculum, attaches to the anterior third of the capsular ligaments, and dynamically tightens this structure. The medial head of the gastrocnemius muscle, although not actually located on the medial side of the knee, does contribute toward medial stability to some extent.

The pes anserinus group of muscles attaches as a weblike structure onto the anterior tibia, and from this structure they derive their name (pes anserinus, or "goose foot"). They are primary flexors of the knee with the secondary function of providing internal rotation of the proximal tibia. Noyes and Sonstegard[57] found that the pes anserinus tendons are 4 to 10 times stronger as flexors than as internal rotators. They dynamically function to assist the static action of the medial capsule and the medial collateral ligament and to assist the ACL in preventing anterior subluxation of the tibia on the femur. The most powerful motor of this group is the semitendinosus muscle. In the surgical procedure of pes anserinus transfer, the semitendinosus muscle is moved from its most distal attachment of the group to a more proximal attachment just beneath the flare of the tibial condyle. This transfer enhances the internal rotational strength of the semitendinosus muscle. Noyes and Sonstegard,[57] in cadaver testing, showed that pes anserinus transplantation reduced flexor power by approximately 30 per cent and enhanced internal rotational power by as much as 50 per cent with the knee at 60° of flexion.

The semimembranosus muscle, although more posteriorly oriented, is a primary dynamic stabilizer in the posteromedial aspect of the joint. It has five distal expansions that enhance its capacity as a posteromedial and posterior stabilizer of the knee.[44] The first limb extends obliquely, laterally, and proximally across the posterior capsule, forming the thickened ligamentous structure called the oblique popliteal ligament. The second tendinous attachment is to the posterior capsule and the posteromedial horn of the medial meniscus. This helps to tighten the posterior capsule below the medial meniscus posteriorly with knee flexion. The anteromedial limb is the third tendinous structure, which continues medially along the flare of the tibial condyle and inserts beneath the medial collateral ligament. This most distinct tendon is often an orientation point on dissections on the medial side of the knee. The direct head of the semimembranosus muscle attaches to the infraglenoid tubercle on the posterior aspect of the medial tuberosity of the tibia just below the joint line posteriorly. The fifth division of the semimembranosus muscle is the continuation distally to form a fibrous expansion over the popliteus muscle and fuses into the periosteum of the medial tibia. The action of the semimembranosus in stabilizing the medial side of the knee is also enhanced by the compressive forces of the quadriceps, as mentioned in the discussion of the quadriceps muscle (Fig. 2–13).

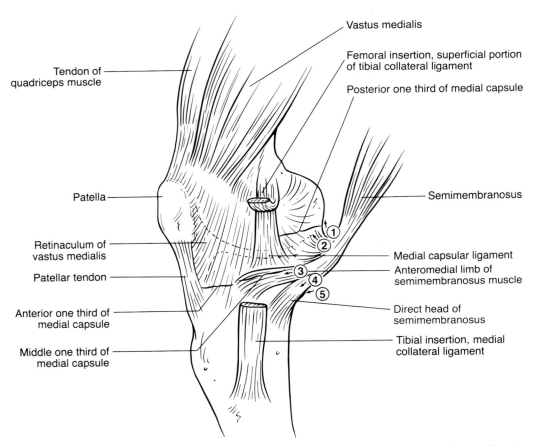

FIGURE 2–13. The five expansions of the semimembranosus. 1, Oblique popliteal ligament; 2, attachment to the posterior horn of the medial meniscus and posterior capsule; 3, the anteromedial tendinous limb; 4, the direct head to the infraglenoid tubercle; 5, continuation as a fibrous expansion over the popliteus muscle.

Posterior Aspect

The important stabilizing capsular, ligamentous, and muscular structures of the posterior aspect of the knee are (1) the posterior capsule; (2) the oblique popliteal ligament (ligament of Winslow), the arcuate ligament, the PCL, and the ligaments of Wrisberg and Humphry; and (3) the popliteus muscle, the semimembranosus muscle, and the medial and lateral heads of the gastrocnemius muscle. Dynamic support is also provided by the quadriceps muscle, particularly as the knee flexes more than 60°. Fischer and colleagues[18] have shown that as the knee flexes more than 60°, the patella describes an arc beginning at a point vertically above the tibial tuberosity and ending behind the point of the tibial tuberosity. As flexion occurs, the vector of force, acting at the level of the tuberosity, generates compression between the articular surfaces of the femur and tibia, as well as working in concert with the PCL, preventing a posterior displacement of the posterior tibia on the femur.

CAPSULAR STRUCTURES. The deep posterior capsule covers the lateral and medial femoral condyles. These condylar capsules are a continuation of the joint capsule and are pulled tightly around the femoral condyles when the knee is in extension. They blend with the medial and lateral tendinous insertions of the gastrocnemius muscle. This thickened posterior capsule over the femoral condyles is the attachment site of the gastrocnemius heads and is called the condylar plate.[42] The lateral condylar capsule is intimately associated with the lateral head of the gastrocnemius muscle and is sometimes reinforced by sesamoid fibrocartilage or bone in the lateral head of the gastrocnemius muscle, called the fabella. The semimembranosus muscle inserts into the medial aspect of the condylar capsule and the posterior aspect of the medial meniscus. Through this attachment, the semimembranosus muscle retracts the meniscus posteriorly and augments the function of the ACL by acting synergistically to prevent anterior subluxation of the tibia from beneath the femur.

LIGAMENTS. The median portion of the posterior capsule is reinforced by the oblique popliteal ligament of Winslow, which is an expansion of the tendon of the semimembranosus muscle directed obliquely across the back of the joint and laterally upward toward the insertion of the lateral gastrocnemius muscle. The semimembranosus muscle helps tighten this structure with contraction. When the oblique popliteal ligament is pulled medially and forward, it tightens the remaining posterior capsule of the knee. This maneuver is used to tighten the posterior capsule and posterior medial corner of the knee in surgical repair.

The arcuate ligament has been described by Basmajian and Lovejoy[5] as the three tendinous origins of the popliteus muscle. These origins form a Y-shaped ligament, the arms being joined together by the capsule and the meniscal origin (Fig. 2–14). The first origin of the popliteus muscle attaches to the lateral femoral condyle just below the attachment to the lateral collateral ligament; the second tendinous origin attaches to the posterior aspect of the fibular head at its styloid process; and the third tendinous origin attaches to the posterior horn of the lateral meniscus. Other authors believe that the arcuate ligament is a thickening of the fascia that comes off the popliteus muscle and blends with the posterior lateral capsule, forming the thickened arcuate ligament itself. The term "arcuate complex" has been used to describe the stabilizing structures in

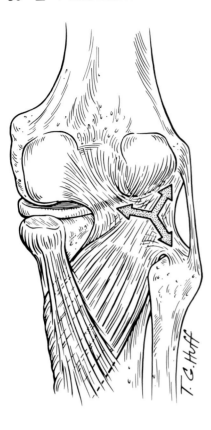

FIGURE 2–14. The three limbs of the arcuate ligament. (See text.) (Redrawn from Basmajian JV, Lovejoy JF Jr: Functions of popliteus muscle in man. J Bone Joint Surg 53A[3]:558, 1971.)

the posterolateral aspect of the knee. These include the arcuate ligament, the popliteal tendon, and the lateral collateral ligament.[31]

The ligamentous layer of the posterior aspect of the knee also includes the ligaments of Wrisberg and Humphry (the meniscofemoral ligaments). These ligaments are not present in all humans (Fig. 2–15). Girgis and associates,[21] in dissections of 44 knees, found 30 per cent of the specimens to have neither ligament. In the remaining 70 per cent, Wrisberg's ligament was more commonly found, but when Humphry's ligament was present, it was more prominent than Wrisberg's ligament. They were not present together in one knee on dissections. The ligament of Wrisberg (posterior meniscofemoral ligament) lies behind the PCL and runs from the posterior aspect of the lateral meniscus to the inner side of the medial femoral condyle. The ligament of Humphry (anterior meniscofemoral ligament) lies in front of the PCL, attaches to the posterior horn of the lateral meniscus, and runs to the inner side of the medial femoral condyle. Both meniscofemoral ligaments act to draw the posterior arch of the lateral meniscus in a medial direction as internal rotation of the tibia occurs with flexion of the knee. Because of the intimate attachment of the popliteus muscle to the posterior horn of the lateral meniscus (the same area as the attachments of Wrisberg and Humphry), some authors believe that these ligaments are a direct extension of the popliteus muscle. The simultaneous function of these ligaments and the contraction of the popliteus muscle provide stability to the tibia and prevent abnormal forward motion. They are thus acting synergistically and with the ACL.

MUSCULAR LAYER. The muscular layer consists of the popliteus

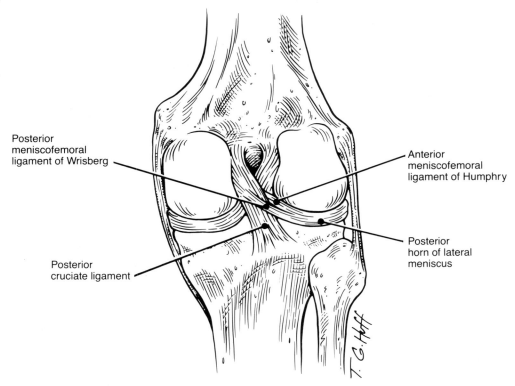

FIGURE 2–15. The ligaments of Wrisberg (posterior) and Humphry (anterior). They are usually not present together in the same knee. (Redrawn from Heller L, Langhams J: The meniscofemoral ligaments of the human knee. J Bone Joint Surg 46B[2]:309, 1964.)

muscle, the semimembranosus muscle, and the lateral and medial heads of the gastrocnemius muscle. The popliteus muscle is unusual in that it has three proximal tendinous origins and a fleshy muscle belly that attaches to the posterior aspect of the tibia at its insertion. The origins under the arcuate ligament are at the lateral femoral condyle below the attachment of the lateral collateral ligament, at the posterior aspect of the fibular head, and at the posterior horn of the lateral meniscus. The popliteus muscle is primarily an internal rotator of the tibia on the femur. In addition, it pulls the posterior horn of the lateral meniscus posteriorly with the flexion of the knee and provides rotatory stability by preventing forward dislocation of the tibia on the femur during flexion. Electromyograms show that the popliteus muscle becomes very active during normal walking from the midpoint of the swing phase, at which time the tibia is internally rotating on the femur, through most of the stance phase. During the early stance phase, with foot strike, the foot pronates in the subtalar joint, which produces an obligatory internal tibial rotation. The position of the tibia in internal rotation is maintained by the activity of the popliteus muscle.[51]

The semimembranosus muscle has been described in the section on the medial muscular layer. The five distal expansions of this muscle act not only to provide medial stability but also to enhance the posterior stability of the knee. Functionally, the semimembranosus muscle is a flexor and an internal rotator of the tibia. It also retracts the posterior rim of the medial meniscus posteriorly in flexion and, through the oblique popliteal ligament, tenses the posterior capsule.

The medial and lateral heads of the gastrocnemius muscle insert into the proximal portions of the respective femoral condyles. The medial gastrocnemius muscle has a more definite tendinous configuration and has been used as a substitute for the PCL. The lateral gastrocnemius insertion is intimately attached to the posterior capsule. Moving the lateral head of the gastrocnemius muscle anteriorly and proximally, as is sometimes done in the treatment of posterolateral instabilities, tightens the posterior capsule as well. When the knee is in full extension, the posterior capsule provides stability to valgus and varus stress even when all other stabilizing structures are cut. This anatomic fact is important clinically in testing of the knee for ligamentous continuity. The knee must be flexed slightly in order to relax the posterior capsule so that the integrity of the other lateral and medial supporting structures can be properly determined.[44]

If injury to the posterior capsular structure has occurred, it is likely that PCL injury, either stretching or disruption, is also present.[30] In injuries to the medial supporting structures, the tears may extend into the posterior capsule, and it is important to look for these extensions so that they can be repaired when acute ligamentous repair is required.[33]

If the posterior capsular injury does occur, it often involves the posteromedial structures or the posterolateral structures.

Lateral Aspect

The lateral structures of the knee can similarly be divided into three layers: the capsular, ligamentous, and muscular layers. The capsular layer is attached to the meniscus anterior to the fibular collateral ligament. Behind this point, the continuity is interrupted by the penetration of the tendinous portion of the popliteus muscle as it rises to attach to the lateral aspect of the femoral condyle. This interruption has been measured in normal subjects and found to vary between 1.2 and 1.5 cm. Such studies suggested that if this area is longer, a tear of the peripheral attachment of the lateral meniscus should be suspected.[9] During arthroscopy, displacement of the meniscus in the joint when the meniscus is pulled may indicate that a tear is present in this area. The lateral capsular ligament is a more tenuous structure than is the medial capsular ligament. It has been shown that in certain injuries, a piece of bone may be pulled from the lateral tibial condylar area (Segond's fracture) at the attachment of the midlateral capsule. When this occurs, there is also an associated ACL tear.[37, 82]

The ligamentous layer on the lateral side of the knee contains the lateral collateral ligament and the arcuate ligament (Fig. 2–16). The lateral collateral ligament inserts proximally into the lateral femoral epicondyle and distally into the fibular head. This ligament is a fibrous cord approximately 5 to 6 cm long, and it reclines slightly backwards as it progresses from the femoral attachment to its insertion in the head of the fibula in front of the styloid process. Passing beneath the fibular collateral ligament is the tendon of the popliteus muscle, which attaches just anteriorly to the lateral collateral ligament on the lateral aspect of the femur (Fig. 2–16B).

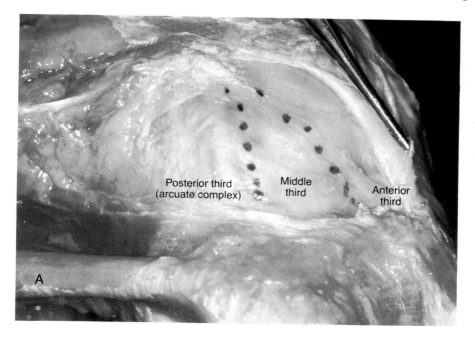

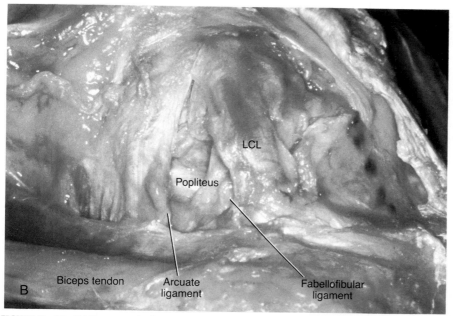

FIGURE 2–16. *(A)* The capsular ligament of the lateral side is divided into thirds. The posterior third is specialized as on the medial side and is called the arcuate complex. *(B)* The arcuate complex consists of the lateral collateral ligament (LCL), the popliteus tendon, the arcuate ligament, and the fabellofibular ligament.

Posterior to the lateral collateral ligament are the arcuate ligament and tendons of the popliteus muscle. The popliteus muscle has been described in the section on the posterior structures. The combination of the arcuate ligament, the popliteal tendon, and the lateral collateral ligament is known as the arcuate complex (posterior lateral apex of Trillat-Dejour-Bousquet).

The short collateral ligament lies deep to the lateral collateral ligament. When a fabella is present, the short collateral ligament attaches to the fabella and is called the fabellofibular ligament. It runs parallel to the lateral collateral ligament and attaches to the fibular head posterior to the tendon of the biceps. It, too, reinforces the posterior capsule and contributes to lateral stability of the knee.[65]

The muscular layer of the lateral side of the knee consists of the iliotibial tract, the biceps femoris, the popliteus muscle, the lateral head of the gastrocnemius muscle, and the vastus lateralis (Fig. 2–17). It should be apparent from the discussion of the structures of the medial and posterior aspects of the knee that there is considerable overlap in the function of the various structures. Arbitrarily assigning them to medial, posterior, or lateral sides of the knee is a matter of convenience for discussion. Kaplan,[43] in describing the attachments of the iliotibial tract, noted that it is attached superiorly at the supracondylar tubercle of the femoral condyle, sends a slip (or band) to the intermuscular septum, and continues downward to attach to Gerdy's tubercle at that anterolateral aspect of the tibia. Kaplan therefore believed that this section of the iliotibial tract is, in fact, a static stabilizer functioning as a ligamentous structure. Müller[55] also described this distal extension of the iliotibial band. He termed it the anterolateral femoral tibial ligament. Terry and colleagues[73] performed a detailed dissection of the area of the iliotibial tract and described five layers: the aponeurotic, superficial, middle, deep,

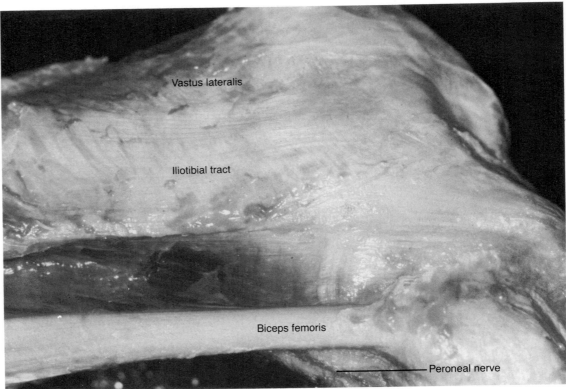

FIGURE 2–17. The muscular layer on the lateral side includes the iliotibial tract, the biceps femoris, and the vastus lateralis.

and capsulo-osseous layers. Terry and colleagues emphasized that the confluence of the deep, capsulo-osseous, and superficial layers of the posterior iliotibial tract provides a functional anterolateral ligament of the knee.

The iliotibial tract moves forward in extension and backward in flexion, but it is tense in both positions[14] (Fig. 2–18). In flexion, the iliotibial band, the popliteal tendon, and the lateral collateral ligament cross each other, enhancing lateral stability. Also during flexion, the iliotibial band and biceps tendon remain parallel with each other as they are in extension, and they enhance lateral stability.

The biceps femoris muscle has three layers of attachment on the lateral aspect. The deep layer is inserted into the edge of the lateral tibial plateau and into Gerdy's tubercle; the middle layer is inserted into the fibula; and the superficial layer expands over Gerdy's tubercle, the head of the fibula, and the aponeurosis of the lateral head of the gastrocnemius muscle. The fibular attachment envelops the distal insertion of the lateral collateral ligament. It is here that the deep layer of the biceps femoris spans the space between the fibula and the tibia, attaching to the posterolateral aspect of the tibia and the lateral capsule.

The biceps femoris muscle is somewhat analogous to the semimembranosus muscle on the medial aspect of the knee. It functions as a flexor of the knee and an external rotator of the tibia on the femur. In addition, it helps to antagonistically control extension of the joint, tenses the lateral and posterior capsules, and works synergistically with the ACL to prevent anterior translation of the tibia on the femur.

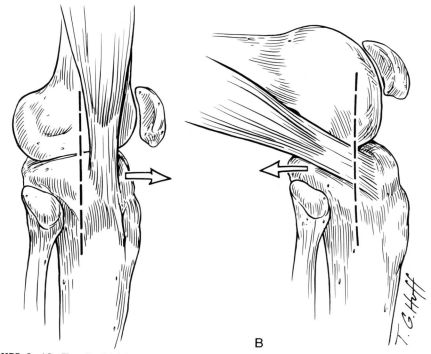

A   B

FIGURE 2–18. The iliotibial band lies anterior to the condyle in extension and does not stabilize the lateral tibial plateau. In flexion, this band slides posteriorly to enhance stability of the tibial plateau. Hence the pivot-shift phenomenon is a reduction of the subluxed tibial plateau as the joint moves from an extended to a flexed position.

The vastus lateralis fascia extends distally as the lateral retinaculum, which attaches to the iliotibial tract and helps tense this tract as the knee extends and the tract moves forward. The vastus lateralis not only functions in extension of the knee but also contributes to lateral stability. The lateral head and the medial head of the gastrocnemius muscle act by providing large forces posteriorly to stabilize the joint, enhancing the work of the extensors and flexors of the knee, which act from above.

The integrated function of the lateral structures has been described both by Johnson[40] and by Kaplan.[44] Kaplan described the quadruple complex as consisting of the iliotibial tract, the lateral collateral ligament, the popliteal tendon, and the biceps femoris muscle. According to Kaplan, stability and nearly normal function are maintained in spite of loss of any two of these four structures. In flexion, the biceps femoris muscle, the iliotibial tract, and the popliteal tendon are the chief lateral stabilizers, whereas the lateral collateral ligament provides its stabilizing action when the knee is in extension.

INTERNAL KNEE ANATOMY

The posterior depression (intercondylar notch) of the distal femur provides the space for the central fixation apparatus of the knee. The cruciate ligaments, which lie in this space, provide stability in the sagittal plane that is enhanced by the flexor and extensor muscles, which are mutually antagonistic to one or the other cruciate ligament. The quadriceps muscle, which is synergistic with the PCL constraint, is antagonistic to the function of the ACL. The flexors of the knee, including the biceps femoris muscle, the semimembranosus muscle, and the pes anserinus group, act synergistically with the ACL, holding the tibia back against forward displacement, and in so doing, they are antagonistic to the PCL.[40]

Anterior Cruciate Ligament

Considerable attention has been given to the importance of the ACL, not only in preventing anterior translation of the tibia on the femur,[7, 20, 21, 56] but also in providing normal helicoid knee action and thus decreasing the chance of meniscal pathology.[8, 17, 47] It has also been shown that if the cruciate ligaments are cut and the anteroposterior load is placed on the menisci, which play an important role in restricting anteroposterior motion, tearing of a meniscus may result. It has been shown that in knees with chronic ACL deficiency, 90 per cent have had meniscal disorder.[36] The pivot shift syndrome is a direct result of the ACL insufficiency.[20]

The synovium enters the posterior intercondylar notch area and covers the entire PCL and the anterior aspect of the ACL. Palmer[60] noted that the inferior portion of the ACL, near its tibial attachment, has a very thin covering of synovium, and the ligament may appear to be bare at this point. The cruciate ligaments are extrasynovial in location, and therefore two clinical subtleties must be recognized. First, in visualization of a cruciate ligament through the arthroscope, the synovium may have remained intact, giving the impression that the underlying ACL is also intact. An incision in the synovium to further inspect the ACL may be necessary to determine the extent of injury. It should also be recognized that a normal-appearing cruciate ligament may be totally incompetent as a result of plastic deformation.[47] The second clinical subtlety of the synovial covering of the ACL is that in the interpretation of imaging studies, the intact synovial band may be interpreted as the cruciate shadow. The assessment of the cruciate shadow in an arthrographic study should include an attempt to ascertain whether there is any breadth to the tissue, which, if present, would indicate a true ACL substance.[74]

Both cruciate ligaments are made up of bundles of fibers that may be taut in various degrees of knee flexion and extension. Girgis and associates[21] described the ACL as having an anteromedial band and a posterior bulk of tissue. Norwood and Cross[56] described three separate divisions: the anteromedial, intermediate, and posterolateral bundles. The anteromedial bundle is the longest, and the posterolateral bundle is the shortest. Norwood and Cross suggested that each of these bundles contributes separately to knee function and stability and that because of their different lengths, they can be torn independently. On the other hand, other investigators believe that the fascicular structure of the cruciate ligaments is a continuum in which some fibers are taut throughout the range of motion (Fig. 2–19). In flexion, the anterior fibers are more taut than the posterior fibers.

The femoral attachment of the ACL is on the most posterior aspect of the medial surface of the lateral femoral condyle. The attachment is crescent-shaped; the anterior side is straight, and the posterior side is convex, which corresponds to the curve of the medial margin of the lateral femoral condyle (Fig. 2–19).[21] Horne and Parsons[27] noted that the posterior capsule separates the femoral attachment of the ACL from the distal end of the lateral intermuscular septum. This septum has two limbs: one passes distally and attaches to the superior margin of the lateral femoral condyle, and the other passes posteriorly, blending into the posterior capsule. The fan-shaped cruciate attachment is approximately 2.3 cm in length. The anteromedial band attaches more posteriorly and superiorly

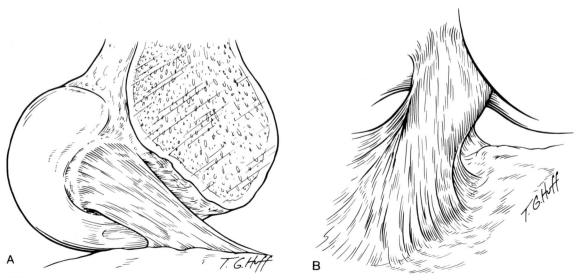

A   B

FIGURE 2–19. *(A)* Anterior cruciate ligament (ACL) as seen from the side, showing its broad femoral attachment. *(B)* ACL as seen from in front, showing the multifascial nature.

on the femur, whereas the bulk of the ligament is attached more anteriorly and inferiorly in this fan-shaped attachment.

The tibial attachment is primarily in front of the anterior tibial spine (medial intercondylar tubercle). Several articles have revealed a discrepancy as to whether the primary attachment is medial or lateral to the tibial spine. According to Horne and Parsons,[27] two thirds of the ACL originates from the tibia immediately anterior and medial to the tibial spine, and the remaining third attaches to the anterior margin of the spine. Norwood and Cross[56] stated that the anteromedial bundle inserts on the medial aspect of the intercondylar eminence, the intermediate bundle inserts lateral to this, and the posterolateral bundle inserts posterior to the lateral bundle, all thereby forming a triangular insertion. Girgis and associates[21] described an attachment to a wide, depressed area in front of and lateral to the tibial spine. At the point of attachment, there is a well-defined slip to the anterior horn of the lateral meniscus.

As the ligament descends from its femoral attachment, it fans out so that the fibers from the convex border of the femoral attachment form the medial side of the ligament and are attached anterior to the anteromedial spine, forming the anteromedial band. Surgeons should bear this anatomic fact in mind when attempting to reattach the femoral attachment of the ACL. The sutures should be directed through the substance of the ACL in a lateral-to-medial direction, and then, because they are attached to the posterior aspect of the intercondylar notch, the most medial sutures should be brought out superiorly in the posterior aspect of the notch and the lateral sutures directed inferiorly. This helps restore the normal twist of the ACL.

The most anterior edge of the tibial attachment of the ACL is approximately 1.5 cm from the anterior border of the tibial articular surface.[21] The average width of the tibial attachment is 3.0 cm. The average length of the ACL is 3.8 cm, and the average width is 1.1 cm.[21] Horne and Parsons[27] attached clips to the femoral and tibial attachments of the ACL and then took radiographs in various amounts of flexion from 0° to 90°. They found that the angle of the ACL and the tibial plateau changed only 25° from 0° to 90° of knee flexion. A greater change—almost 90°—was noted in the angulation between the ACL direction and the femoral shaft. As the knee flexes, the vertical femoral attachment of the ACL becomes horizontal. This enables the posterior bulk of the ACL to become more relaxed in flexion and the anteromedial bundles to remain taut. The studies of Girgis and associates[21] also showed that the femoral attachment was weaker than the tibial attachment, which may be one of the reasons why the femoral attachment is more frequently torn (Fig. 2–20).

The ACL is vascularized chiefly by the middle genicular artery. This artery enters from the posterior aspect of the knee, and a branch of this artery, the tibial intercondylar artery, passes along the dorsal surface of the ACL.[64, 81] Vascularity is also supplied by surrounding synovium and fatty tissue, which provide fasciculi separated by spaces containing loose connective tissue, tortuous blood vessels, and nerve fibers. The central portion of the ACL has the most limited vascular supply. Kennedy and colleagues[47] stated, "The vascular supply, though not profuse . . . ., was by no means sparse . . . and appeared to be adequate for healing of ligaments. . . ."

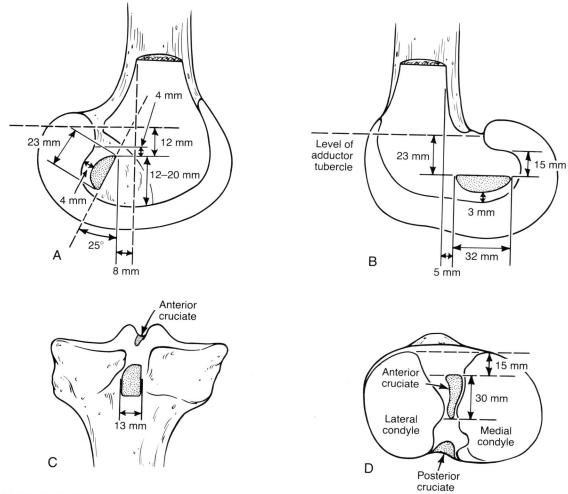

FIGURE 2–20. The femoral and tibial attachments of the anterior and posterior cruciate ligaments. *(A)* Femoral attachment of ACL. *(B)* Femoral attachment of PCL. *(C)* Posterior view of the tibia, showing PCL attachment. *(D)* Superior view of tibial plateau showing attachment sites of ACL and PCL. *(A, C,* and *D* redrawn from Girgis FG, Marshall JL, Monajem ARS: The cruciate ligaments of the knee joint; anatomical, functional, and experimental analysis. Clin Orthop 106:216–231, 1975. *B* redrawn from Arnoczky SP: Anatomy of the anterior cruciate ligament. Clin Orthop 172:19–25, 1983.)

Posterior Cruciate Ligament

The major control of knee stability has been ascribed to the PCL. This strong ligament, which according to tensile testing is approximately two times stronger than any other ligament around the knee,[46] is the axis about which knee rotation occurs. Hughston and collaborators[32] stated that when the PCL has been torn, no rotatory instability can be demonstrated because the axis of rotation has been lost in the grossly unstable knee. This loss is manifest as a posterior translation movement of the entire tibia on the femur. The PCL is the primary stabilizer against posterior displacement of the tibia on the femur. It is almost vertical in its alignment in the sagittal plane. In the coronal plane, it passes obliquely upward and medially to its femoral attachment. This ligament, like the ACL, is also extrasynovial but intracapsular.[21, 32]

The femoral attachment of the PCL is on the lateral aspect of the medial femoral condyle in the intercondylar notch area (Fig. 2–20*B*). It too attaches as a semicircle in a horizontal orientation in the extended position. The distalmost portion of the attachment is convex and parallel to the lower articular margin of the condyle. The width of the fan-shaped insertion is approximately 3.2 cm. This ligament also consists of bundles. The posterior fibers and the bulk of the ligament were described by Girgis and associates.[21] The posterior fibers attach at the proximalmost portion of the femoral attachment, whereas the anterior fibers, or the bulk of the ligament, attach mainly to the convex portion of the femoral attachment. The tibial attachment is to the depression behind the interarticular upper surface of the tibia and extends for 3 mm onto the adjoining superior surface of the tibia (Fig. 2–20*C*). Near its tibial attachment, a separate slip arises to blend with the posterior horn of the lateral meniscus. The ligaments of Wrisberg (posterior meniscal femoral) and Humphry (anterior meniscal femoral) were absent in 30 per cent of the knees studied by Girgis and associates. In their dissection, they did not find these two ligaments to occur together and found the ligament of Wrisberg to be more common than the ligament of Humphry.[21] Both of these accessory ligaments pass obliquely downward and laterally, attaching to the posterior horn of the lateral meniscus. Dissection studies showed the PCL to be approximately the same length (3.8 cm) as the ACL but slightly wider (approximately 1.3 cm) and more robust. It is narrowest in its midportion, fanning out at each end. The femoral attachment is in an anteroposterior direction, whereas the tibial attachment is in a lateromedial orientation, which provides a spiral orientation of the fibers.

In flexion, the bulk of the PCL is taut, but the posterior band is loose. In extension, the posterior portion tenses, and the bulk of the ligament becomes lax. Because of its more posterior position in the intercondylar notch area and more abundant surrounding soft tissues, the vascular supply to the PCL appears to be more abundant than the supply to the ACL.[32]

Tensile testing has been conducted by Kennedy and colleagues[46] and others to show the relative strength of the various ligaments of the knee. These studies show the PCL to be the strongest ligament in resisting distraction forces. The ACL and the medial collateral ligament were of equal strength. The cruciate ligaments are the secondary restraints to the function of the collateral ligaments for their half of the joint; thus the PCL is the lateral border of the medial joint compartment, and the ACL is the medial border of the lateral joint compartment. The cruciate ligaments also prevent excessive rotatory motion. With external rotation of the tibia on the femur, the cruciates unwind. As this excessive external rotation continues, the ACL is wrapped around the medial side of the lateral femoral condyle, limiting further external rotation.[21] With internal rotation, the cruciate ligaments twist on each other and help limit internal rotation.

This crossing of the ligaments in space was studied by Müller.[55] The lateral collateral ligament runs from an anterior attachment on the femur to a more posterior position on the fibular head. The medial collateral ligament has a slightly forward inclination from its femoral attachment to its tibial attachment. This alternation of orientation from one side of the knee to the other provides additional mechanical enhancement to stability. Because the collateral ligaments are in different planes of obliquity as the knee undergoes external rotation, the collateral ligaments cross in space and tighten as the cruciate ligaments unwind and relax. The reverse occurs with internal rotation. Thus the two sets of ligaments work synergistically to maintain the contact of the joint surfaces.

Some portion of the cruciate complex is taut in all degrees of knee motion. Therefore, the cruciate ligaments maintain contact pressure between the femoral and tibial condyles in all degrees of knee motion. This pressure is enhanced when a compressive load that helps increase the stabilizing function of the condylar surfaces is applied. Walker,[75] in explaining the biomechanical principle, stated that when a horizontal force tends to move the femur forward on the tibia, the PCL and the collateral ligaments and capsule come under an increasing tension, the posterior capsule being the dominant restraint. The ligamentous tension produces a pressing together of the joint surfaces, which results in a force that is approximately equal to the sum of the ligament forces. When there is a vertical compressive force in addition, the reaction force is increased, and its contribution to restraint may be larger than that of the PCL.

The Menisci

The medial meniscus is attached at its anterior horn to the articulating surface of the tibia and extends slightly below this front edge. From this anterior attachment, the ligamentum transversum attaches to the anterior horn of the medial and lateral menisci. This attachment limits the motion of the cartilages at the anterior aspect. The posterior horn of the medial meniscus is attached to the excavation just posterior to the intercondylar tubercle of the tibia. This attachment is anterior to the PCL, which attaches to the depression between the two tibial condyles beneath the articular surface. The posterior horn of the medial meniscus is wider than the anterior horn. Recognition of this point is important in interpreting arthrographic studies, because if the posterior horn of the medial meniscus appears to be the same width as the anterior horn, there may be a bucket-handle tear that has diminished the width of the posterior horn.

The lateral meniscus is more circular and of a more uniform width from anterior to posterior. This meniscus covers more of the articular surface of the tibia than does the medial meniscus. Both the anterior and posterior horns of the lateral meniscus are inserted near a common attachment posterior to the intercondylar tubercle of the tibia and near the attachment of the posterior horn of the medial meniscus.

The peripheral areas of the medial meniscus are attached to the medial capsule; this attachment divides this structure into the meniscofemoral and meniscotibial portions. On the lateral side, the lateral capsule attaches to the meniscus as far posteriorly as the recess for the popliteal tendon. This recess has been found to be 1.2 to 1.5 cm in length.[9] Posterior to this recess are (1) the attachment of the arcuate ligament, the popliteus muscles, and the ligaments of Wrisberg and Humphry, and (2) a small slip from the PCL. A discoid lateral meniscus with an inadequate posterior tibial attachment has been termed a Wrisberg ligament type of discoid lateral meniscus. Because there is only one posterior attachment, the meniscofemoral ligament (ligament of Wrisberg), there is hypermobility of the posterior horn of the lateral meniscus, causing the syndrome of a "snapping" knee.[12] On the medial aspect, the semimembranosus muscle provides tendinous insertion to the posterior capsule and the posterior horn of the medial meniscus (Fig. 2–21).

Ligamentous struts run from the anterior horns of the menisci to the patella. The patellomeniscal ligaments help to draw the menisci forward as the knee is extended. This occurs in concert with the rolling action of the femoral condyles. With flexion, the menisci move posteriorly under the action of the semimembranosus muscle on the medial side and the action of the popliteus muscle and the ligamentous attachments on the lateral side.[26, 42]

The menisci are wedge-shaped pieces of fibrocartilage, the inner three quarters of which are avascular. More peripheral fiber zones contain capillaries and fuse with the parameniscal zone, which is the vascular connection between the capsule and meniscus. Even the peripheral quarter, in which most of the vascularity is present, shows some areas of avascularity.[4]

Microscopic evaluation reveals the meniscus to have three collagen patterns within different zones. The majority of the collagen fibers are oriented in a circumferential fashion, which suggests that the meniscus is designed to resist forces that tend to elongate it.[6] Rotary motions also cause change in position in relation to the tibial condyle. It is believed that motion with flexion and extension occurs between the menisci and the femur, whereas rotary motion of the knee occurs between the meniscus and the tibia. Because the lateral meniscus is less firmly attached, when the tibia is externally rotated the lateral meniscus is held backward, and the tibial condyle protrudes slightly anterior to the meniscal border. During internal rotation, the procedure is reversed. The motion of the

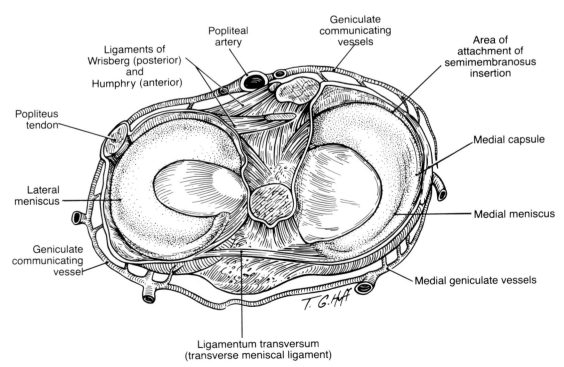

FIGURE 2–21. The anatomic relationships of the medial and lateral menisci, viewed from above.

lateral meniscus in following the rolling forward of the lateral femoral condyle as the knee extends causes a section of the tibial condyle to lie behind the lateral meniscus.

The medial meniscus moves slightly with internal-external rotation, but because of its firmer peripheral attachment and the decreased motion of the medial tibial plateau in rotation, its movements are not as excessive. The elastic fibrous tissue of the medial meniscus at the peripheral attachment causes it to return to the peripheral position after displacement with joint motion. When an uncontrolled flexion or extension movement blocks the normal rotation, the menisci may become trapped between the condyles of the tibia and femur. The tension produced as the meniscus attempts to return to its normal position may cause a tear. Tears of the menisci may also occur when they become crushed between the femoral and tibial condyles or when their peripheral attachments are torn as a result of distractive forces.[71]

The functions that have been attributed to the menisci include nutrition, by moving the synovial fluid around the joint;[50] shock absorption;[48] stability (deepening of the joint);[28] weight bearing;[66, 69] control of motion;[55, 76] enlargement of contact area;[48, 75] and prevention of synovial impingement.[39] Many of these functions have been investigated with regard to their validity. The three major functions of the menisci are stability, enlargement of the contact area, and joint lubrication.

The synovial fluid acts to provide nutrition to the articular cartilage surfaces, which are, for the most part, avascular. The elasticity of the menisci has long been recognized. The menisci can be compressed from 5.0 to 2.5 mm. Such elasticity provides a gentle breaking action that stores energy that is released upon movement in the opposite direction. Krause and collaborators[48] found the menisci to absorb energy most efficiently at relatively low loading rates. Palmer[60] described the menisci as being "like mobile lips in the joint cavities improving the fit of the articular surfaces and protecting the margins in the joint." In this regard, the space-filling effect of the menisci has given rise to the function of preventing impingement of the synovium between the articular surfaces.[39] The elasticity also enables the menisci to conform to the femoral condyles, improving the congruency of the contact of the femoral condyles with the tibia.

The studies by Krause and collaborators[48] also showed that there is a two- to threefold increase in stress across the joint when the menisci are absent. These studies were conducted on cadaver knees with strain transducers in order to note elongating as meniscal loading occurred. The experiments showed that the menisci transmit weight and protect the articular cartilage and the subcondylar bone. In humans, the menisci transmit between 30 and 55 per cent of the load.

The menisci also help disburse the synovial fluid, thus aiding in lubrication of the joint. MacConaill[50] found a 20 per cent increase in joint friction when the menisci were absent.

Contact stress, which is a measurement of the load per unit area, was found to increase threefold after meniscectomy. Studies showed that with no load, the contact area was on the menisci. With loads up to 50 kg, the medial meniscus and exposed cartilage shared the load. It was also noted that the lateral meniscus carried a greater load than did the medial meniscus.[39, 48]

Contributions that the menisci make to joint stability are also recognized. Markolf and colleagues[52] showed that removal of menisci increased anteroposterior laxity approximately 2 mm. This is in addition to the normal 2-mm laxity. Wang and Walker[77] concluded that the menisci serve to restrict both primary and secondary rotary laxity. The primary rotary laxity, which occurred before any significant resistance of the soft tissue was encountered, was increased 14 per cent after meniscectomy; secondary laxity, which occurred after significant resistance of the soft tissue, was increased 2 per cent after meniscectomy. Hsieh and Walker[28] found that meniscectomy had little effect on anteroposterior laxity; however, if the cruciate ligaments were sectioned and the menisci were also removed, large differences in anteroposterior stability were noted. They thus concluded that the menisci play an important role in providing stability when cruciate ligament function has been lost.

Cox and co-workers[10] demonstrated the development of severe degenerative changes in dogs after removal of undamaged menisci. Johnson and associates,[38] in the follow-up of 99 patients who had undergone a meniscectomy an average of 17 years previously, showed that 37 patients had readily demonstrable anteromedial instability. Fairbank,[16] in 1948, described the radiologic changes after meniscectomy as being osteophytic ridges on the femoral condyle and joint space narrowing with flattening of the femoral condyle on the side of meniscectomy. Johnson and associates[11] showed that 77 per cent of the 99 postmeniscectomy patients had at least one of the changes described by Fairbank, whereas the opposite unoperated knee showed these changes in only 6 per cent. It cannot be stated with certainty whether the removal of the meniscus increases contact stress (as a result of the attendant decreased energy absorption) or increases instability, or whether a combination of both effects produces the degenerative changes within the knee. It is, however, becoming more evident that meniscectomy is not an entirely benign procedure.[2, 11]

Synovial Folds and Sheaths

The synovial membrane lines the capsule and covers the cruciate ligaments on their anterior aspect. The peripheral attachment of the synovium overlaps the margin of the articular cartilage for 2 to 4 mm but does not cover the surface of the menisci. The synovial membrane has been classified as fibrous, fatty, or areolar, depending on the nature of the synovial tissue. The synovium around the popliteal tendon, the medial collateral ligament, the patellar ligament, and the anterior wall of the suprapatellar bursa is a type of fibrous synovium. The synovium covering the intracapsular fat pads is a fatty type of synovium. Such fat pads are seen beneath the patellar tendon at its juncture with the inferior pole of the patella. Another fat pad conceals the femoral attachment of the PCL, and a third pad covers the posterior surface of the suprapatellar pouch.

Also located along the synovial lining are small pedunculated synovial villi. These occur at the chondrosynovial junctions on synovial folds and along the course of the cruciate ligaments.

More prominent synovial folds may be seen producing plicae, or shelves, and are examples of the areolar type of synovial tissue.[25, 61] The most commonly described are (1) plica synovialis suprapatellaris, (2) plica synovialis medial patellaris (medial shelf), (3) chorda obliqua synovialis, and (4) the synovial fringes on the infrapatellar fat pad. The plica synovialis suprapatellaris is a remnant of the septum separating the suprapatellar bursa from the knee joint cavity and persists in 10 per cent of human knee joints. In the extended position, it lies in the horizontal direction and runs from the upper pole of the patella toward the synovial lining of the joint. Plicae, or peripheral remnants, occur in about 70 per cent of humans as crescent outlines more commonly formed on the medial side. Other folds may be vertically directed from the medial fat pad to the parapatellar fat pad extending from the medial and superior corridors of the infrapatellar fat pad to the undersurface of the suprapatellar plica. These shelves have been implicated as a cause of catching and of medial joint pain, particularly after a traumatic episode. Oblique synovial folds (chorda obliqua synovialis) are sometimes noticed during full extension of the knee when medial and lateral retinacula are under tension. They extend from the margins of the patella distally to the tibial femoral joint line, delineating the lateromedial margins of the infrapatellar fat pad.

BLOOD VESSELS AND NERVES ABOUT THE KNEE

The capsule and ligamentous tissue are well supplied by nerves. The ligamentomuscular reflex, as described earlier, is produced by the myelin-free nerve endings in the ligamentous tissue. The muscle spasms that frequently accompany injuries to the knee are a result of the pathologic irritation of these nerve endings. Sympathetic nerve fibers around the joint produce a vasomotor response to injury that results in edema.

Two nerves are of particular importance in surgical dissection about the knee. On the lateral aspect, the peroneal nerve descends from the tibial nerve and passes beneath the biceps femoris around the fibular head and into the anterior tibial muscle mass. It may be injured with varus stresses to the knee, and its location should be verified in surgical approaches to the lateral aspect in order to protect it from harm. The other nerve important in knee surgery is the saphenous nerve,[35, 70] which gives off two branches: the infrapatellar branch and the sartorial branch. The infrapatellar branch begins beneath the sartorial muscle and proceeds beneath the tibial condylar flare to the region of the tibial tubercle. It is frequently cut in incisions medial to the patella and the patellar tendon, and this cut creates an area of decreased sensitivity around the anterior aspect of the tibial tubercle.[35] It is occasionally injured in surgical dissection to the point that a neuroma develops in this area, creating an area of exquisite tenderness in response to pressure.

The sartorial branch of the saphenous nerve begins beneath the sartorial muscle near its musculotendinous junction and proceeds distally underneath the pes anserinus group of muscles. Care should be taken to protect this nerve when the pes anserinus area is dissected because this nerve supplies the sensitivity to the anteromedial aspect of the calf. It, too, should be identified and dissected in this area so that it is neither injured nor constricted by transplanted tissue (Fig. 2–22).

The knee has a rich vascular anastomosis consisting of the superior, middle, and inferior genicular arteries on both the medial and lateral

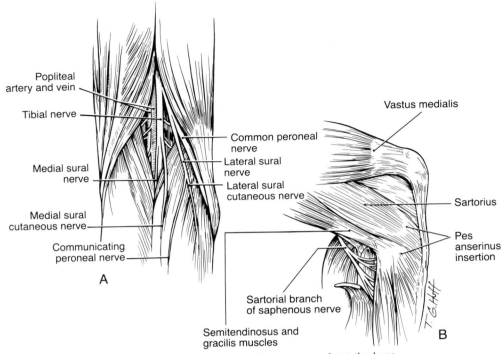

FIGURE 2–22. Neurovascular structures about the knee.

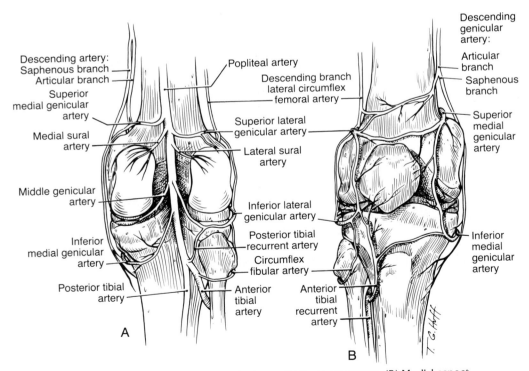

FIGURE 2–23. Blood supply to the knee. *(A)* Posterior aspect. *(B)* Medial aspect.

aspects.[3, 81] The inferior lateral genicular artery runs within the substance of the lateral capsule, just below the joint line (Fig. 2–23). It may be injured during a lateral meniscectomy, and care should be taken to protect it or, if it is cut, to coagulate or tie it. Because of the rich vascular network around the knee, hematoma after injury or surgical approach may occur. In reconstructive surgery about the knee, hemostasis is important, although complete hemostasis is often difficult to obtain. It is wise, therefore, to use suction drainage in any major reconstructive procedure on either the medial or the lateral aspect of the knee.

SUMMARY

The study of knee joint anatomy cannot be relegated to a static joint or divided into isolated segments with any hope of understanding the complex physiology of joint mechanics that enables the functional use of this joint. The interplay of all of the structures supporting the joint, as well as the complexity of the joint motion, highlights the difficulties in reconstructive knee joint surgery. This problem must be recognized and the surgical limitations realized if knee surgery is to be approached in a realistic manner.

REFERENCES

1. Alm A, Liljedahl SE, Stromberg B: Clinical and experimental experience in reconstruction of the anterior cruciate ligament. Orthop Clin North Am 7:181–189, 1976.
2. Appel H: Late results after meniscectomy in the knee joint: a clinical and roentgenologic follow-up investigation. Acta Orthop Scand (Suppl) 133:1, 1970.
3. Arnoczky SP: Blood supply to the anterior cruciate ligament and supporting structures. Orthop Clin North Am 16:15–28, 1985.
4. Arnoczky SP, Warren RF: Microvasculature of the human meniscus. Am J Sports Med 10:90–95, 1982.
5. Basmajian JV, Lovejoy JV: Functions of the popliteus muscle in man: a multifactorial electromyographic study. J Bone Joint Surg 53A:557–562, 1971.
6. Bullough PG, Munuera L, Murphy J, Weinstein AM: The strength of the menisci of the knee as it relates to their fine structure. J Bone Joint Surg 52B:564–570, 1970.
7. Butler DL, Noyes FR, Grood ES: Ligamentous restraints to anterior-posterior drawer in the human knee. J Bone Joint Surg 62A:259–270, 1980.
8. Cabaud HE, Slocum DB: The diagnosis of chronic anterolateral rotary instability of the knee. Am J Sports Med 5:99–105, 1977.
9. Cohn AK, Mains DB: Popliteal hiatus of the lateral meniscus. Am J Sports Med 7:221–226, 1979.
10. Cox JS, Nye CE, Schaefer WW, Woodstein IJ: The degenerative effects of partial and total resection of the medial meniscus in dogs' knees. Clin Orthop 109:178–183, 1975.
11. Dandy DJ, Jackson RW: The diagnosis of problems after meniscectomy. J Bone Joint Surg 57B:349–352, 1975.
12. Dickhaut SC, Delee SC: The discoid lateral meniscus syndrome. J Bone Joint Surg 64A:1068–1073, 1982.
13. Dye SF: An evolutionary perspective of the knee. J Bone Joint Surg 69A:976–983, 1987.
14. Ellison AE: Distal iliotibial-band transfer for anterolateral rotatory instability of the knee. J Bone Joint Surg 61A:330–337, 1979.
15. Eriksson E: Reconstruction of the anterior cruciate ligament. Orthop Clin North Am 7:167–179, 1976.
16. Fairbank TJ: Knee joint changes after meniscectomy. J Bone Joint Surg 30B:664–670, 1948.
17. Feagin JA, Curl WW: Isolated tear of the anterior cruciate ligament, 5 year study. Am J Sports Med 4:95–100, 1976.
18. Fischer LP, Guyot J, Gonon GP, et al: The roles of the muscles and ligaments in stabilization of the knee joint. Anat Clin 1:43–53, 1978.
19. Fulkerson JP, Gosling HR: Anatomy of the knee joint lateral retinaculum. Clin Orthop 153:183–188, 1980.

20. Galway RD, Beaupre A, MacIntosh DL: Pivot shift: a clinical sign of symptomatic anterior cruciate instability. J Bone Joint Surg 54B:763–764, 1972.
21. Girgis FG, Marshall JL, al Monajeh ARS: The cruciate ligaments of the knee joint. Anatomical, functional and experimental analyses. Clin Orthop 106:216–231, 1975.
22. Goodfellow J, Hungerford DS, Zindel N: Patellofemoral joint mechanics and pathology. J Bone Joint Surg 58B:287–290, 1976.
23. Grood ES, Noyes FR: Diagnosis of knee ligament injuries: Biomechanical precepts. *In* Feagin IA (ed): The Crucial Ligaments, pp. 245–260. New York: Churchill-Livingstone, 1988.
24. Hallen LG, Lindahl D: Rotation in the knee joint in experimental injury to the ligaments. Acta Orthop Scand 36:400–407, 1965.
25. Hardaker WT, Whipple TL, Bassett FH III: Diagnosis and treatment of the plica syndrome of the knee. J Bone Joint Surg 62A:221–225, 1980.
26. Helfet AJ: The Management of Internal Derangements of the Knee. Philadelphia: JB Lippincott, 1965.
27. Horne JG, Parsons CJ: The anterior cruciate ligament: its anatomy and a new method of reconstruction. Can J Surg 20:214–220, 1977.
28. Hsieh HH, Walker RS: Stabilizing mechanisms of the loaded and unloaded knee joint. J Bone Joint Surg 58A:87–93, 1976.
29. Hughston JC: Subluxations of the patella. J Bone Joint Surg 50A:1003–1026, 1968.
30. Hughston JC, Andrews JR, Cross MJ, Moschi A: Classification of knee ligament instabilities, part I: The medial compartment and cruciate ligaments. J Bone Joint Surg 58A:159–172, 1976.
31. Hughston JC, Andrews JR, Cross MJ, Moschi A: Classification of knee ligament instabilities, part II: The lateral compartment. J Bone Joint Surg 58A:173–179, 1976.
32. Hughston JC, Bowden JA, Andrews JR, Norwood LA: Acute tears of the posterior cruciate ligament. J Bone Joint Surg 62A:438–450, 1980.
33. Hughston JC, Eilers A: The posterior oblique ligament in the repair of acute medial (collateral) ligament tears of the knee. J Bone Joint Surg 55A:923–940, 1973.
34. Hungerford DS, Barry M: Biomechanics of the patellofemoral joint. Clin Orthop 144:9–15, 1979.
35. Hunter LY, Louis DS, Ricciarbe JR, O'Connor GA: The saphenous nerve: its course and importance in medial arthrotomy. Am J Sports Med 7:227–230, 1979.
36. Jackson RW: The torn ACL: natural history of untreated lesions and rationale for selective treatment. *In* Feagin IA (ed): The Crucial Ligaments, pp. 341–348. New York: Churchill-Livingstone, 1988.
37. Johnson LL: Lateral capsular ligament complex: anatomical and surgical considerations. Am J Sports Med 7:156–160, 1979.
38. Johnson RJ, Kettlecamp DB, Clark D, Leaverton R: Factors affecting late meniscectomy results. J Bone Joint Surg 56A:719–729, 1974.
39. Johnson RJ, Pope MH: Functional anatomy of the meniscus. *In* American Academy of Orthopaedic Surgeons (ed): Symposium of Reconstructive Surgery of the Knee, pp. 3–13. St. Louis: CV Mosby, 1978.
40. Johnson RJ, Pope MH: Knee joint stability without references to ligamentous function. *In* American Academy of Orthopaedic Surgeons (ed): Symposium of Reconstructive Surgery of the Knee, pp. 14–25. St. Louis: CV Mosby, 1978.
41. Jones KG: Reconstruction of the anterior cruciate ligament: a technique using the central one-third of the patellar ligament. J Bone Joint Surg 45A:925–932, 1963.
42. Kapandji IA: The Physiology of Joints: Annotated Diagrams of the Mechanics of the Human Joints, vol 2, pp. 72–135. London: Churchill-Livingstone, 1977.
43. Kaplan EB: Factors responsible for the stability of the knee joint. Bull Hosp Joint Dis 18:51–59, 1959.
44. Kaplan EB: Some aspects of the functional anatomy of the human knee joint. Clin Orthop 23:18–29, 1962.
45. Kennedy JC, Fowler PJ: Medial and anterior instability of the knee: an anatomical and clinical study using stress machines. J Bone Joint Surg 53A:1257–1270, 1971.
46. Kennedy JC, Hawkins RJ, Willis RB, Danylchuk KP: Tension studies of human knee ligaments. J Bone Joint Surg 58A:350–355, 1976.
47. Kennedy JC, Weinberg HW, Wilson AS: The anatomy and function of the anterior cruciate ligament. J Bone Joint Surg 56A:223–237, 1974.
48. Krause WR, Pope MH, Johnson RJ, Wilder DE: Mechanical changes after meniscectomy. J Bone Joint Surg 58A:599–604, 1976.
49. Laurin CA, Dussault R, Levesque HP: The tangential x-ray investigation of the patellofemoral joint: x-ray technique, diagnostic criteria and their interpretation. Clin Orthop 144:16–20, 1979.
50. MacConaill MA: The movements of bones and joints: the synovial fluid and its assistants. J Bone Joint Surg 32B:244–252, 1950.
51. Mann RA, Hagy JL: The popliteus muscle. J Bone Joint Surg 59A:924–927, 1977.

52. Markolf KL, Mensch JS, Amstutz HC: Stiffness and laxity of the knee—the contributions of the supporting structures. J Bone Joint Surg 58A:583–594, 1976.

53. McLeod WD, Mioschi A, Andrews JR, Hughston JC: Tibial plateau topography. Am J Sports Med 5:13–18, 1977.

54. Merchant AC, Mercer RL, Jacobsen RH, Cool CR: Roentgenographic analysis of the patellofemoral congruence. J Bone Joint Surg 56A:1391–1396, 1974.

55. Müller W: The Knee: Form, Function, and Ligament Reconstruction, pp. 8–12. New York: Springer-Verlag, 1982.

56. Norwood LA, Cross MJ: Anterior cruciate ligament: Functional anatomy of its bundles in rotatory instabilities. Am J Sports Med 7:23–26, 1979.

57. Noyes FR, Sonstegard DA: Biomechanical function of the pes anserinus at the knee and the effect of its transplantation. J Bone Joint Surg 55A:1225–1241, 1973.

58. O'Donoghue DH: A method for replacement of the anterior cruciate ligament of the knee: report of twenty cases. J Bone Joint Surg 45A:905–924, 1963.

59. Palmer I: On the injuries to the ligaments to the knee joint: a clinical study. Acta Chir Scand (Suppl 53) 81:3–282, 1938.

60. Palmer I: Injuries to the crucial ligaments of the knee joint as a surgical problem. Reconstruct Surg Trauma 4:181–196, 1957.

61. Patel D: Arthroscopy of the plicae—synovial folds and their significance. Am J Sports Med 6:217–225, 1978.

62. Ross R: A quantitative study of rotation of the knee joint in man. Anat Rec 52:209–223, 1932.

63. Ruetsch H, Morscher E: Measurement of the rotatory stability of the knee joint. *In* Chapchal G (ed): Injuries of the Ligaments and their Repair; Hand-Knee-Foot, pp. 116–122. Stuttgart: PSG Publishing, 1977.

64. Scapinelli R: Studies on the vasculature of the human knee. Acta Anat 70:305–331, 1968.

65. Seebacher JR, Inglis AE, Marshall JL, et al: The structure of the posterolateral aspect of the knee. J Bone Joint Surg 64A:536–541, 1982.

66. Seedhom BB, Dowson D, Wright V: Functions of the menisci: A preliminary study. J Bone Joint Surg 56B:381, 1974.

67. Semlak K, Ferguson AB Jr: Joint stability maintained by atmospheric pressure: an experimental study. Clin Orthop 68:294–300, 1970.

68. Shaw JA, Murray DG: The longitudinal axis of the knee and the role of the cruciate ligaments in controlling transverse rotation. J Bone Joint Surg 56A:1603–1609, 1974.

69. Shrive N: The weight bearing role of menisci of the knee. J Bone Joint Surg 56B:381, 1974.

70. Slocum DB, Larson RL: Pes anserine transplantation: a surgical procedure for control of rotatory instability of the knee. J Bone Joint Surg 50A:226–242, 1968.

71. Smillie IS: Injuries of the knee joint, 4th ed. Baltimore: Williams and Wilkins, 1970.

72. Steindler AL: Kinesiology of the Human Body Under Normal and Pathologic Conditions. Springfield, IL: Charles C Thomas, 1955.

73. Terry GC, Hughston JC, Norwood LA: The anatomy of the iliopatellar band and iliotibial tract. Am J Sports Med 14:39–45, 1986.

74. Tonque JR, Larson RL: Limited arthrography in acute knee injuries. Am J Sports Med 8:19–23, 1980.

75. Walker PS: Contact areas and total transmission in the knee. *In* American Academy of Orthopaedic Surgeons (ed): Symposium on Reconstructive Surgery of the Knee, pp. 26–36. St. Louis: CV Mosby, 1978.

76. Wang CJ, Walker PS: The effects of flexion and rotation on the length patterns of the ligaments of the knee. J Biomech 6:587–596, 1973.

77. Wang CJ, Walker PS: Rotatory laxity of the human knee. J Bone Joint Surg 56A:161–170, 1974.

78. Warren LF, Marshall JL, Gigis F: The prime static stabilizers of the medial side of the knee. J Bone Joint Surg 56A:665–674, 1974.

79. White AA, Raphael IG: The effect of quadriceps loads and knee position on strain measurements of the tibial collateral ligament. Acta Orthop Scand 43:176–186, 1972.

80. Wiberg G: Roentgenographic and anatomic studies on the femoral patellar joint. Acta Orthop Scand 12:319–410, 1941.

81. Wladmirov D: Arterial sources of blood supply of the knee joint in man. Acta Med 47:1–10, 1968.

82. Woods GW, Stanley RF, Tullos HS: Lateral capsular sign: x-ray clue to a significant knee instability. Am J Sports Med 7:27–33, 1979.

CHAPTER 3

Physiologic

and

Biomechanical

Considerations

WILLIAM A. GRANA, M.D.

■

The management of any disorder of the knee must begin with an understanding of the basic properties and function of the joint. This basic knowledge includes the comprehension of physiologic responses of the tissues as well as their chemical and mechanical interaction. The clinical manifestation of an injury or a disease depends on a sequential response by the joint to a stimulus. In addition, the treatment imposed places additional consequences on the effects of this injury or disease and thereby alters the ultimate result. Therefore, it is critical to know the physiologic processes and the biomechanics of the knee in order to appropriately evaluate and treat any problem. The pathophysiologic processes of osteoarthritis, as well as the effects of infection and other inflammatory problems, are determined by the response of the synovium and the articular surface and their interrelationship. The biochemical and physiologic characteristics of the joint determine the short- and long-term implications of the disease process and the effects of any treatment. The knee is a link between the hip and the ankle and, therefore, must provide for sufficient motion with adequate stability in order to transmit the load through the lower extremity. These functions place an enormous mechanical burden on the joint. In addition, the physical requirements and effects of these forces and functions must be considered in reconstructive surgery for ligament insufficiency or for implant design in resurfacing procedures for articular surface damage.

The anatomic configuration of the tibia and the femur provide for little inherent stability. The ligaments and the menisci not only provide for stability but also guide normal joint motion.[5, 11, 23, 29, 35, 36, 40] This is a passive control of the knee (Fig. 3–1). However, active control is provided by the muscles about the joint, principally the quadriceps, hamstring, adductor, and gastrocnemius muscles. Together, these tissues determine the overall load-bearing qualities of the joint.[11, 23, 29, 30, 39, 42]

The kinematics of the knee are important because the three-dimensional motion of the knee and the loads applied during these motions are the ultimate determinants of the load on the articular surface, the ligaments, and the menisci. The ability of the knee to withstand load during activity results in a signature relationship between the tibia and the femur that determines the physical and physiologic needs of the tissues. With

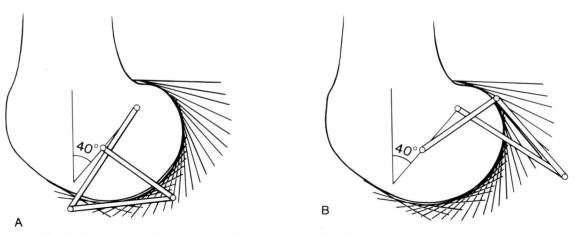

A   B

FIGURE 3–1. The cruciate ligaments provide a passive control of knee motion through the four-bar linkage.

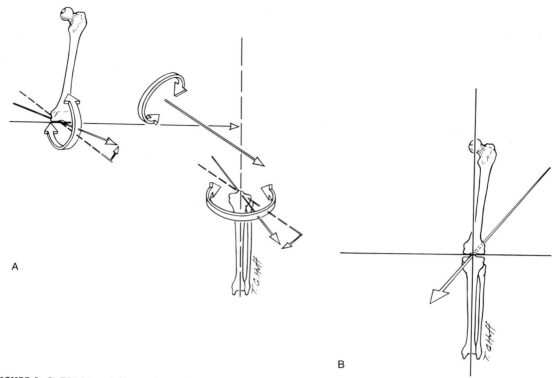

FIGURE 3–2. Tibial translation and rotation on the coordinates of the three-dimensional axes (*B*) allows six degrees of freedom for the tibia with relation to the femur (*A*).

regard to motion, the relationship between the tibia and the femur is described by the science of kinematics, which relates rigid bodies to each other by the use of mathematical relationships.[17, 29, 35] Simply stated, this means that the femur and the tibia can move in a relationship to each other that is described by translation back and forth on the three axes (X, Y, and Z) of the three-dimensional plot of motion or by rotation about these axes (Fig. 3–2). This results in side-to-side, front-to-back, flexion, extension, rotational, and compressive (axial) motion. These six motions are allowed by the osseous structures and the control or guide function of the ligaments, the menisci, and the muscles.[11, 17, 23, 29, 35, 36, 40, 41]

The purpose of this chapter is to give an understanding of the interconnection between the forces on the knee and the tissues that support it: the articular cartilage, the ligaments, the muscles, the menisci, and the extensor mechanism.

TIBIOFEMORAL JOINT

The knee serves as a link between the hip and the ankle. Together, these anatomic structures support the body through the lower extremity. Therefore, the knee must provide support for a variety of loads that may be measured in toto by a force plate as the force applied to the foot (ground reaction force) in stance or gait (Fig. 3–3). This force is balanced by a combination of articular contact force, ligamentous force, muscular force, and inertial force. In single-leg stance, the loaded knee supports more

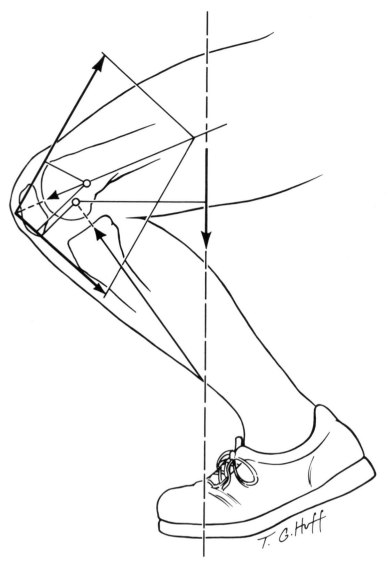

FIGURE 3–3. Forces exerted on the knee of a subject when squatting. P, partial body weight; P_a, force exerted by the patella tendon; R_4, reaction force to the resultant of forces P and P_a or femorotibial compressive force; M_v, force exerted by the quadriceps tendon; R_5, reaction force to the resultant of forces P_a and M_v or patellofemoral compressive force; e, lever arm of force P; c, lever arm with which force P_a acts on the femorotibial joint; k, lever arm with which force P_a acts on the patellofemoral joint; q, lever arm with which force M_v acts on the patellofemoral joint. These complex forces result in an enormously complex response from the anatomy of the knee.

than twice the body weight. In walking, these loads increase to six times the body weight, depending on the phase of gait.[5, 17, 29, 35, 40, 41] How such loads affect the joint is determined by the integrity of the anatomic structure and its ability to function normally. In this section, the ability of the tibiofemoral joint to respond to these large loads and the nature of the response in the normal knee and injury are examined.

The loads just described are distributed over the surface of the knee during impact as a compressive force (contact force). The alignment of the knee determines how equally these forces are distributed. If there is a displacement of the force on the knee as a result of muscle imbalance, there is not only a compressive force but also a shearing force, and these stresses affect the surface of the joint in an unequal way (Fig. 3–4). The side of the joint to which the load is shifted bears more of the stress. Therefore, in varus angular deformity of the knee, more load is borne on

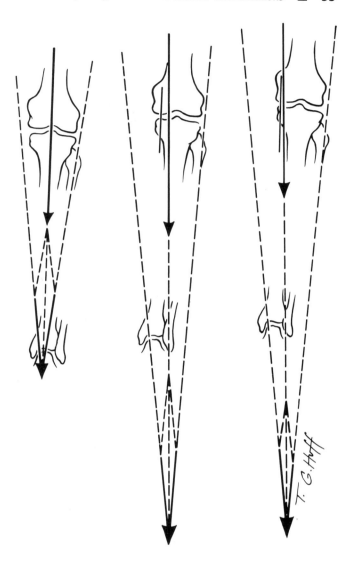

FIGURE 3–4. The normal mechanical axis falls medial to the anatomic axis of the knee, placing a varus movement on the joint.

the medial compartment, and in genu valgum, more of the load is on the lateral compartment of the knee.[10, 11, 25, 29, 31, 35, 41]

The normal anatomic axis of the knee is about 5° of valgus.[10] The normal mechanical alignment (a line from the center of the femoral head to the center of the ankle) is medial to the center of the knee and is therefore a varus moment (Fig. 3–5). In normal stance 75 to 90 per cent of the load is borne on the medial portion of the knee.[25, 31] Hence with this degree of load on the medial side, angular deformity, especially varus deformity, can predispose the joint to more rapid deterioration of the articular surface and menisci on the medial portion. (Coventry[10] and other authors[11, 31] have noted that with increasing body weight, increasing age, or increased physical stress resulting from decreased strength or sports participation, this angular deformity increases the risk of wear and tear change.)

Much of the understanding of the mechanical effects of stress on the

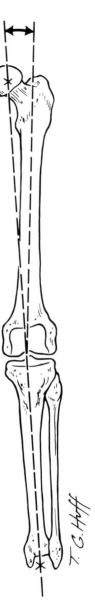

FIGURE 3–5. Varus deformity and weakened musculature shift the weight bearing load farther medially.

knee comes from analysis in stance or normal gait. It appears reasonable to assume that with running or the cutting of certain structures, these stresses are simply accentuated. As the demands on the joint change, the muscles and the ligament action compensate for these increasing loads.[30, 42, 49] The muscles about the knee—the quadriceps, hamstring, and gastrocnemius muscle groups—resist the effect of body weight to induce flexion or extension of the knee when the load falls outside the flexion axis of the knee. This flexion axis is the mechanical center of gait in the sagittal plane. If the ground reaction force is anterior to the flexion axis, the knee extends, and if it is posterior, the knee flexes.[29, 35, 49] The muscles work with the cruciate and collateral ligaments to stabilize this effect. For example, the knee is balanced in extension by the forward pull of the quadriceps muscle and the backward pull of the anterior cruciate ligament, the gastrocnemius muscle, and the collateral ligaments. On the other hand, the hamstring muscles have a similar antagonistic action with the posterior cruciate ligament and the posterior capsule. The action of these three muscles can effectively unload the cruciate ligaments (Fig. 3–6).[23, 36, 39] These findings have important implications for rehabilitation after injury and reconstruction. In addition, when the muscles and the ligaments work in concert, the knee is protected from injury. However, if the forces overcome the effects of muscular control or if antagonistic muscles are unbalanced, injury to the knee may occur, especially in the cruciate-meniscus complex.[5, 11, 19, 23, 39, 40]

When the muscles and the ligaments do not function normally, the result is excessive load on the articular cartilage. Articular cartilage has a remarkable ability to withstand compressive load with great efficiency,[7, 31, 43] in spite of poor blood supply, poor healing ability, and minimal tissue thickness. Fortunately, the structure of articular cartilage of the knee is well suited to these limitations and functions.[32, 34] The collagen, proteoglycan, and water provide pressurization in the structure, which is anchored to the bone in such a way that the changes in configuration occur at the surface. The small pores in the collagen at the surface admit water but not larger molecules. The proteoglycan maintains the water pressure, and

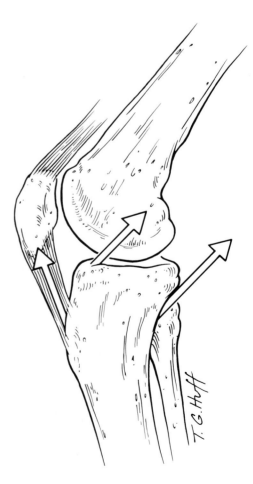

FIGURE 3–6. Muscle pull can load or unload the cruciate ligaments. For example, the hamstrings with the anterior cruciate ligament resist the pull of the quadriceps.

the arrangement of the collagen fibers resists expansion of the pressurized matrix, acting in tension but resisting these compressive loads.[7, 18, 33, 34, 43]

The ability of articular cartilage to hold water is attributable to the proteoglycan matrix. These repetitive disaccharide units of chondroitin sulfate and keratin sulfate bind to hyaluronic acid to form large aggregates. The anionic groups of the proteoglycan attract cationic molecules, which generate osmotic pressure that is responsible for the large swelling pressures. The compressive stiffness of articular cartilage arises from this osmotic pressure and is constrained by the integrity of the collagen structure. Stress applied to the cartilage is dissipated by driving fluid through the porous structure of the cartilage, holding it in the proteoglycan matrix until the stress is withdrawn, and then releasing it back into the joint (Fig. 3–7).[18, 26, 33, 50]

When injury to the articular cartilage is penetrating, it disrupts the

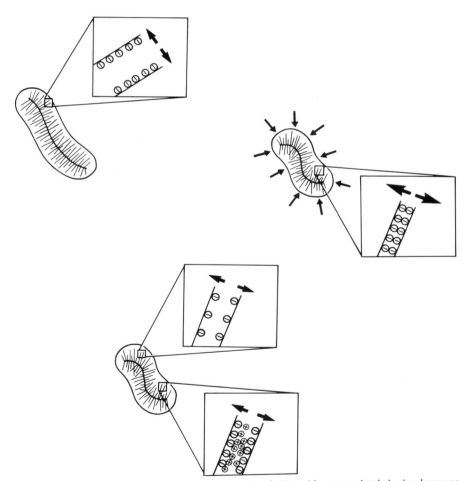

FIGURE 3–7. Schema of proteoglycan aggregate in solution with appropriately ionized groups. Repelling forces are associated with the fixed negative charge groups on the glycosaminoglycan chains. Compressive stresses decrease the aggregate solution domain, which in turn increases the charge density and thus the osmotic pressure and intermolecular charge repulsive forces. Decreasing solution pH or increasing the solution ionic concentration decreases the osmotic pressure and intermolecular charge repulsive forces. The compressive stiffness arises from this osmotic pressure held in place by the integrity of the collagen.

function of the proteoglycan, which affects the mechanism for support of compressive load. As long as the collagen network is intact, the chondrocytes can regenerate the proteoglycan matrix. When there is trauma without disruption of the collagen structure and without death of chondrocytes, as in repetitive impact loading (running or jumping), full healing theoretically should occur.[46] However, penetrating injury that is of full thickness heals, depending on the size of the defect, with a tissue that is fibrocartilage and does not have the type or content of normal proteoglycan. The result is that more than half of such defects undergo degenerative changes 6 to 12 months after injury.[6, 7, 28] No current method of treatment of partial- or full-thickness articular cartilage defects results in a lasting realizable healing response, and therefore the approach to treatment is to relieve mechanical symptoms, not to effect repair.

Earlier in this chapter, the role of ligaments in dissipation of load was noted. This function is related to the role of ligaments in containing the motion of the knee. In this section, the control of motion, the individual functions of ligament complexes, and the physical proprietor of individual ligaments are considered.

The ligamentous structure of the knee guides the motion of the knee through six potential motions (degrees of freedom) along or around the X, Y, and Z coordinates of the three-dimensional space that describe the relationship of motion between the femur and the tibia (Fig. 3–8).[25, 35] The ligaments provide the linkage that controls this motion and its potential degrees of freedom. Most authors have assumed that the linkage between the cruciate ligaments is the most importance of these guides to motion of the knee. The relationship between the anterior and posterior cruciate ligaments is called a four-bar linkage, in which the central axis of these ligaments does not change length (Fig. 3–9).[17, 41] The result is that this

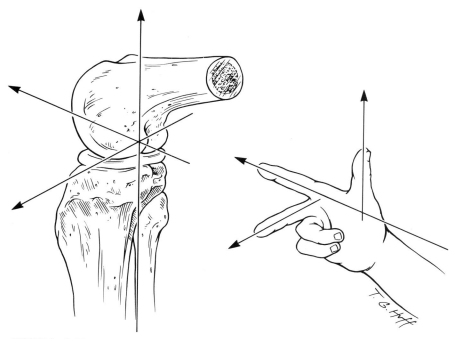

FIGURE 3–8. The three-dimensional axes for the knee form a so-called right-hand system.

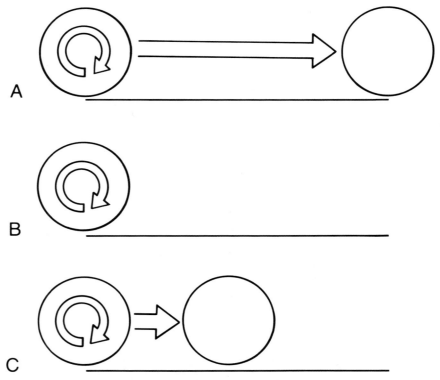

FIGURE 3–9. The rolling and gliding motion of the femur on the tibia is a complex relationship. *(A)* With pure rolling, the wheel travels its circumference. *(B)* In pure gliding, the wheel does not change position. *(C)* In rolling and gliding, the wheel travels less than its circumference but a distance proportionate to the rolling component. Therefore, 50 per cent rolling equals 50 per cent of the circumference. These relationships are controlled and guided by the ligaments.

relationship defines the flexion axis of the knee by the point of intersection of the cruciate ligaments.[35] Hence the concept of restoration of the usual constraints to joint motion relies on maintaining the isometry (anatomic positioning) of the individual ligament complexes, but especially the cruciate ligaments (Fig. 3–10).

Individual ligaments have complex roles in stabilizing the motion of the knee. Butler and colleagues[9] described the interrelationship among the various ligament complexes and the concept of primary and secondary restraints to motion in each of the degrees of freedom of the knee. A primary restraint is the structure that accounts for the majority of ligamentous force that resists an externally applied force in a specific direction. Table 3–1 summarizes the current knowledge of the primary and secondary restraints to the limitation of knee motion in each direction. Figure 3–11 also depicts the effects of isolated ligament disruption.

The important physical properties of ligaments for treatment of injury include ultimate strength, elongation, and stiffness. Figure 3–11 describes this information for the anterior and posterior cruciate ligament complexes.[36] This information is obviously important for reconstruction when biologic autografts are used and eventually will have greater application in the use of allografts and the development of prosthetic replacements. In addition, the information on these physical properties is important for

TABLE 3–1. Primary and Secondary Restraints to Limits of Knee Motion Based on Quantitative In Vitro Studies: ACL, PCL, and Medial and Lateral Structures

Motion	Anterior Cruciate Ligament (ACL)	Posterior Cruciate Ligament (PCL)	Medial Structures				Lateral Structures		
			Superficial Medial Collateral Ligament	Anterior Medial Capsule	Middle Medial Capsule	Posterior Medial Capsule	Lateral Collateral Ligament	Posterior Lateral Capsule	Popliteal Tendon
Anterior displacement	Primary	0	Minor secondary	0	Major secondary	Unknown	Minor secondary	Minor secondary	Unknown
Posterior displacement	0	Primary	Minor secondary	0	0	0	Minor secondary (full extension)	Minor secondary (full extension)	Unknown
Varus	Minor secondary (full extension)	Minor secondary (full extension)	0	0	0	0	Primary	Major secondary	Unknown
Valgus	Minor secondary	Minor secondary	Primary (full extension to 90°)	Unknown	Primary (full extension to 30°)	Unknown	0	0	0
Internal rotation	Major secondary	0	Primary (full extension to 90°)	Unknown	Primary (full extension to 30°)	Unknown	0	0	0
External rotation	Minor secondary	Major secondary (90°)/minor secondary (full extension)	0	0	0	0	Primary (full extension to 90°)	Primary (full extension to 45°)	90°

From Shoemaker SC, Daniel DM: The limits of knee motion. *In* Daniel D, Akeson W, O'Conner J (eds): Knee Ligaments: Structure, Function, Injury, and Repair, Chap 9. New York: Raven Press, 1990.

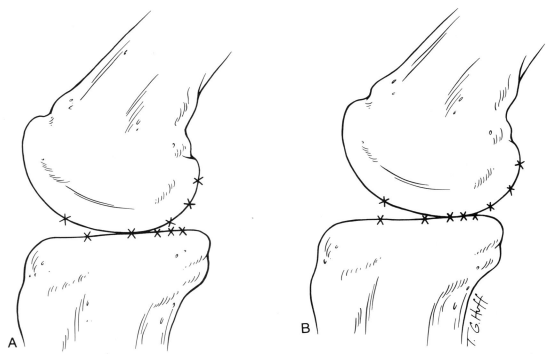

FIGURE 3–10. This diagram shows what happens to the relationship between the rolling and gliding motions with ligament loss (anterior cruciate ligament [ACL] insufficiency). In the normal knee *(A)*, the contact points match as they should, but in the ACL-deficient knee *(B)*, the points no longer match as a result of anterior tibial subluxation.

the autografts used in reconstruction. Table 3–2 contains this information for the commonly used autografts.

The meniscal function is part of the load-bearing mechanism of the knee. These two C-shaped structures transmit 30 to 70 per cent of the load across the knee. Complete meniscectomy reduces the contact area by 50 to 70 per cent and with greater reduction, less load is borne by the meniscus.[32, 34, 45] As long as the outer meniscal rim is left intact, this effect is reduced; hence the benefit of partial meniscectomy. In addition, the shock absorption capacity is also significantly reduced (20 per cent or more), and the load per unit area (stress) is increased by two or three times in the human cadaver knee. Finally, the meniscus improves lubrication by distributing the fluid extended during weight bearing. Meniscectomy results in a 20 per cent increase in due coefficient of function of the joint.[51] The overall effect of meniscectomy is to increase the load borne by the articular cartilage and the ligaments in compression load.[48]

The menisci play an important role in the stability of the knee. With the cruciate ligaments, the menisci contribute to rotary and anteroposterior stability. With muscles about the joint (the quadriceps, popliteus, and semimembranosus muscles), the menisci contribute to the dynamic stability of the joint. The menisci limit joint motion in extreme flexion and extreme extension, and through the functional range of motion, they provide congruity. The meniscus responds to compressive load by viscoelastic changes similar to those of articular cartilage but with different coefficients of friction. The menisci bear compression load in tension just

Combined Medial Structure–ACL Disruption

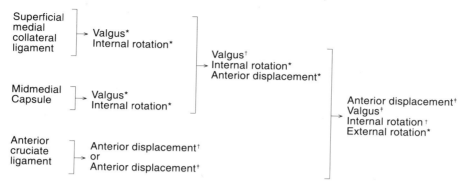

Combined Lateral Structure–ACL Disruption

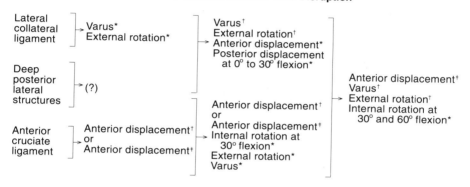

Combined Lateral Structure–PCL Disruption

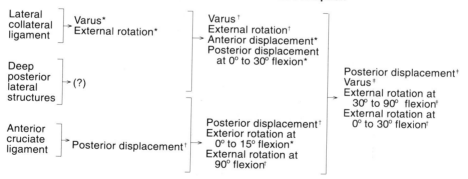

FIGURE 3–11. Three types of ligament disruption. ACL, anterior cruciate ligament; PCL, posterior cruciate ligament. *Demonstrable increase in vitro but probably too small to detect clinically. †Clinically apparent, small increase. ‡Clinically apparent, large increase. (From Shoemaker SC, Daniel DM: The limits of knee motion. *In* Daniel D, Akeson W, O'Conner J [eds]: Knee Ligaments: Structure, Function, Injury, and Repair, Chap. 9. New York: Raven Press, 1990.)

TABLE 3–2. Comparison of Structural Properties of Various Autograft Tissues Commonly Used for Reconstruction of the Anterior Cruciate Ligament (ACL)

Tissue	Number of Specimens	Width (mm)	Ultimate Load (N)	Ultimate Load as % of ACL	Stiffness (N/mm)	Energy Absorbed to Failure (N − m)
ACL	6	—	1725 ± 269	100	182 ± 33	12.8 ± 2.2
Bone–patellar tendon–bone						
Central third	7	13.8 ± 1.4	2900 ± 260	168	685 ± 86	12.8 ± 2.4
Medial third	7	14.9 ± 1.1	2734 ± 298	159	651 ± 85	12.8 ± 2.2
Semitendinosus muscle	11	—	1216 ± 50	70	186 ± 9	8.9 ± 0.5
Fascia lata	18	15.6 ± 0.8	628 ± 35	36	118 ± 5	3.0 ± 0.4
Gracilis muscle	17	—	838 ± 30	49	171 ± 11	3.5 ± 0.4
Distal iliotibial tract	10	18.0 ± 1.6	769 ± 99	44	—	—
Quadriceps–patellar retinaculum–patellar tendon						
Medial	7	14.4 ± 1.9	371 ± 46	21	—	—
Central	6	16.3 ± 3.5	266 ± 74	15	—	—
Lateral	7	13.7 ± 1.8	249 ± 54	14	—	—

From Shoemaker SC, Daniel DM: The limits of knee motion. *In* Daniel D, Akeson W, O'Conner J (eds): Structure, Function, Injury, and Repair, chap 9. New York: Raven Press, 1990.

as the articular cartilage does. This is accomplished by the circumferentially oriented collagen fibers of the meniscus (Fig. 3–12).[4, 8, 12, 51]

PATELLOFEMORAL JOINT

Extensor mechanism disorders may result from intrinsic, congenital, or developmental abnormality in the bone or in the soft tissue structure of the patellofemoral joint. Incongruous motion or increased load may result

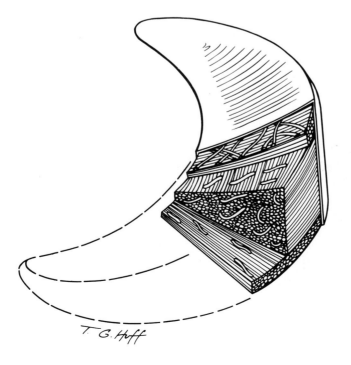

FIGURE 3–12. The collagen fiber orientation determines the ability of the menisci to bear compressive loads.

T. G. Huff

in localized stress and be the first step in articular cartilage damage. Therefore, in order to understand extensor mechanism abnormality, the factors that affect tracking and contact force must be examined.

Normal patellar motion follows a concave lateral curve, which begins laterally, proceeds medially as the patella enters the trochlear groove and the tibia de-rotates, and follows the course of the groove until the knee has flexed to 90°.[15] The bony determinants of this motion include the location, the size, and the configuration of the patella. The soft tissue determinants include the active effect of the quadriceps and hamstring muscles and the passive effect of the capsule and of its specialized expansions.

Wiberg[52] defined patellar shapes as seen on the tangential view of the patella. The types are classified by the width and shape of each facet. The smaller the medial facet, the more likely the association with instability and articular cartilage damage.

Because of the tendency toward lateral tracking during the first 20° of flexion, there is increased load on the lateral facet but only small areas of increased load on the medial side. Therefore, the forces applied during the function are localized to the lateral patellofemoral joint, whereas the medial facet of the patella is relatively free of load during flexion (Fig. 3–13).[22]

A flattening or hypoplasia of the trochlear groove allows the patella more than the normal lateral excursion, particularly in a knee with a weak vastus medialis and a tight lateral retinaculum. Hypoplasia of the lateral condyle enables more lateral excursion of the patella.

Several alignment abnormalities of the lower extremity may increase the valgus vector (described by Ficat and Hungerford[14, 15]) from the pull of the quadriceps muscle and the patellar tendon on the patella. The

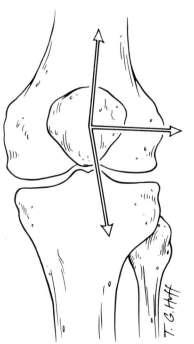

FIGURE 3–13. The normal valgus vector on the patella creates the lateral tracking seen in the first 20° of flexion.

standing alignment of the extremity is such that the width of the pelvis creates this valgus vector and the tendency for the patella to shift or track laterally. The effect of alignment is reflected in the Q-angle (described in Chapter 4) which in turn depicts the degree of real or relative lateral insertion of the patellar tendon. Genu valgum, external tibial torsion, and femoral anteversion have all been implicated as causes of such lateral insertion, which produces an increase in the Q-angle.

Extension of the knee is accomplished by the quadriceps muscle through the patella. This muscle functions as a unit with the oblique fibers of the vastus medialis, providing the main counteraction to the valgus vector of patellar motion and to the larger bulk of the vastus lateralis.[22] In addition, the vastus medialis is the weakest portion of the muscle, the first portion to atrophy, and the last portion to be rehabilitated. Therefore, disuse or any trauma that produces an effusion may lead to relative weakness of the vastus medialis, which allows an excessive amount of lateral tracking of the patella.

On the lateral side, there is an expansion of the vastus lateralis with a superficial layer and a deep layer; this expansion forms the lateral retinaculum. The deep layer forms the lateral patellofemoral ligament, which is a static guide for the patella as it moves through the trochlear groove. If it is too tight, it may contribute to the occurrence of lateral tracking and increased lateral patellofemoral compressive forces. There also may be decreased medial excursion of the patella owing to this tightness on physical examination.[22, 27]

The hamstring muscles act synergistically with the quadriceps muscle. There is a normal flexion:extension strength ratio for these muscles that varies with the velocity of activity. If the hamstring:quadriceps ratio is higher than normal or if there is hamstring tightness, increased load may be applied to the patellofemoral joint. Acute trauma or effusion may produce alterations in this ratio by reflex decrease in quadriceps strength, resulting in patellar compression and lateral tracking.

The different areas of contact between the patella and the distal end of the femur have been reported by several authors. Goodfellow and associates[21] described the patellofemoral contact areas through the range of motion of the knee. In full extension, the patella is not in contact with the distal femur; rather, it sits above the trochlear fat pad without significant compressive load. Initial contact between the articular cartilage of the patella and the distal femur occurs between 10° and 20° of flexion, depending on the length of the patellar tendon. The initial contact occurs between the lateral femur and a narrow band extending across both the medial and lateral facets of the distal patella. The area of contact (extending from the lateral border of the patella to the ridge separating the medial and odd facets) moves proximally on the patella with *increasing* flexion. The proximal border of the patella is reached at 90° of flexion. Therefore, during the first 90° of flexion, all of the patellar articular cartilage, except for the odd facet, comes into contact with the trochlea. The area of contact between the patella and the trochlea also increases with increasing flexion, which helps to distribute the forces of the associated increasing compressive load.

The patella has both a tensile force, caused by the pull of the quadriceps muscle and patellar tendon, and a patellofemoral compressive force acting on it during motion. The magnitude of this patellofemoral compressive force, called the patellofemoral joint reaction (PFJR) force depends on the angle of knee flexion, the quadriceps muscle tension, and the patellar tendon tension.[15, 24] PFJR force may be represented graphically at any angle of flexion[22] (Fig. 3–14). More quadriceps tension is required in order to resist the flexion moment of body weight as knee flexion increases and the resultant PFJR force also increases. Reilly and Martens[44] showed that the PFJR force reached 2.5 to 3.0 times the body weight in a person performing knee bends to 90° of flexion; during ascent and descent of stairs, the force is 3.3 times the body weight, and during deep knee bends to 130°, the force is 7.8 times the body weight. These data help explain why patients with patellofemoral pain experience an increase in symptoms during the performance of activity with knee flexion beyond 45° to 60°. The PFJR force was initially zero at 90°, increased rapidly to a maximum of 1.4 times the body weight at 36° of flexion, and then decreased rapidly to approximately 0.5 times the body weight at full extension. However, the quadriceps tension continues to increase in this situation to its maximal value at full extension. This explains why straight leg raising and short-arc to (20° 0°) knee extension exercises provide maximal stress to the quadriceps muscle while at the same time producing minimal compression on the patellofemoral joint.

Hungerford and Barry[24] compared the unit-load contact stress for flexion of the knee under body weight load and extension against 9-kg

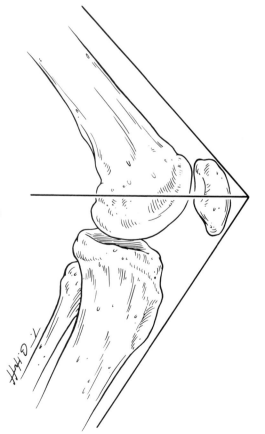

FIGURE 3–14. The patellofemoral joint reaction (PFJR) force can be calculated for any angle of flexion of the knee.

boot resistance. Extension with a 9-kg boot exceeds physiologic compression at 52° of flexion. This occurs because the contact areas of the patella increase with increasing knee flexion, which distributes the increasing PFJR force over a large area to minimize contact stress. This is the situation that exists in flexion under body weight. However, in extension against resistance, the increasing PFJR force is distributed over a smaller area, and therefore contact stress is increased. For this reason, patients with patellofemoral pain who perform extension exercises against resistance from 90° of flexion experience increased pain and worse symptoms.

Several authors have discussed increased contact stress on the patella caused by tightness of the lateral structures and lateral tracking of the patella.[14, 27, 29, 31] Minns and collaborators[31] demonstrated that in a patient with chondromalacia patellae, an increase in the valgus vector produced greater stresses on the patella and articular cartilage. The stress on the patella was reduced 50 per cent when the Q-angle was reduced from 15° to 5° at 30° of flexion.

EFFECTS OF MOTION AND IMMOBILIZATION

Stress and joint motion are important in maintaining the functional integrity of connective tissues and cartilage. The effects of joint immobility on these tissues are deterioration in cartilage, ligament, and tendon structure, biochemical characteristics, and biomechanics.[1, 2, 3, 13] These changes produce significant increases in joint stiffness and contracture.[37] These effects begin immediately and can be irreversible.[16, 55, 56] Decreases in water content and proteoglycans mirror these mechanical changes.[1, 2, 3] The underlying bone becomes osteoporotic and is susceptible to failure. Fibrofatty connective tissue infiltrates the joints. The bony insertion sites of tendons, ligaments, and capsules show a rapid decline in junctional strength.[3, 38, 55, 56] Failure at these sites is more apt to occur through bone after prolonged immobilization. Remobilization or increased activity after immobilization reverses most of the detrimental changes at insertion sites after 4 months to 1 year.[54]

Muscle and the myotenositis junction are adversely affected by immobilization. Muscle sarcomeres are deleted, and length changes to a new, shortened position. Muscle develops less force and fails at a shorter length when stretched, in comparison with nonimmobilized muscle.[53] Failure usually occurs at the myotendinous junction.

Articular cartilage requires synovial fluid for nutrition and metabolic activity. Immobilization decreases the flow of synovial fluid to all portions of articular surface. There is what Salter and associates called "obliterative degeneration" of articular cartilage with adherence of the synovial membrane to the joint surface.[47] Along with this scar formation is a decrease in the volume of the joint capsule and fibroarthrosis. Subchondral bone requires weight-bearing stresses to maintain biomechanical integrity. When the mechanical stress and motion are eliminated, there is an alteration in cartilage fluid dynamics. Subchondral bone atrophy occurs along with chondrocyte clumping.[13] These changes are noted on histologic studies to begin within days of immobilization and can become permanent after 8 weeks.[20]

An exercise program should be designed to minimize immobility but protect against overloading the healing tissues. Early mobilization after injury or surgery should initially consist of controlled passive motion. It is during the inflammatory phase of healing when immobilization can have the most deleterious effects on the joint surface. How this early motion is achieved depends on the individual patient. However, most patients can be taught to perform passive motion. The ability to perform heel slides obviates the need for a continuous passive motion machine. Controlled passive motion need not be continuous. This early motion prevents the formation of adhesions between the synovium and the articular surface. Active assisted and active unassisted motion should proceed as early as the injury or reconstructive procedure allows.

SUMMARY

Anatomic integrity is vital for the integrated function of the knee. Disruption of an anatomic unit places excessive demand on other parts of this complex unit that results in deleterious effects. An understanding of the mechanical and physiologic interactions of these structures better enables the physician to make decisions for treatment and to understand the trade-offs made in each instance.

REFERENCES

1. Akeson WH, Amiel D, LaViolette D: The connective tissue response to immobility: a study of chondroitin 4- and 6-sulfate and detmatin sulfate changes in periarticular connective tissue in control and immobilized knees of dogs. Clin Orthop 51:183–197, 1987.
2. Akeson WH, Amiel D, Mechanic GL, et al: Collagen cross-linking alterations in joint contractions: changes in the reducible cross links in periarticular connective tissue collagen after nine weeks of immobilization. Connect Tissue Res 5(1):15–20, 1977.
3. Akeson WH, Woo SLY, Amiel D, et al: The connective tissue response to immobility: biochemical changes in periarticular connective tissue of the immobilized rabbit knee. Clin Orthop 93:356–362, 1973.
4. Annoczky S, Adams ME, DeHaven K, et al: Meniscus. *In* Woo SLY, Buckwalter JA (eds): Injury and Repair of the Musculo-Skeletal Soft Tissue, pp. 487–537. Park Ridge, IL: American Academy of Orthopaedic Surgeons, 1988.
5. Askew MJ, Melby A, Brower RS: Knee mechanics: a review of in vitro simulations of clinical laxity tests. *In* Ewing JW (ed): Articular Cartilage and Knee Joint Function, pp. 249–266. New York: Raven Press, 1990.
6. Buckwalter JA, Rosenberg LC, Coutto R, et al: Articular cartilage: injury and repair. *In* Woo SLY, Buckwalter JA (eds): Injury and Repair of the Musculo-Skeletal Soft Tissue, pp. 465–482. Park Ridge, IL: American Academy of Orthopaedic Surgeons, 1988.
7. Buckwalter JA, Rosenberg LC, Hunziker EB: Articular cartilage: composition, structure, response to injury and methods for facilitating repair. *In* Ewing JW (ed): Articular Cartilage and Knee Joint Function, pp. 19–56. New York: Raven Press, 1990.
8. Bullough PG, Munuera L, Murphy J, Weinstein AM: The strength of the menisci of the knee as relates to their fine structure. J Bone Joint Surg 52B:564–570, 1970.
9. Butler DL, Noyes FR, Grood E: Ligamentous restraint to anterior-posterior drawer in the human knee. J Bone Joint Surg 62A:259–270, 1980.
10. Coventry MB: The effect of axial alignment of the lower extremity on articular cartilage of the knee. *In* Ewing JW (ed): Articular Cartilage and Knee Joint Function, pp. 311–318. New York: Raven Press, 1990.
11. Crowninshield R, Pope MH, Johnson RJ: An analytical model of the knee. J Biomech 9:397–405, 1976.
12. DeHaven KE: The role of the meniscus. *In* Ewing JW (ed): Articular Cartilage and Knee Joint Function, pp. 103–116. New York: Raven Press, 1990.
13. Evans EB, Eggers GWN, Butler M, et al: Experimental immobilization and remobilization of rat knee joints. J Bone Joint Surg 42A:737–758, 1960.
14. Ficat RP: Degeneration of the patellofemoral joint. *In* Inguierson B (ed): The Knee Joint. New York: Excerpta Medica, 1974.

15. Ficat RP, Hungerford DS: Disorders of the Patellofemoral Joint. Baltimore: Williams and Wilkins, 1977.
16. Finsterbush A, Friedman B: Reversibility of joint changes produced by immobilization in rabbits. Clin Orthop 111:290–298, 1975.
17. Frankel VH, Burstein AH: Kinematics, pp. 118–144. Philadelphia: Lea and Febiger, 1970.
18. Fulkerson JP, Edwards CC, Chrisman OD: Articular cartilage. *In* Albright JA, Brand RA (eds): The Scientific Basis of Orthopaedics, 2nd ed. East Norwalk, CT: Appleton and Lange, 1987.
19. Gillquist J: Knee stability: its effect on articular cartilage. *In* Ewing JW (ed): Articular Cartilage and Knee Joint Function, pp. 267–272. New York: Raven Press, 1990.
20. Ginsberg JM, Eyring EJ, Curtiss PH: Continuous compression of rabbit articular cartilage producing loss of hydroxyproline before loss of hexosamine. J Bone Joint Surg 51A:467–474, 1969.
21. Goodfellow JW, Hungerford DS, Woods C: Patello-femoral joint mechanics and pathology: 1. Functional anatomy of the patello-femoral joint. Bone Joint Surg 58A:287–290, 1976.
22. Grana WA, Kuegshauser LA: Scientific basis of extensor mechanism disorders. Clin Sports Med 4(2):247–257, 1985.
23. Hsieh HH, Walker PS: Stabilizing mechanisms of the loading and unloaded knee joint. J Bone Joint Surg 58A:87–93, 1976.
24. Hungerford DS, Barry M: Biomechanics of the patellofemoral joint. Clin Orthop 144:9–15, 1979.
25. Kettelkamp DB, Wenger DR, Chao EYS, Thompson C: Results of proximal tibial osteotomy: the effects of tibiofemoral angle, stance-phase, flexion-extension, and medial-plateau force. J Bone Joint Surg 58A:952–960, 1976.
26. Kwan MK, Lai WM, Mow VC: Fundamentals of fluid transport through cartilage in compression. Ann Biomed Eng 12:537–558, 1984.
27. Larson RL, Cabaud HE, Slocum DB, et al: The patellar compression syndrome: surgical treatment by lateral retinacular release. Clin Orthop 134:158–167, 1978.
28. Mankin HJ: The response of articular cartilage to mechanical injury. J Bone Joint Surg 64A:460–466, 1982.
29. Maquet PGJ: Biomechanics of the Knee, pp. 1–14. Berlin: Springer-Verlag, 1984.
30. Markolf KL, Mensch JS, Amstutz HC: Stiffness and laxity of the knee—the contributions of the supporting structures: a quantitative in vitro study. J Bone Joint Surg 58A:583–594, 1976.
31. Minns RJ, Birnie AJM, Abernethy PJ: A stress analysis of the patella and how it relates to patellar articular cartilage lesions. J Biomech 12:699–711, 1979.
32. Mow VC, Fethian DC, Kelly MA: Fundamentals of articular cartilage and meniscus biomechanics. *In* Ewing JW (ed): Articular Cartilage and Knee Joint Function, pp. 1–18. New York: Raven Press, 1990.
33. Mow VC, Holmes MH, Lai WM: Fluid transport and mechanical properties of articular cartilage: a review. J Biomech 17:377–394, 1984.
34. Mow VC, Rosenwasser MP: Articular cartilage: biomechanics. *In* Woo SLY, Buckwalter JA (eds): Injury and Repair of the Musculo-Skeletal Soft Tissues, pp. 427–563. Park Ridge, IL: American Academy of Orthopaedic Surgeons, 1988.
35. Müller W: The Knee: Form, Function, and Ligament Reconstruction. Berlin: Springer-Verlag, 1983.
36. Noyes FR, Butler DL, Grood ES, et al: Biomechanical analysis of human ligament grafts used in knee ligament repairs and reconstructions. J Bone Joint Surg 66A:344–352, 1984.
37. Noyes FR, Touik PJ, Hyde WB, et al: Biomechanics of ligament failure: II. An analysis of immobilization, exercise and reconditioning effects in primates. J Bone Joint Surg 56A:1406–1418, 1974.
38. O'Conner J, Biden E, Bradley J, et al: The muscle stabilized knee. *In* Daniel D, Akeson W, O'Conner J (eds): Knee Ligaments: Structure, Function, Injury, and Repair, pp. 239–277. New York: Raven Press, 1990.
39. O'Conner J, Goodfellow JW, Young S, et al: Mechanical interactions between muscles and the cruciate ligaments of the knee. Trans Orthop Res Soc 31; 140, 1985.
40. O'Conner J, Shercliff T, Fitzpatrick D, et al: Mechanics of the knee. *In* Daniel D, Akeson W, O'Conner J (eds): Knee Ligaments: Structure, Function, Injury, and Repair, pp. 201–238. New York: Raven Press, 1990.
41. O'Conner J, Shercliff T, Fitzpatrick D, et al: Geometry of the knee. *In* Daniel D, Akeson W, O'Conner J (eds): Knee Ligaments: Structure, Function, Injury, and Repair, pp. 163–200. New York: Raven Press, 1990.
42. Piziali RL, Seering WP, Nagel DA, Schurman DJ: The function of the primary ligaments of the knee in anterior-posterior and medial-lateral motions. J Biomech 13:777–784, 1980.
43. Radin EL, Paul IL, Lowy M: A comparison of dynamic force transmitting properties of subchondral bone and articular cartilage. J Bone Joint Surg 52A:444–451, 1970.
44. Reilly DT, Martens M: Experimental analysis of quadriceps muscle force and patellofemoral joint reaction force for various activities. Acta Orthop Scand 43:16–37, 1972.

45. Renstrom P, Johnson R: Anatomy and biomechanics of the menisci. Clin Sports Med 9(3):523–538, 1990.
46. Repo RU, Finlay JB: Survival of articular cartilage after controlled impact. J Bone Joint Surg 59A:1068–1076, 1977.
47. Salter RB, Simonond DF, Malcolm DW, et al: The biological effect of continuous passive motion of healing of the full-thickness defects in articular cartilage. J Bone Joint Surg 62A:1232–1251, 1980.
48. Seedholm BB, Hargreaves DJ: Transmission of the load in the knee joint with special reference to the role of the menisci: II. Experimental results, discussion and conclusions. Eng Med 8:220–226, 1979.
49. Shoemaker SC, Daniel DM: Limits of knee motion: in vitro studies. *In* Daniel D, Akeson W, O'Conner J (eds): Knee Ligaments: Structure, Function, Injury, and Repair, pp. 153–161. New York: Raven Press, 1990.
50. Torzilli P: Influence of cartilage conformation on its equilibrium water partition. J Orthop Res 3:473–483, 1985.
51. Voloshin AS, Wosk J: Shock absorption of meniscectomized and painful knees: a comparative in vivo study. J Biomed Eng 5:157–161, 1983.
52. Wiberg G: Roentgenographic and anatomic studies of the femoralpatellar joint. Acta Orthop Scand 12:319–410, 1941.
53. Williams PE, Joldspink G: Connective tissue changes in immobilized muscle. J Anat 138:343–350, 1984.
54. Winston TB, Walmsley R: Some observations on the reaction of bone and tendon after tunneling of bone and insertion of tendon. J Bone Joint Surg 42B:377–386, 1960.
55. Woo SLY, Gomez MA, Sites TJ, et al: The biomechanical and morphological changes in the medial collateral ligament of the rabbit after immobilization and remobilization. J Bone Joint Surg 69A:1200–1211, 1987.
56. Woo SLY, Gomez MA, Woo YK, Akeson WH: Mechanical properties of tendons and ligaments II: the relationships of immobilization and exercise on tissue remodeling. Biorheology 19:397–408, 1982.

CHAPTER 4

Clinical

Evaluation

ROBERT L. LARSON, M.D.

■

All components of the knee work in harmony to provide the stability and the range of motion that enable the activities of daily living as well as walking, running, jumping, kicking, and pivoting. When such function is compromised by limited motion, lack of stability, muscle weakness, or pain, the patient usually seeks medical evaluation and diagnosis so that proper treatment or advice can be rendered.

Although injury is the most frequent initiator of knee dysfunction, it is not the only one. A recent event that causes knee discomfort may also unmask problems within the knee that the patient did not know existed or paid little heed to until a functional problem developed. It is therefore necessary to evaluate a knee problem with a systematic and consistent method that reveals all possible conditions that beset the knee because they may occur concomitantly.

It is helpful to use a knee evaluation form that elicits the important details of the history and physical findings that lead to a proper diagnosis of any pathologic problem that exists (Fig. 4–1).

HISTORY

The personal demographic characteristics of the patient, including sex, age, occupation, height, and weight, may provide important clues as to possible causes of the knee problem. For instance, a patient over 60 years of age very likely has a problem related to degenerative joint disease; a young athlete more likely has a problem related to injury or overuse.

The chief complaint is ascertained. A checklist of pain, swelling, limitation of motion, deformity, instability, catching, locking, or other symptoms is used. Multiple problems are often present but should be sorted out as to which are more disabling, frequent, and severe. The date of onset or the duration of symptoms is recorded.

How the problem occurred is asked: injury, spontaneous, gradual, or sudden? If an injury—sport, work, vehicular—is determined, the details as to the mechanism of injury are elicited. These details are particularly important in possible ligamentous injury because they may provide a clue as to which ligaments are injured. Also important in this regard is the onset of swelling (immediate or delayed), whether a pop was heard (possible injury to the anterior cruciate ligament), ability to continue the activity, loss of motion (immediate, late, locked), and preceding treatment (aspiration, brace, crutches, injection).

A history of any knee injury, condition, or surgery and any residual problems that still exist are determined. A general questionnaire relating to the patient's health history is also filled out by the patient in order to evaluate whether any systemic problems relate to or amplify the knee problem.

The patient's current status is investigated in detail. Specific questions must be asked because the patient may forget or think that some pertinent information is not worthy of mentioning. Again, a checklist with room for explanation is used. The following questions are asked: Are the symptoms acute, chronic, or intermittent? What are the location, type, and severity of the pain, and is it related to activity, postactivity, or night? Is the swelling persistent, does it occur with activity, and what is the degree? Are there problems with sitting, arising, squatting, or kneeling?

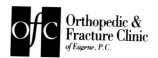

KNEE HISTORY

DATE: _____

M.D.   3   4   5   6   7   8   9

NAME _____ AGE _____

OCCUPATION/POSITION _____

                                                        M   F   Right   Left   Both

CHIEF COMPLAINTS: Pain   Swelling   Limitation Motion   Deformity   Instability   Catching   Locking

                    Other _____

DATE OF INJURY/ONSET: _____

Onset: Injury   Spontaneous   General

If injury: Sport   Occupational   Vehicular

         Other _____

         Pop   Swelling: 0-6, 6-24, 24-48 hrs.   Minimal

– PRESENT STATUS –

SYMPTOMS: Acute   Chronic   Intermittent

PAIN: Location _____

         Type _____ Severity _____

         Activity related _____

         Post-activity _____ Nite _____

SITTING   Y____ N____   ARISING   Y____ N____

SQUATTING   Y____ N____   KNEELING   Y____ N____

LIMITATION OF MOTION: Extension _____   Flexion _____

SWELLING   Y____ N____

STANDING: _____ Pain _____ Tolerance _____

WALKING GAIT:

    Level ground _____   Uneven ground _____

    Tolerance _____

    Stairs: Up _____   Down _____   FOF _____   Unable _____

    Hills: Up _____   Down _____

WEAKNESS _____ GIVE WAY _____

                   INSTABILITY _____

RUNNING GAIT: Speed _____   Endurance _____

CUTTING _____   PIVOTING _____   TWISTING _____

JUMPING: Take-off _____ Landing _____

CATCHING _____

LOCKING _____ No. of Times _____

POPPING _____

GRINDING _____

LOOSE BODY _____

PATELLAR DISLOCATION _____ SUBLUXATION _____

OTHER _____

COMPENSATION: Y____ N____   LITIGATION: Y____ N____

PAST HISTORY: Related   Nonrelated

PREVIOUS SURGERY:

FORM #312

FIGURE 4–1. Form used by the author for recording the history and the physical examination in evaluation of knee problems.

Illustration continued on following page

Orthopedic & Fracture Clinic *of Eugene, P.C.*

KNEE EXAMINATION FORM

BODY BUILD: Endomorphic **CONDITIONING:** Hard
Mesomorphic Medium
Meseoctomorphic Soft
Ectomorphic Flabby

HEIGHT _____

WEIGHT _____

ENTERS: Walking   Cane   Crutches   Limp

	RIGHT	LEFT	NOTES
STANDING ALIGNMENT:			
Varus: cms between knees °			
Valgus: cms between ankles °			
Tibial Torsion: Int. Ext.			
Hyperextension			
FUNCTIONAL TEST:			
Gait			
Stationary Jog			
Leaning Hop Test			
Squat			
Kneeling			
Duck Waddle			
MEASUREMENTS:			
Leg Length			
Mid calf			
Mid patella			
7 cms above joint			
KNEE MOTION: Hyperextension ° to °			
Extensor lag			
PAIN:			
On Forced Extension			
On Forced Flexion			
Motion Valgus Stress/Crepitus			
Motion Varus Stress/Crepitus			
SWELLING: Intra-articular			
Extra-articular			
MUSCLE STRENGTH: Quadriceps			
(5 to 0) Hamstrings			
Hip Flexors			
EXTENSOR MECHANISM:			
Patellar Position: Standing			
Sitting			
Patellar Tracking: Smooth Y ☐ N ☐			
Deviation Y ☐ N ☐			
Vastus Medalis Dysplasia			
Quadriceps			
Quadriceps Tendon			
Patella:			
Height: normal; increased			
Mobility: normal; increased supine ☐			
prone ☐			
Subluxates; dislocates			
Pain on forced lateral luxation (45°)			
Tenderness: Peripatellar ☐ Retropatellar ☐			
Facet ☐			
Retropatellar grating with ☐			
without ☐ pain			
Medial Retinaculum			
Lateral Retinaculum			
Patellar Tendon			
Q-Angle			
Tibial Tubercle: Prominent ☐ Swollen ☐			
Tender ☐			

FORM #313

FIGURE 4–1 *Continued*

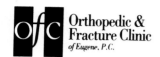

Orthopedic &
Fracture Clinic
of Eugene, P.C.

Page 2

TENDERNESS	RIGHT	LEFT
Anteromedial Joint Line		
Mid-medial Joint Line		
Posteromedial Joint Line		
Anterolateral Joint Line		
Mid-lateral Joint Line		
Posterolateral Joint Line		
Medial Capsule		
Tibial Collateral Ligament - where		
Lateral Capsule		
Fibular Collateral Ligament		
P.O.L.		
Pes Anserinus		
PALPABLE OSTEOPHYTES		
A. Femoral ☐ B. Tibial ☐		
LIGAMENTOUS LAXITY ON		
Forced Valgus at 0° Flexion		
Forced Valgus at 30° Flexion		
Forced Anteromedial		
Forced Varus at 0° Flexion		
Forced Varus at 30° Flexion		
Forced Hyperextension		
ROTATION INSTABILITY TEST		
Lachman Test		
FRD Test		
Anterior drawer Neutral		
Internal Rotation		
External Rotation		
Pivot Shift Test		
Posterior Drawer Test		
Posteolateral Instability Sign		
Recurvatum Sign		
Reverse Pivot Shift		
McMURRAY TEST		
External Rotation Pop/Pain		
Internal Rotation Pop/Pain		
CATCH OR POP		
POPLITEAL SPACE		
Swelling		
Tumor – Baker's Cyst		
Tenderness		
TIBIAL EXT. ROT. @ 90°		
HIP ROM F/E		
AB/AD		
ER/IR		
ANKLE ROM DF/PF		
DIAGNOSIS/NOTES		

RIGHT

LEFT

FORM #313

FIGURE 4–1 *Continued*

Is limitation of motion in flexion, extension, or both? Is there pain in standing, and what is the patient's tolerance? Does walking cause pain on level and uneven ground, stairs, and hills (up, down, foot over foot; unable), and what is the patient's tolerance? Is there weakness, giving way, or instability? How is running gait in terms of speed, endurance, stopping, starting, cutting, pivoting, and twisting? In jumping, is there pain in take-off or landing? Is there catching, locking, popping, or grinding? Is there a loose body? Is there patellar dislocation or subluxation? Additional information that may be determined from discussion with the patient includes the patient's motivation for following the necessary treatment program and whether worker's compensation or litigation is involved.

PHYSICAL EXAMINATION

The physical examination of the knee is often compromised by many factors. Pain that causes the patient to guard the knee may make evaluation of motion and ligament stability difficult. Swelling may limit motion and interfere with palpation. The size of the extremity may make grasping and testing for stability strenuous and formidable (alternative methods may be necessary). Considerable adipose tissue around the knee makes a precise examination impossible.

The proper examination becomes a learning experience that may be modified by some of the extenuating circumstances just listed. A systematic and methodical examination includes inspection; palpation; measurements for motion, muscle strength, leg lengths, and muscle girth; functional tests for assessing walking gait, stationary running, hopping, and squatting; tests for mechanical or meniscal problems such as McMurray's test, Apley's test, or LeMaire's test; evaluation of ligament stability; evaluation of the extensor mechanism; and evaluation of the popliteal space. These procedures provide the examiner with a nearly complete inventory of knee function. Modifications or omissions may be desirable. A patient with obvious degenerative joint disease with swelling, deformity, and pain obviously would not be tested for the functional abilities of jogging in place, hopping, and so forth.

The physical examination recommended is a compendium of the most efficient methods learned through the author's experience and by other surgeons interested in knee surgery. The patient wears shorts so that both extremities can be visualized in their entirety.

Standing Alignment

The patient is viewed from the front and the side so that any deformity or malalignment present in either extremity is seen. Valgus or varus angle is measured as distance between the knees or ankles or is determined with the goniometer, and the degree of tibial torsion is noted. Equality of extremity lengths is noted by comparing the levels of each side of the pelvis.

Functional Tests

The walking gait is evaluated for any limp or abnormality. The patient performs stationary jogging and high-knee stationary jogging, and any uncertainty of support, limitation of knee motion, weakness, or pain is noted. Asymmetry of motion, if present, is evident to the examiner. In the leaning hop test (Fig. 4–2), the patient hops up and down on one leg at a time with the other leg abducted to the side. Deficiency of strength or uncertainty of support is evident from decreased pushing off of the affected extremity. The patient also rotates the leg both inward and outward during hopping in order to elicit any uncertainty of support or actual instability. This test can also be conducted with the patient's opposite leg crossed over the leg being tested in order to put different stress to the ligament structures in an attempt to produce signs or symptoms of instability.[1] The squat test reveals any limitation of knee flexion and may produce impingement symptoms if meniscal pathologic

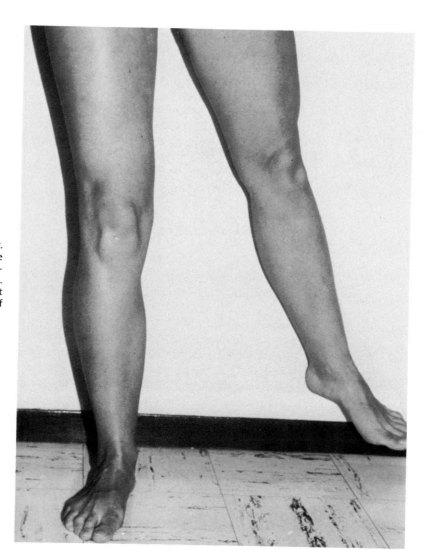

FIGURE 4–2. Leaning hop test. Hopping on the leg with the other extremity abducted produces a valgus stress to the knee. Rotating the leg as the patient hops accentuates the feeling of instability.

processes are present. The duck waddle test can be used to place additional stress and impingement to the menisci and the ligaments.

The patient then sits on the examining table, and tests (such as muscle strength testing) are conducted, patellar position and its tracking are evaluated, and evidence of tibial rotation is noted. As active flexion and extension are performed, the knee is palpated in order to feel for any crepitation of the joint or patellofemoral articulation.

Muscle Strength

Quadriceps, hamstring, and hip flexor strengths are clinically estimated by manual resistance to their action and graded on a scale of 5 (high strength) to 0 (no strength). The patient then lies supine on the examining table for other tests.

Measurements

Leg lengths and midcalf, midpatella, and thigh circumferences (measured at equal distances above the patella on each leg) are recorded. Knee motion is measured, with checks to see whether there is any hyperextension or extensor lag. A goniometer is used to measure full knee extension and flexion.

PAIN. Evidence of any pain with knee motion—either active or passive—is noted. While this test is being manually performed by the patient, the examiner feels for any crepitus with passive motion and valgus and varus stress.

SWELLING. Presence and degree of both intra-articular and extra-articular swelling are noted.

Extensor Mechanism

The patellar position is noted in both the standing and sitting positions. As the patient squats during the functional testing, the examiner palpates both knees to check for crepitation and grinding. In order to check patellar tracking, the patient, in the sitting position, extends and flexes the knee while the examiner observes the movement of the patella for smoothness or any deviation. During active and passive movement, the patella is also palpated for crepitation or any catching or clicking. To check for vastus medialis dysplasia, the patient extends the knee against firm resistance, and any difference in the symmetry of the two sides is noted. The quadriceps muscle is also observed for any evidence of atrophy, and the quadriceps tendon is palpated as quadriceps contraction occurs in order to see whether any tenderness or defect is present.

The patella itself is checked with the patient in the supine position. Its height (whether it is high or low), its mobility (normal or increased), whether it can be manually subluxated or dislocated, and any apprehension with side-to-side movement, particularly lateral luxation (apprehension sign), are noted. The examiner also checks for tenderness (peripatellar, retropatellar, facet) and for retropatellar grating with both pressure and manual movement and whether this grating occurs with or without pain. The medial and lateral retinacular structures are palpated for any thickening, bands, snapping with motion (plica), or tenderness. (A history of a blow to the front of the knee with subsequent snapping and a tender palpable band may indicate a symptomatic medial plica.)

The patellar tendon is palpated for any tenderness, thickening, or defect. The area around the patellar tendon is where the infrapatellar fat pad is located and should be palpated for any thickening or tenderness. The Q-angle (the angle formed by an imaginary line through the antero-superior iliac spine, the center of the patella, and the center of the tibial tubercle) is determined as a measure of proneness for lateral subluxation or recurrent dislocation. The tibial tubercle is assessed for any prominence, swelling, or tenderness.

Tenderness

Tenderness to pressure around the joint is carefully elicited by firm palpation. Joint line tenderness is defined as anteromedial, midmedial, posteromedial, anterolateral, midlateral, or posterolateral. The examiner checks for tenderness in the medial and lateral capsules, over the medial and lateral collateral ligaments, over the posterior oblique ligament, around the pes anserinus area (pes anserinus bursitis or sartorial branch of the saphenous nerve irritation), and in the area medial to the tibial tubercle (infrapatellar branch of saphenous nerve neuroma). Tenderness over the popliteal tendon should be differentiated from posterolateral joint line tenderness.

Palpation

Evidence of thickening of the synovium and the presence of palpable osteophytes of the femur or the tibia are noted. Stability and tenderness of the fibular head can be checked.

Ligament Laxity and Rotatory Instability Testing

This important aspect of the knee examination is discussed later in this chapter. The ligament laxity is graded on a scale of 0 (normal, very slight elasticity of the ligament) to 3+ (a marked opening or displacement of the joint with no definite endpoint discernible).

Tests for Meniscal Pathology

McMurray's test and Apley's test are done with the knee in both internal and external rotation in order to see whether any impingement, catch, pop, click, or pain is produced. In McMurray's test, the physician manually flexes and extends the knee with the foot in the internally and externally rotated positions while first a valgus stress and then a varus stress are placed on the knee. In *Apley's test*, the patient is prone. The physician flexes the knee and performs the maneuver of extending the knee with the foot in both the internally and externally rotated positions but with downward compression on the joint. *LeMaire's test* is conducted to evaluate laxity of the posterior oblique ligament. If this ligament is torn or stretched, the medial tibial plateau can be displaced anteriorly with the knee flexed to 90° and the foot externally rotated. Anterior stress on the tibia may produce a click, indicating incompetency of the peripheral attachment of the medial meniscus, which causes the meniscus to be pulled forward underneath the medial femoral condyle.

Popliteal Space

The patient is turned to the prone position, and Apley's test is completed. The space is then palpated for any swelling, mass (possible Baker's cyst), or tenderness.

Tibial external rotation with the knee flexed to 90° can be assessed for symmetry.

Hip and ankle ranges of motion should also be recorded because both may play a role in knee function.

TESTS FOR LIGAMENTOUS LAXITY AND ROTATORY INSTABILITY[12]

"Laxity" and "instability" are terms that are often mistakenly used interchangeably. Laxity is a slackness of ligament support that allows a discernible amount of joint displacement to occur when the joint is stressed. This may be normal for one individual or excessive, depending on the type of laxity, the degree of laxity, and the variation in comparison with the opposite knee. Instability is the condition that produces an uncertainty of joint support as a result of displacement of joint structures (produced by abnormal laxity of one or more ligaments). Although there may be physiologic laxity that does not produce a disabling problem, instability is a pathologic condition that affects joint use and may produce a disability.

Variations in the degree of physiologic laxity present in a joint exist among individuals. Some people have very lax joints, whereas others have very tight joints. To appreciate this fact, the examiner must compare the uninvolved knee with the involved knee. Caution should also be exercised because previous injuries to ligament structures in the "uninvolved knee" may have left residual pathologic laxity.

Testing for isolated ligament support requires the knee to be put in positions that allow secondary restraints to slacken so that the individual ligament can be more precisely evaluated. Such testing must be conducted with the realization that the knee performs a complex of movement involving translational as well as rotational freedom of movement. Abnormal ligament laxity may cause excessive displacement in more than one plane of motion. Ligament laxity must therefore be analyzed in terms of three dimensions whereby portions of the joint displace with both translational and rotational components.[17] A more detailed and biomechanical explanation of the concepts of primary and secondary restraints is given in the chapters on specific ligament instabilities.*

Valgus and Varus Laxity Tests

Stress testing for valgus and varus laxity or instability must be conducted with the knee in full extension; this may be hyperextension in a lax joint, or it may be hyperextension caused by ligamentous injury. The knee is also stressed at 0° and 30° of flexion. The patient must be relaxed in order for the test to be reliable because any guarding of the muscles helps splint the knee. Guarding may be prevented by leaving the thigh supported on the examining table while the knee is brought out over the side. Valgus and varus stress to the patient's knee can then be applied by the examiner with one hand while the patient's foot is held with the examiner's other hand with the patient's leg at the proper position. This is particularly helpful in a patient with an acute injury in which any extra movement causes pain and causes the patient to reflexively guard the knee from movement. Another method used when the patient can relax is to cradle the patient's foot in the examiner's axilla (Fig. 4–3) while the examiner uses the hands to palpate the patient's knee while stress is being applied by the examiner's body.

Joint opening at hyperextension or at 0° indicates a significant ligamentous injury that probably involves one or both cruciate ligaments. A knee with hyperextension on only the injured side that opens with varus stress testing indicates rupture of the posterior cruciate ligament (PCL) as well as of the arcuate complex. Such a situation with a valgus stress indicates a medial capsular and cruciate ligament disruption. With the knee at 30° of flexion, the cruciate ligaments are relaxed, and the use of valgus and varus stress constitutes more accurate testing of the corresponding collateral ligament integrity. Slight laxity may be noted in comparison with the test at 0°, but any opening more than a few millimeters wider than that in the opposite side indicates a pathologic laxity. In tests for varus laxity at the 30° position of flexion, the opening is slightly wider on the lateral side than on the medial side. This degree of laxity is the physiologic laxity of the lateral side.

Tests for Anterior Cruciate Laxity

LACHMAN'S TEST. Lachman's test[21] is one of the more accurate and sensitive tests for assessing anterior cruciate ligament (ACL) deficiency.[3, 11] A positive finding suggests laxity of this ligament but does not necessarily mean that an instability is present. The test is conducted with the patient in the supine position and the knee resting on the examining table (Fig. 4–4A). The knee is passively flexed to 15° to 30°, or the distal thigh is placed on a bolster to provide this position. The examiner grasps the patient's distal femur with one hand and the patient's proximal tibia with the other. An anterior stress is placed on the tibia while the femur

---

*A very precise form for recording the results of laxity testing was developed by Noyes and Grood.[17] A committee composed of members of the American Orthopaedic Society of Sports Medicine and the European Society of the Knee and Arthroscopy developed a standardized form for reporting the evaluation for knee instability. This form is described in Chapter 18.

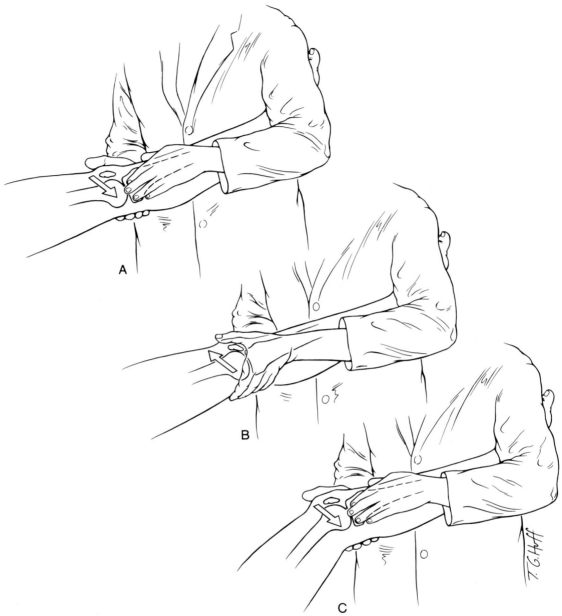

FIGURE 4–3. Abduction (valgus) stress test. *(A)* A valgus stress is placed on the patient's foot by the examiner's body while the examiner's hands palpate the patient's medial joint line for any opening while stabilizing the knee. *(B)* A similar test is done by providing a varus stress and palpating the lateral joint line for any opening. *(C)* These tests are repeated with the knee flexed to 30°.

is stabilized. When the ACL is intact, minimal motion occurs, and a definite endpoint is appreciated. If the ACL is deficient, the tibia moves forward excessively, and the contour of the patellar tendon, normally concave, becomes convex. The degree of displacement is graded as 0 (no displacement), 1+ (displacement of up to 5 mm), 2+ (6 to 10 mm), and 3+ (11 to 15 mm). As noted, a comparison with the opposite knee is

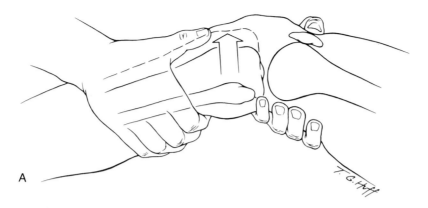

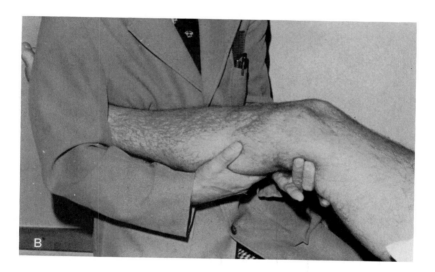

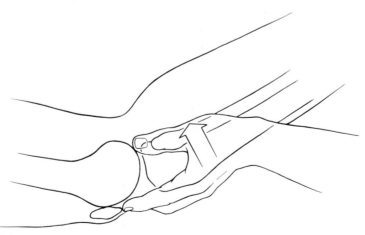

FIGURE 4–4. See text. *(A)* Lachman's test with the patient supine. *(B)* Alternative method when largeness of the leg prevents grasping the distal femur or the proximal tibia. *(C)* Prone Lachman's test. The patient's femorotibial relationship is palpated by the examiner's fingers. (Redrawn from Feagin JA: Introduction: principles of diagnosis and treatment. *In* Feagin JA [ed]: The Crucial Ligaments, p. 11. New York: Churchill Livingstone, 1988.)

made in order to determine whether the displacement is indeed pathologic for the affected knee.

Alternative methods of performing this test may be necessary when the girth of the patient's extremity is so large that the examiner cannot comfortably grasp the patient's distal femur or proximal tibia. One method is to cradle the patient's distal leg in the examiner's axilla, leaving the examiner's hands free to provide alternating anterior pressure to the posterior condyles of the patient's femur and tibia (Fig. 4–4B). The examiner feels for excessive anterior motion of the tibia and observes any loss of contour of the patella and patellar tendon as the tibia is pushed anteriorly. A second alternative method was described by Feagin[4] (Fig. 4–4C). The patient lies prone, and the knee is flexed to 30°. Pressure is applied to the tibial tubercle in order to see whether it can be displaced posteriorly, which would negate the gravitational effect of the tibia's displacement anteriorly from the ACL deficiency.

A test for differentiation between posterolateral and posteromedial laxity is conducted in a similar manner. With the patient prone and the knee flexed 30°, pressure is applied to the tibial tubercle. The direction in which the foot rotates indicates the laxity present. If the foot rotates externally, more posterolateral laxity is present. If it rotates internally, more posteromedial laxity is demonstrated.

FLEXION-ROTATION-DRAWER (FRD) TEST. The knee is flexed and extended while the physician alternately performs Lachman's test as it is extended and a posterior drawer test (described in the next section) as it is flexed (Fig. 4–5). As the knee is extended, the weight of the thigh causes the femoral condyle to drop back into a subluxated position as the lateral tibial plateau is pulled forward with Lachman's test. The examiner watches for the femoral condyle to roll into external rotation as this action occurs. When the knee is flexed with a posterior push on the tibial condyle, the femoral condyle rolls into internal rotation as the subluxation is reduced when the lateral tibial condyle is pulled posteriorly by the iliotibial tract. Noting the direction in which the patella moves helps in monitoring the rotation of the femoral condyles. According to Noyes and Grood,[17] this test assesses the function of the ACL in controlling both translation and rotation.

ANTERIOR DRAWER TEST. This test is performed in three positions of tibial rotation[20] (Fig. 4–6). The patient's knee is flexed between 60° and 90° with the foot resting on the examining table. The author prefers to sit on the patient's foot in order to maintain the position and stabilize the patient's leg. The foot is in neutral rotation, and the amount of anterior displacement of the tibia is estimated in millimeters (recording in this manner, rather than as 1+, 2+, or 3+, more accurately defines the translation of the tibia). The lateral tibial plateau comes slightly more forward than the medial plateau when the anterior drawer test is performed with the patient's foot in the neutral position. This is because of the shapes of the respective tibial plateaus (the lateral plateau is convex; the medial plateau is concave). If the medial tibial plateau comes forward equally to the lateral tibial plateau, some laxity of the posterior oblique ligament may be present. The foot is then placed in 15° of external rotation, and the anterior drawer test is repeated. Note is made of the anterior displacement of the medial tibial plateau. A greater degree of anterior displacement on the affected side than on the opposite side

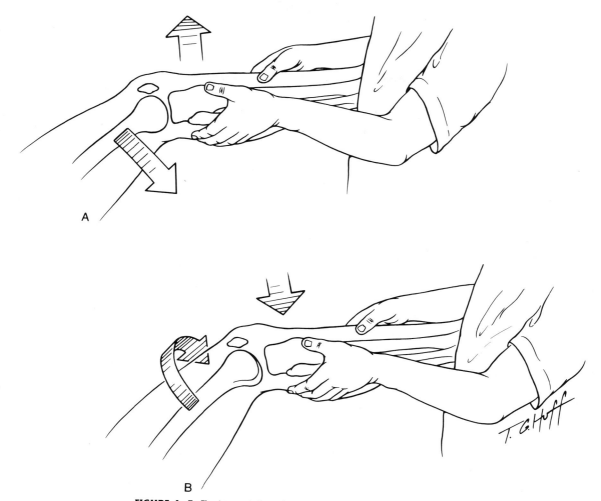

FIGURE 4–5. Flexion-rotation-drawer test. (See explanation in text.)

suggests stretching of the medial capsular ligament support. If the ACL has been torn, an anterior translation of the tibia occurs with the rotation, indicating a more global type of instability. The foot is then internally rotated 30°, and the anterior drawer test is again performed. This rotation tightens the iliotibial tract, the lateral structures, and the PCL. Anterior displacement of the tibia in this position indicates laxity of these structures and is often indicative of a PCL injury.

Test for Anterolateral Rotatory Instability

PIVOT-SHIFT PHENOMENON.* This event, first described by MacIntosh and Galway,[6, 15] has many variations. All are devised to allow the

---

*Although in North America MacIntosh is usually credited with first describing the pivot-shift phenomenon, many earlier investigators described a similar situation. The earliest reference was by Hey Groves[7] in a paper published in 1920: "In active exercise, when the foot is put forward and the weight of the body is pressed on the leg, then the tibia slips forward. Sometimes this forward slipping of the tibia occurs abruptly with a jerk."

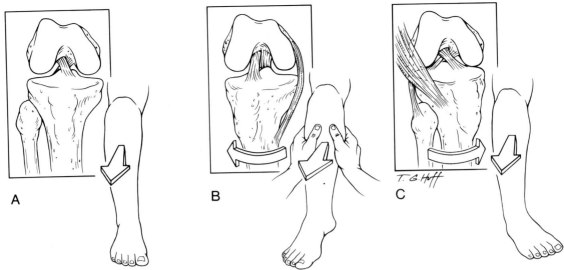

FIGURE 4–6. Anterior drawer test. (See explanation in text.) Anterior stress on the proximal tibia with the foot in neutral rotation *(A)*, with the foot in 15° of external rotation *(B)*, and with the foot in 30° of internal rotation *(C)*.

tibia to subluxate forward and the lateral femoral condyle to slip posteriorly onto the posterior slope of the lateral tibial condyle as the knee reaches extension (Fig. 4–7). This action is allowed because of the inadequacy of the ACL in restraining forward motion of the tibia. As the knee is flexed, a reduction occurs as the iliotibial tract moves posteriorly past the center of the axis of rotation of the knee and pulls the tibia into the reduced position (Fig. 4–7C).

MacINTOSH'S PIVOT-SHIFT TEST. As originally described, this test begins with the knee in full extension. The knee is in the "locked home" position. With the foot in internal rotation, a valgus anterior stress is applied to the lateral tibial condyle as the knee is slowly flexed (Fig. 4–8A). The tibia displaces forward as a result of the ACL loss, and the lateral femoral condyle slides off the convex surface of the lateral tibial plateau and onto the slope of the posterior lateral condyle (Fig. 4–8B). When the knee reaches 20° to 40° of flexion, there is a sudden reduction of the tibia (Fig. 4–8C). The valgus thrust to the knee enhances the velocity of the reduction and accentuates the jerk that occurs, as does weight bearing.

JERK TEST. This test, as described by Hughston and associates,[8] begins with the knee in the flexed position. The tibia is in the reduced position. With the foot in internal rotation and a valgus stress to the lateral tibial plateau, the knee is gradually extended. As the knee approaches 20° to 40° toward extension, a sudden "jerk" occurs as the tibia moves anteriorly and the lateral femoral condyle subluxates posteriorly. The patient often states that this is the same sensation produced as when the "knee goes out" during activity.

ANTEROLATERAL ROTARY INSTABILITY (ALRI) TEST. This, too, is a modification of the MacIntosh test as described by Slocum and colleagues[19] (Fig. 4–9). It is helpful for detecting the pivot-shift phenomenon when the extremity is very heavy or when the patient has trouble relaxing. The patient rolls onto the unaffected side with the medial side of the foot of the affected extremity on the table and the pelvis rolled posteriorly

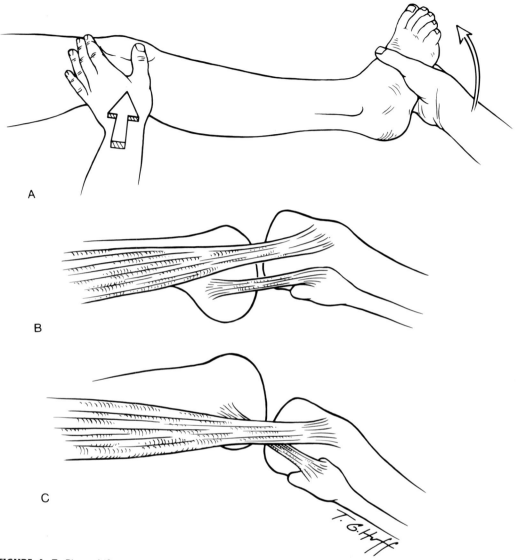

FIGURE 4–7. Pivot-shift test. *(A)* Valgus anterior thrust placed against the proximal tibia with the foot in internal rotation and the knee extended. *(B)* In the nearly extended position, the tibia is anteriorly subluxated as a result of insufficiency of the anterior cruciate ligament. The iliotibial tract lies anterior to the central axis of knee rotation. *(C)* As the knee is flexed, the iliotibial tract moves posterior to the central axis of knee rotation and pulls the tibia into its reduced position. Valgus stress accentuates the "jerk" of reduction.

approximately 30°. The unaffected hip is flexed in order to get the knee out of the way. With the patient's involved knee extended, the examiner grasps above and below the patient's knee to apply a valgus stress. The patient's knee is passively flexed. A positive response is one in which the tibia suddenly reduces at 20° to 40° of flexion.

LOSEE'S TEST.[14] This test is a refinement of MacIntosh's test when the iliotibial tract is insufficient and may not produce the sudden reduction noted in other tests (Fig. 4–10). With the patient supine, the tibia internally rotated, and the knee flexed at 20°, gravity causes the unsupported lateral femoral condyle to fall into an externally rotated subluxed position. With

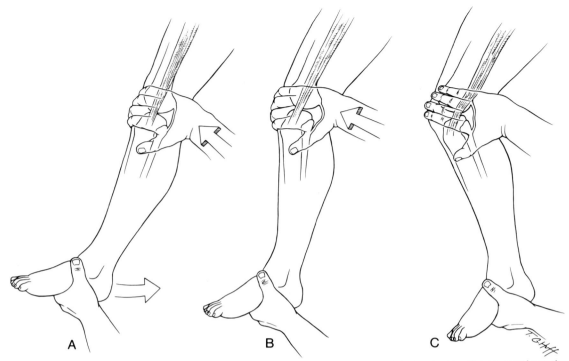

FIGURE 4–8. Pivot-shift test as described by MacIntosh. *(A)* Knee in extension with the foot in slight internal rotation. Anterior valgus stress to the lateral tibial condyle. *(B)* As the knee flexes, the tibia moves forward and the lateral femoral condyle slides off the posterior tibial slope. *(C)* As the knee reaches 20° to 40° of flexion, the tibia reduces as the iliotibial tract moves posterior to the central axis of rotation.

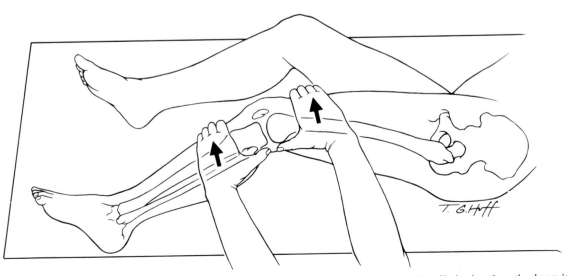

FIGURE 4–9. Anterolateral rotary instability (ALRI) test. Valgus stress is applied over the fibular head as the knee is passively extended and flexed in the range of 0° to 40°. Subluxation on extension and reduction on flexion of the tibia occur with deficiency of the anterior cruciate ligament.

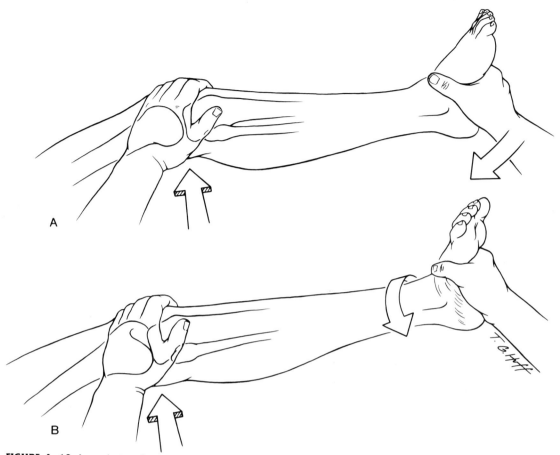

FIGURE 4–10. Losee's test for impingement reduction by tibial rotation. *(A)* With knee in 10° to 20° of flexion, the foot is held in internal rotation. Gravity causes the lateral femoral condyle to sublux posteriorly. *(B)* Valgus thrust to the lateral proximal tibia is applied as the foot is forcibly externally rotated, causing an impingement reduction of the lateral joint compartment.

one hand the examiner exerts a valgus thrust to the lateral side of the patient's proximal tibia and, with the other hand, externally rotates the patient's foot (Figure 4–10B). This action causes a reduction with impingement, which reproduces the clinical situation in which the foot is fixed and the knee is flexed 10° to 20° as the tibia subluxes.

Losee earlier described a similar variation of MacIntosh's test in which the foot is held in external rotation and the knee in 45° of flexion[13] (Fig. 4–11). Pressure is applied with the examiner's opposite hand with the fingers over the patient's patella and the examiner's thumb over the patient's fibular head. While the examiner maintains a valgus thrust, the patient's knee is slowly extended as forward pressure is exerted by the examiner's thumb on the patient's fibular head. The tibia should be allowed to twist internally as the lateral tibia subluxates. When the knee is just short of full extension, the lateral tibial plateau subluxates anteriorly, and the patient recognizes this as a reproduction of the instability.

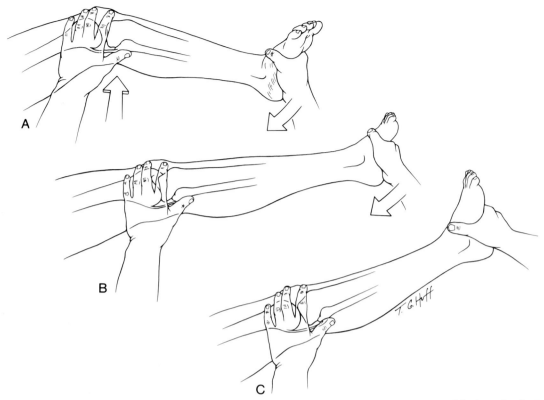

FIGURE 4–11. Losee's original test. *(A)* The test begins with the patient's knee in 45° of flexion, the foot externally rotated, and the examiner's hand over the lateral aspect of the patient's knee. The examiner's fingers are placed over the patient's patella and the examiner's thumb over the patient's fibular head. *(B)* With valgus pressure and the examiner's thumb exerting an anterior thrust, the patient's knee is extended, causing the tibia to move into internal rotation as the tibia subluxates anteriorly. *(C)* As full extension is achieved, the subluxation gently reduces.

TESTING FOR POSTERIOR AND POSTEROLATERAL INSTABILITIES

Posterior Drawer Test

The posterior drawer test is performed with the foot in two positions: neutral and external rotation. Each provides specific information. As previously mentioned in the description of the anterior drawer test with the foot in internal rotation of 30°, the lateral structures as well as the PCL are tightened. Applying an anterior stress in this position helps determine the adequacy of the PCL and may be helpful in the acute situation in determining whether there is PCL involvement. With the patient's foot in a neutral position, the posterior stress applied to the proximal tibia helps test for PCL stability (Fig. 4–12*A*). Secondary structures, if intact, may mask significant posterior displacement.

In the chronically unstable knee, stretching of the secondary structures and loss of the PCL cause the tibia to sag posteriorly (Fig. 4–12*B*). If the anterior displacement of the tibia from its *abnormal* position is not recognized during the anterior drawer test, it may be mistakenly inter-

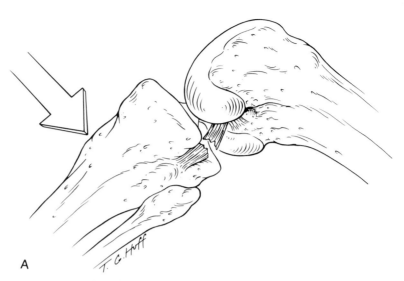

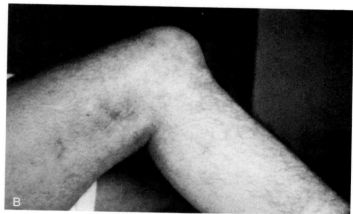

FIGURE 4–12. Posterior drawer test. *(A)* Posterior stress to the proximal tibia with the knee in 90° of flexion. *(B)* Chronic posterior cruciate ligament insufficiency with marked posterior sag of the tibia. *(C)* Palpation of anterior edge of the tibial plateau in relation to the femoral condyles. In the normal knee, the tibial plateau is approximately 1 cm anterior to the femoral condyles. If the anterior tibia is at the same level as the anterior femoral condyle and displaces forward with an anterior drawer test, posterior laxity is present.

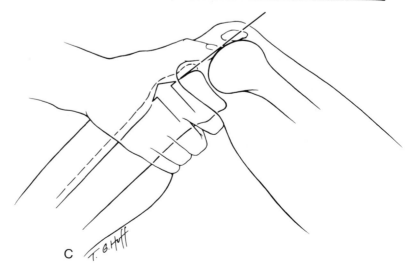

preted as an ACL deficiency. To avoid this mistake, the examiner should palpate with his or her fingers the edge of the patient's anterior tibial plateau with the patient's knee flexed to 90° and the foot resting on the examining table (Fig. 4–12C). The tibial plateaus should be palpable approximately 1 cm anterior to the femoral condyles. If the anterior tibial edge and the femoral condyles lie on the same plane and the tibia moves forward 1 cm with an anterior drawer, a posterior laxity is present. The sagging tibia has merely been pulled forward to its normal position.

When the secondary structures are intact and there is a deficiency of the PCL, a posterior stress on the proximal tibia produces a posterior displacement of 5 to 10 mm. A displacement more extensive than this suggests involvement of the secondary supporting structures. Noyes and Grood[17] believed that any posterior drawer of more than 15 mm involves the medial structures. A subtlety of this test was recognized by Fukubayaski and collaborators,[5] who showed that if a posterior force is applied to an intact knee, an external tibial torque is generated, and external rotation occurs. This phenomenon disappears when the PCL is sectioned. This occurs because of the stability of the medial side of the joint with its concave medial tibial plateau, which helps fix the medial femoral condyle and enables the lateral compartment to rotate. Also, the PCL, which arises in the transverse plane at an angle of 50° to 60°, enables the posterior forces to be directed posterolaterally, producing the external rotation.

With the foot in external rotation, a posterior drawer test (also called the posterolateral drawer test[9]) is also conducted. If an increase in the external rotation of the affected knee, in comparison with the opposite knee, accompanies a posterior displacement, the posterolateral structures and the PCL are involved. A concavity of the normal contour of the anterior aspect of the knee that is produced by the posterior force or merely by external rotation of the foot demonstrates the insufficiency of these structures (Fig. 4–13A). With the knee in 30° of flexion (as in Lachman's test), a posterior force applied to the proximal tibia with the foot externally rotated produces increased external rotation in the affected knee, in comparison with the opposite knee, when posterolateral insufficiency is present. This increase in rotation may be elicited when the PCL is intact, which indicates involvement of only these structures (Fig. 4–13). Combining these tests with the knee in the 60°-to-90° and the 30° flexed positions helps to delineate isolated posterolateral involvement and such involvement associated with a PCL loss.

EXTERNAL ROTATION RECURVATUM TEST. Posterolateral instability can sometimes be detected by holding the patient's extended extremities by the toes and observing whether recurvatum or tibial external rotation occurs (Fig. 4–14). If either does, it is because of laxity of the posterolateral structures. This recurvatum or rotation must be differentiated from the hyperextension that results from generalized ligamentous laxity or from a torn or stretched ACL, which involves the entire knee rather than just the posterolateral corner.

REVERSE PIVOT-SHIFT TEST.[10] In this situation, the tibia is reduced in extension and subluxates posteriorly with flexion of the knee (Fig. 4–15). The test is conducted by producing a valgus stress to the flexed knee. As the knee is extended with the foot in external rotation, there is a sudden reduction as the lateral tibial plateau moves from its subluxated posterior position. Flexing the knee reproduces the subluxation. It is sometimes

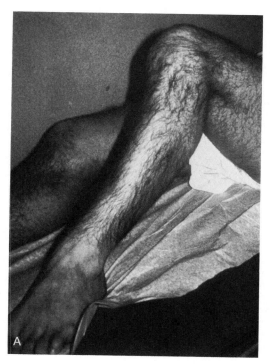

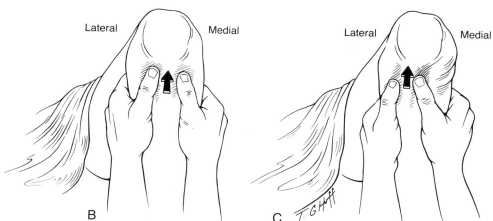

FIGURE 4–13. *(A)* Foot in external rotation with knee flexed 90°. Note the concavity of the anterior aspect of the knee, which is produced by the posterior sag of the tibia and increased external rotation. *(B)* Posterolateral drawer test. With the examiner's thumbs palpating the patient's anterior tibial edge, a posterior drawer test is conducted in neutral rotation. *(C)* The foot is placed in 15° external rotation, and a posterior thrust on the proximal tibia is applied. If the posterior cruciate ligament is intact and a deficiency of the posterolateral structures is present, the lateral tibial plateau externally rotates excessively around the intact posterior cruciate ligament. If there is also insufficiency of the posterior cruciate ligament, this may be less pronounced because the whole proximal tibia displaces posteriorly.

difficult to determine whether the event occurring is a true anterior pivot shift or a reverse pivot shift. The other tests for laxity or instability help differentiate these shifts. The patient can occasionally demonstrate this type of instability by standing on the involved leg and moving the knee into flexion and extension with the foot externally rotated. Visual movement of the tibia posteriorly and the femur anteriorly may be noted. If

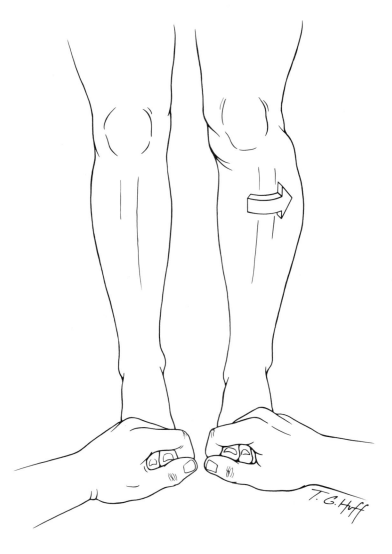

FIGURE 4–14. External rotation recurvatum test. The legs are suspended in extension by the toes. Any increased recurvatum of knee and external rotation of tibia that may be present with posterolateral laxity should be noted.

combined ACL laxity and posterolateral laxity are present, the examiner may find an anteriorly subluxated tibial plateau in extension that reduces with flexion and then goes into a posterior subluxed position.

Shelbourne and associates[18] described the dynamic posterior shift test (Fig. 14–16) for assessing posterior and posterolateral instability. The patient is supine, and the hip and the knee are flexed to 90°. In this position with posterior or posterolateral laxity, the tibia is subluxated posteriorly by gravity and the action of the hamstring muscles. The supported heel is then used to gently extend the knee while keeping the hip flexed at 90°. (If this is painful, the hip flexion can be decreased slightly as the knee reaches extension in order to decrease the loading force.) If the PCL is injured, the subluxated tibia suddenly reduces with a palpable and sudden jerk or "clunk" as full knee extension occurs. This action is produced by axial loading of the tightened hamstring muscles as the knee is extended. With straight posterior instability, both tibial plateaus reduce simultaneously. With posterolateral instability, the lateral tibial plateau reduces, and the increased tibial rotation can be detected

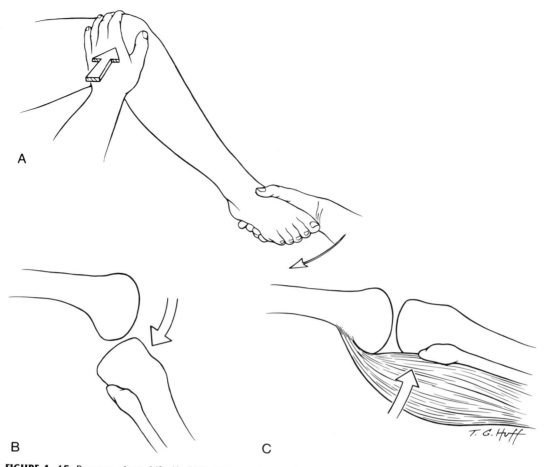

FIGURE 4–15. Reverse pivot shift. *(A, B)* Deficiency of posterior cruciate ligament and posterolateral structures allow the tibia to subluxate posteriorly with knee flexion. *(C)* When the knee reaches extension, tightening of the posterior capsule and the lateral gastrocnemius muscle produces reduction, often with a snap.

visually by the examiner. This test is a variation of the reverse pivot-shift test described earlier.

ACTIVE QUADRICEPS TEST FOR PCL DEFICIENCY.[2] With the knee flexed at 90° and the foot on the examining table, the patient slides the foot forward while it is resisted by the examiner. Anterior translation of the tibia occurs when there is a PCL deficiency and a posterior sag. The vector of force produced by the quadriceps contraction pulls the tibia from its posterior position (Fig. 4–17).

INSTRUMENTED TESTING

Several instruments for measuring the anterior or posterior translation of the tibia on the femur are currently available. All involve the use of pressure on the patella as the femoral reference point and a movable arm on the tibial tubercle for recording the displacement of the tibia with anterior or posterior forces. The accuracy can be influenced by the patient's failure to relax, by improper application of the device, and by some variability among examiners in performing the test or in ability to perform

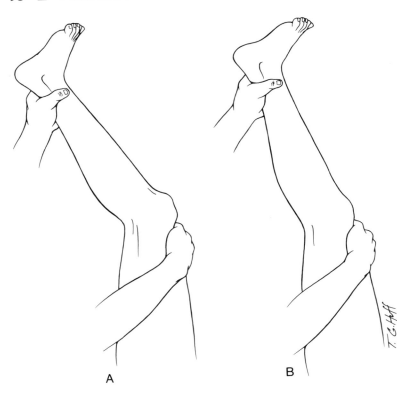

FIGURE 4–16. Dynamic posterior shift test. *(A)* In flexion, the tibia is posteriorly subluxated by the pull of the tightened hamstring tendons. *(B)* With extension, a sudden reduction occurs as the posterior capsule and the lateral gastrocnemius muscle tighten. (Redrawn from Shelbourne KD, Benedict F, McCarroll JR, et al: Dynamic posterior pivot shift test. Am J Sports Med 17:276, 1989.)

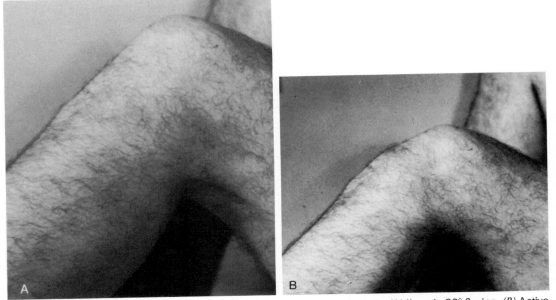

FIGURE 4–17. Active quadriceps test for posterior cruciate ligament deficiency. *(A)* Knee in 90° flexion. *(B)* Active quadriceps resisted by the examiner shows anterior displacement of the patient's tibia (note increased prominence of the tibial tubercle). Abnormal posterior sag is pulled forward by contracting the quadriceps muscle.

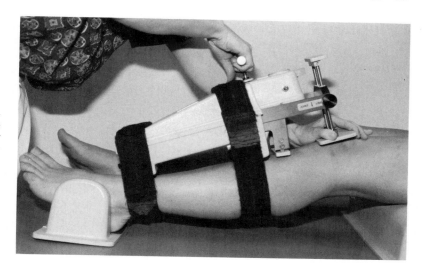

FIGURE 4–18. KT-1000 Arthrometer, a device for measuring the amount of anterior and posterior displacement of the tibia in relation to the femur (see text).

the test. Comparisons of the magnitudes of movement in each leg and the side-to-side differences are usually the measurements that determine whether an abnormal laxity exists.

One such instrument, the KT-1000, measures the anterior displacement by a determined 15-, 20-, and 30-pound pull on the proximal tibia, a maximal anterior pull by the examiner, and an active quadriceps muscle contraction by the patient (Fig. 4–18). The posterior displacement is determined by placing the uninvolved knee in the degree of flexion at which quadriceps muscle contraction does not cause either an anterior or a posterior translation (called the quadriceps neutral angle).[2] The involved knee is placed at this angle, and the active quadriceps test is conducted. The measured amount of forward displacement of the tibia is the posterior laxity that is present.

DIAGNOSIS AS DETERMINED BY THE CLINICAL EVALUATION

After the history and the physical examination have been completed, the physician should be able to place the problem into a specific category of knee problems. Additional evaluation such as radiographs, magnetic resonance imaging, arthrography, arthroscopy, or various laboratory tests may be required before an exact diagnosis can be rendered. The following are broad categories that help narrow the diagnosis and form the basis for further study. They are listed in order of the relative frequency with which they are seen in the usual orthopaedic practice. Fracture and dislocations about the knee are not included in this outline of diagnostic problems because they do not require the careful clinical evaluation described earlier; they are discussed in Chapter 7. Each of the categories to be described is discussed in detail in its respective chapter.

Degenerative Conditions

Wear and tear changes in the joint produce symptoms ranging from recurrent swelling with no pain to severe pain without significant swelling.

A history of either gradual onset of symptoms or an injury to the joint, as well as the age of the patient, gives insight into the possibilities of articular changes as a cause of the problem. A recent insult to the joint such as overuse, a twist, or weakening of the muscles from inactivity may lead to the onset of the symptoms.

Mechanical Derangement

Conditions that produce a mechanical derangement of knee function include meniscal lesions, articular lesions, loose bodies, and osteochondritis dissecans. The presence of such a problem is suspected on the basis of the patient's history. The testing for meniscal impingement may determine whether the problem is meniscal in origin. Loose bodies may be palpated or may be suspected on the basis of the history of intermittent catching or the patient's explanation that he or she can feel a loose body. Often they are detected on radiographs, but if cartilaginous, they may not be seen.

Instability

The history of a functional problem described as the knee's "going out" or "giving way" provides a clue as to the problem. This description is not confirmatory, however. The mechanical derangements described earlier may be interpreted by the patient as a "giving way" when the knee catches. The feeling of the knee buckling may be caused by quadriceps weakness, quadriceps inhibition as a result of a painful stimulus, or actual ligamentous instability. The examination for ligamentous laxity and true instability usually provides the clinician with a definitive diagnosis. Inability of the patient to relax may preclude an adequate evaluation.

Extensor Mechanism Problems

Problems of the extensor mechanism relate to pain or instability. The diagnosis is often difficult because pathologic processes do not always correlate with symptoms. The problem is often seen in the adolescent years when increased activity puts further demands on the knee. Congenital abnormalities relating to the alignment of the extremities, to formation and development of the femoral sulcus or patellar configuration, and to muscle imbalances play a part in producing the symptoms.

Extra-Articular Problems

Many conditions about the knee are not related to the joint itself. Bursitis is an example. Prepatellar bursitis occurs as a swelling over the patellar area and may be interpreted by the patient to be "swelling in the knee." Many bursae are present around the knee and may become inflamed or tender and produce discomfort. Careful palpation may help establish the diagnosis by clinical means. Neuromas, iliotibial band syndrome, and muscular problems are usually detected from the history and by means of physical examination. These problems are discussed in detail in Chapter 12.

Inflammatory or Infectious Problems

The physical condition of the joint that is swollen, warm, and painful usually makes the category clear. The differentiation between an inflammatory problem relating to irritation within the joint (disease or mechanical process) and an infection certainly requires specific tests.

Congenital Problems

Problems relating to the development of the joint may be evident at birth or may not become obvious until the patient begins to walk. Some problems do not become manifest until more strenuous activities such as running or athletic activities are undertaken. The physical examination for detecting any deformity, alignment problems, or muscle imbalance thus becomes important for placing the problem in this category.

Tumors

The rarity and the insidious onset of this category of problems often cause them to be overlooked or the diagnosis delayed. Benign and malignant tumors can occur in the bone, the muscles, and the synovium, as well as in other soft tissues. Only because of a physician's awareness that they can occur and through a proper evaluation when their presence is suspected will an early diagnosis be forthcoming.

Although the clinical evaluation may enable the physician to place the problem only in broad categories, it forms the rationale for the use of other diagnostic modalities. The importance of a proper history and a careful physical examination cannot be overemphasized.

REFERENCES

1. Arnold JA, Coker TP, Heaton LM, et al: Natural history of anterior cruciate tears. Am J Sports Med 7:305–313, 1979.
2. Daniels DM, Stone ML: Diagnosis of knee ligament injury: tests and measurements of joint laxity. *In* Feagin JA (ed): The Crucial Ligaments, pp. 287–300. New York: Churchill-Livingstone, 1988.
3. DeHaven KE: Diagnosis of acute knee injuries with hemarthrosis. Am J Sports Med 8:9–14, 1980.
4. Feagin JA: Introduction: principles of diagnosis and treatment. *In* Feagin JA (ed): The Crucial Ligaments, pp. 3–154. New York: Churchill-Livingstone, 1988.
5. Fukubayaski T, Torzilli PA, Sherman MF, et al: An in vitro biomechanical evaluation of anterior-posterior motion of the knee. J Bone Joint Surg 64A:258–264, 1982.
6. Galway HR, MacIntosh DL: The lateral pivot shift: a symptom and sign of anterior cruciate insufficiency. Clin Orthop 147:45–50, 1980.
7. Hey Groves EW: The crucial ligaments of the knee joint: Their function, rupture, and the operative treatment of the same. Br J Surg 7:505–515, 1920.
8. Hughston JC, Andrews JR, Cross MJ, et al: Classification of knee ligament instabilities: Part I. J Bone Joint Surg 58A:159–172, 1976.
9. Hughston JC, Norwood LA: The posterolateral drawer test and external rotational recurvatum test for posterolateral rotatory instability of the knee. Clin Orthop 147:82–87, 1980.

10. Jakob RP, Hassler H, Staeubli HU: Instability of the lateral compartment of the knee. Acta Orthop Scand 52(Suppl 191):1–32, 1981.
11. Jonsson T, Althoff B, Peterson L, et al: Clinical diagnosis of ruptures of the anterior cruciate ligament: a comparative study of the Lachman test and the anterior drawer sign. Am J Sports Med 10:100–102, 1982.
12. Larson RL: Physical examination in the diagnosis of rotatory instability. Clin Orthop 172:38–44, 1983.
13. Losee RE, Johnson TR, Southwick WO: Anterior subluxation of the lateral tibial plateau. J Bone Joint Surg 60A:1015–1030, 1978.
14. Losee RE: Concepts of the pivot shift. Clin Orthop 172:45–51, 1983.
15. MacIntosh DL, Galway HR: The lateral pivot shift: a symptomatic and clinical sign of anterior cruciate insufficiency. *Presented at* the Annual Meeting of the American Orthopaedic Association. Tucker's Town, Bermuda: American Orthopaedic Association, 1972.
16. Noyes FR, Basset RW, Grood ES, et al: Arthroscopy in acute traumatic hemarthrosis of the knee. J Bone Joint Surg 62A:687–695, 1980.
17. Noyes FR, Grood ES: Diagnosis of knee ligament injuries. *In* Feagin JA (ed): The Crucial Ligaments, pp. 261–286. New York: Churchill-Livingstone, 1988.
18. Shelbourne KD, Benedict F, McCarroll JR, et al: Dynamic posterior shift test: an adjuvant in evaluation of posterior tibial subluxation. Am J Sports Med 17:275–277, 1989.
19. Slocum DB, James SL, Larson RL, et al: Clinical test for anterolateral rotary instability of the knee. Clin Orthop 118:63–69, 1976.
20. Slocum DB, Larson RL: Rotatory instability of the knee: its pathogenesis and a clinical test to determine its presence. J Bone Joint Surg 50A:211–225, 1968.
21. Torg JS, Conrad W, Kalen V: Clinical diagnosis of anterior cruciate ligament instability in the athlete. Am J Sports Med 4:84–93, 1976.

CHAPTER 5

Diagnostic

Evaluation

WILLIAM A. GRANA, M.D.

■

Evaluation of the knee is based on a careful history and a thorough physical examination, as elaborated in Chapter 4. There is simply no substitute for this basic information when handled by an experienced orthopaedic surgeon. Such an evaluation is without question the most cost-effective method for defining a patient's problem and beginning a plan of management. To substitute tests as a means for defining a problem without specific therapeutic benefit is a disservice to the patient and is soundly condemned. The current craze for magnetic resonance imaging (MRI) is a perfect example of a potentially valuable technique for specific diagnostic and research needs that is misused as a screening device for the clinician. There is no substitute for reading, for studying, and for examining patients. However, some additional diagnostic information should be part of the initial evaluation. Certain specific, standard, inexpensive plain radiographs are part of the initial evaluation. These basic radiographs are part of a systematic evaluation needed for an adequate differential diagnosis of an individual knee problem. If the initial evaluation does not provide sufficient information for classifying a clinical problem, additional imaging studies may be needed. The purpose of this chapter is to review those diagnostic evaluations, both specific and screening tests, that pinpoint the diagnosis and direct therapeutic methods.

PLAIN RADIOGRAPHS

O'Donoghue (personal communication) believed that the initial evaluation of the knee required a basic radiographic evaluation of the joint as well as the history and the physical examination. The basic views are a standing anteroposterior (AP) view of both knees together, a lateral view at 45° of flexion, an intercondylar notch view, and a patellofemoral (sunrise) joint view. These views constitute a complete initial radiographic evaluation of the knee. The most common reason to fail to make a diagnosis, aside from an inadequate history and physical examination, is failure to obtain the basic screening radiographic evaluation. Moreover, too often primary care physicians bypass these basic radiographs and move directly to more expensive, needless imaging techniques.

Plain Radiographs[3]

BASIC VIEWS

STANDING ANTEROPOSTERIOR PROJECTION. This projection is accomplished as a series of bilateral weight-bearing AP radiographs. The patient is positioned before the cassette with the knees toward the tube, and a 10 × 12 inch film is used. The patient stands with weight evenly borne on both feet and with toes straight ahead. The film is centered at the level of the inferior pole of the patella, and the tube is positioned between the knees and centered on the inferior pole of the patella (Fig. 5–1).

This film is most useful as a general screen to define varus or valgus angulation of the knee as well as unicompartmental or bicompartmental collapse of the tibiofemoral joint, as in osteoarthritis.

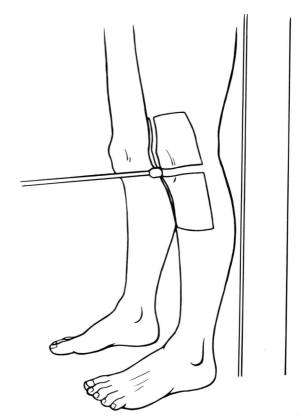

FIGURE 5–1. Positioning for the standing anteroposterior film. (See text for description of film.)

LATERAL PROJECTION. The patient is positioned on the affected side with the knee in 45° of flexion unless a suspected fracture or pain prevents this position. The film is centered on the joint line, and the leg is horizontal. The patella is perpendicular to the film. The tube is angled 5° cephalad (Fig. 5–2).

The lateral view is in 45° of flexion to enable determination of patella alta or baja by relation of the inferior pole of the patella to Blumensaal's line or in order to determine the patella/patellar-tendon index as a measure

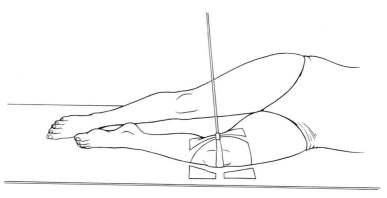

FIGURE 5–2. Positioning for the lateral view at 45° of flexion. (See text for description of film.)

of patellar height. In addition, osteochondral lesions are identified in this lateral projection. These lesions usually occur in the medial femur or the medial condyle in an area bounded by Blumensaal's line and a line projected to the joint surface from the posterior cortex of the femur. The contours of the patella and the presence of osteoarthritic spurs are also best identified in this projection.

INTERCONDYLAR NOTCH PROJECTION. The patient is positioned prone with the leg in neutral rotation. The knee is flexed 45° on the film with the knee in the upper half of the film. The tube is angled 45° from the perpendicular to the film. This projection opens the intercondylar notch (Fig. 5–3).

This view is useful for identifying a femoral osteochondral lesion or a loose body and for sizing the notch area. This projection is also used for assessing flattening of the femoral condyles, as in osteoarthritis.

PATELLOFEMORAL JOINT PROJECTION (SUNRISE VIEW). The patient is positioned supine with the knee flexed 45°. The film is held firmly behind the knee, and the tube is directed at 5° to 10° from perpendicular to the cassette to direct the x-ray through the patellofemoral joint (Fig. 5–4).

This view is used to measure the trochlear groove and to assess the size and configuration of the patella. Merchant's congruence angle, Laurin's assessment of patellar tilt, and lateral patellar overhang are all determined from this view. In addition, a patellar fracture, an osteochondral lesion, or an osteophytic spurring is also identified.

WEIGHTED FLEXED ANTEROPOSTERIOR PROJECTION

This film is taken with the knees flexed 45°, and in the osteoarthritic patient, it may be a better assessment of joint collapse and flattening of the femoral condyles.

LOWER EXTREMITY STANDING ANTEROPOSTERIOR PROJECTION

A special cassette is used to show the extremity from hip to ankle, or two standard cassettes are used. The view is used to define the mechanical and anatomic axis of the knee, as defined in Chapter 3. This view is used

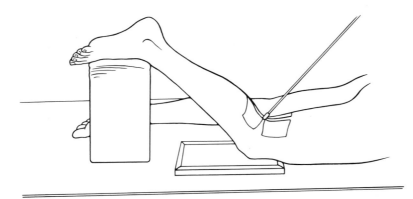

FIGURE 5–3. Position for intercondylar notch view. (See text for description of film.)

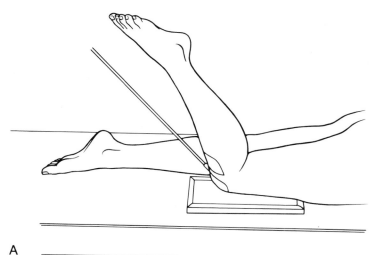

FIGURE 5–4. Two methods (*A*, *B*) of positioning for the patellofemoral (sunrise) view.

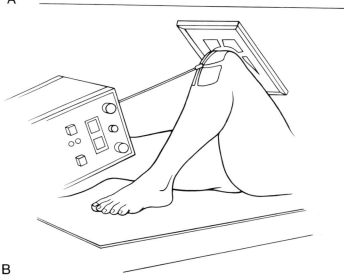

B

in planning osteotomy of the femur and the tibia and in total knee replacement.

Comparison Stress Radiographs

AP stress radiographs are accomplished with the knee flexed 20° over a bolster and equal stress applied firmly in the appropriate direction to produce the pathologic laxity. Grade III injuries produce a difference of 8 to 10 mm or more (Fig. 5–5). The greatest value of these stress films is to differentiate physeal injury from ligamentous injury in the skeletally immature patient (Fig. 5–6). They are mandatory in the evaluation of such a patient with clinical varus or valgus laxity.

Lateral stress radiographs are useful in the evaluation of the patient with complex laxity of the knee. If the clinician is uncertain of the severity of laxity, two lateral films are made with the knee flexed at 90° and with anterior and posterior stress applied to the proximal tibia. These views

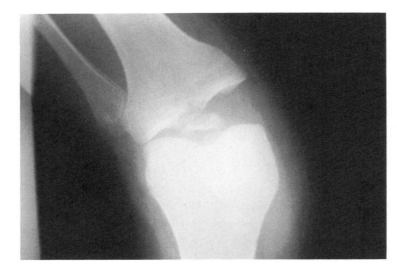

FIGURE 5–5. An anteroposterior stress radiograph delineates a complete medial collateral ligament injury and an intercondylar eminence fracture, not evident on the plain anteroposterior radiograph.

are compared with the normal side, and combined anterior or posterior laxity is then differentiated. The use of aspiration followed by injection of 10 to 15 mL of 1 per cent lidocaine (Xylocaine) for analgesia is helpful for evaluating the acute injury.

Plain Tomography of the Knee

This technique has been replaced in most situations by the more detailed evaluation provided by computed tomography (CT) or MRI. However,

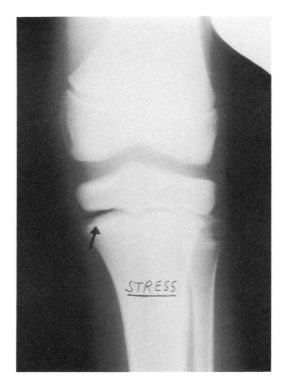

FIGURE 5–6. A proximal tibial physeal injury is demonstrated by a valgus stress radiograph with the laxity apparent at the physeal line (*arrow*).

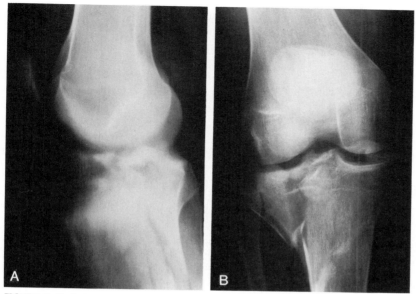

FIGURE 5–7. Plain tomogram *(A)* demonstrates the depressed and split portions of the type III tibial plateau fracture, as demonstrated in the plain radiograph *(B)*.

for certain tumors such as osteoid osteoma, tomography provides the information needed for planning or assessing surgical technique. It is most efficiently performed with the thinnest sections available, usually 3 to 5 mm (Fig. 5–7).

ARTHROGRAPHY

Although arthrography has been replaced in most cases by MRI, it is still useful when MRI is not available or cost effective.

The technique includes aspiration of the knee from a superolateral puncture site with appropriate synovial fluid analysis when indicated. Ten milliliters of metrizamide and 50 mL of air are instilled in the knee. A series of plain AP and oblique lateral radiographs are made to evaluate the internal anatomy. In certain acutely injured patients, the discomfort of the evaluation is mitigated by local instillation of lidocaine (Xylocaine), but in other such patients, the evaluation must be limited.

The patient is in the semiprone position, and the knee receives valgus stress from the medial side and varus stress from the lateral side. The film is beneath the knee, and the tube is centered on the compartment to be studied. The patient rotates 30° toward the supine position for each of six exposures. The opposite compartment is filmed in a similar manner. The cruciate ligaments are visualized by positioning the patient with the knee at 90° and a bolster behind the tibia. The patient holds the cassette with the tube in the position for a lateral radiograph.

This technique is best used for assessment of the menisci and the cruciate ligaments, and when it is combined with plain tomography or computed axial tomographic scan, it is useful for osteochondral lesions as well. In total knee replacement, aspiration (for culture fluid analysis) followed by arthrography is used to document gaps at the interfaces between bones and prostheses.

The reliability of arthrography has been well documented in the past. The area of most difficulty in assessment is the posterolateral corner of the lateral meniscus. The popliteal hiatus and its folds are difficult to define as normal or representative of a meniscal tear. Furthermore, an intrasynovial rupture of a cruciate ligament may be mistaken for an intact ligament (Fig. 5–8).

The author uses arthrography in the assessment of a popliteal mass to demonstrate a communication with the joint and to document the size of such a mass.[14, 16, 38] Otherwise, the clinical value and use of arthrography have been superseded by those of MRI when it is available.

SCINTIGRAPHY (BONE SCAN)

This technique has been available since the 1970s, but it was not until the relatively high dose of radiation administered was reduced with the use

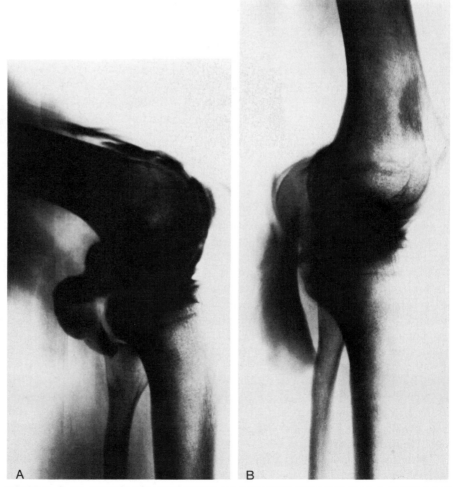

A　　　　　　　　　B

FIGURE 5–8. An example of normal double-contrast arthrograms that show a popliteal cyst *(A)* and the same cyst ruptured into the calf *(B)*.

of technetium phosphate isotopes that this imaging technique became more widely used. Currently, technetium phosphate is used for its bone-seeking capability, gallium compounds are used for imaging soft tissues, and indium-labeled leukocytes are used for the evaluation of infection.[40] A radioisotope accumulates in the appropriate target tissue, and then appropriate images are made. Spot film capability is mandatory for adequate assessment of the knee.

Technetium (Tc) scans are most useful for localization of osseous disease, such as osteomyelitis or tumor, or of osteochondral injury, such as osteochondritis dissecans. Tc scans have also been used to identify osteonecrosis but are being replaced by MRI, which is more sensitive for this use. In the past, Tc scans were used to evaluate loosening in total knee replacement. However, gallium and indium scans are more sensitive means for identifying loosening with or without sepsis. When MRI is not available, Tc scintigraphy with standard radiographs (including weight-bearing projections) is a sensitive way to evaluate the severity of involvement of the three compartments of the knee by osteoarthritis.[39] In osteochondritis dissecans, the Tc scan is used to follow the maturation or the healing of the lesion.

Gallium- and indium-labeled leukocytes are used in the evaluation of infection of the joint, especially after total knee replacement or in combination with Tc scans, to differentiate bone from soft tissue or synovial involvement. These leukocyte scans are most sensitive in the evaluation of painful prosthetic replacements. In one series, all 18 patients with confirmed sepsis had positive scans, and 20 of 22 sterile arthroplasties had negative scans.[32]

The author uses scintigraphy to screen the patient whose pain does not fit the usual clinical patterns. If the scintigram is positive, CT is used to characterize the problem. Suspected stress fracture of the patella and osteochondritis dissecans are specific problems for which this technique provides diagnostic information (Fig. 5–9). The gallium or indium scan was used by the author to evaluate one patient with a painful prosthetic knee.

ULTRASONOGRAPHY

Diagnostic ultrasonography in the evaluation of the knee has limited application. The thickness of articular cartilage of the knee and the degree of effusion are well defined. Soft tissue masses can be differentiated into solid and cystic tumors.[15]

In diagnostic ultrasonography, sonic waves are used to produce a digitized image on a screen. The technique is used in a fashion similar to that of fluoroscopy without the risk of radiation. The sound wave strikes a transducer and is then converted to a real-time image on a monitor.

Ultrasound waves are produced by a transducer that converts electrical energy into ultrasound wave energy and then back again. The principle makes use of the piezoelectric effect, in which a suitable crystal expands or contracts, depending on the polarity of the electric signal. If the signal oscillates, the alternating expansion and contraction produces mechanical motion that results in ultrasound waves. The reverse is possible as well. The crystal element is lead zirconate titonate, quartz, or lithium sulfate.

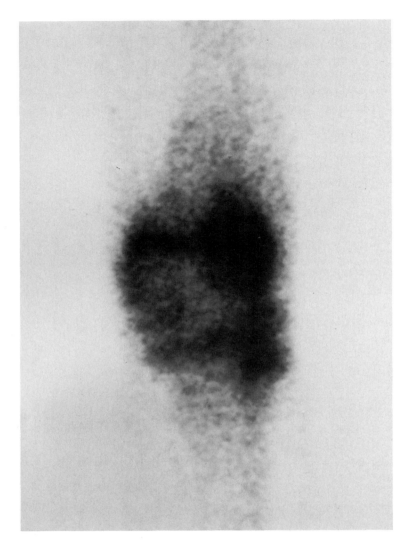

FIGURE 5–9. A bone scan showing increased uptake in the patella as a result of an osteochondral lesion.

The ultrasound wave is pulsed and then reflected back to the transductor by each tissue layer that it passes through. The tissue required for the pulse to be reflected to the transductor determines the position of the interface on a cathode ray tube screen. If a series of scanners is linked, a real-time image is produced by movement of the scanners over the body to be imaged.

In the knee, patellar tendon abnormality, osteoarthritis, and popliteal cysts are problems that are effectively differentiated.[1, 10, 20, 24] In addition, tears of the muscles about the knee, such as quadriceps, hamstring, or gastrocnemius strain, are all well identified both actively and passively.[8, 11, 23, 25] This method is cost effective for documenting or confirming a clinical diagnosis when a specific diagnosis is considered, and the greater volume of information of the more costly MRI is not needed. Photographic permanent prints are made of the real-time sonographic images. The use of this diagnostic modality depends on the availability of skilled technicians and a radiologist with experience in the evaluation of the knee (Fig. 5–10).[28]

COMPUTED TOMOGRAPHY

The CT scan is the most widely used cross-sectional imaging method for musculoskeletal disorders. It is similar to MRI in spatial resolution but inferior as to contrast resolution. It is superior to MRI for the evaluation of osseous detail, especially cortical bone, ossification, and calcification. The technique is most useful for the assessment of high-density tissue such as bone.[2]

By "reconstruction" of a series of transverse slices of the knee with the appropriate computer software, a three-dimensional representation of the knee in any plane can be accomplished for total knee reconstruction or tumor surgery for implant design and surgical planning. Over the long term, this technique may be coupled with machine instruments in order to make the cuts for prosthetic implants. This application is promising, particularly for press-fit porous designs.

In CT, an x-ray beam is directed on the patient, and the radiation that passes through the object in a detector connected to a computer is measured. The software of the computer then analyzes the signal and reconstructs a visual image, which is displayed on a television monitor. This image is photographed in order to produce a permanent hard copy

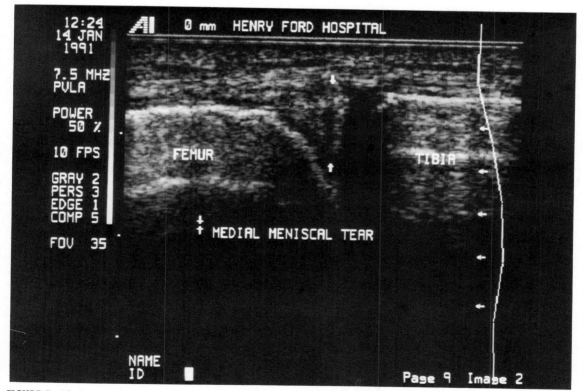

FIGURE 5–10. A normal ultrasonogram of the knee demonstrates the tendons and spaces around the joint. (Courtesy of Joseph Introcuso and Marnix van Holsbeeck.)

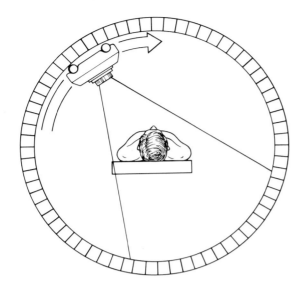

FIGURE 5–11. A diagrammatic representation of the computed tomographic (CT) scanner. The multiple blocks are the detectors, and the tube rotates to complete the evaluation.

to store. In modern CT scanners, the x-ray source rotates, and a series of detectors are arranged in a fixed circle. The beam itself is fan-shaped and provides for varied thickness in the axial slice. In this type of scanner, the radiation dose is somewhat higher, which is a disadvantage (Figs. 5–11, 5–12).[5]

The use of CT scans for examining disorders of the knee is best suited to the evaluation of fractures and bone tumors. However, they are also useful in the assessment of the patellofemoral relationship and in the planning of patellar reconstructive procedures. Aside from the evaluation of fractures and tumors, CT scans about the knee have value in the assessment of muscle tendon injury. Garrett and colleagues evaluated 10 college athletes with clinical hamstring muscle injury and documented low-density changes on CT scan in the affected muscle. Two additional

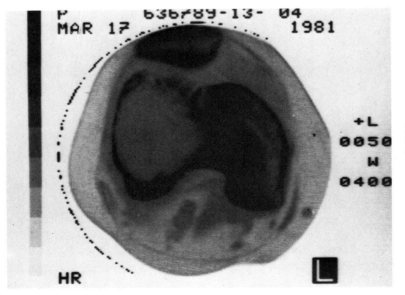

FIGURE 5–12. Giant cell tumor of the lateral femoral condyle seen on CT scan.

athletes had clinical findings, but no abnormality was detected on CT. The original 10 patients had delayed recovery, which signified more severe injury.[12] However, the routine use of CT in this type of injury was not recommended. In the problem case, it may be useful to document the severity of injury.

Several investigators[7, 17, 27, 34, 35] have used CT scans to characterize the patellofemoral relationship with a high degree of sensitivity and specificity. No method of evaluation is entirely satisfactory, but CT combined with clinical and arthroscopic findings may offer the most information for making surgical decisions and planning.

MAGNETIC RESONANCE IMAGING

MRI is based on the principle that the nucleus of an atom has inherent magnetization as a result of its spinning and orientation in space. If an external magnet is applied to the nuclear magnetic spin, a slight "wobble," called precession, is used. The frequency of this precession is determined by the strength of the external magnet and the type of nucleus involved. Normally, in clinical MRI, the hydrogen nucleus is used for study. The nuclei in response to the external magnet react in a precession in which they are out of phase with each other. However, if a radiofrequency that matches the unique frequency of precession of the hydrogen nucleus is applied, then all hydrogen nuclei in the object resonate in phase or with the same frequency and then align with the external magnet. The number of hydrogen nuclei present is the spin density and determines the size of the magnetization vector. The larger this vector is, the more intense is the signal and the brighter is the magnetic resonance image. When the radiowave is turned off, the nuclei return to the out-of-phase state. This state is called relaxation, and when this occurs, a radiofrequency signal is emitted. As the nuclei relax or return to equilibrium, they give off energy to the tissue as a whole. This energy released to the tissue is a characteristic of the tissue itself and is called the spin-lattice relaxation time, or T_1. A second kind of relaxation occurs as the individual nuclei go out of phase, and there is a decrease in the magnetic vector. The decay in this vector is the T_2 relaxation time. T_2 is always less than T_1, and both are characteristic for various tissues. By variation in the imaging techniques, either of these relaxations or spin density may be emphasized. Thus there may be a T_1-weighted image, a T_2-weighted image, or spin density–weighted image.[21]

For the knee it is essential that a saddle type of surface coil be used, and the pulse sequences for the radiowaves are inversion recovery (IR) and spin echo (SE). Which pulse sequences are used depends on the specific clinical problem and the tissues involved (joint, tumor, muscle, and so forth). The most commonly used sequence for the knee is spin echo. In T_1 images, cortical bone, tendon, ligament, and fibrocartilage are black. Muscle is of intermediate signal, fibrocartilage is brighter, and fat and bone marrow are white. In T_2 images, fluid such as an effusion or a cyst appears bright.[12, 21, 22, 30]

The examination is performed with the patient supine, with the extremity extended, and with a circumferential coil. The slices should be 5 mm thick and the magnetic field at least a 1.5-tesla system (Figs. 5–13 to 5–17).[6]

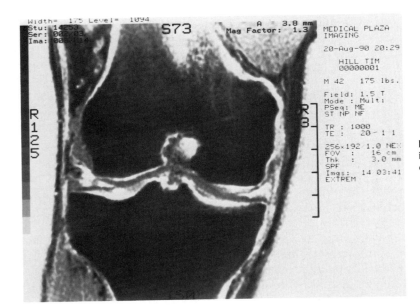

FIGURE 5–13. The abnormal signal intensity in these menisci confirm degenerative tears.

MRI is most useful for evaluating soft tissue problems. In the knee, it is most effective for evaluating tumors in order to differentiate tissue type or tissue of origin. There is no question of its value in the evaluation of such problems from the standpoint of both cost and safety. However, it is in the evaluation of acute intra-articular and ligamentous problems that this diagnostic modality has become most popular and most controversial.[26] In teenage and young adult patients with an acutely injured knee, primary care physicians, orthopaedists, and insurance companies are using MRI to decide whether surgery is indicated.[29] Radiologists encourage this trend, and perhaps the eponym MRI best stands for *more radiologic income* when it is used as a screening device in a young athletic

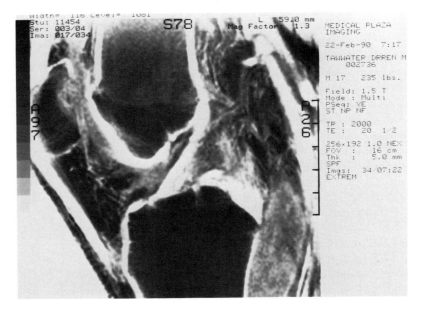

FIGURE 5–14. A normal signal for the anterior cruciate ligament.

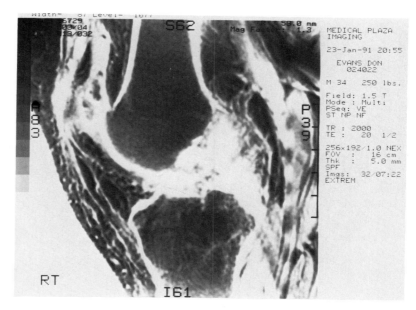

FIGURE 5–15. A disrupted anterior cruciate ligament after acute injury.

population. This concept was documented by Boden and associates in a study to assess the cost effectiveness of MRI for acute knee problems.[4] The conclusion was that MRI is useful for patients with chronic or nonspecific symptoms and signs, but it is not cost effective for young patients with acute knee injuries because a high percentage of these patients (87%) undergo arthroscopy. These findings were reinforced by Senghas, who noted that MRI is not indicated if it will not affect treatment no matter what the result.[36] The experienced observer is a more effective diagnostic tool than any test. Too often the inexperienced observer uses the MRI to retain control of the patient rather than providing a judicious referral.

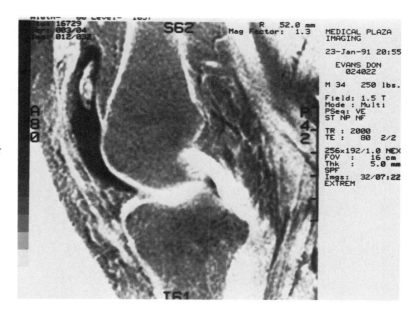

FIGURE 5–16. A normal signal for the posterior cruciate ligament.

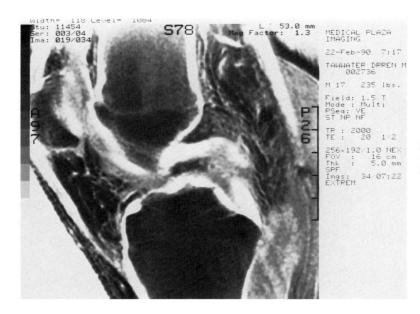

FIGURE 5–17. A disrupted posterior cruciate ligament after acute injury.

With regard to meniscal disorder, Jackson and others have established that the MRI signal from the meniscus must be classified and that treatable lesions were primarily grade III lesions with extension of the signal abnormality to the edge of the meniscus.[18, 37] Even with strict criteria in a large multicenter study, Fischer and co-workers noted a quality ranging from 64 to 95 per cent for the medial meniscus and 83 to 94 per cent for the lateral meniscus. In addition, 17 per cent of grade II lesions of the meniscus were seen as unstable, grossly torn lesions on arthroscopy, and yet on the basis of MRI, these lesions were not thought to be surgically treatable.[9] Raunest and colleagues, in a double-blind study, found a diagnostic accuracy of 72 per cent and a specificity of 57 per cent.[33] These studies and others indicate that unless there is a specific need for information about the problem patient or confirmation of clinical diagnosis, MRI is not indicated. As a screening device, MRI is not cost effective or 100 per cent accurate even in radiologists' studies of this technique.[13, 21, 29, 31]

In the author's practice, MRI is used for evaluating the personal injury or compensation case to provide documentation that would justify avoiding surgery, but even in this setting, a patient should undergo arthroscopy for absolute certainty of diagnosis.[19] There is no need to use MRI in the routine assessment of meniscal and ligamentous injury of the knee.

OTHER ADJUNCTS IN EVALUATION

Aspiration of Effusion

In the patient with chronic effusion, aspiration is essential for diagnosis. In 80 per cent of acute injuries, the presence of gross blood means injury to the anterior cruciate ligament. The presence of fat means osteochondral injury or fracture and may be associated with patellar dislocation. In chronic effusion, there may be some blood, but more important is the clarity and color of the fluid. The white blood cell count and differential are critical for differentiating inflammatory from infectious disorders. In general, all counts of fewer than 100,000 cells are seen in inflammatory problems with a preponderance of lymphocytes, whereas in sepsis, the white blood cell count is more than 100,000, with a majority of polymorphonuclear cells.

In addition to cell count, microscopic analysis for crystals under regular and polarized light demonstrates urate, pyrophosphate, and oxalate crystals seen in gout and pseudogout, respectively. Finally chemistry determinations of protein and sugar plus rheumatoid factor (RF) and antinuclear antibody (ANA) help distinguish inflammatory and infectious causes.

In screening the patient with chronic effusion, peripheral blood analysis includes complete blood count with differential; measurements of sedimentation rate and uric acid levels; and RF, ANA, and HLA B-27 antigen test. In addition, serum calcium phosphorus, alkaline phosphatase, blood urea nitrogen, and creatinine levels, as well as protein electrophoresis, are useful in the evaluation of certain tumors and metabolic problems. These tests form a basis for the evaluation of inflammatory problems caused by sepsis, collagen vascular disease, tumor, and metabolic problems.

TECHNIQUE OF ASPIRATION

The patient is supine and relaxed. The anterior and lateral portion of the knee is prepared with betadine in a formal scrub and then wiped with alcohol in the area of aspiration. Using sterile gloves, the examiner palpates the "soft spot" on the lateral aspect of the knee, and the patient's skin is anesthetized with 1% plain lidocaine (Xylocaine) with a 25-gauge needle. If the local anesthetic is injected slowly, the only discomfort is with the penetration of the synovium. When the skin and subcutaneous tissue are infiltrated, a No. 16 or No. 18 gauge needle is used to aspirate the effusion. For comfort, the joint is aspirated as completely as possible, and if needed, pressure is applied to the medial aspect of the joint in order to force fluid to the site of aspiration. The fluid is then segregated for analysis by hematology, chemistry, and microbiology laboratories. The aspiration site is cleaned with alcohol and dressed with an adhesive bandage.

For suspected infection, aerobic and anaerobic cultures and, in difficult or chronic cases, fungal and acid-fast cultures as well should be taken. Gram staining is conducted for immediate assessment of infection, and the cultures are followed for at least 72 hours.

ISOKINETIC TESTING

The value of isokinetic strength testing in the evaluation of a patient both before and after treatment is in providing baseline and longitudinal information about the patient's strength, power, and endurance. This information, combined with simple extremity measurements of the thigh and the calf, aids the clinician in the determination of muscular adequacy and its role in diagnosis and rehabilitation. The patient's progress in regaining these muscular parameters is documented and provides assistance in determining return to function. The author generally uses the value of 80 per cent strength and power in the affected extremity in comparison with the unaffected side as a criterion for return to running activity. In addition, for anterior cruciate ligament and patellofemoral problems, this testing is of value to maintain an appropriate quadriceps:hamstring strength ratio. Concentric and eccentric testing is of value because isolated deficits in one or the other form of muscular strength can be present. Finally, for return to sports, the author prefers that the strength of the affected side be 90 per cent that of the unaffected side. In addition, this isokinetic testing is invaluable for objectively assessing and comparing the results of treatment.

Ligament Laxity Testing

With the advent of simple mechanical laxity testing devices for anterior or posterior cruciate ligament laxity, there is an objective means to quantify laxity in patients with suspected injury to these ligaments. The key to accurate assessment is test-retest reliability and comparison of side-to-side differences. With regard to these parameters, the most reliable testing devices are the KT-1000 by Med-Metric and the Stryker Ligament Laxity Testor. Side-to-side differences with a 30-pound force or maximal manual drawer must be compared. In addition, with the latter, measurements from testing with the two devices are comparable and the numbers of false-positive and false-negative results are very small. A number of studies have documented the reliability of these two testing devices.

With regard to anterior laxity, normal values for right-left differences are 1 to 2 mm. In patients with anterior cruciate ligament injury, 3- to 5-mm differences between the affected and unaffected sides are generally tolerated well. Differences of more than 5 mm are poorly tolerated, and instability is a symptom for such patients.

Again, to objectively assess results after reconstructive surgery or to follow the success or failure of a therapeutic regimen in the initial evaluation of the patient with suspected pathologic processes or laxity of the knee ligament, laxity testing is essential for confirming the clinical assessment. The testing device is inexpensive, is easy to use in the office setting, and provides reliable data. Its use should be an essential part of any experienced practitioner's office evaluation.

SUMMARY

Some or many of these diagnostic evaluations are clearly a part of the initial workup in the patient with a disorder of the knee. However, the decision to use these additional tests is based on the essential initial physical examination, which provides a differential diagnosis and therefore a rationale for the use of these tests. Without this rationale, the choice of such tests cannot be specific or cost effective. Experience and an understanding of the purpose and the limitations of each additional diagnostic evaluation enable the clinician to choose wisely for each patient.

REFERENCES

1. Aisen AM, McCune WJ, MacGuire A, et al: Sonographic evaluation of the cartilage of the knee. Radiology 153:781–784, 1984.
2. Alfidi RJ, Haaga JR: Computed Tomography of the Whole Body, vol 1. St. Louis: CV Mosby, 1983.
3. Ballinger PW: Radiographic Positions and Radiologic Procedures, 5th ed. St. Louis: CV Mosby, 1982.
4. Boden SD, Labropoulos PA, Vailas JC: MR scanning of the acutely injured knee: sensitive, but is it cost effective? Arthroscopy 6(4):306–310, 1990.
5. Bushong SC: Computed tomography. *In* Bushong SC (ed): Radiologic Science for Technologists—Physics, Biology, and Protection, 4th ed. St. Louis: CV Mosby, 1988.
6. Bushong SC: Physical principles of magnetic resonance imaging. *In* Bushong SC (ed): Radiologic Science for Technologists—Physics, Biology, and Protection, 4th ed. St. Louis: CV Mosby, 1988.
7. Delgado-Martins H: A study of the position of the patella using computerized tomography. J Bone Joint Surg 61B(4):443–444, 1979.
8. Doppman JL: Baker's cyst and the normal gastrocnemiosemimembranosus bursa. Am J Radiol 94:646–652, 1965.
9. Fischer SP, Fox JM, Del Pizzo W, et al: Accuracy of diagnoses from magnetic resonance imaging of the knee. J Bone Joint Surg 73A:1–10, 1991.
10. Fornage BD, Rifkin MD, Touche DH, et al: Sonography of the patellar tendon: preliminary observations. AJR 143:179–182, 1984.
11. Fornage BD, Touche DH, Segal P, et al. Ultrasonography in the evaluation of muscular trauma. J Ultrasound Med 2:549–554, 1983.
12. Garrett WE Jr, Rich FR, Nikolaou PK, Vogler JB III: Computed tomography of hamstring muscle strains. Med Sci Sports Exerc 21:506–514, 1989.
13. Glashow JL, Katz R, Schneider M, Scott WN: Double-blind assessment of the value of magnetic resonance imaging in the diagnosis of anterior cruciate and meniscal lesions. J Bone Joint Surg 71A:113–119, 1989.
14. Gristina AG, Wilson PD: Popliteal cysts in adults and children: a review of 90 cases. Arch Surg 88:357–363, 1964.
15. Harcke HT, Grissom LE, Finkelstein MS: Evaluation of the musculoskeletal system with sonography. AJR 150:1253–1261, 1988.
16. Hermann G, Yeh HC, Lehr-Janus C, et al: Diagnosis of popliteal cyst: double-contrast arthrography and sonography. AJR 137:369–372, 1981.
17. Inoue M, Shino K, Hirose H, et al: Subluxation of the patella. J Bone Joint Surg 70A:1331–1336, 1988.
18. Jackson DW, Jennings LD, Maywood RM, Berger PE: Magnetic resonance imaging of the knee. Am J Sports Med 16:29–38, 1988.
19. Johnson LL: Impact of diagnostic arthroscopy on the clinical judgment of an experienced arthroscopist. Clin Orthop 167:75–83, 1982.
20. Kaufman RA, Towbin RB, Babcock DS: Arthrosonography in the diagnosis of pigmented villonodular synovitis. AJR 139:396–398, 1982.
21. Konig H, Sauter R, Deimling M, Vogt M: Cartilage disorders: comparison of spin-echo, CHESS, and FLASH sequence MR images. Radiology 164:753–758, 1987.
22. Kursunoglu-Brahme S, Resnick D, Dalinka MK (guest eds): Magnetic resonance imaging of the knee. Orthop Clin North Am 21(3):561–572, 1990.
23. Laine HR, Harjula A, Peltokallio P: Experience with real-time sonography in muscle injuries. Scand J Sports Sci 7(2):45–49, 1985.
24. Laine HR, Harjula A, Peltokallo P: Ultrasound in the evaluation of the knee and patellar regions. J Ultrasound Med 6:33–36, 1987.
25. Lehto M, Alanen A: Healing of a muscle trauma: correlation of sonographical and histological findings in an experimental study in rats. J Ultrasound Med 6:425–429, 1987.
26. Mandelbaum BR, Finerman GAM, Reicher MA, et al: Magnetic resonance imaging as a tool for evaluation of traumatic knee injuries: anatomical and pathoanatomical correlations. Am J Sports Med 14:361–370, 1986.
27. Martinez S, Korobkin M, Fondren FB, et al: Diagnosis of patellofemoral malalignment by computed tomography. J Comput Assist Tomog 7:1050–1053, 1983.
28. Meire HB, Lindsay DJ, Swinson DR, et al: Comparison of ultrasound and positive contrast arthrography in the diagnosis of popliteal and calf swellings. Ann Rheum Dis 33:221–224, 1974.
29. Mink JH, Levy T, Crues JV III: Tears of the anterior cruciate ligament and menisci of the knee: MR imaging evaluation. Radiology 167:769–774, 1988.
30. Pettersson H, Springfield DS, Enneking WF (eds): Diagnostic imaging modalities: technical comments. *In* Radiologic Management of Musculoskeletal Tumors. New York: Springer-Verlag, 1987.
31. Polly DW, Callaghan JJ, Sikes RA, et al: The accuracy of selective magnetic resonance

imaging compared with the findings of arthroscopy of the knee. J Bone Joint Surg 70A:192–198, 1988.

32. Pring DJ, Henderson RG, Rivett AG, et al: Autologous granulocyte scanning of painful prosthetic joints. J Bone Joint Surg 68B:647–652, 1986.
33. Raunest J, Oberle K, Loehnert J, Hoetzinger H: The clinical value of magnetic resonance imaging in the evaluation of meniscal disorders. J Bone Joint Surg 73A:11–16, 1991.
34. Schutzer SF, Ramsby GR, Fulkerson JP: Computed tomographic classification of patellofemoral pain patients. Orthop Clin North Am 17:235–248, 1986.
35. Schutzer SF, Ramsby GR, Fulkerson JP: The evaluation of patellofemoral pain using computerized tomography: a preliminary study. Clin Orthop 204:286–293, 1986.
36. Senghas RE (ed): Indications for magnetic resonance imaging. J Bone Joint Surg 73A(1), 1991.
37. Stoller DW, Martin C, Crues JV III, et al: Meniscal tears: pathologic correlation with MR imaging. Radiology 163:731–735, 1987.
38. Swett HA, Jaffe RB, McIff EB: Popliteal cysts: presentation as thrombophlebitis. Radiology 115:613–615, 1975.
39. Thomas RH, Resnick D, Alazraki NP, et al: Compartmental evaluation of osteoarthritis of the knee. Radiology 116:585–594, 1975.
40. Wukich DK, Abreu SH, Callaghan JJ, et al: Diagnosis of infection by preoperative scintigraphy with indium-labeled white blood cells. J Bone Joint Surg 69A:1353–1360, 1987.

CHAPTER 6

Congenital and Developmental Problems of the Knee

J. ANDY SULLIVAN, M.D.

■

The lower extremities go through a normal sequence of development that is generally complete by age 7 years, at which time the normal adult gait pattern is established.[5, 10] Most angular deviations that occur about the knee are normal and do not require treatment. The physician must be aware of this development and of the conditions that do not self-correct spontaneously in order to adequately counsel parents. A working knowledge of the conditions that do not self-correct is also necessary.

PHYSIOLOGIC BOWING AND GENU VALGUM

At birth most children have mild genu varum that probably results from intrauterine positioning. Ordinarily, this angulation reaches a maximum at age 18 months. Most children then develop genu valgum around age 3 years and achieve normal adult knee angulation between approximately 5 and 8 years of age. Normal adult genu valgum is approximately 6°. It is not unusual to see 20° of genu varum in children less than 2 years of age, and genu valgum may reach 20°.

Salenius and Vankka measured the tibiofibular angle in children from birth through 4 years of age.[19] They noted pronounced genu varum that tended to self-correct at about 18 months of age. They noted that genu valgum developed during the second and third years and decreased spontaneously until approximately age 6 or 7, at which point adult angulation was reached. In their study of 1480 normal children, genu varum averaged 15°. During the second and third years, the change was toward marked genu valgum of 12° (Fig. 6–1).

Of importance is to notice whether the lower extremities are symmetric. In most instances, if there are no other underlying medical conditions such as metabolic disease or renal abnormalities, radiographic evaluation is not necessary. If a radiograph is obtained, it is important to look carefully at the contour and the symmetry of the physes (Figs. 6–1*B*, 6–1*D*). Mild bowing and some beaking medially on both the femur and the tibia are not unusual in children less than 24 months of age.

Both genu varum and genu valgum are seen in older children with underlying metabolic diseases or skeletal dysplasias, such as achondroplasia, spondyloepiphyseal dysplasia, rickets, and renal osteodystrophy. These children may present in early adolescence with knee pain and obvious angular deformity (Fig. 6–2). Corrective osteotomies are indicated to restore normal skeletal alignment.

Rickets in its various forms can cause angular deformity at the knee. True rickets and vitamin D–deficient rickets cause genu varum, usually with accompanying internal tibial torsion. Patients with chronic renal disease who develop hypophosphatasia develop genu valgum deformity (Fig. 6–3).

BLOUNT'S DISEASE

The most common cause of nonphysiologic bowing is Blount's disease, in which there is abnormal growth in the medial tibial physis that results in growth suppression on the medial side, which in turn leads to progressive genu varum deformity if not treated. Thompson and colleagues' study suggested three specific forms of tibia vara on the basis of age of clinical

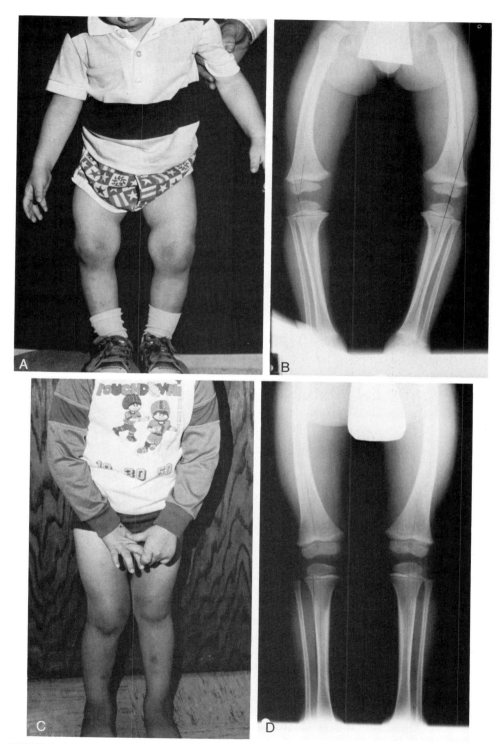

FIGURE 6–1. Photographs and radiographs of a patient with genu varum at 18 months of age (*A, B*) and genu valgum at 4 years of age (*C, D*). Note the metaphyseal beaking in the medial femurs and tibias *(B)*, which is a normal finding.

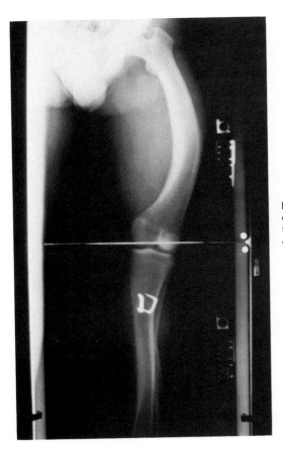

FIGURE 6–2. Anteroposterior (AP) radiograph of a 12-year-old male with vitamin D–resistant rickets. Note the staples in the tibia from a previous osteotomy. This film was taken before a femoral osteotomy.

onset: in the infantile type, onset is 0 to 3 years; in the juvenile type, 4 to 10 years; and in the adolescent type, after 10 years (Fig. 6–4).[23] The juvenile type is characterized by a higher rate of recurrence after surgical correction, whereas children with the other types tend to do well if there is no physeal bar or if the disease has not reached an advanced stage. Blount's disease is more common in children who are black or are obese than in white or normal-weight children. It has both familial and geographic influences.

The etiologic process of infantile tibia vara is obscure. Langenskiold and Riska examined biopsies from nine patients.[11] There were islands of densely packed cells and acellular fibrous cartilage with abnormal groups of capillary cells. There was no evidence of avascular necrosis. It has been suggested that some children may have physiologic genu varum and are overweight, which produces more stress on the medial physis and suppresses growth. Left untreated, this condition may result in a bony bridge.

Wenger and collaborators suggested that adolescent tibia vara is a physiologic disturbance of growth in the medial or posteromedial portion of the proximal tibial metaphysis rather than a bridge.[24] They postulated that a child with residual physiologic genu varum could develop the adolescent form of Blount's disease during the teenage growth spurt as a result of obesity, extreme activity, or repetitive trauma. They evaluated seven cases of adolescent tibia vara in which they were able to review the

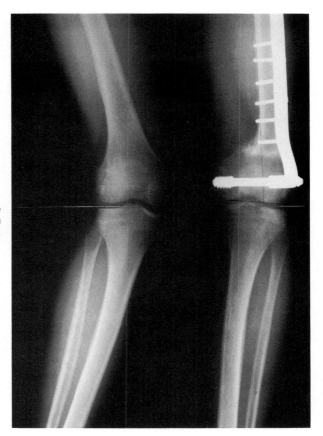

FIGURE 6–3. Standing radiograph of a patient who has chronic renal disease and renal rickets. The film was taken before his second distal femoral osteotomy.

histopathologic findings. There was a loss of orderly cartilage columns, and the overall picture resembled a growth arrest line rather than a bony bridge. A large amount of fibrovascular repair tissue was noted in the metaphysis at the cartilage-bone junction. The authors postulated that these children had a physiologic genu varum in childhood rather than a partial or an unresolved type I or type II infantile tibia vara.

Treatment of tibia vara is based on the severity of the process and on the age of the patient. The severity is best graded by using the method of Langenskiold and Riska in which six stages of severity are described on the bases of the degree of growth disturbance and the maturity of the skeleton.[11] Grade I is the mildest form, and in grade VI there is complete closure of the physis. It has been suggested that bracing is the treatment of choice for grades I and II. The efficacy of bracing is questionable; however, no treatment other than observation or bracing is indicated for these mild forms. Orthotic treatment is very difficult in small children because it is difficult to obtain cooperation from both the parents and the child. If an orthosis is used, it must be a long leg brace that can apply three-point bending pressure to create a valgus force at the knee. It is difficult to achieve much force if the knee is allowed to bend. For these reasons, this author rarely uses a brace in young children with Blount's disease.

In children over age 3 years with progressive deformity, tibial and fibular osteotomy in which the leg is placed in mild genu valgum may

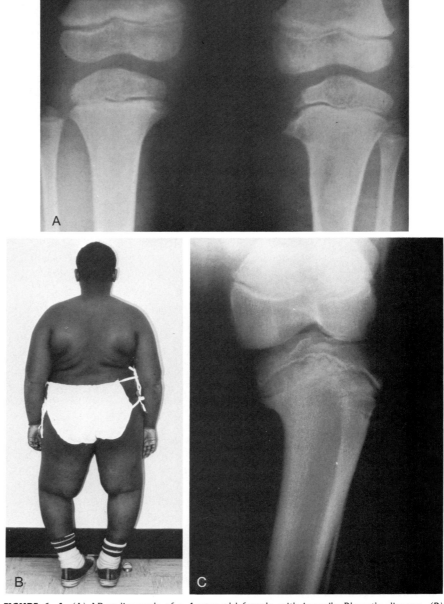

FIGURE 6–4. *(A)* AP radiograph of a 4-year-old female with juvenile Blount's disease. *(B)* Clinical photograph of a patient with adolescent Blount's disease. *(C)* AP radiograph of the knee of the patient in *B*.

reverse the process. Figure 6–5 demonstrates the author's preferred method of performing the osteotomy. In grades III and IV, the condition is believed to be reversible if osteotomy is performed before age 4 years. In the more severe forms (grades V and VI), the only treatment is operative correction, which may include a variety of procedures. Physeal bridge resection and interpositional material may address the underlying problem. Osteotomy may be required in order to correct the deformity caused by the process. In some children who are at the end of growth or in

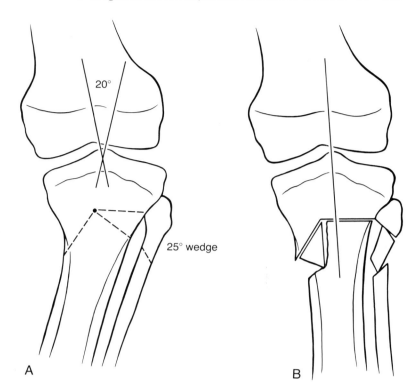

FIGURE 6–5. Line drawings (A, B) of the author's preferred method of performing proximal tibial and fibular osteotomies to correct genu varum.

whom the bridge is too extensive, epiphyseodesis may be necessary. Unless it is performed bilaterally, epiphyseodesis causes or accentuates a discrepancy in leg lengths. The deformity caused by Blount's disease can be complex and three-dimensional. The deformity may not be correctable with a single-plane osteotomy. This is an area in which there is a high complication rate from peroneal nerve injury and compartmental syndrome. The procedure must be carefully performed, and the neurovascular status must be monitored closely postoperatively.

Schoenecker and associates examined 32 patients with a diagnosis of Blount's disease treated at the St. Louis Shriner's Hospital and made specific treatment recommendations.[20] Thirty-one patients had the infantile type, whereas only 1 of the 32 was of the adolescent variety. The authors recommended bracing for children more than 2 years of age who have grade I or II Blount's disease and a varus deformity of more than 15°. If the deformity does not resolve with brace treatment, surgical correction is the treatment of choice. The authors suggested that such children undergo definitive surgical treatment before 5 years of age. They concluded from their retrospective review that correction to within 5° of neutral predictably resulted in satisfactory outcome if the osteotomy was performed before the patient's fifth birthday.

Thompson and colleagues reviewed late-onset tibia vara.[23] The clinical characteristics of the populations studied were a consistent preponderance of black patients (two to every white patient), a predominance of males, normal height, marked obesity, and knee pain as the primary complaint.

Genu varum averaged 19° (the range was 10° to 45°). On radiographs, the epiphyses appeared wedged-shaped with medial flattening. The physes were irregular in thickness, and there was minimal, if any, increased prominence of the proximal medial metaphysis. Among children with clinical onset at less than 10 years of age, the recurrence rate was 50 per cent, which was suggestive of the three forms of the disease.

Bracing has not proved effective in children with the adolescent form of Blount's disease. Early corrective osteotomy to place the leg in 6° to 10° of valgus angulation may restore normal alignment to the leg and prevent further physeal damage.

ANGULAR DEFORMITY OF THE KNEE FROM TRAUMA

Trauma is an important cause of angular deformity about the knee. Physeal injuries can cause cessation of growth, which may result in discrepancy in leg lengths or in angular deformity that at times is very complex. It has long been recognized that physeal fractures, particularly of the Salter III and Salter IV varieties, are accompanied by a high incidence of problems unless they are anatomically repaired and held. Articles have also stressed that all physeal injuries of the distal femur may be associated with such injury and need to be followed until skeletal maturity (Figs. 6–6A, 6–6B, 6–6C).[13, 17] In the series by Lombardo and Harvey, two thirds of the patients had an angular discrepancy of 1 cm or more or an angular deformity requiring operative procedures.[13] Prognosis is more dependent on the amount of initial displacement than on the Salter-Harris classification. Proximal tibial physeal injuries may also be associated with closure (Fig. 6–6).

Long bone fractures of the femur and the tibia may be associated with injuries to the physis, which sometimes are unrecognized. Fractures of the femur may be accompanied by distal physeal injuries and, in some patients, proximal tibial physeal injuries as well. In an automobile accident in which unrestrained patients are thrown forward, the knee may be struck, and in the skeletally immature patient, the tibial tubercle and the anterior portion of the physis can be damaged, resulting in physeal closure, patella baja, and genu recurvatum (Fig. 6–7). At the time of injury, the only recognized injury may be the fracture of the femur. In other instances, fractures of the femur are associated with unrecognized physeal injuries. These injuries often require complex solutions such as combinations of physeal resection, physeal closure of the contralateral side, corrective osteotomy, and, sometimes, ipsilateral lengthening (Figs. 6–8, 6–9).

Genu valgum deformity can also occur after mildly displaced fractures of the tibial metaphysis. These fractures characteristically are minimally displaced fractures through the proximal tibial metaphysis with an intact or plastically deformed fibula in a child less than 5 years of age (Fig. 6–10). The etiologic process is unknown, but the deformity may result from overgrowth of the tibia in relation to the fibula. Other authors have thought that the deformity results from soft tissue interposition. The physician must be aware of the sequence of events involving a minimally displaced fracture in which progressive valgus deformity develops after healing. This deformity may progress over a 2- to 3-year period. The best

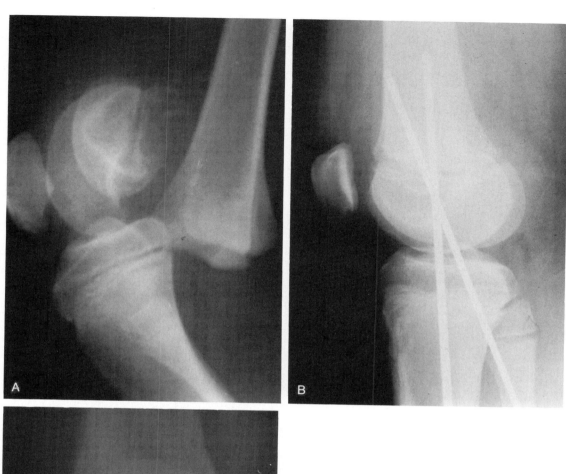

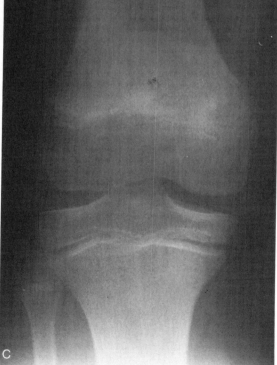

FIGURE 6–6. *(A)* Lateral radiograph of a Salter-Harris II distal femoral physeal separation. *(B)* Postmanipulation and percutaneous radiograph. *(C)* Two-year follow-up radiograph demonstrating distal femoral physeal closure. The closure was symmetric so that there was no angular deformity, but there was a 2.8-cm discrepancy in leg lengths.

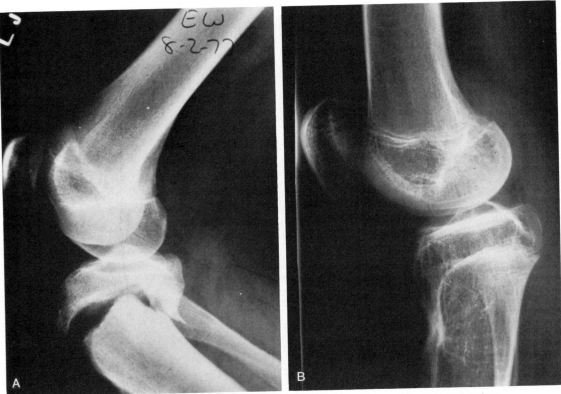

FIGURE 6—7. *(A)* Proximal tibial physeal fracture. *(B)* Physeal closure with genu recurvatum.

treatment is observation until the child is 7 to 8 years of age because spontaneous recovery almost always occurs. There is an exceedingly high recurrence rate, even after osteotomy of both tibia and fibula with correction of the deformity. Most authors now recommend waiting until the patient reaches puberty to correct the deformity.

Zionts and MacEwen reviewed cases of seven children with posttraumatic tibia valga.[25] These children were between the ages of 11 months and 6 years 4 months at the time of the injury. In all the children, the most rapid progression of the deformity was in the immediate postfracture period, but it continued to develop during the first year after injury, in some instances for as long as 17 months. Overgrowth of as much as 1.7 cm accompanied this deformity. In six of the seven patients, correction was sufficient that no treatment was necessary.

CONGENITAL DISLOCATION OF THE KNEE

Infants may manifest a spectrum of knee hyperextension, including mild correctable hyperextension, subluxation, and true congenital dislocation of the knee (Fig. 6–11).[3, 8, 9, 15] Some of these conditions are associated with other conditions such as myelomeningocele or arthrogryposis, but they can occur as isolated entities. If true anterior dislocation of the tibia on the femur is seen, other anomalies should be sought. The condition is bilateral in 21 per cent of patients. Clubfoot (41 per cent), breech presen-

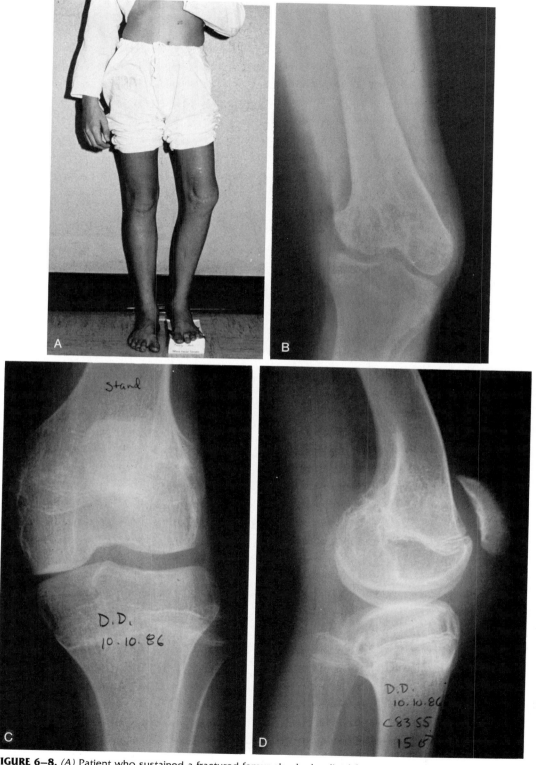

FIGURE 6–8. *(A)* Patient who sustained a fractured femur also had a distal femoral physeal injury that was not recognized until 4 years later. *(B)* Radiograph of the patient in *A.* *(C, D)* AP and lateral radiographs of another patient with an unrecognized physeal injury associated with femur fracture.

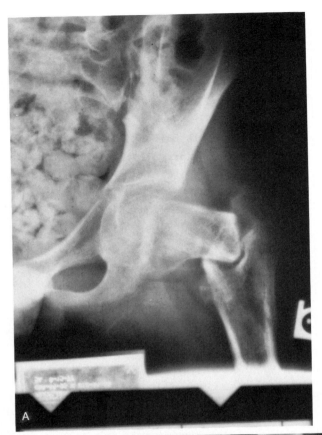

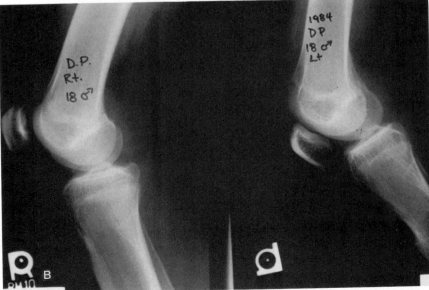

FIGURE 6–9. *(A)* AP radiograph of a patient who sustained a comminuted proximal femur fracture that required internal fixation and bone grafting for the nonunion. *(B)* Lateral knee radiographs of the knees taken 8 years later when the patient complained of knee pain with jogging. The left knee radiograph shows an irregular tibial tubercle and patella alta.

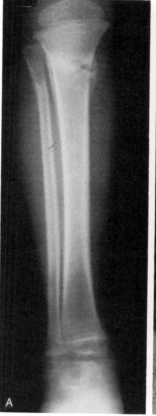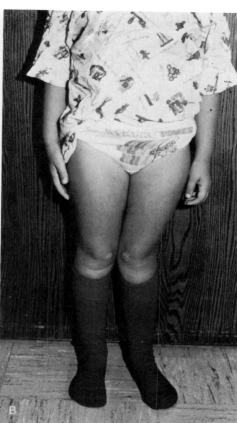

FIGURE 6–10. *(A)* Radiograph of a minimally displaced proximal tibial fracture with an intact fibula. *(B)* Photograph 1 year later demonstrating tibia valgum.

tation (30 per cent), congenital dislocation of the hip, and craniofacial, hand, and spine anomalies are all common among such patients.[1, 8] Congenital dislocation of the hip must be carefully sought because it may be difficult to detect and will influence the sequence of treatment.

Congenital dislocation of the knee is readily apparent. The hips are acutely flexed, and the knees are hyperextended, usually with an increased number of skin folds anterior to the knee. All the structures anterior to the knee, including the quadriceps muscle and the knee joint capsule, are contracted, whereas the posterior structures are lengthened.

Leveuf and Pais divided congenital dislocation of the knee into grade I (severe recurvatum), grade II (subluxation), and grade III (complete dislocation).[12] In grade III there is often loss of the patellar pouch, which carries a worse prognosis. The cruciate ligaments may be absent. The pathologic anatomy includes contracture of the quadriceps muscle and of the iliotibial band. There may be anterior translation of the tibia and the hamstring tendons.

In all varieties, an initial period of conservative management is indicated. These include attempts at stretching the contracted structures and reducing the subluxation and dislocation by a series of casts. Although in some patients the long leg cast may be sufficient, a spica may be necessary in a small infant with marked dislocation. Just as with an interphalangeal joint dislocation, simple traction is not sufficient to reduce

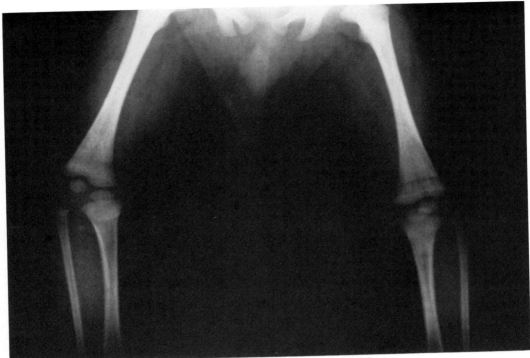

FIGURE 6–11. AP lower extremity radiograph of an infant with complete, bilateral knee dislocation.

the deformity, and accentuation of the deformity with stretching is sometimes necessary for adequately repositioning the tibia on the femur.

Some children have hyperextension without anterior displacement on the femur. In general, this deformity can be flexed and reduced.

In the series by Nogi and MacEwen, an average of 6 weeks was required in order to achieve reduction, and then the children were maintained in bivalved casts or a Pavlik harness.[15] The harness was discontinued when 120° of knee flexion was obtained. Of the 17 patients, closed management was successful in 14, but three required open reduction. Surgery consisted of lengthening the quadriceps muscle, relocating the hamstring muscles posteriorly, and releasing the anterior knee capsule. The medial and lateral knee ligaments were left intact. In the three children treated surgically, reduction and more than 90° of flexion were maintained. In this series, 47 per cent of these children had normal clinical or x-ray evaluation of the hip. Two children had frank bilateral hip dislocations, and both had been in breech presentations at birth. In five others, there was mild residual acetabular dysplasia, bilateral in two and always on the ipsilateral side in the other three.

If satisfactory range can be obtained by casting and if radiographs indicate a normal relationship of the tibia on the femur, the patient may be managed by maintenance in casting or conversion to some type of orthotic device, such as the Pavlik harness, that maintains the hips and knees in flexion. Exercises conducted by a physical therapist and by the parents may be beneficial for maintaining range of motion. In the young infant, it may be preferable to confirm the reduction with arthrography. This outlines the femoral condyles and may also give information about the presence or absence of the cruciate ligaments, as well as the presence or absence of the suprapatellar pouch.

Lack of ability to achieve satisfactory reduction and range of motion, which probably should be at least 60° to 90° in the first 4 to 6 months of life, is an indication for operative intervention. A frequently performed procedure is a V-Y lengthening of the quadriceps muscle with mobilization of other structures as necessary to achieve reduction. The knee should be reduced to a minimum of 90° of flexion; 120° is preferable. Roy and Crawford reported that percutaneous recession of the quadriceps muscle is effective in the treatment of some cases of congenital hyperextension deformities of the knee in neonates.[18]

Bensahel and colleagues studied 56 knees in 46 babies.[1] Grade III was the most common form of hyperextension. In 24 patients, the goal of 120° of flexion was achieved with conservative means alone. There were only two bad results in the entire group.

Johnson and associates reviewed 23 cases.[8] Serial casting was successful in 10 patients, whereas 13 required surgery. The authors believed that the prognosis was better for patients with unilateral involvement and for patients in whom surgery was performed before age 2 years. In their series, 17 patients required a total of 75 operations on the musculoskeletal system. Eighty-eight per cent had other anomalies that influenced the treatment of the knees. The authors suggested that the feet and the knees be corrected before reducing the dislocation in the hips.

CONGENITAL ABSENCE OF THE CRUCIATE LIGAMENTS

Absence of the cruciate ligaments has been reported in association with a variety of conditions, including congenital short femur, congenital dislocation of the knee, congenital changes in the menisci, and the TAR syndrome (thrombocytopenia and absent radius).[3, 7, 9, 22] Thomas and collaborators examined 10 patients, all of whom had at least one other congenital abnormality in a lower extremity.[22] Fifty per cent of the patients were asymptomatic. The patients had positive results in anterior drawer and grade III Lachman tests, as well as complex instability. Radiographs yielded a variety of findings. There was hypoplasia of the tibial spine, femoral condyles, and patellae (Fig. 6–12). The intercondylar notch was V-shaped. In some patients, the fibular head was hypoplastic or absent. In all patients the absence of the anterior cruciate ligament was confirmed arthroscopically. Three of the patients had an abnormality of the posterior cruciate ligament as well. No treatment recommendations were made. Half the patients were asymptomatic, and so it would be hard to recommend treatment. The authors stated that the natural history was unknown, but they suspected that it was the same as that of persons who experience traumatic loss of the cruciate ligaments.

CONGENITAL DISLOCATION OF THE PATELLA

This is an unusual condition in which there is an irreducible lateral subluxation or a dislocation of the patella.[6, 21] Commonly associated features include a hypoplasia of the femoral condyle and excessive mobility

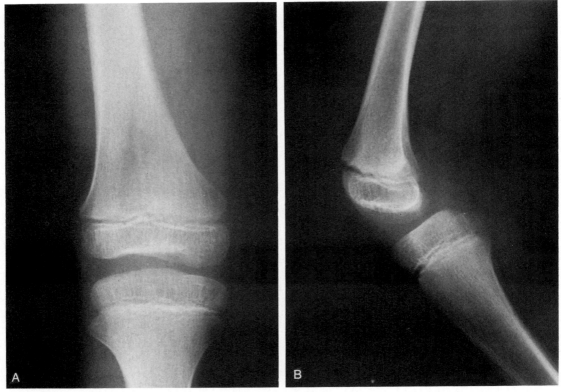

FIGURE 6–12. Knee radiographs (*A, B*) of patient with congenital short femur and clinical evidence of cruciate ligament laxity. Note the absence of the tibial spines and the hypoplasia of the femoral condyles.

of the patella accompanied by thickening of the lateral capsule and tethering to the iliotibial band.

Treatment includes complete immobilization of the quadriceps muscle with adequate lateral release, medial plication, and movement of half of the patellar tendon medially.

Other children manifest chronic subluxation or dislocation of the patella each time the knee is flexed.[2] This is sometimes seen in children with hypoplastic femoral condyles, Down's syndrome, and other skeletal dysplasias (Fig. 6–13). Treatment involves medial plication and lateral release, which sometimes requires an extensive release of the vastus lateralis and the vastus intermedius and lengthening of the rectus femoris. In the author's experience, this condition has been difficult to manage. The combination of contracted soft tissues, hypoplasia of the femoral condyle, and abnormality of the patella makes surgical treatment unpredictable. Patellectomy may be required if all else fails.

BIPARTITE PATELLA

Bipartite patella is frequently discovered as an incidental finding in the child who obtains a radiograph because of knee pain. It occurs in a variety of forms and should be recognized lest it be mistaken, as often occurs in emergency rooms, for a fracture. It is thought to be a developmental

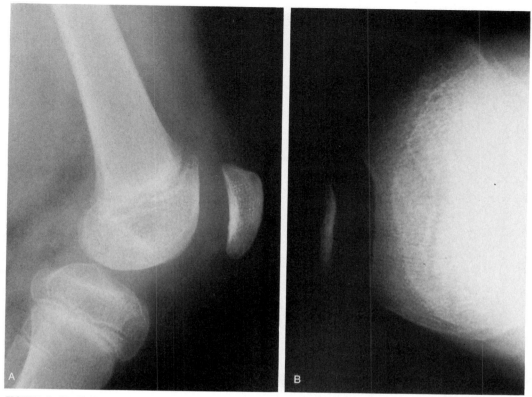

FIGURE 6–13. Radiographs (A, B) of a patient with persistent patellar dislocation of the patella with flexion. Note the hypoplasia of the lateral femoral condyle.

condition in which a portion of the patella fails to coalesce with the remainder or a separate ossification center. The most usual location is the superior lateral portion of the patella, but it has been found in a variety of other locations (Fig. 6–14). It is exceedingly unusual for such patients to be symptomatic. Many patients do manifest knee pain and a bipartite patella, but careful physical examination usually reveals that the pain is not in the location of the bipartite lesion.

The absence of knee effusion, of crepitation, of hematoma, or of evidence of direct trauma helps to rule out an acute fracture. In most instances, acute fracture can be easily recognized through a combination of history, clinical examination, and review of the radiograph. If there is any doubt about the diagnosis, short-term immobilization may be indicated to rule out the possibility of an acute fracture. In some rare instances, such fractures are symptomatic, and removal of the bipartite fragment may be required. In these instances, the undersurface of the patella is usually uneven.

OSGOOD-SCHLATTER DISEASE

Osgood-Schlatter disease is thought to be one of the osteochondroses involving a traction apophysis. In this instance, the tibial tubercle becomes painful and enlarged. The etiologic process of Osgood-Schlatter disease is

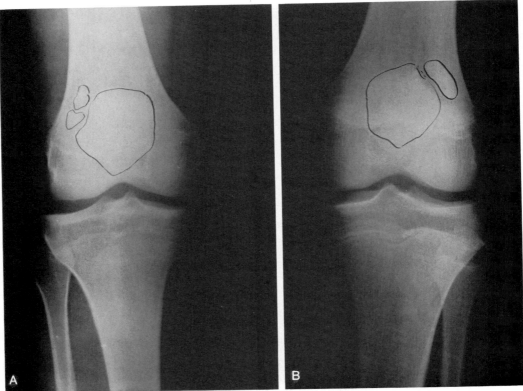

FIGURE 6–14. Two patients with bipartite patella show different presentations (*A, B*).

uncertain. Vascular damage, trauma, and structural changes have all been suggested. Ogden and Southwick discussed the various etiologic processes and evaluated the tibias from autopsies of fetuses and children whose ages ranged from a few days to 16 years.[16] On the basis of their study and literature review, they thought the cause was an avulsion of the portion of the developing ossification center and the overlying hyaline cartilage. The fibrocartilaginous growth plate appears to be a structural adaptation to prevent avulsion of the tibial tuberosity away from the anterior tibial metaphysis. The growth plate of the tibial tuberosity is an apophysis and subject to tension stresses rather than to compression forces. This area is also primarily fibrocartilage and fibrous tissue. Osgood-Schlatter disease tends to be a result of the repetitive exertion of these tensile forces on the tibial tuberosity.

Patients present with a history of knee pain. Clinical findings include tenderness, swelling, and enlargement of the tibial tubercle with pain on direct palpation. Radiographic findings include irregular fragmentation within the tibial tubercle. The physician must be aware that the normal tibial tubercle often has irregular ossification.

The diagnosis of Osgood-Schlatter disease should be reserved for patients with a clinical history and a physical examination that confirm a painful tibial tubercle. This condition is more prevalent among males than among females and tends to occur during early adolescence. It is common in patients who are involved in activities that repetitively stress the extensor mechanism and the tibial tubercle.

Treatment involves limitation of activities, anti-inflammatory medicines, and, in the recalcitrant case, immobilization in a cast. The author's experience has been that immobilization in a cast for a week to 10 days is usually enough to convince the patient that self-limitation of activities is sufficient treatment. The author has rarely had to resort to a cast. In a rare patient in late adolescence, a large, prominent ossicle with an overlying bursa may persist and cause pain, especially if repetitive kneeling is necessary. In these cases, which are fairly uncommon, simple excision of the ossicle is necessary.

SINDING-LARSEN-JOHANSSON SYNDROME

This condition is in the spectrum of chronic strains of the extensor mechanism of the knee. These include Osgood-Schlatter disease of the tibial apophysis, patellar tendinitis, jumper's knee at the junction of the patellar tendon and patella, and Sinding-Larsen-Johansson syndrome, which is a traction apophysitis at the junction of the patella with the patellar tendon. It commonly manifests in early adolescent children and usually more commonly in males, who tend to place repetitive stress on the extensor mechanism of the knee. It resolves spontaneously, usually within a year. Irregular calcification or ossification may be apparent on radiographs if the contrast is adjusted in order to enhance these fine differences in density. Like the other conditions involving repetitive stress, it responds best to limitation of activities, occasionally to anti-inflammatory medicines, and, on rare occasions in the difficult case or in patients who refuse to otherwise limit activity, to immobilization. No long-term morbidity is associated with the condition.

Medlar and Lyne conducted a prospective study of children with pain in the knee.[14] They were able over a 14-month period to identify eight patients (10 knees) with the clinical and roentgenographic findings of Sinding-Larsen-Johansson disease. All children were otherwise healthy and were vigorous athletes. The pain in the knee was accentuated by activities involving forceful knee extension. In five of the patients, the problem was managed by limitation of activities. The other three patients wore a cylinder cast for a brief period of time because of severe pain. All patients eventually became symptom free, and most were able to return to athletics.

The criterion for clinical diagnosis was point tenderness at the anterior pole of the patella. Roentgenographic findings included calcification near the inferior pole of the patella. These patients were in a younger age category than those with Osgood-Schlatter disease, in which the range is 10 to 13. In most patients with Sinding-Larsen-Johansson syndrome, the disease ran its course in 3 to 12 months.

BAKER'S (POPLITEAL) CYST

Baker's cyst is a small synovial cyst most often in the lateral popliteal space. In children, these cysts can appear at almost any age and are not ordinarily associated with intra-articular disorder. They are usually asymptomatic, nontender, and discovered incidentally by the patient's parents. Popliteal cysts are probably an enlargement of the bursa between the semimembranosus and gastrocnemius muscles. In Dinham's series, boys outnumbered girls by 2 to 1.[4] Children in his series presented between ages 2 years 4 months and 14 years; the mean age was about 6 years. The incidence of popliteal cysts is decreased after age nine, which suggests spontaneous remission.

If there is concern about the diagnosis, it can at times be confirmed by aspiration with a large-bore needle, which will draw out viscous, ganglionic, clear yellow fluid. Often the families of patients are quite concerned about these cysts, and the patients have been referred for evaluation of a possible tumor. The physician must spend enough time to convince them that the best course is to do nothing other than continue observation.

In Dinham's review of the natural history of 120 popliteal cysts in children, 51 of 70 untreated cysts disappeared spontaneously during a mean period of 1 year 8 months. Of the 50 that were treated surgically, 21 recurred in a mean period of 7 months. Seventy-three per cent of untreated cysts and 24 per cent of recurrent cysts resolve in 5 years. The best advice is to leave them alone.

REFERENCES

1. Bensahel H, Dal Monte A, Hjelmstedt A, et al: Congenital dislocation of the knee. J Pediatr Orthop 9:174–177, 1989.
2. Bergman NR, Williams PF: Habitual dislocation of the patella in flexion. J Bone Joint Surg 70B:415–419, 1988.
3. Curtis BH, Fisher RL: Congenital hyperextension with anterior subluxation of the knee: surgical treatment and long term observations. J Bone Joint Surg 51A:255–269, 1969.
4. Dinham JM: Popliteal cysts in children: the case against surgery. J Bone Joint Surg 57B:69–71, 1975.
5. Engel GM, Staheli LT: The natural history of torsion and other factors influencing gait in childhood: a study in angle of gait, tibial torsion, knee angle, hip rotation, and development of the arch in normal children. Clin Orthop 99:12–17, 1974.
6. Green JP, Waugh W, Wood H: Congenital lateral dislocation of the patella. J Bone Joint Surg 50B:285–289, 1968.
7. Johansson E, Aparisi T: Missing cruciate ligament in congenital short femur. J Bone Joint Surg 65A:1109–1115, 1983.
8. Johnson E, Audell R, Oppenheim WL: Congenital dislocation of the knee. J Pediatr Orthop 7:194–200, 1987.
9. Katz MP, Grogono BJ, Soper KC: The etiology and treatment of congenital dislocation of the knee. J Bone Joint Surg 49B:112–120, 1967.
10. Kling TF Jr, Hensinger RN: Angular and torsional deformity of the lower limbs in children. Clin Orthop 176:136–147, 1983.
11. Langenskiold A, Riska EB: Tibia vara (osteochondrosis deformans tibiae): survey of seventy-one cases. J Bone Joint Surg 46A:1405–1420, 1964.
12. Leveuf J, Pais C: Les dislocations congénitales du genou. Rev d'Orthop 32:313–350, 1946.
13. Lombardo SJ, Harvey JP Jr: Fractures of the distal femoral physis: factors influencing prognosis. A review of 34 cases. J Bone Joint Surg 59A:742–751, 1977.
14. Medlar RC, Lyne ED: Sinding-Larsen-Johansson disease: its etiology and natural history. J Bone Joint Surg 60A:113–116, 1978.
15. Nogi J, MacEwen GD: Congenital dislocation of the knee. J Pediatr Orthop 2:509–513, 1982.
16. Ogden JA, Southwick WO: Osgood-Schlatter's disease and tibial tuberosity development. Clin Orthop 116:180–190, 1976.
17. Riseborough EJ, Barrett IR, Shapiro F: Growth disturbances following distal femoral physeal fracture-separations. J Bone Joint Surg 65:885–893, 1983.
18. Roy DR, Crawford AH: Percutaneous quadriceps recession: a technique for management of congenital hyperextension deformities of the knee in the neonate. J Pediatr Orthop 9:717–719, 1989.
19. Salenius P, Vankka E: The development of the tibiofemoral angle in children. J Bone Joint Surg 57A:259–261, 1975.

20. Schoenecker PL, Meade WC, Pierron RL, et al: Blount's disease: a retrospective review and recommendations for treatment. J Pediatr Orthop 5:181–186, 1985.
21. Stanisavljevic S, Zemenick G, Miller D: Congenital, irreducible, permanent lateral dislocation of the patella. Clin Orthop 116:190–199, 1976.
22. Thomas NP, Jackson AM, Aichroth PM: Congenital absence of the anterior cruciate ligament: a common component of knee dysplasia. J Bone Joint Surg 67B:572–575, 1985.
23. Thompson GH, Carter JR, Smith CW: Late-onset tibia vara: a comparative analysis. J Pediatr Orthop 4:185–194, 1984.
24. Wenger DR, Mickelson M, Maynard JA: The evolution and hisopathology of adolescent tibia vara. J Pediatr Orthop 4:78–88, 1984.
25. Zionts LE, MacEwen GD: Spontaneous improvement of post-traumatic tibia valga. J Bone Joint Surg 68A:680–687, 1986.

CHAPTER 7

Regional

Fractures of

the Knee

H. David Moehring, M.D.

■

Regional fractures of the knee are a potential source of significant disability largely related to residual deformity, loss of motion, and articular injury. The goal of treatment is to prevent these complications by restoration of anatomic structure and function. Joint congruity must be obtained and rendered secure so that motion can be initiated early. The appropriate manner of achieving this goal is controversial, and a review of the literature reveals excellent supportive studies for both nonoperative and surgical treatment of these fractures.

Comparative analysis of the two methods is difficult because of the many treatment variables, the length of follow-up, and differences in evaluating results. There has been a decided tendency toward operative treatment of articular fractures, especially those involving weight-bearing joints. Much of this enthusiasm is attributable to the development of an improved technology and surgical methodology devised by the Association for Osteosyntussis (AO) group. The resultant improvement in surgical results has been most welcome but has been associated with a declining experience with or knowledge of nonoperative methods in many teaching institutions. These methods can provide good results when appropriately used.[25] In addition, they provide a back-up form of treatment in cases in which surgery is refused or contraindicated. Orthopaedic surgeons in developing countries often lack the institutional support and logistics to safely carry out sophisticated surgical procedures. Nevertheless, they have learned to satisfactorily treat their patients with less invasive and nonoperative techniques. Conversely, the orthopaedist who practices in a modern high-volume trauma center has a distinct advantage by virtue of surgical volume, experience, and available resources.

In the multitrauma setting, treatment of articular fractures is second in importance only to the stabilization of long bones. After treatment of life-threatening systemic injuries and stabilization of diaphyseal fractures, articular fractures may be addressed. If prioritization of systemic injuries precludes the increased anesthetic time, operative treatment may have to be deferred, but it should be accomplished as soon as possible. Exceptions to this guideline are open intra-articular fractures and the presence of associated vascular injury that requires repair. Displaced fractures associated with acute compartmental syndrome should also be surgically stabilized. The most effective way to treat the soft tissue is to reduce the fracture. If multiple fractures are stabilized, the patient's pain and the incidence of cardiopulmonary complications are greatly diminished. These goals are more readily attained in trauma centers geared specifically for treating patients with multiple injuries. Many patients are young, active persons who have sustained high-energy injuries as a result of motor vehicle accidents. In general, the quality of the bones is good, and the patients respond more favorably to aggressive surgical treatment.

The surgical treatment of displaced articular fractures about the knee can be technically difficult. However, the requisite skills can be acquired by the interested and qualified orthopaedic surgeon. The wisdom regarding selection of surgical candidates, proper timing, and specific procedures is perhaps more slowly acquired. It is important to know which patient requires an operation, but it is even more important to identify those patients who do not. The dictum "primum non nocera" (first do no harm) should be observed. For patients with significant medical complications, patients with severe osteoporosis, or nonambulatory patients, nonoperative treatment is often appropriate.

Articular surgery requires preoperative planning, respect for the soft tissues, and restoration of anatomic structure. Operative treatment should provide frigid internal fixation. However, the importance of avoiding excessive fixation, especially on subcutaneous bone in which the hazard of skin slough and subsequent infection can be disastrous, has been emphasized. Supplemental external fixation, cannulated screws, or dynamic orthoses or a combination of these often provides security with less risk. The continued improvement in metallurgy will result in stronger atraumatic implants and less invasive surgical techniques. Arthroscopic treatment of amendable articular fractures will no doubt become more common. Limited or biologic fixation may become increasingly more applicable if healing accelerants and compounds that protect articular cartilage and promote union are produced.

Finally, it must be realized that the destiny of many severe articular injuries is determined at the time of injury. Not all fractures are fixable. Articular surgery is dedicated first to the restoration of joint congruency, but secondary goals of axial alignment, preservation of bone stock, and prevention of shortening are extremely important for future reconstruction. The orthopaedist should always strive to be the "last surgeon," but if this is not possible, the "next surgeon" must be considered.

SUPRACONDYLAR FRACTURES OF THE FEMUR

Fractures of the distal femur, including those with articular extension, are generically termed supracondylar fractures. This area corresponds anatomically to the diaphyseal-metaphyseal junction proximally and to the articular level distally;[28] in general, it corresponds to the distal 10 to 12 cm of the femur. Transverse and minimally comminuted fractures in the proximal supracondylar region may essentially be treated as shaft fractures. Those that are more distal and especially those that extend to the joint remain therapeutic challenges and are the main focus of this discussion.[25, 26] Motor vehicle accidents account for the majority of supracondylar fractures. Low-energy fractures are associated with falls and athletic injuries.

These fractures have historically resulted in great disability, characterized by Sir Astly Cooper as "evil results." Treatment of comminuted fractures by various forms of splints and immobilization frequently led to excessive shortening, angular deformity, and loss of motion. Before the advent of antibiotics, open fractures frequently led to above-knee amputation or death as a result of septic complications. The modern era of treatment began with the use of skin traction popularized by Gurdon Buck and later mechanically improved by Russell in the early 19th century.[28] Skeletal traction was a vast improvement and was described in 1907 by Fritz Steinmann and later by Martin Kirschner. Despite this, there were still problems in controlling the supracondylar fracture in traction, and various modifications such as the two-pin technique were developed. The two-pin technique was described by Modlin in 1945 but no doubt was used before that time. In this technique, a second pin was placed in the distal femoral fragment to overcome the posterior and flexed position commonly encountered. Results were improved but still suboptimal; thus the initial enthusiasm for various forms of internal fixation turned to disillusionment as inconsistent results were obtained. In the mid-1960s, Stewart and colleagues and Neer and associates, in separate papers, retrospectively compared the results of nonoperated and surgically treated patients and found better results among those treated nonoperatively.[24, 35] Subsequently, Connolly and colleagues, Mooney and associates, Rockwood and Green, and others advocated a shorter time in traction followed by the use of a cast-brace that allowed early motion and ambulation.[6, 22, 28]

From a review of the literature, it is clear that the natural history of this fracture is one of potential extreme disability and that the leading cause of this disability was inability to obtain and maintain fracture reduction with enough security to begin early motion.[24, 35] Surgery nowadays is much safer because of improvements in anesthesia, the use of prophylactic antibiotics, and the use of regimes for prevention of pulmonary embolism. This is generally perceived by the public, and more patients prefer the shorter hospitalization, the decreased expense, and especially the resultant increased mobility provided by operative treatment. There is no doubt that conservative treatment can produce satisfactory results. However, it seems that the appropriate use of traction is becoming a lost art. Patients' expectations continue to rise, and in the United States, lawsuits are initiated over what were once considered acceptable or minimal residual deformities. Although both surgical and nonoperative methods may produce satisfactory results, it is evident that nonoperative treatment cannot consistently produce the same numbers of good and excellent results as can rigid internal fixation and early mobilization. Thus this section is devoted mainly to the various surgical methods, their indications, complications, and postoperative care.

Clinical Assessment

The diagnosis of supracondylar fracture is usually not difficult. The characteristic signs of pain, swelling, deformity, and inability to bear weight are usually present. Problems in diagnosis may occasionally arise in multitraumatized patients with minimally displaced fractures. These patients need frequent reassessment and radiographic screening of all suspicious areas. Supracondylar fractures are fixed at the time when the other injuries are stabilized or as soon as possible thereafter.[23] Before surgery, the patient can be placed in balanced skeletal traction through a proximal tibial pin. The presence of other fractures and the priority of their treatment need to be considered. Stabilization of the spine and the long bones takes precedence over other treatments. The skin and soft tissues must be examined carefully for the presence of occult open fractures, abrasions, or burns, which may modify or dictate timing or surgery and placement of incisions. Neurovascular status must to be recorded and reassessed appropriately. When there is any question of arterial injury, angiograms should be obtained without hesitation. When an arterial repair has been performed, stabilization of the bone should usually also be accomplished. With gross contamination or devitalized or missing soft tissue, external fixation should be used.

Current hospital organization at most trauma centers emphasizes a team approach whereby the treatment of nonorthopaedic injuries and general systemic care are dictated by general surgeons and other surgical disciplines as indicated. Nevertheless, the careful orthopaedist should not be a mere spectator to these events and must ensure that the patient's general assessment and care are appropriate and ongoing.

Open Fractures

In addition to irrigation and debridement in the operating room, open articular fractures should be surgically stabilized wherever possible.[4] Definitive internal fixation can usually be accomplished with grade I, grade II, and certain grade III fractures. If there has been extensive abrasion, burn, or soft tissue loss, as in grade IIIB fractures, definitive treatment must be delayed until the soft tissue situation is benign. In these instances, the patient may be treated briefly in traction or external fixation across the knee. However, the latter, if prolonged, may compromise the safe use of subsequent internal fixation. When contamination or soft tissue injury precludes the safe use of definitive internal fixation, limited fixation of the articular surface can usually be accomplished with smooth Kirschner wires or screws. Definitive internal fixation is then carried out either at delayed primary closure or at such a time that the soft tissue condition safely permits. The use of antibiotic-impregnated beads in association with systemic antibiotics may offer additional protection against infection. They are, of course, removed at the time of definitive fixation. Bone grafting may have to be deferred in these situations. The open fracture involving the knee is much more likely to be problematic in direct proportion to the soft tissue injury or development of infection.

Classification

Classifications are an attempt to standardize fracture evaluation so that appropriate treatment may be inferred and outcomes reliably compared. When they are straightforward and logical, useful information can be derived. It should be remembered that classifications are basically gradations of injury severity and are not a substitute for accurate anatomic description of the pathologic process involved. The system developed by the AO group fulfills the requirements requisite for useful classification.[23] It is based on the anatomic location of the fractures and the degree of comminution, which to a significant degree dictate the type of surgical treatment. This classification is shown in Figure 7–1.

Nonoperative Treatment

Impacted or incomplete supracondylar fractures of the femur may be treated with immobilization.[3, 28] This may take the form of a long leg cast or a cast-brace, depending on the patient's body habitus, age, and tolerance for immobilization. Stable fracture patterns permit early weight bearing. For nonambulatory patients who have sustained fracture, the goals are to make the patient comfortable and to obtain fracture healing

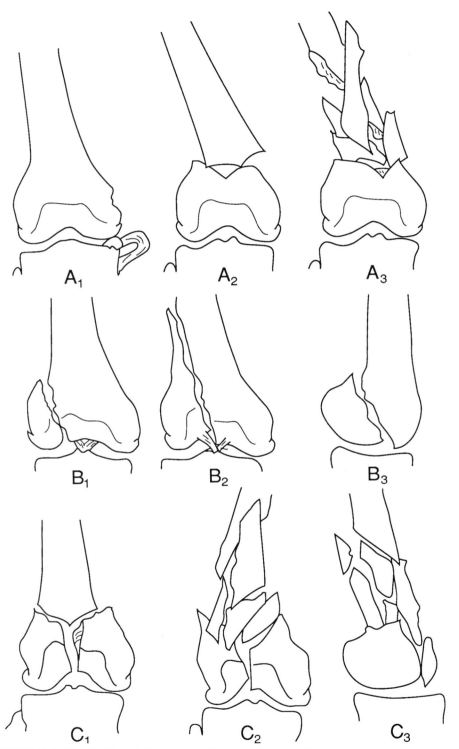

FIGURE 7–1. Classification of distal femoral fractures. (Redrawn from Müller ME, Allgower M, Schneider R, Willenegger H: Manual of Internal Fixation, 2nd ed. New York: Springer, 1979.)

without severe deformity. Paraplegic patients or others with insensate skin should have adequate padding in order to prevent skin breakdown. Patients with displaced fractures treated by traction should be protected from thromboembolism with low doses of sodium warfarin (Coumadin), with sequential stockings, or with other acceptable prophylactic regimes. Skeletal traction is instituted with a smooth Kirschner wire in the proximal tibia and the knee in the amount of flexion that best reduces the fracture. Because of gravity and the pull of the gastrocnemius muscles, the distal fragment tends to displace and angulate posteriorly. Despite this, excessive flexion often does not improve the position and may cause problems in evaluating rotation and angulatory position.[28] A second pin placed in the distal fragment is occasionally helpful. An appropriate amount of weight, usually 15 to 20 pounds, is necessary to prevent excessive shortening. However, excessive weight may cause angulation, not infrequently valgus deformity as a result of tightening of the iliotibial band. Manipulation at the patient's bedside while the patient is under anesthesia or appropriate sedation is also occasionally helpful.

If adequate reduction is not obtained within the first 7 to 10 days, it is unlikely to be successfully obtained. Radiographs should be obtained at appropriate intervals in order to assess healing. When there are signs of healing, indicated by diminution of tenderness and early callous formation, the patient can be placed in a dynamic orthosis or a cast brace. Progressive active and actively assisted range-of-motion exercises should be encouraged, and weight bearing should progress in accordance with fracture characteristics. Limbs with extremely comminuted fractures require longer periods in traction and delayed weight bearing because they have a propensity for shortening (Fig. 7–2). Residual angulatory deformities are common and not infrequently may result in valgus angulation, in contradistinction to more proximal fractures, which invariably angulate into varus formation with weight bearing. Delayed union may occur with resultant increase in deformity.

In the majority of fractures, advanced healing is in progress by 12 weeks. The presence of gross motion at the fracture and absence of radiographic healing are characteristic of nonunion. This should be treated by surgical stabilization and bone graft before the development of progressive deformity. Displaced intra-articular fractures, malposition, and nonunion are all indications for abandonment of this method in favor of surgical treatment.

Surgical Indications

Proponents of conservative and operative treatment of supracondylar fractures agree on the need for reduction, maintenance of alignment, and early motion. Any method that achieves these goals is capable of producing good results. Discussion with the patient of the advantages and disadvantages, or the risk/benefit ratio, is mandatory. Thus familiarity and experience with both methods are necessary if optimal care is to be provided.[3, 5, 6, 28, 35] Assuming that these criteria are present, the following indications for operative treatment are generally accepted:

1. Joint incongruity.
2. Failure of closed treatment.

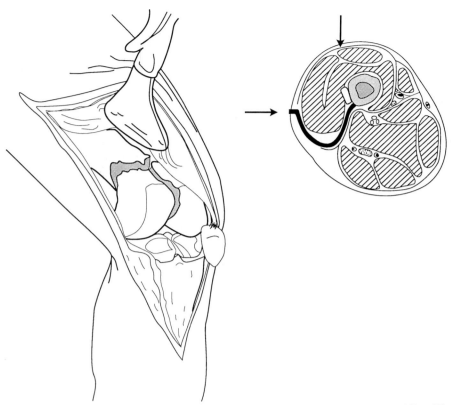

FIGURE 7–2. Surgical approach to fractures of the distal femur. (Redrawn from Mize RD, Bucholtz RW, Grogan DP: Surgical treatment of displaced, comminuted fractures of the distal end of the femur. J Bone Joint Surg 64A:878, 1982.)

3. Segmental or ipsilateral fractures.
4. Vascular injury with repair.
5. Multitrauma/multiple fractures.
6. Extreme obesity of the patient.

Surgical Contraindications

The only absolute contraindications for surgery are gross sepsis and uncorrected hemorrhagic diaphysis. Relative contraindications are as follows:

1. Nonambulatory status of the patient.
2. Extensive soft tissue abrasion, burn, or swelling.
3. Extreme comminution.
4. Severe osteoporosis.
5. Uncontrolled diabetes or other systemic disease.
6. Skeletal immaturity.
7. Late presentation.

Principles of Operative Treatment

The goal of fracture treatment is recovery of maximal function for the injured extremity. It has been said that life is movement and movement is life. When fractures have been rendered stable, progressive mobilization can be initiated, with all its physiologic benefits to both soft tissues and bone. The achievement of this general goal is best met by the following dictums:

1. Restoration of anatomic structure.
2. Atraumatic surgery.
3. Stable internal fixation.
4. Early motion.

R. Salter, in his elegant experiments, demonstrated the beneficial effects of motion on articular cartilage, and it is now well recognized that failure to appropriately mobilize surgically treated articular fracture often results in greater loss of motion than does nonoperative treatment. (Fig. 7–3). The recognition of this fact must of course be tempered with the knowledge of the security of fixation. Extensively comminuted fractures may require more cautious mobilization or the use of a postoperative dynamic orthosis until early healing and stability have been achieved.[3, 5, 40] In the majority of articular fractures, good stability can be obtained by internal fixation, and brief support or splinting is necessary only for the patient's postoperative comfort and soft tissue healing.

In order to achieve success, logistical support for accomplishing the surgical goal is essential. In addition to the instruments and implants, this also means the availability of personnel and necessary institutional support for achieving the goal. Good preoperative planning takes this into account in the selection of an appropriate form of treatment.[23] Members of the AO group are proponents of making tracings of the fracture or using plastic overlays of the injured and uninjured limbs in order to plan the specific details of the surgical fixation. This is more useful for dealing with fixed deformities such as malunion and for the planning of subsequent osteotomies. Although it may be applicable to certain fractures, in general, it is not practical for dealing with fractures that must be treated on an urgent basis.

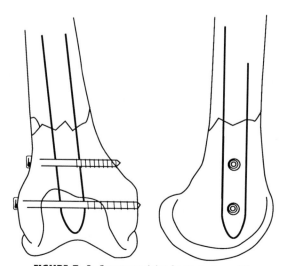

FIGURE 7–3. Supracondylar fracture, type A2.

Internal Fixation Devices

Intramedullary Fixation

Intramedullary fixation may be used for transverse fractures in the proximal supracondylar region. The fixation of choice for fractures in this location is an interlocked rod seated in the subchondral bone of the distal fragment. Theoretically, distal interlocking should be sufficient because of the intramedullary hold of the nail in the proximal isthmic portion of the femur. From a practical standpoint, however, proximal locking yields predictable results and is quickly accomplished, ensuring maintenance of reduction.

If interlocking techniques or instruments are unavailable, an acceptable alternative is flexible intramedullary (Ender) rods inserted proximally from the greater trochanter (Fig. 7–4). They are inserted through a small incision over the trochanter with the patient in the supine position and under image intensifier control. At least three flexible rods are inserted: usually one in the medial femoral condyle and two in the lateral condyle. With this arrangement, torsional stability is obtained. If the fracture is relatively transverse and noncomminuted, shortening does not occur.

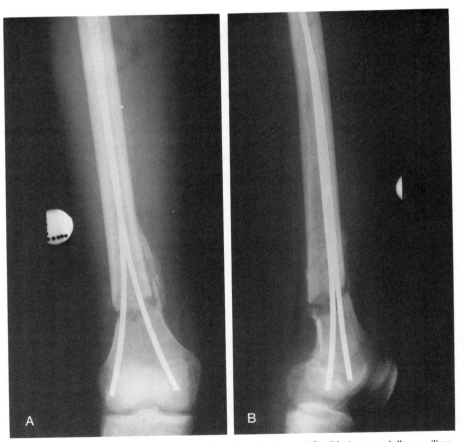

FIGURE 7–4. *A.* Five-week postoperative closed reduction and flexible intramedullary nailing. *B.* Lateral radiograph 5 weeks postoperative flexible intramedullary fixation. Full weight bearing was begun, and ultimate healing with normal function was obtained.

Caution must be used in extending this method to comminuted fractures because excessive shortening and angulation may occur and may be accompanied by the backing out of the pins and further loss of fixation.

DYNAMIC COMPRESSION SCREW

The devices most commonly used to treat supracondylar fractures are the dynamic compression screw (DCS) and the side plate or fixed supracondylar blade plate. The latter is preferred in European countries, whereas the DCS is preferred in the United States.[13, 21, 23, 30] Both devices must be inserted accurately; however, there is slightly more tolerance with the DCS. In addition, interfragmental compression can be obtained when a frequently associated intercondylar fracture is present.

BUTTRESS PLATE

The supracondylar buttress plate may be necessary because of excessive comminution, especially with condylar fractures in the coronal plane.[24] These fractures preclude or render difficult insertion of the more stable DCS or supracondylar blade plate. Bicortical fixation is used to secure the proximal portion of the plate to the lateral femoral shaft, and 6.5-mm cancellous screws are inserted in the condyles in the most efficacious manner. This device will not withstand the varus compressive forces acting on the fracture in the presence of excessive medial comminution. Although initial radiographic findings often are satisfactory, there is an inexorable tendency toward varus deformation. Therefore, when this device is used, medial comminution should be accompanied by iliac crest bone graft and, if necessary, a bridging medial plate. A well-fitting postoperative dynamic orthosis in a physiologic degree of valgus angulation is useful. This plate should always be available because it may be the only efficient fixation device for the bicondylar fracture with medial comminution or intercondylar coronal fracture (type C3, to be described).

MODULAR SYSTEM

The Alta Supracondylar System consists of a 95° side plate and sliding dynamic screw, much like the AO implant described earlier (Fig. 7–5). It is made of titanium, which is biologically inert, and theoretically produces less stress shielding than does the AO implant because of a lower modulus of elasticity. An additional advantage is its modularity, which enables correction or adjustment in the frontal plane, if this is necessary, by slightly bending the modular extension plate and then slotting it into the 95° plate. The condylar screw usually achieves good fixation; however, in unusual instances of severe osteoporosis, augmentation with polymethyl methacrylate can be performed. This requires that the cement be inserted in a doughy stage just before the condylar screw is seated. Alternatively, the dome and plunger that are unique to this system can be used. The dome can be filled with doughy cement and inserted on the plunger, after which the screw and the side plate are inserted over the guide pin. As the dome is pulled down on the plunger and expanded, the soft cement is extruded in a rosette or flower-petal pattern in the medial femoral condyle, greatly enhancing fixation. Use of cement should be reserved for those cases in which implant removal is not envisioned. Subsequent need

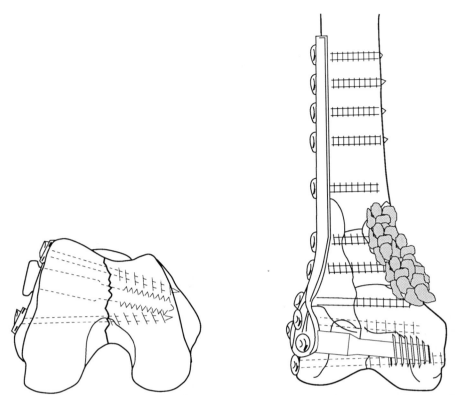

FIGURE 7–5. Internal fixation with dynamic compression screw (DCS). Bone graft areas of medial comminution. (Redrawn from Müller ME, Allgower M, Schneider R, Willenegger H: Manual of Internal Fixation, 2nd ed. New York: Springer, 1979.)

for total knee arthroplasty must be considered because it might be complicated by the inability to safely remove this construct.

The Alta 6.5-mm cancellous screws are self-tapping and should be used with washers when the condylar cortical bone is weak. The Alta supracondylar buttress plate is very useful and molds well to the contour of the anterolateral aspect of the femur (Fig. 7–6). The three slots distally allow for placement of two screws in each and enable more variation and direction than with the conventional buttress plate.

When two screws are inserted in the same slot, they should be directed at different exit points in order to avoid weakening fixation in the opposite cortex. If a medial plate is necessary, the buttress plate designed for the opposite femur often fits well on the medial supracondylar region (see Fig. 7–3). Because these plates are modular, they offer the opportunity for additional correction by slightly bending the proximal side plate before connecting it with the supracondylar buttress plate. Buttress plates are invaluable for treating the comminuted C3 type of fracture for which it is impossible to satisfactorily use the transcondylar bolt or screw.

Surgical Technique

The patient is placed in the supine position, and the fracture is exposed. Traditionally, a lateral skin incision has been described; however, with

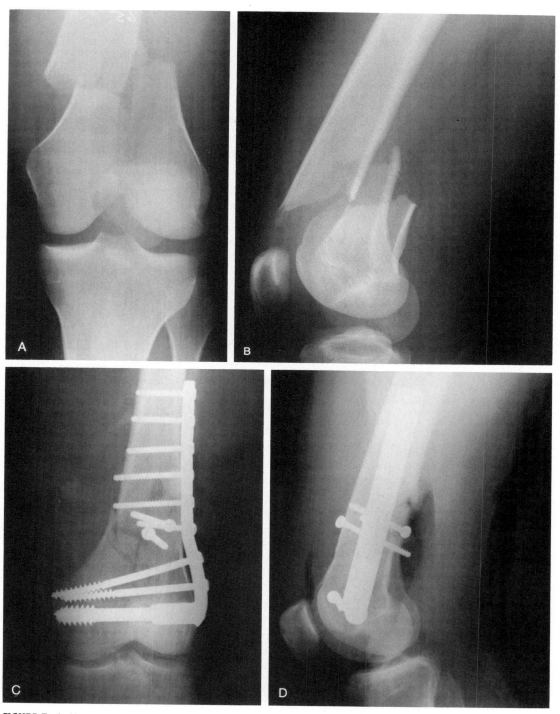

FIGURE 7–6. *(A)* Anteroposterior radiograph of type C1 supracondylar fracture of the femur. *(B)* Lateral radiograph of type C1 fracture. *(C)* Internal fixation of C1 type fracture with DCS, anteroposterior view. *(D)* Posteroperative lateral view of type C1 supracondylar fracture of the femur.

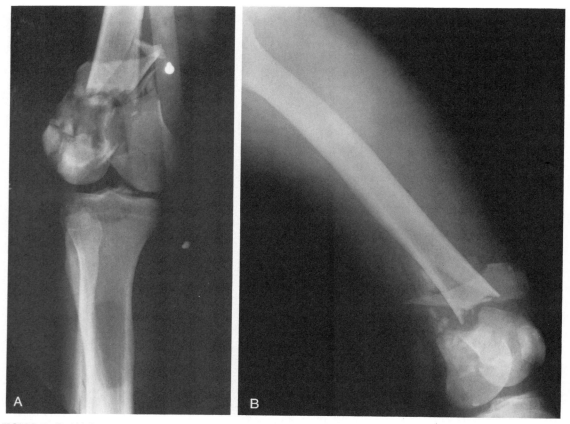

FIGURE 7–7. *(A)* Anteroposterior view of grade IIIB, open type C2 supracondylar fracture of the femur. Patient has associated grade I open tibial fracture. *(B)* Lateral radiograph of open C2 fracture.

excessive comminution or wherever a second medial plate is planned, an anterior incision should be used (Fig. 7–7). This avoids the need for making an accessory medial incision and renders subsequent secondary reconstructive procedures such as total knee arthroplasty much safer. Regardless of the skin incision, the vastus lateralis is elevated off the lateral intermuscular septum and reflected medially in classic fashion.[21] When necessary, the tibial tubercle can be osteotomized, which provides wide exposure of the distal femur and joint by reflecting the quadriceps mechanism proximally. The tibial tubercle should be predrilled and subsequently replaced.

The foot piece on the operating table is lowered, allowing 90° of knee flexion. A large bolster can be placed behind the knee to gain additional flexion and facilitate exposure of the posteriorly displaced condylar fragments. With intercondylar fractures, the next step is realigning the articular surfaces after first clearing the fracture of small bone fragments, soft tissue, and hematoma. The fracture is held in the reduced position with tenaculum forceps, after which provisional K-wire fixation is obtained. Then 6.5-mm lag screws are used to secure the articular fragments. Cannulated screws can be used effectively in this situation. They should be placed so as not to interfere with subsequent placement of the dynamic condylar screw and side plate. The screws should cross the fracture and not enter the intercondylar notch.

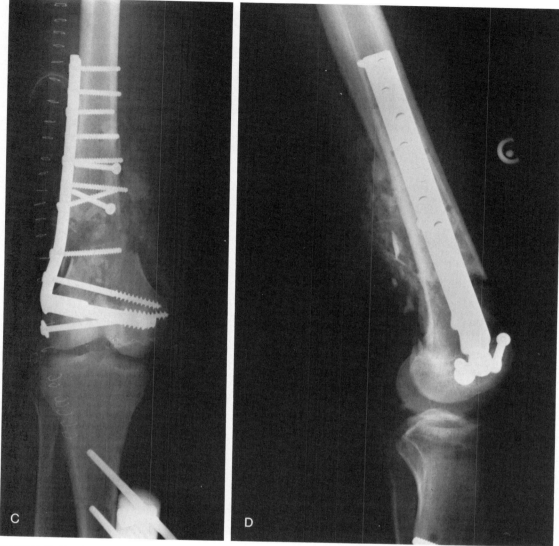

FIGURE 7–7. *Continued. (C)* Postoperative anteroposterior view. Note abundant medial bone graft and early healing. *(D)* Lateral postoperative follow-up radiograph. Ultimate good result with 0° to 115° range of motion, normal alignment, and minimal symptoms.

On occasion, initial fixation is begun on the proximal side when a large cortical fragment can be reduced anatomically to the shaft and secured with interfragmentary cortical lag screws. This aids greatly in the subsequent reduction and assessment of alignment when the condylar fragments are secured to the shaft. Small fragments should be ignored and left with their soft tissue attachments undisturbed. A femoral distractor may be helpful in obtaining alignment via ligamentotaxis and tensioning of the soft tissues. The disadvantage is that it is sometimes awkward to work around the distractor, and it does not permit the flexion of the knee.

The condylar screw is accurately inserted into the reduced distal condylar fragments, and the side plate is reduced to the lateral femoral

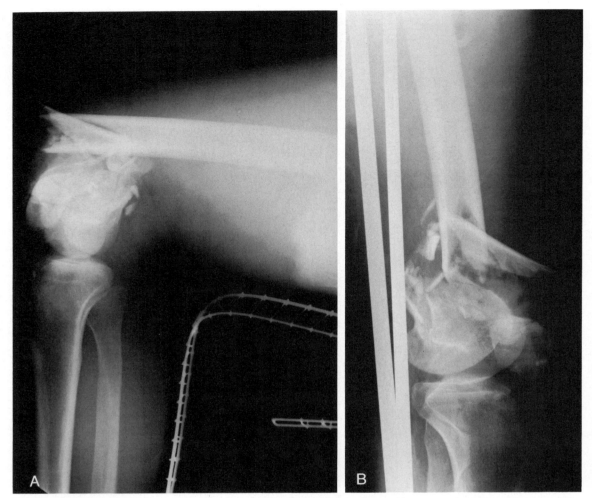

FIGURE 7–8. *(A)* Grade III, open type C3 supracondylar fracture of the femur. Note comminution and inappropriate splinting. *(B)* Lateral radiograph obtained after aligning of leg and splinting in extension.

shaft under appropriate tension. The plate is then secured with a provisional screw proximally. Correct alignment and reduction are confirmed at this time by anteroposterior and lateral radiographs. The iliac crest bone is then harvested, and the comminuted medial cortex is liberally grafted. Additional cancellous lag screws may be directed through the plate into the condyles as necessary. When a condylar buttress plate is used, it is often advantageous to slip the plate over appropriately placed condylar K-wires, where it can be best assessed for optimal placement before it is secured to the condyles with lag screws.

ASSOCIATED SOFT TISSUE INJURY

On occasion, the shaft or comminuted fragments are impaled through the iliotibial band or the quadriceps tendon; this necessitates small longitudinal incisions to free them. These injuries should be repaired with absorbable sutures after completion of internal fixation. The knee ligaments and menisci are usually spared. Any portions of the iliotibial band incised

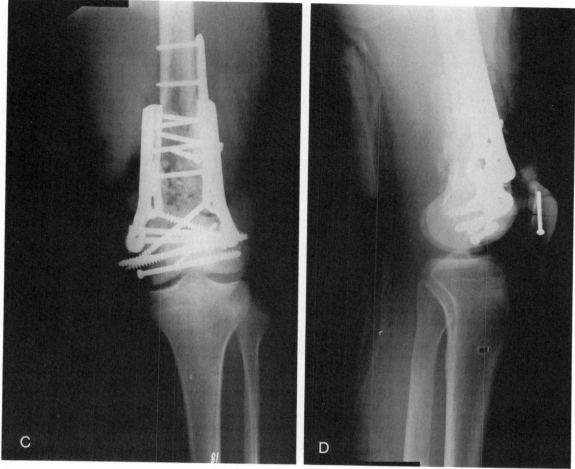

FIGURE 7–8. *Continued.* (C) Postoperative radiograph showing bicondylar fixation with Alta buttress plate. (D) Postoperative lateral radiograph of the same fracture. Note bone graft posteriorly and associated patellar fracture.

during exposure should be repaired. On infrequent occasions, the quadriceps mechanism is avulsed and must be securely reattached to the patella and the retinaculum. This poses significant problems for knee mobilization. With adequate repair, the knee can usually be placed in 30° or 40° of passive flexion without undue tension on the repair. Further flexion in a dynamically controlled orthosis can be attempted with caution over the next 6 weeks as soft tissue healing proceeds. The combination of quadriceps disruption and comminuted supracondylar fracture has a higher potential for disability because of loss of motion or residual quadriceps weakness.

If extensive soft tissue loss is encountered, muscle pedicle flaps, fasciocutaneous flaps, or local rotational flaps can be used. In rare instances in the knee region, there is extensive soft tissue loss, which results in wide exposure of the knee joint and requires a remote microvascular free flap. It is important to conduct these procedures without delay so that desiccation of bone or joint structures does not occur. If the orthopaedic surgeon is not experienced in these techniques, it is wise to obtain consultation with a plastic surgeon.

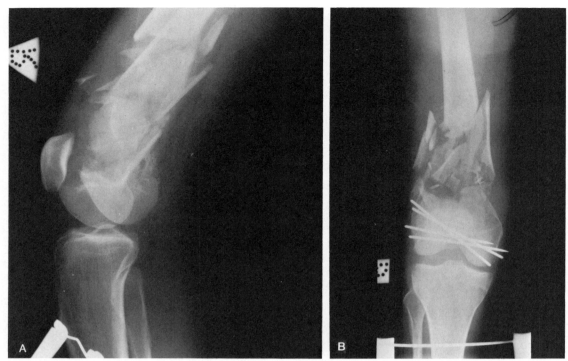

FIGURE 7–9. *(A)* Markedly comminuted grade I open supracondylar fracture of the femur. Note displaced coronal intra-articular fracture (type C3). *(B)* Anteroposterior postoperative view. Anatomic articular reconstruction was obtained and followed by balanced skeletal traction for 8 weeks and a cast-brace.

Fracture-Specific Treatment

A1 – A displaced fracture of the adductor tubercle and the origin of the medial collateral ligament can be secured after reduction by an appropriate-sized cancellous or malleolar screw and washer.[23] When the fragment is linear in nature or too small to accommodate a screw, staple fixation may be required. Undisplaced fractures can be treated with a knee immobilizer or an appropriate dynamic orthosis. In a preoperative physical examination, the likelihood for associated injury to the cruciate ligaments or the menisci should be assessed. These injuries can usually be addressed arthroscopically, often on a delayed basis. Preoperative magnetic resonance imaging (MRI), when available, can provide valuable information.

A2 – Transverse fractures at the proximal level can be satisfactorily treated with an interlocked, intramedullary rod (Fig. 7–8). Fixation of distal fragment requires two well-placed bicortical interlocking screws. If an interlocking rod is not available, transverse fractures at this level can also be treated with flexible intramedullary fixation (see Fig. 7–4). In order to insert the Ender rod in the medial femoral condyle from the supine position, the tail of the rod should be straightened, and the rod should be driven across the fracture site (directed laterally), rotated 180°, and seated in the subchondral bone of the medial femoral condyle. Two additional nonmodified C-shaped rods

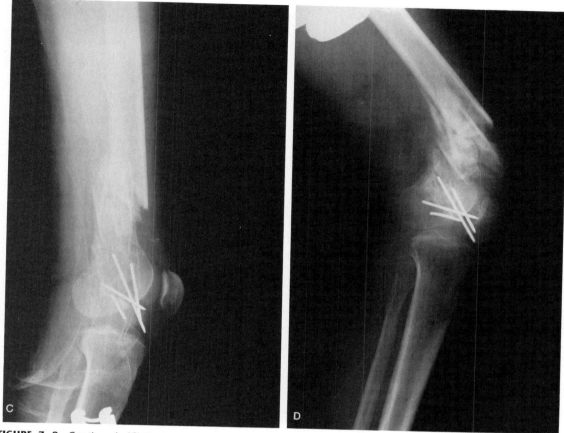

FIGURE 7–9. *Continued. (C)* Postoperative lateral radiograph in traction. *(D)* One-year postoperative radiograph showing malunion and posterior displacement of femoral condyles.

Illustration continued on following page

are then placed in the lateral femoral condyle. Elderly patients with a larger intramedullary canal may require additional flexible rods for providing stability.

A3 – Traditionally, the distal fracture was best fixed with a dynamic condylar screw or an angled blade plate. Because it is rendered stable by virtue of reduction, a condylar buttress plate could also be used, but it would be less secure. Certain distal A2 and A3 fractures may be amenable to interlocking intramedullary fixation. The advantage of the closed rodding technique is the avoidance of additional surgical trauma, diminished adhesions between the quadriceps mechanism and the fracture site, and more rapid healing. The disadvantage is less secure fixation and the possibility of loss of reduction with the early motion necessary for healing of the fracture.

A4 – In the comminuted supracondylar fracture, the articular surface is spared, but the fracture extends into the metaphyseal-diaphyseal junction. Fixation is accomplished with the dynamic condylar screw and the side plate (Fig. 7–9). Autogenous iliac crest bone grafting

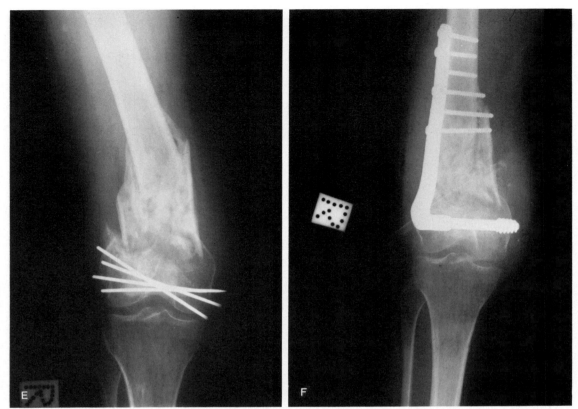

FIGURE 7–9. *Continued. (E)* Anteroposterior radiograph 1 year after operation showing valgus malunion. Note preservation of joint space. *(F)* Anteroposterior radiograph 1 year after injury and after corrective osteotomy and bone graft.

is performed in order to promote union of the comminuted medial cortex and diminish the likelihood of cyclic fatigue failure of the implant. With comminuted fractures, appropriate length must be restored. Excessive lengthening should also be avoided because it can result in significantly delayed healing and diminished knee motion secondary to quadriceps tensing and relative shortening. Length can best be assessed by palpating or visualizing the posterior cortex, which is often intact. With excessive comminution, the surgeon may have to rely on the tension in the quadriceps muscle. In anticipation of this problem with an extremely comminuted fracture, it is wise to have the opposite uninvolved extremity prepared and draped so that it can be used as a reference. Rotational alignment must also be ensured. On occasion, a narrow bridge plate may be necessary on the medial side in order to provide additional security and prevent late varus deformity.

B1 – Fracture of the lateral condyle is unicondylar, and a good buttress is obtained with lag screw fixation into the opposite condyle; large 6.5-mm cancellous screws and washers should be used. In healthy bone, this is all that is necessary. Older patients or osteoporotic bone may require a buttress plate. This may be a small dynamic

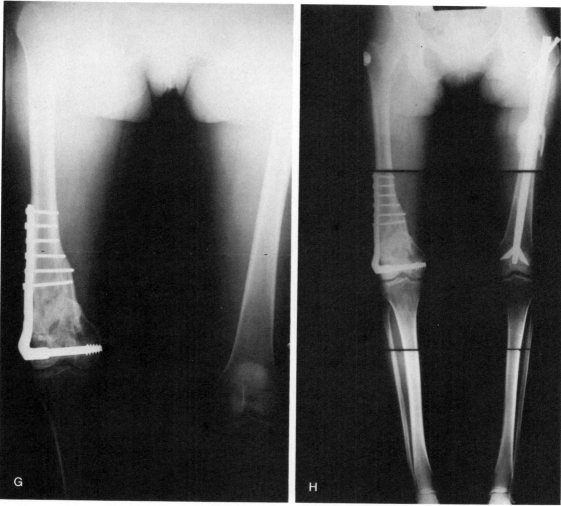

FIGURE 7–9. *Continued. (G)* Resultant union with 5.5 cm of shortening, but preservation of joint space and 0° to 100° range of motion. *(H)* Radiograph after equalization of leg lengths by closed femoral shortening of opposite femur. The ultimate result was satisfactory, with normal gait, 0° to 110° range of motion, and minimal symptoms secondary to patella baja. Lessons learned: (1) Articular reconstruction is mandatory. (2) Comminuted supracondylar fractures have a propensity to shorten. (3) A buttress plate could have been used effectively in this situation in conjunction with bone grafting. (4) Secondary reconstruction procedures (corrective osteotomy, leg length equalization) are capable of producing satisfactory results if articular integrity is preserved.

compression plate, a T-plate, or an Alta supracondylar buttress plate.

B2 – Proximal extension of a lateral condyle fracture requires more secure fixation. In addition to interfragmental screws, the long dynamic compression plate, or the Alta plate may be necessary if the weaker T-plate does not provide good fixation.

B3 – Coronal fracture of one or both condyles is referred to by the AO groups as the Hoffa fracture.[23] It usually involves the lateral condyle but can also involve the medial condyle. It should be fixed with 6.5-mm cancellous lag screws perpendicular to the fracture. The screws should be placed from anterior to posterior and should avoid the patellofemoral groove and the articular surface if possible. On occasion, a 4.0-mm cancellous screw can be inserted in the intercondylar notch in a non–weight-bearing portion of the articular surface. These screws should be countersunk well below the articular cartilage but should not be inserted so deeply that the subchondral purchase is weakened.

C1 – Supracondylar fracture with intercondylar extension, or the T-Y type (Fig. 7–10), is commonly the result of high-energy injuries and requires anatomic restoration of the articular surface followed by secure fixation of the condyles to the shaft so that early motion may be initiated. Temporary fixation is carried out with Kirschner wires that reduce the articular surface and fix the two condyles together. They are then secured with 6.5-mm cancellous screws. If the Kirschner wires are placed in optimal position, cancellous lag screws can be used to great advantage. The interfragmentary screws should be placed in such a fashion that they do not interfere with subsequent insertion of a blade plate or a DCS. A washer should be used for providing additional purchase in the relatively thin cortical bone of the condyle. A guide wire is then inserted in the lateral condyle 2 cm distal to the articular surface and in the approximate midpoint of the anterior half of the lateral femoral condyle. The appropriate

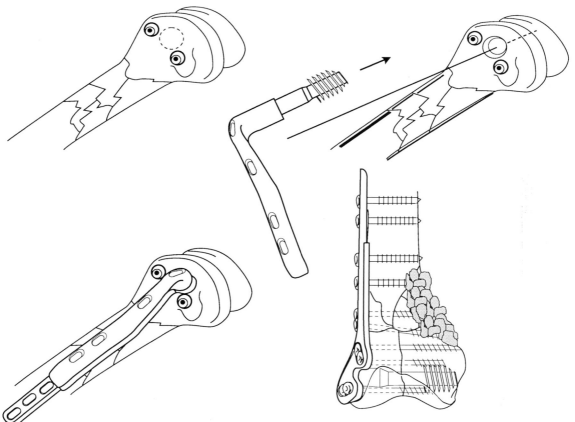

FIGURE 7–10. Alta supracondylar 95° plate.

site for placement is usually easily determined. It is important to ascertain that the guide pin is parallel to the joint line, and an image intensifier is helpful for confirming appropriate placement. The reamer is inserted over the guide pin, and the condyle is reamed to the appropriate depth, which is in the subchondral bone of the medial femoral condyle. The DCS is then inserted over the guide pin. Additional fixation is obtained by engaging the opposite cortex without excessive penetration, which can often be determined by palpation. This fracture is relatively stable once it is secured.

C2 – For bicondylar fracture with comminution of the distal shaft, fixation proceeds as for the C1 fracture but may be more difficult because of excessive comminution (Fig. 7–11). It is important to ascertain that appropriate length and rotational alignment have been obtained before the plate is secured to the side plate, as in the comminuted A3 type fractures. Fixation is then carried out as described for the C1 fracture, with the addition of liberal cancellous bone graft to the comminuted medial surface.

C3 – This fracture is the most challenging and represents comminution of the femoral condylar articular surface in more than one plane

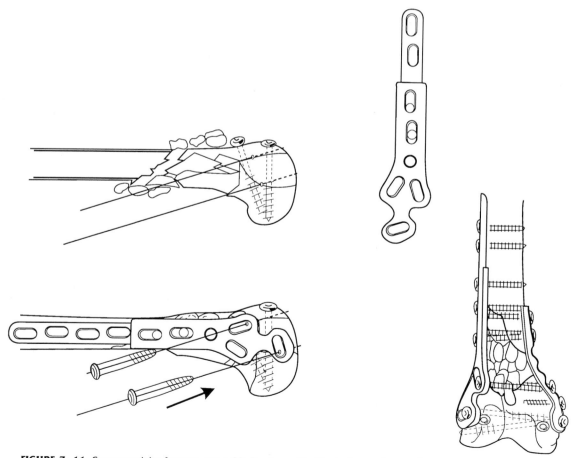

FIGURE 7–11. Supracondylar fracture, type C3. Fixation with Alta buttress plate and small medial bridge plate.

(Fig. 7–12; see also Fig. 7–2). Usually there is a tangential fracture that runs obliquely in the coronal plane, necessitating the insertion of screws in an anterior-to-posterior direction. This precludes or renders difficult the insertion of the 95° condylar plate or screw. In this situation, stabilization must be achieved with the buttress plate. Bone grafting of the comminuted medial cortex should be accomplished. On occasion, a second narrow bridge plate anchored with two screws proximally and distally is necessary for increasing stability and preventing a tendency toward varus drift. If more secure fixation is deemed advisable, substantial bicondylar fixation may be necessary. The C3 fracture is a high-energy injury with much articular damage and a greater propensity for delayed union, late varus drift, and loss of knee motion. Because the articular damage is usually more extensive than in other fractures, there is a higher incidence of posttraumatic arthritis as well. For an acceptable degree of motion to be obtained, fixation should be secure enough to begin immediate continuous passive motion (CPM) exercises followed by graduated range-of-motion exercises, as described previously.

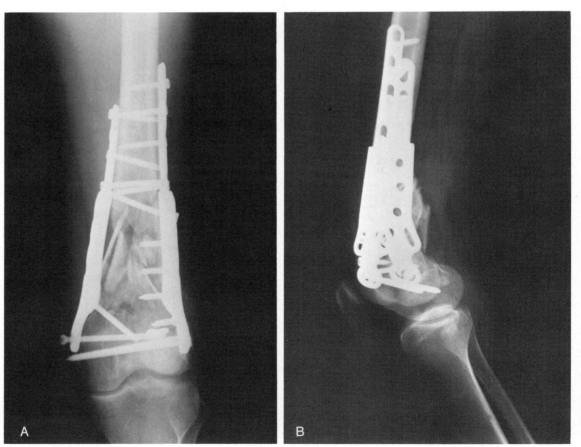

FIGURE 7–12. (A) Postoperative anteroposterior radiograph of comminuted type C3 supracondylar fracture of the femur. (B) Postoperative lateral radiograph of the same fracture. The ultimate result was poor because of failure to mobilize early and poor compliance despite anatomic articular reconstruction.

Postoperative Care

The single most important aspect of postoperative care is the prompt institution of early motion. CPM exercises are begun followed by actively assisted motion and active range-of-motion exercises progressively as permitted by other injuries, degree of local swelling, and soft tissue trauma. As a general rule, CPM exercises can be started within the first 24 to 48 hours postoperatively from a range of 0° to 30° of flexion and progresses to 90° of flexion over the next 7 to 10 days, as tolerated. Usually within the first week the patient can begin some general active-assist exercises and by the time of discharge should be able to raise the leg straight satisfactorily and should initiate active motion. This can be done in a dynamic orthosis such as a Bledsoe brace. CPM can be continued on an intermittent basis while the patient is an outpatient over the next several weeks. If this modality is not available, the knee should be initially supported in 60° to 90° of flexion as is comfortable for the patient postoperatively, and gentle passive and active range-of-motion exercises should be performed several times a day by the nursing staff or the physical therapist. Early on, the patient should actively participate in rehabilitation, which must be ongoing and progressive in terms of strengthening and range of motion over the first several months. Failure to mobilize the surgically stabilized knee results in more loss of motion and more stiffness than does nonoperative treatment.[5, 6, 21, 22, 26, 35] Careful scrutiny of the papers in which authors retrospectively compared operative and nonoperative treatment, with a preference for the latter, reveals that inadequate fixation and failure to mobilize were often important determinents of outcome.[24, 35]

Suction drainage should be used for the first 24 to 48 hours postoperatively. When the tourniquet has not been used, hemostasis is usually more secure, and less postoperative bleeding and swelling are noted. If CPM exercises are undertaken, bandages should not be tight and sterile strips should not be used, because the combination of swelling and motion may cause blistering of the skin. As soon as the wound has healed and seepage has stopped, it may be left open. If there are no other contraindicating injuries, progressive ambulation may begin within the first few days, with only light touchdown weight bearing. Weight bearing should be restricted for a minimum of 10 to 12 weeks in cases of comminuted fractures.[6, 21, 25, 30] In the stable pattern, such as A2 and C1 fractures, partial weight bearing may begin earlier. After fracture healing, any residual muscle weakness or atrophy should be vigorously treated with muscle-strengthening exercises. Significant residual loss of knee motion may in rare instances require gentle manipulation while the patient is under anesthesia or arthroscopic lysis of adhesions. On occasion, dynamic corrective splinting (Dyna splint) may be helpful.

Complications and Evaluation of Results

Early complications include wound hematoma, infection, and postoperative peroneal nerve palsy. Arterial injury accompanying the fracture is less common than might be expected. Open type C3 fractures often dictate above-knee amputation. Compartmental syndrome in the calf is uncommon but should be diagnosed and treated promptly by fasciotomy. In the presence of early infection, the indications are irrigation and debridement, antibiotic-impregnated beads, suction irrigation systems, or a combination of these. Intravenous antibiotics specific for the offending organisms are administered and continued until the infection is quiescent. Such quiescence is determined mainly on clinical grounds and is characterized by absence of drainage, of erythema, and of induration. It usually coincides with the return of the erythrocyte sedimentation rate to normal. It is essential that stable internal fixation be retained, although late infection and chronic or focal osteomyelitis often requires removal of hardware for eradication. The incidence of infection is low after closed fractures (3 to 5 per cent) but increases significantly with open fractures of high grade.

Deep venous thrombosis is common after any type of extremity surgery, and the incidence has been estimated to be as high as 50 per cent. Propagation of a calf thrombus into the thigh or the pelvic system is potentially lethal, and prophylactic regiments therefore must be instituted in all patients undergoing major surgery about the knee. Early mobilization, the use of sequential compression stockings, low doses of sodium warfarin (Coumadin), or other accepted prophylactic regimes are mandatory. When these precautions are followed, fatal pulmonary embolus is uncommon.

The most common late complications have to do with residual fracture deformity (see Fig. 7–2). In rare instances, reflex sympathic dystrophy may occur. Valgus deformity is generally well tolerated if it does not exceed 12° to 14° and is unassociated with shortening or malrotation. Varus angulation of any degree is undesirable and often results in symptomatic degenerative joint disease. This may necessitate a corrective osteotomy or total knee replacement in the appropriate age group.

In general, results are satisfactory if the fracture has healed in normal alignment with a functional range of motion and is nonpainful. Most supracondylar fractures are healed by 12 to 16 weeks, although it may be difficult to ascertain the degree of healing in fractures that have been rigidly fixed surgically. Fractures with no evidence of healing at this point may be classified as delayed union, and beyond 6 months, as frank nonunion. Repeat bone grafting or electrical stimulation or both may be necessary in order to achieve union. Knee motion should also have essentially returned by the time of fracture healing, although small increases in flexion or in terminal extension may be gained for as long as a year or so after injury.

A number of criteria have been suggested for evaluation. The scale devised by Neer and associates accounts for both subjective and objective aspects.[26] Schatzker and colleagues established a similar system for analyzing five separate variables and that lends itself well to evaluation and comparison of results (Table 7–1).[32] Few long-term studies have been published, and a biologic price will likely be exacted for many of the more severe intra-articular fractures at some future point. Nevertheless, by accurately restoring the anatomic structure and initiating motion, the surgeon provides the optimal potential for recovery.

TABLE 7–1. Functional Evaluation (Worst Measurement Is Determinant of Result)

Parameter	Score*
Motion	
Flexion	
>125° (Able to squat and perform all activities of daily living) (ADL)	3
110° to 124° (Able to tie shoes)	2
100° to 109° (Can sit and climb stairs)	1
<100° (Has difficulty with sitting and ADL)	0
Extension	
0°	3
<5°	2
6° to 10°	1
>10°	0
Pain	
No pain	3
Occasional or weather pain or both	2
Pain with fatigue	1
Constant pain	0
Deformity	
Angulation	
0°	3
<10°	2
>10°, <15°	1
>15°	0
Shortening (cm)	
0	3
<1.5	2
>1.5, <2.5	1
>2.5	0
Ambulation	
Walking	
Unrestricted	3
>30 minutes, <60 minutes	2
<30 minutes	1
Home ambulation, wheelchair, or bedridden	0
Stairs	
No limitation	3
Holds rail	2
One at a time	1
Elevator only	0
Return to Work	
Employed Before Injury	
Returned to preinjury job	3
Returned to preinjury job with difficulty	2
Altered full-time job	1
Part-time or unemployed	0
Retired Before Injury	
Returned to preinjury lifestyle	3
Needs occasional help with shopping/laundry	2
Needs assistance at home for ADL	1
Moved in with family/nursing home	0

From Schatzker J, Lambert L: Supracondylar fractures of the femur. Clin Orthop 138:77–83, 1979.
*3, excellent; 2, good; 1, poor; 0, failure.

Caveats

1. Consider alternative treatment for patients with multiple medical complications, nonambulatory patients, and patients with advanced osteoporosis.

2. Preoperative planning includes careful assessment of patients for associated injury, neurovascular compromise, or unrecognized medical problems. Review radiographs carefully, plan sequential surgical steps, and ensure that medical equipment and personnel are available.

3. Avoid use of tourniquets, excessive stripping, prolonged muscle retraction, and desiccation of bone and soft tissues.

4. Bone graft comminuted fractures.

5. Comminuted fractures requiring buttress plates are prone to develop varus drift unless supported with a medial bridge plate or a well-fitting dynamic orthosis preventing varus, or both.

6. Mobilize fractures early, using CPM and aggressively progressing to actively assisted and active-motion exercises.

TIBIAL PLATEAU FRACTURES

Fractures that extend into the proximal tibial weight-bearing articular surface are known as tibial plateau fractures. The caveats just discussed regarding supracondylar fractures of the femur apply equally to fractures of the tibial articular surface. Conservative treatment consisting of traction, manipulation of the fracture, and ligamentotaxis has been advocated by J. J. Fahey, Hohl and Luck, Apley, and others.[1, 9, 14] When a fracture was reducible by strong traction and manipulation, patients were treated with cast immobilization for several weeks until early consolidation would permit a graduated range of motion exercises. For extremely comminuted fractures of the proximal tibia that were deemed to be unsuitable for this method and nonfixable by operation, traction through a distal tibial pin and early passive motion was used to restore alignment and help the condylar fragments mold themselves to "acceptable position."[1, 28] Historically, early attempts to fix the articular surfaces operatively were met with varying degrees of success primarily because of the limited surgical experience and the unavailability of appropriate instruments and implants. Displaced fractures of the tibial plateau are now treated operatively by methods for restoring anatomic structure, bone grafting subarticular defects, and rigidly internal fixation of displaced articular fractures.[4, 15, 32] The AO group has developed a classification, a surgical methodology, and an implantation technology that have resulted in greatly improved outcomes for these fractures.[23]

Tibial plateau fractures can be categorized in two general groups. Low-energy fractures occur in osteoporotic bone as a result of falls or relatively trivial injury. Higher energy injuries occur in younger patients often as a result of motor vehicle accidents or pedestrian injuries in which other fractures or systemic injuries have been sustained. In general, the lower energy injuries tend to involve the lateral tibial plateau and are less likely to be severely displaced, and thus they have a relatively favorable prognosis.[2, 8, 27] In addition, should reconstruction ultimately be necessary, patients with these injuries are often in the age bracket in which total knee arthroplasty can be performed predictably. In contradistinction, the high-energy injuries occurring in younger patients are often more severe injuries that mandate open reduction and internal fixation when the bones are displaced.

When a medial tibial plateau or a bicondylar injury is present, the prognosis is less favorable. Like the supracondylar fracture, these fractures also must be securely stabilized so that motion can be initiated early.[23] It is essential that open fractures of the proximal tibia be stabilized internally whenever possible.[4, 32] If the soft tissue injury is too severe or the possibility of infection is high, external fixation can be used (Fig. 7–13). This usually necessitates bridging the knee joint. In general, fractures of the tibial plateau and the proximal tibia heal relatively rapidly, and so partial weight bearing can usually be started 8 to 10 weeks after injury. The ultimate prognosis is dependent on the severity of the articular damage and the individual deformity. Therefore, therapeutic efforts must address appropriate means for restoring anatomic structure and maximal functional potential.

Clinical Evaluation

The causes of these injuries have been discussed earlier. The mechanism of injury is usually axial impaction accompanied by a valgus, or occasionally a varus, stress on the semiflexed knee. Severe injuries are caused by direct trauma and along with comminution and displacement may be associated with significant soft tissue trauma.

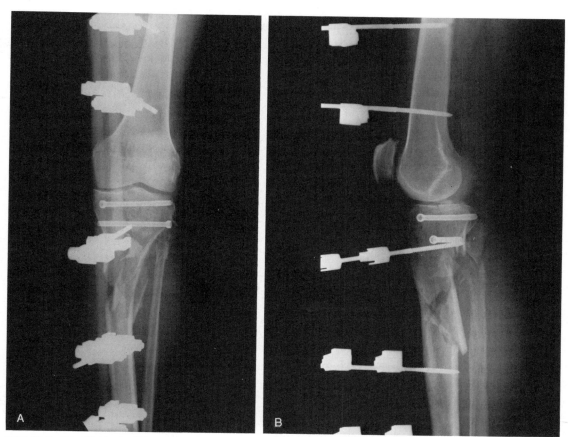

FIGURE 7–13. *(A)* Grade IIIB open degloving injury. Intra-articular fracture of the proximal tibia with diaphyseal extension. Treatment with cannulated screws for articular portion and external fixation across the knee. *(B)* Lateral view of open proximal tibial fracture.

The typical findings are swelling, tenderness, deformity, and inability to bear weight. In the initial assessment, any break in skin, presence of an open fracture, or neurovascular injury should be noted carefully. Gentle stress testing of the knee is performed with the leg in extension in order to evaluate stability of the medial ligamentous restraints as well as the propensity for fracture displacement. Until definitive treatment is initiated, the patient should be placed in a comfortably padded posterior splint. In contradistinction to supracondylar fractures of the femur, for which routine radiographs are usually sufficient, computed tomographic (CT) evaluation or anteroposterior and lateral tomography are often helpful in assessment of tibial plateau fractures. Routine radiographs frequently do not show fully the actual extent of articular depression in apparently minimally displaced fractures. It is often surprising to see the extent of depression when anteroposterior and lateral tomography are used. CT evaluation has added another dimension to the investigation of these fractures but does not offer any distinct advantage over tomography and is considerably more expensive (Fig. 7–14).

The information obtained from these studies determines the necessity

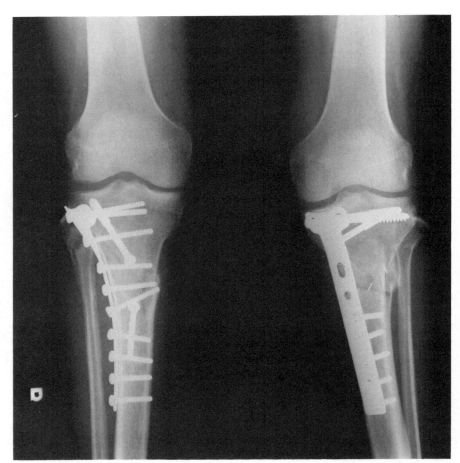

FIGURE 7–14. Bilateral proximal tibial fractures. Medial T-plate used for bicondylar fracture of the left proximal tibia with associated popliteal artery disruption. Successful arterial repair and ultimate healing bilaterally with excellent range of motion. Several screw heads eroded through the skin over the medial subcutaneous plate. Fortunately, no infection ensued.

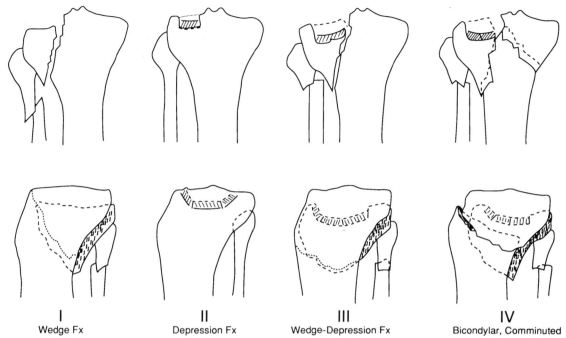

I
Wedge Fx

II
Depression Fx

III
Wedge-Depression Fx

IV
Bicondylar, Comminuted

FIGURE 7–15. Classification of tibial plateau fractures. (Redrawn from Müller ME, Allgower M, Scneider R, Willenegger H: Manual of Internal Fixation, 2nd ed. New York: Springer, 1979.)

for and the type of operative treatment. Severely displaced bicondylar or medial condylar fractures of the proximal tibia may be associated with neurovascular injury, and they should be investigated promptly with arteriograms (Fig. 7–15). Once a decision has been made to operate, the procedure should be undertaken as soon as possible.

Classification

The AO classification for tibial plateau fractures is as shown in Figure 7–16. This classification is succinct and clearly defines the major differentiating features and appropriately directs treatment accordingly. It is being revised to conform with a universal system of classification.

Nonoperative Treatment

Nonoperative treatment is appropriate for undisplaced fractures and may consist of a cast followed by a cast-brace or a dynamic orthosis as healing progresses over 4 to 6 weeks.[2, 28] Weight bearing should be restricted in all cases of articular fractures until fracture consolidation is well under way. For wedge, compression, and wedge-compression fractures of the tibial plateau with minimal displacement, closed reduction with traction and manipulation may be attempted.[8, 9] The articular surface can be somewhat difficult to evaluate on the image intensifier. If adequate reduction is obtained, the patient can be immobilized in a well-fitting long-leg cast, which can be converted to a cast-brace or an orthosis. For

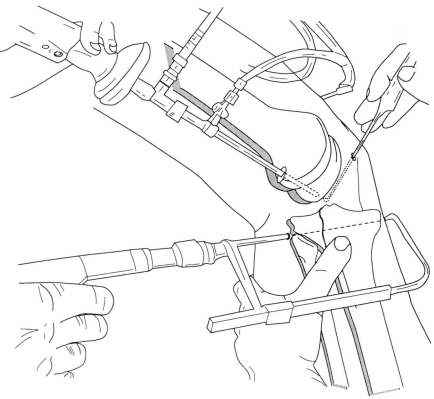

FIGURE 7–16. Arthroscopic assisted reduction of tibial plateau fracture: fixation with cannulated screws.

severely comminuted fractures not deemed fixable, traction by means of a distal tibial pin can be instituted for 4 to 6 weeks, during which time the patient uses a sling to passively flex the knee and mold the articular surface.[1] Satisfactory results with this method can be obtained if articular integrity is reasonably restored and if angulatory deformity is not present.[4, 33, 34] Varus angulation of any degree is undesirable, whereas up to 10° to 12° of valgus angulation is compatible with a satisfactory result. Knee stiffness can be avoided or minimized by early institution of motion. Comparative studies have shown that nonoperative treatment produces better results than does nonrigid internal fixation followed by failure to mobilize the knee.[11, 18, 32]

Operative Treatment

The indication for operative treatment is articular displacement of more than 5 mm in an active patient with normal bone. This is only a guideline inasmuch as injuries of lesser degrees of displacement or nondisplaced fractures "at risk" in active people are occasionally amenable to closed reduction and percutaneous screw fixation. In elderly or marginally ambulatory patients, more depression of the lateral condyle in the absence of valgus instability is acceptable. Ipsilateral femoral fractures, or so-called floating knee injuries, require fixation of both fractures.

Fixation begins with the most unstable lesion, which is usually the femoral fracture. Operative treatment of specific fracture types proceeds as described earlier and basically follows the AO principles, which have been well established and used in trauma centers for many years. The tenets of this philosophy have withstood the test of time; however, there have been some subtle changes emphasizing the biologic processes of fracture healing and the importance of atraumatic surgery. This has led to the more restrictive use of metal implants, especially in subcutaneous locations in which a small external fixator or a narrow bridge plate can be substituted (called biologic fixation). In addition, the use of fluoroscopically guided cannulated screws inserted percutaneously and arthroscopically assisted reduction of articular fractures provide an atraumatic way to treat amenable fractures (Fig. 7–17). When this method is extended to

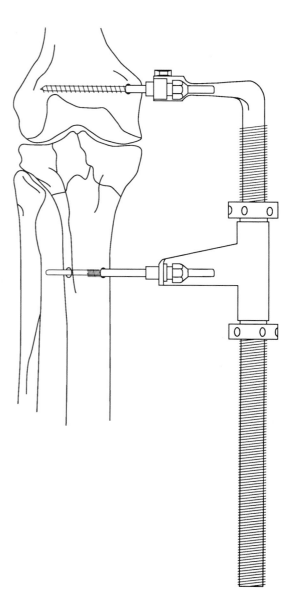

FIGURE 7–17. Reduction with use of a distractor. Good exposure is provided, but flexion of the knee and maneuverability are limited. Avoid axial malalignment when using. (Redrawn from Mast J, Jakob R, Ganz R, Willenegger H: Planning and Reduction Technique in Fracture Surgery. New York: Springer Verlag, 1989.)

grades II and III fractures, bone grafting can be accomplished through a limited exposure of the subcondylar cortex.

SURGICAL EXPOSURE

A straight anterolateral incision of sufficient length to provide exposure of the joint is used for fractures involving the lateral plateau. In medial plateau fractures or in extensive bicondylar injuries, a straight midline or medial patellar incision is used. In this instance, it may be necessary to perform Z-plasty of the patellar tendon in order to reflect the extensor mechanism proximally and thereby widely expose the proximal tibial articular surface. It is important to keep the incisions close to the midline so that subsequent reconstructive surgery is not compromised. In addition, should a plate be necessary on the proximal subcutaneous border, it will not come to lie directly under the suture line.

With incisions of sufficient length and flexion of the knee, posterior aspects of the condyles can be reached for manipulation and reduction. These fragments can be secured with lag screws directed posteriorly. A distractor can be used to facilitate exposure (Fig. 7–18). However, it limits knee flexion and is somewhat awkward to work around. When this device is used, axial malalignment should be avoided.

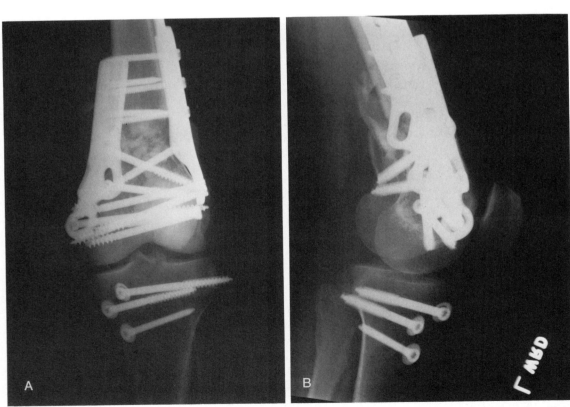

FIGURE 7–18. *(A)* Wedge fracture of the proximal tibia, type 1: fixation with cancellous lag screws and washer. Note bicondylar fixation of supracondylar femur fracture with Alta buttress plates. *(B)* Lateral radiograph of same fracture. Note good articular restoration on both views.

Fracture-Specific Treatment

TYPE I. Type I fractures can often be treated by closed techniques if an anatomic reduction can be obtained. The patient is placed on the fracture table, and an appropriate amount of traction is applied. Manual pressure, varus stress, and reduction tenaculums are all useful in obtaining a reduction. This fracture is amenable to arthroscopic treatment, but this method is more invasive, is likely to be more time consuming, and is no more accurate than fluoroscopy, on which the displaced cortical spike and split fragment provide excellent clues as to the adequacy of reduction. If closed reduction is successful, percutaneous or cannulated screws are inserted.

Open treatment involves exposure of the joint as described previously, inspection or removal of small osteochondral fragments in the joint, and anatomic reduction and internal fixation of the split fragment. This may be accomplished with cancellous screws (Fig. 7–19), including an apex screw and washer or, when additional security is required, L- or T-shaped buttress. The L-shaped plate fits nicely on the lateral condyle in most instances.

TYPE II. Depression of the articular portion of the tibial plateau requires

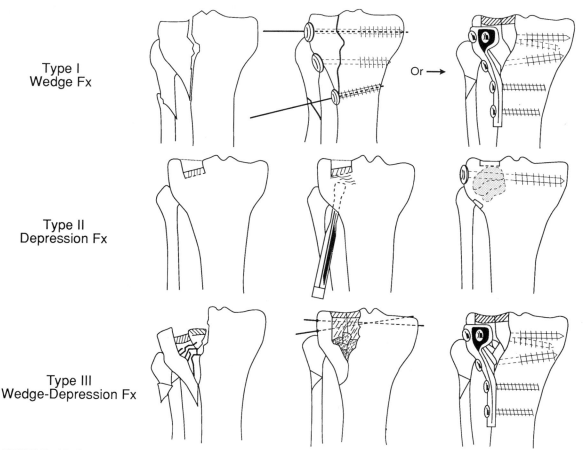

FIGURE 7–19. Operative treatment of tibial plateau fractures, types I, II, and III. (Redrawn from Müller ME, Allgower M, Schneider R, Willenegger H: Manual of Internal Fixation, 2nd ed. New York: Springer, 1979.)

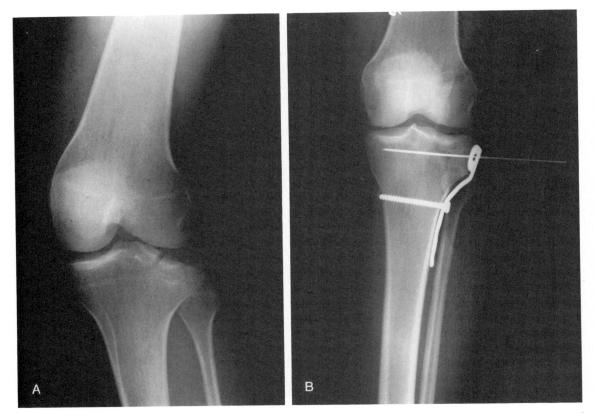

FIGURE 7–20. *(A)* Wedge-depression type fracture of lateral tibial plateau. Note valgus instability. *(B)* Provisional fixation after elevation and bone graft of subarticular defect.

elevation, bone grafting, and rigid internal fixation and buttressing (Fig. 7–20). Alternatively, arthroscopic-percutaneous techniques may be used effectively with lesser degrees of depression and comminution. It is likely that small depressions can be elevated and held up with 6.5-mm screws alone, but any sizable depression leaves a large subarticular defect after elevation, and this defect is best packed tightly with cancellous bone graft.

On some occasions, cortical cancellous graft is more advantageous and provides better support. After exposure of the joint, the first step is careful lavage and inspection of the joint. The meniscus is usually spared. The graft can be incised at the coronary ligament and reflected upward with the femoral condyle. It can be transected near the attachment of the anterior horn but is more difficult to repair with this method and usually does not provide any more advantage in terms of exposure. In order to elevate the depressed portions of the lateral tibial plateau, a fenestration should be made 2 to 3 cm below the articular surface in the anterolateral cortex below the defect.

It is very important to carefully tease the depressed fragments up en masse. Smaller instruments are more likely to abruptly penetrate the joint. Usually this can be accomplished without difficulty, but with extreme comminution, gentle arranging of the fragments without disturbing the depression mass itself is necessary. On occasion, the depressed fragments can be gently molded into place against the femoral condyle. The de-

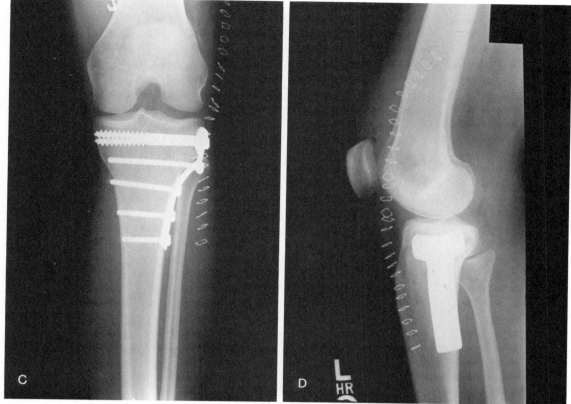

FIGURE 7–20. *Continued. (C)* Postoperative anteroposterior view showing final internal fixation and anatomic restoration of the joint. *(D)* Lateral radiograph of same fracture.

pressed portion should be brought up at least to the articular level or overreduced by a few millimeters because there some settling will occur. Transcondylar K-wires are then inserted transversely from lateral to medial in the subcondylar bone. The exact positioning of the wires is usually obvious but can be verified by image intensifier. When optimal position has been obtained, the L-plate can be slipped over the Kirschner wires and assessed along the lateral cortex (Fig. 7–21).

Usually some minor amount of modification of the plate is necessary for ensuring a snug fit. The surgeon should avoid overbending the plate so that the distal portion does not snugly appose the cortical bone of the shaft. In this instance, as the distal screws are tightened, proximal fixation and reduction may be lost. Once adequate reduction and positioning of the plate has been ensured, 6.5-mm cancellous screws are used in the metaphyseal portion, and 4.5-mm bicortical screws in the distal portion secure the plate to the shaft. The tourniquet should be released as soon as the fracture is internally fixed, and hemostasis should be obtained before closure. Clinical alignment is usually fairly easy to assess but should be confirmed by long anteroposterior and lateral standard radiographs obtained in the operating room before closure. The image intensifier has a narrow field that is usually satisfactory for evaluating the articular surface but does not give adequate information regarding alignment.

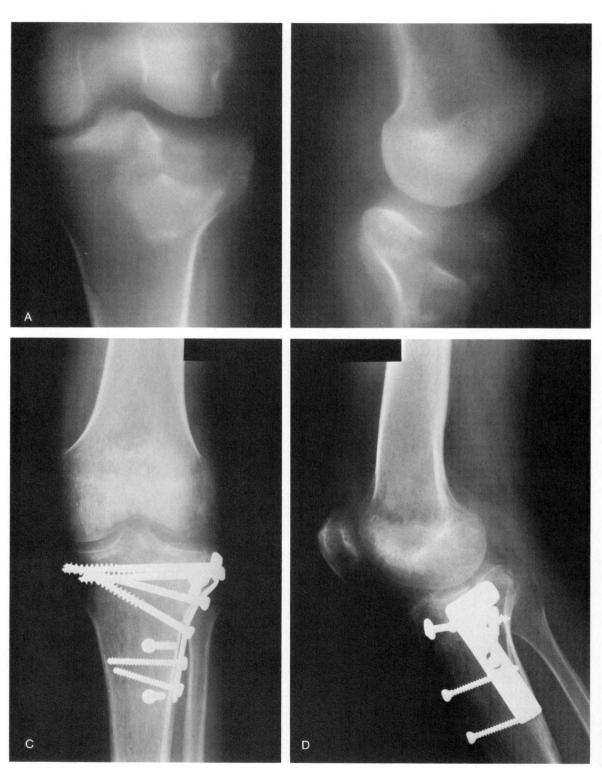

FIGURE 7–21. *(A)* Anteroposterior tomogram of bicondylar proximal tibial fracture with severe depression and comminution of lateral plateau. *(B)* Lateral tomogram of same fracture. *(C)* Postoperative anteroposterior radiograph showing provisional fixation and joint restoration. *(D)* Lateral radiograph of same fracture.

TYPE III. This fracture is a combination joint depression and wedge-type fracture. Treatment is with open reduction, elevation of depressed fragments, subarticular bone graft, and rigid internal fixation with inter-fragmentary screws and a buttress plate. The medial collateral ligament occasionally may be torn but generally is stretched or held intact by descent of the lateral condyle and deformation of the tibial plateau. Also, in rare instances, the meniscus may be caught or trapped in the fracture, but usually it descends or is retained with the wedge fragment. Taking advantage of the wedge, the surgeon opens it to gain access to the depressed articular fragments, which are again elevated en masse and supported with tightly packed cancellous bone graft. Internal fixation then proceeds as described earlier.

After completion of internal fixation, the meniscus is resutured to the coronary ligament or bone with heavy absorbable sutures, and if necessary, the medial ligament is repaired. The need for ligamentous repair is determined by the degree of instability after fracture fixation.

TYPE IV. This is a high-energy injury and results in bicondylar fracture with varying degrees of displacement and soft tissue injury (Figs. 7–22, 7–23). If displacement is extreme, neurovascular damage can accompany this fracture. A fracture of the medial plateau often includes the intercondylar eminence or a portion of it and is usually noncomminuted. In extremely displaced or complex fractures, a midline incision with Z-plasty of the patellar tendon that reflects the extensor mechanism proximally

Type IV - Bicondylar Fracture

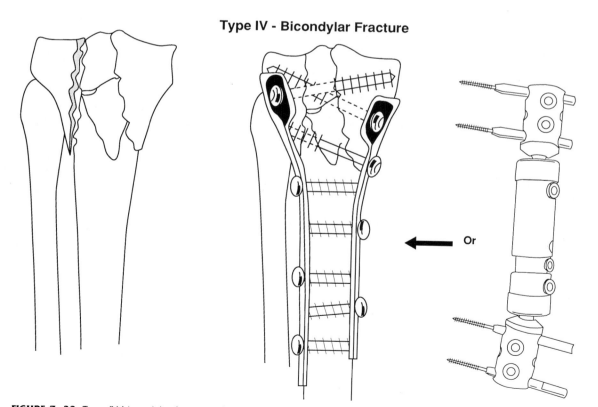

Or

FIGURE 7–22. Type IV bicondylar fracture of the proximal tibia: operative treatment. Medial plate should be used with caution. An external fixator may be substituted.

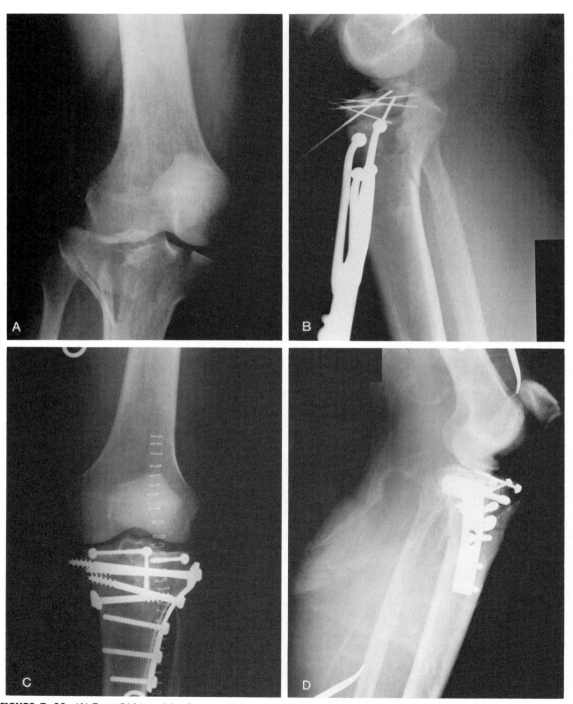

FIGURE 7–23. *(A)* Type IV bicondylar fracture dislocation of the knee. *(B)* Interoperative lateral radiograph showing K-wire fixation of articular surface and intercondylar eminence. *(C)* Postoperative radiograph showing final fixation and satisfactory restoration of joint congruency. *(D)* Lateral radiograph before reattachment of patellar tendon.

provides the wide exposure necessary.[4, 32] Very often the tibial tubercle is in close juxtaposition and, therefore, cannot safely be osteotomized.

Although bicondylar plate fixation provides secure fixation, it does so at a distinct biologic price secondary to the extensive stripping of the bone of the proximal tibia. In addition, should skin slough occur over the subcutaneous plate, a very serious situation ensues, with significant potential for infection, delayed union, and secondary loss of fixation. A medial gastrocnemius muscle flap should be performed to cover the exposed bone and plate in this case.

Whenever possible, the medial plateau should be secured by noninvasive interfragmentary fixation or a small external fixator, which achieves good purchase in the subcondylar bone proximally and the intact shaft distally. An associated arterial injury should be repaired before fracture stabilization, which then usually can be carried out without danger to the anastomosis if excessive traction or tension on the vascular repair does not occur. The usual wide vascular exposure posteriomedially provides ample access to the medial plateau, but the temptation to place a large subcutaneous plate in this location should be avoided if the fracture can be secured medially with less invasive methods.

The general principles of surgery are the same as described previously, with elevation of the pressed articular fragments, bone grafting, and secure internal fixation. In general, the prognosis is not quite as good as in types 1, 2, and 3 fractures, and the incidence of complications are higher.

FRACTURES WITH DIAPHYSEAL EXTENSION

Comminuted fractures of the articular surface of the proximal tibia that extend into the diaphysis are some of the most challenging injuries to be encountered (Fig. 7–24).[4, 32] Unfortunately, this combination presents the dual problems of difficult union associated with diaphyseal fractures and the necessity for articular reconstruction of the plateau and the requisite early motion. Unless the shaft fracture lines are incomplete and can be easily stabilized with interfragmentary screws, this fracture pattern is extremely unstable.

In order to provide rigid enough fixation to begin motion and prevent angulation or skin problems, a 3.5-mm or a 4.5-mm dynamic compression plate must be used along the lateral diaphysis, extending well onto the metaphyseal flair. The plate acts as a secure buttress for the interfragmentary fixation of the diaphyseal fragments. Usually this results in an anatomic reduction of the shaft. The incision often must be extended to the distal third of the tibia and should be over the anterolateral portion of the calf, avoiding the crest and subcutaneous medial border. It is difficult to mold the large dynamic compression plate to the contour of both shaft and condylar regions. In this situation, the L- or T-plate can be fitted over the dynamic compression plate and molded appropriately to the contour of the condylar surface proximally. A good fit is necessary for avoiding displacement of the fracture as the screws are tightened. Because of the instability involved, the diaphysis often must be stabilized first.

This fracture can present formidable technical problems. If surgery cannot be performed safely, it may be best to fix the condyles in a limited fashion and to treat the diaphyseal fracture with an external fixator. This

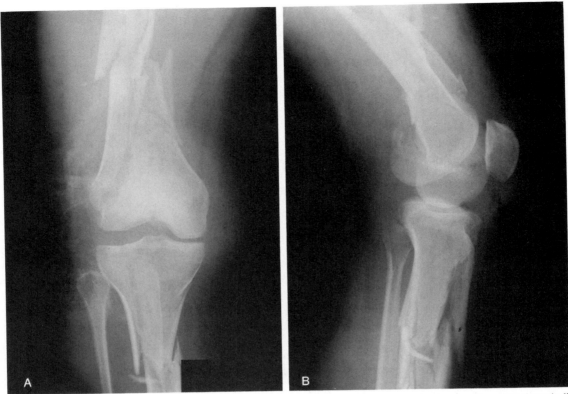

FIGURE 7–24. *(A)* Comminuted intra-articular fracture of proximal tibia with diaphyseal extension. Associated grade III open supracondylar fracture ("floating knee"). *(B)* Lateral radiograph of same fracture.

method may be followed by conversion to a cast-brace at the appropriate time. On occasion, the surgeon may have to resort to traction treatment.

Postoperative Care

Prophylaxis for deep venous thrombosis is instituted. Drains are removed at 24 hours, and CPM exercises are begun. Usually full extension to 90° can be achieved within the first postoperative week. On occasion, because of swelling or excessive bleeding, modification or reduction in progression may be necessary. Alternatively, passive motion as well as actively assisted range-of-motion exercises can be instituted under the guidance of the physical therapist or the nursing staff.

Quadriceps muscle exercises and straight-leg raising are begun immediately, and the patient is taught to participate in a progressive rehabilitation program. Comminuted or bicondylar fractures with less secure fixation require a dynamic orthosis that allows controlled flexion and extension. The patient should be mobilized rapidly and allowed ambulation with touchdown weight bearing on the involved side. Partial weight bearing may begin at the eighth to tenth week of treatment, depending on fracture characteristics; however, full weight bearing is prohibited for 12 weeks. With a thorough understanding of the rehabilitation goals, the patient is discharged, and progress is monitored clinically and radiographically as appropriate.

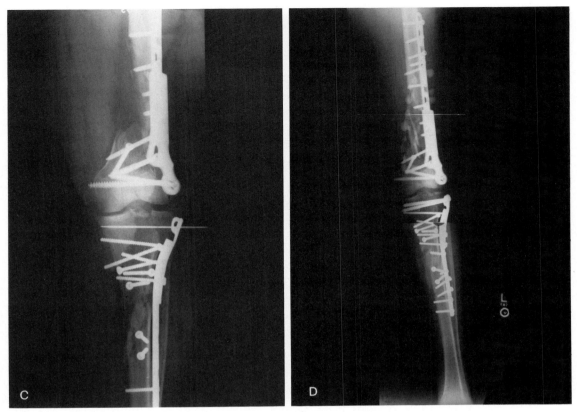

FIGURE 7–24. *Continued. (C)* Provisional fixation. Note condylar T-plate placed over tibial dynamic compression plate. Provisional Alta buttress plate and modular extension used for supracondylar fracture. Note missing bone. *(D)* Final fixation of both fractures. Note bone grafting of supracondylar femur fracture and prophylactic antibiotic impregnated beads.

Illustration continued on following page

Complications

Early complications include neurovascular injury, skin slough, and infection. All of these generally are avoidable by careful atraumatic technique, appropriately placed incisions, and internal fixation screws. Tourniquet time should be kept to a minimum. In most cases, fracture reduction and internal fixation are accomplished at least provisionally by 1 hour. The tounniquet is released at that time. Absolute hemostasis can be ensured as the soft tissues are repaired and the wound carefully is closed over a drain. Early infection is treated by irrigation and debridement in addition to intravenous antibiotics. Late infection often requires the removal of metal implants.

Loss of fixation usually occurs late in treatment and often indicates that there is a problem with healing or that initial fixation was inadequate. Fixation is occasionally lost early because of additional injury secondary to fall or to premature weight bearing. In these instances, it should be promptly reapplied. In late loss of fixation or metal failure, the risks of reoperation may have to be weighed against the benefits of allowing for consolidation and delayed reconstruction. Reflex sympathetic dystrophy is uncommon and can be prevented by early mobilization, which is also

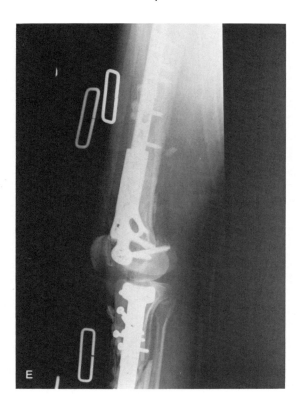

FIGURE 7–24. *(E)* Lateral radiograph of same fracture.

effective in diminishing the incidence of deep venous thrombosis and pulmonary embolism.

Residual knee stiffness and decreased range of motion are more easily prevented than treated. Vigorous range-of-motion exercises, occasional manipulation while the patient is under anesthesia, or the application of dynamic splints in order to regain terminal extension may be useful. Excessive residual deformity can be treated with subcondylar osteotomy. Patellofemoral symptoms can be bothersome. In rare instances, with excessive valgus angulation, lateral subluxation of the patella may require surgical treatment. With extensive degenerative changes, total knee arthroplasty is a sound and satisfactory method of relieving pain. Knee fusion is not often indicated and is less likely to be accepted by younger patients. Nevertheless, it remains a viable alternative in selective cases of young patients with destroyed joints and severe pain.

Conclusions and Evaluation of Results

Several grading systems exist for evaluation of results. The system of Hohl and Luck (Table 7–2), with various modifications or additions, has been used by many authors to evaluate results of tibial plateau fractures.[14] In most published series, authors report good results in 75 to 85 per cent of patients. These series include studies that encompassed a variety of treatment modalities as well as those treated exclusively by either surgical or nonoperative methods. Although it is difficult to analyze objectively all of the variables involved in comparative studies, several important common factors emerge. As might be expected, nondisplaced or minimally

TABLE 7–2. Criteria of Grading

Anatomic Grade	
Excellent (all of the following)	Not more than 5° increased valgus angulation; restoration of displacement within 3 mm; no degenerative joint changes
Good (not more than one of the following)	5° to 10° increased valgus angulation; minimal degenerative joint changes
Fair (not more than two of the following)	More than 10° increased valgus angulation; moderate degenerative joint changes; lack of fracture reduction; loss of physiologic valgus angulation
Poor (all of the following)	More than 10° increased valgus angulation; moderate and severe degenerative joint changes; lack of fracture reduction; any valgus angulation
Functional Grade	
Excellent (all of the following)	Full extension of the knee; 120° range of motion or more; no abnormal abduction rocking; normal strength and endurance; occasional ache permissible
Good (not more than one of the following)	Lack of knee extension beyond 170°; excessive lateral mobility; mild aching each day; 90° total range of motion; weakness or easy fatigue
Fair (not more than one of the following)	Lack of knee extension beyond 170°; 75° range of motion; discomfort for ordinary activity; excessive lateral mobility
Poor (any of the following)	Severe pain; instability and giving way; motion arc <75°

From Hohl M, Luck JV: Fractures of the tibial condyle; clinical and experimental study. J Bone Joint Surg 38A:1001–1018, 1956.

displaced fractures heal well regardless of the type of treatment. Also, lateral-sided injuries have a significantly better prognosis than do medial injuries because valgus deformity is better tolerated than varus deformity and lateral compartment degenerative changes are slow to evolve.

Fractures associated with suboptimal or poor results are comminuted, displaced, and usually involving both condyles or the medial plateau. An important determinant of the outcome is the extent of soft tissue injury and instability. Blokker and collaborators found that the most important prognostic indicator was adequacy of reduction regardless of the means of achieving it.[2]

Finally, as mentioned earlier, tibial plateau fractures, like supracondylar fractures of the femur, must be mobilized early after surgical stabilization. Failure to do so results in loss of motion and suboptimal results.

FRACTURES OF THE PATELLA

Fractures of the patella are not uncommon injuries that occur by one of two mechanisms.[4] Direct trauma is the usual cause, often the result of high-energy motor vehicle accidents. These injuries are frequently comminuted or stellate in nature and may be associated with soft tissue injury or associated ipsilateral fractures. The fracture fragments are usually not widely separated as the retinaculum is intact. It is less common for the patella to fracture during the act of falling or stumbling, in which case the strong pull of the quadriceps mechanism tears the retinaculum, which results in a transverse fracture of the patella with wide separation of the fragments. Regardless of the mechanism of injury, the treatment goals are restoration of articular congruency and preservation of quadriceps muscle integrity.[4, 23, 28]

Diagnosis

Diagnosis is usually not difficult; the characteristics are pain, swelling, and difficulty or inability to extend the knee. Palpation may reveal crepitus or wide separation of the fracture fragments. Small abrasions are common when the injury is a result of a direct blow, and on occasion a frank open fracture is present. There may be associated injuries or fractures of the ipsilateral extremity that should be stabilized simultaneously. Standard radiographic views reveal the patella fracture in a vast majority of cases. If the history is suggestive of patellar dislocation with spontaneous reduction, a sunrise view is helpful for ruling out osteochondral fracture of the medial facet or the lateral femoral condyle. This view is not routinely necessary and has the potential for fracture displacement.

Classification

Patellar fractures may be classified as transverse, polar, comminuted, or longitudinal. Longitudinal fractures are uncommon, are usually minimally displaced, and require operative treatment less frequently. Osteochondral fractures usually occur in adolescents often as isolated injuries, in contradistinction to such fractures adults, in whom there often exist other associated pathologic processes.

Patellofemoral Biomechanics

Historically there has been some controversy over the contribution and the importance of the patella and the consequences of excision. Hey Groves and Watson-Jones believed that the patella inhibited quadriceps action and that extensor function was satisfactory after patellectomy.[17, 38] Brooke showed experimentally that following patellectomy there was an increase in the speed of knee extension lending credence to this point of view. In addition, West, Boucher, and Geckeler and Quaranta demonstrated good quadriceps function in the majority of patients undergoing patellectomy.[12, 38]

In contradistinction, DePalma and Flynn, Smillie, McKeever and others believed that the patella was an essential and important component of the knee extensor mechanism.[7, 16] This viewpoint is supported by the experimental work of Kaufer and Haxton and also by the clinical studies of Lieb, Perry, and others.[16, 17, 19] Kaufer demonstrated a progressively increasing contribution of the patella to the quadriceps moment arm as the knee moved into full extension. The patella is an important link in the quadriceps mechanism, providing continuity between the quadriceps muscle above and the patellar ligament below. In addition, it functions as a fulcrum, producing significant anterior displacement of the patellar tendon with progressive knee extension. Patellar contact pressures increase with knee flexion. Thus it is not surprising that varying degrees of quadriceps atrophy, loss of strength, and symptoms of weakness or instability are common after excision of the patella. Range of motion is affected little, and cosmetic deformity is usually insignificant.

Nonoperative Treatment

Nonoperative treatment is indicated for undisplaced fractures or for fractures with less than 2 mm of articular displacement. A cylinder or long leg cast is applied with the knee in 0° to 15° of flexion. Straight-leg raising exercises should be initiated as soon as the patient is comfortable, and full weight bearing is allowed as tolerated. Immobilization is continued for approximately 4 to 6 weeks, at which time the cast is removed and progressive range-of-motion exercises are begun. The knee needs to be protected against sudden flexion forces until full range of motion is obtained and healing is complete. In selected instances, a dynamic orthosis may be used to provide additional security after cast removal.

Surgical Treatment

Whenever possible, the articular surface of displaced patella fractures should be restored. This is accomplished without difficulty in transverse fractures and in fractures with minimal small fragment comminution. Comminuted fractures are more difficult to treat but are usually amenable to cerclage wiring or modifications of interfragmental fixation and wiring techniques.[23, 37]

A transverse or vertical incision may be used. The vertical incision provides good exposure of the knee, is extensile, and simplifies subsequent reconstructive surgery should it be necessary. The fracture is readily encountered, and in cases in which the retinaculum is torn, the joint is widely exposed. Usually there is no damage to the subjacent articular cartilage of the femoral condyles or other structures of the knee. After irrigation of the knee and removal of the small detached loose fragments, the surgical treatment is dictated by the injury pattern and is described for specific fractures as follows.

TRANSVERSE FRACTURES

The patellar fragments are reduced through the use of tenaculum forceps. If the retinaculum is torn, the articular surface can be visualized or inspected digitally. If the retinaculum is not torn, a small accessory parapatellar incision is made for inspection. The fracture is then internally fixed with either interfragmentary lag screws or AO tension band techniques. Excellent results are possible with both methods (Fig. 7–25). The use of cancellous lag screws provides interfragmentary compression and is in harmony with contemporary concepts of fracture treatment. The additional security of a figure-eight tension band may be provided by placing the wire around the screws. This necessitates their exiting the superior pole by 3 or 4 mm, so that satisfactory purchase for the figure-eight tension band is obtained.

In the AO method, parallel Kirschner wires are inserted from the proximal pole of the reduced fracture and exit inferiorally. The patella can be predrilled if desired in order to enable smooth passage of the wires and subsequent ease of seating them in the proximal pole. The Kirschner wires should be slightly above the midcoronal plane of the patella so that an anterior tension band is created. A No. 18 gauge wire is then placed close to the bone under the Kirschner wires and tightened. A small loop

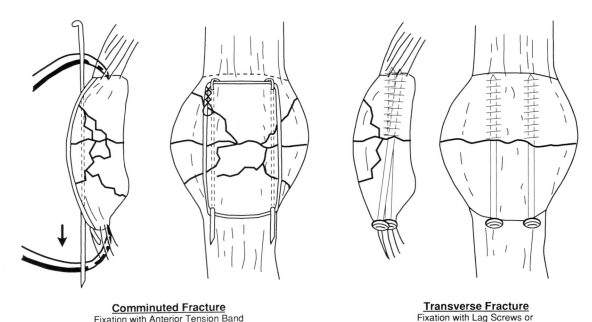

Comminuted Fracture
Fixation with Anterior Tension Band

Transverse Fracture
Fixation with Lag Screws or
Figure-8 Tension Band

FIGURE 7–25. Patellar fractures. (Redrawn from Müller ME, Allgower M, Schneider R, Willenegger H: Manual of Internal Fixation, 2nd ed. New York: Springer, 1979.)

can be placed in the tension band before it is passed around the Kirschner wires. This allows an additional locus for evenly tightening the tension band. The Kirschner wires are then bent 180° proximally, and the short hook formed is seated in the superior patellar fragment and buried in the quadriceps insertion. The distal 1 cm of the Kirschner wires is then bent down into the patellar tendon. A No. 14 or No. 16 gauge needle can be inserted transversely at the superior and inferior poles of the patella in order to ensure that the wire passes close to the bone and to avoid excessive kinking. Either circumferential or figure-eight wiring can be used. The figure-eight wiring technique provides a more stable configuration. (Fig. 7–26). With this technique, the patellar fragments are loaded in compression with knee flexion.

POLAR FRACTURES

DISTAL POLE. Distal pole fractures are common and usually have some degree of comminution. If a sizable fragment remains, it can be secured with a 4.0-mm cancellous screw and washer in association with tension band wiring, as described earlier (Fig. 7–27). Whenever possible, the fragments of the inferior pole should be retained because bone-to-bone healing is more secure than ligament-to-bone healing. The distal pole occasionally contains no salvageable patellar fragments, and in this case, direct suturing of the patellar tendon to the remaining proximal portion of the patella is performed. It has classically been advised that this be done by approximating the tendon to the articular surface.[10, 29] However, cadaver studies have shown that approximation of the tendon

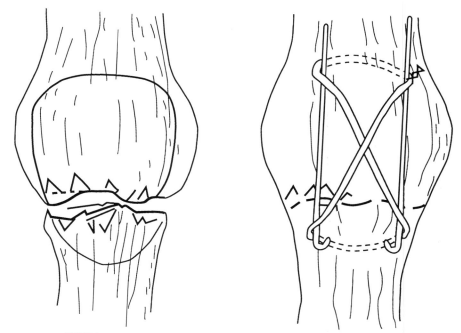

FIGURE 7–26. Distal pole fracture of the patella: tension band fixation.

to the dorsal surface is more physiologic and does not result in excessive tilting of the proximal fragment if at least 50 per cent of the patella remains.[36]

It is likely that the surgical technique and quality of retinacular repair are more important than the site of approximation (Fig. 7–28). Heavy,

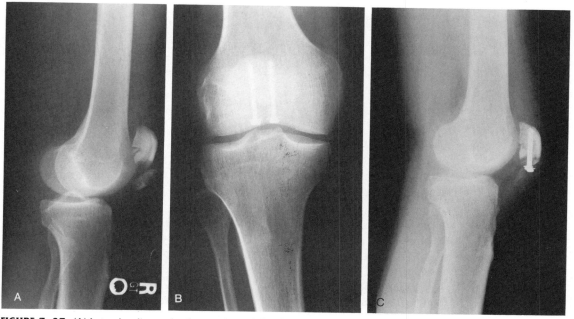

FIGURE 7–27. (A) Lateral radiograph of comminuted distal pole patellar fracture. (B) Repair of distal pole fracture with Lag screws and washer. (C) Lateral view of same fracture.

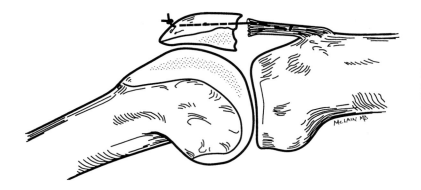

FIGURE 7–28. Comminuted distal pole patellar fracture: Excision of fragments and suturing of patellar tendon to proximal fragment.

absorbable polyglactin 910 (Vicryl) sutures are weaved through the patellar tendon in Bunnell fashion and inserted through secure drill holes entering the fracture near its midcoronal plane and exiting the proximal patella dorsally. Usually three or four separate pairs of sutures in the tendon are pulled through drill holes in the patella and then tied over the dorsal bony bridge. For any retinacular tears, the surgeon should preplace sutures that are progressively tied in figure-eight fashion from the periphery to the midline; the patellar tendon sutures are usually tied last. In good retinacular repair, the central patellar tendon anastomosis is secure. Nonabsorbable sutures, such as Tevdek, can be used if preferred.

PROXIMAL POLE. Proximal fractures are less common but are treated in a fashion similar to that described for distal pole fractures. Often less bone is involved, and treatment is essentially the same as for quadriceps rupture, ensuring that the central rectus tendon is anchored to bone and that the quadriceps expansion is sutured into the retinaculum securely. After repair of polar fractures, immobilization in extension is indicated for the first 10 to 14 days, after which the sutures are removed and the swelling has receded. At this point, with cooperative patients, gentle passive range-of-motion exercises may be begun, but they are best done in a protective fashion with the use of a dynamic orthosis when flexion can be controlled. If the security of repair is in doubt, immobilization in a cylinder or a long leg cast for 4 to 6 weeks is indicated.

COMMINUTED FRACTURES

Comminuted fractures of the patella are more challenging, but often reasonably good reduction is obtained with the use of cerclage wire and tension band techniques as described earlier. On occasion, a dual-tension band technique can be used with an initial figure-eight configuration through the patella tendon and quadriceps tendon. This wire is tightened while digital palpation of the articular surface guides the fragments into a reasonable order. Kirschner wires are then placed through the assembled fragments in the best mechanical position, and a second cerclage wire is passed beneath them, as described earlier. This procedure carries a higher possibility of postoperative discomfort secondary to prominent fixation unless careful technique is used. Nevertheless, as demonstrated by Pauwels many years ago, it is possible to treat extensively comminuted fractures with resultant satisfactory outcomes. Thus indiscriminate patellectomy for comminuted fractures should be avoided.

Numerous studies have shown that total patellectomy is associated with a higher incidence of knee dysfunction and a higher percentage of fair or poor results after patella fracture.[7, 16, 17] However, this procedure is no doubt performed for the more severe injuries for which fracture fixation is not possible. A significant portion of the extensor mechanism is disrupted when the patella is removed, and therefore surgical repair and reconstruction of the remaining ligament, the retinaculum, and the quadriceps tendon must be performed carefully. If this is not done, extensor lag and significant weakness will be evident.[19] It has been the author's experience that if these problems have been avoided, properly performed patellectomy leads to a good range of motion and a satisfactory result.

Postoperative Care

At the completion of surgery, the tourniquet should be released and hemostasis ensured. Use of a suction drain for 24 hours is recommended. Initial immobilization is in a removable posterior splint or a knee immobilizer until swelling has receded and sutures have been removed. The timing of mobilization is dependent on the type of fracture and repair. As noted in the discussion of specific fracture treatment, it is desirable to initiate motion early in treatment whenever possible. Transverse fractures and those securely fixed with an interfragmentary screw or a tension band are ideal for this method. Straight-leg raising and isometric quadriceps exercises are initiated 24 to 38 hours after treatment begins. Controlled passive range-of-motion exercises through a 30° to 60° arc, followed by actively assisted exercises then follows. A dynamic orthosis, such as a Bledsoe brace that controls the amount of flexion and extension, is often of benefit. CPM can be used but is not often necessary for isolated patella fractures. If the repair is less secure, immobilization in a cylinder or a long leg cast for 4 to 6 weeks is indicated. Comminuted fractures and tendon-to-bone repair should be mobilized more cautiously. After patellectomy, controlled mobilization can be initiated in 3 to 4 weeks but should be advanced gradually.

Complications

Infection is uncommon after operative treatment of closed patellar fractures, but it is a serious complication. It is treated in the usual fashion with irrigation, debridement, and antibiotics. Arthroscopic irrigation and debridement are also effective and less traumatic than is open treatment. Stable internal fixation should not be removed in these instances. Loss of fixation early in treatment may be treated by reoperation. Loss that occurs late in treatment is best accepted and may necessitate eventual patellectomy.

Nonunion of patellar fractures is distinctly unusual but has been reported to occur in a small percentage of patients. Some elongation and minor degrees of displacement are not uncommon, especially in comminuted fractures. Avascular necrosis of the proximal pole may occur because the main nutrient arteries arise from branches of the geniculate vessels in the region of the inferior pole and near the midpatellar region.[31] The appearance of a radiographically dense proximal pole does not necessarily signify a failure or indicate that irreversible avascular necrosis has occurred. Long-term follow-up may reveal variable posttraumatic radiographic changes involving the patellofemoral joint or either compartment of the knee in approximately one third of patients.[29] Such changes do not preclude a satisfactory outcome.

Prognosis

The prognosis is good even in the presence of significant comminution. Most investigators have reported good results in approximately 80 per cent of patients. The remaining 20 per cent have varying symptoms related primarily to pain. This pain is increased with activities that require repetitive extension and full flexion of the knee. Results are more favorable for less comminuted fracture patterns and for patients who achieve full or nearly normal return of motion and strength. Quadriceps muscle function is somewhat slow to return, and rehabilitation may take 8 to 10 months or longer. As noted earlier, some permanent quadriceps atrophy and weakness may remain. Patients with significant pain and articular incongruity may eventually require patellectomy. In general, good results closely follow accurate reduction.

FRACTURES OF THE INTERCONDYLAR EMINENCE OF THE TIBIA

These injuries are more common in children and adolescents.[20, 28, 39] The mechanism of injury in these patients is often relatively low-energy torsional forces acting on the flexed knee. In this respect, it is not dissimilar from the mechanism that causes disruption of the anterior cruciate ligament in older patients and adults. Before skeletal maturation, the surface of the intercondylar eminence is largely cartilaginous. The bone is weaker than the ligament in children in comparison with adults, and thus the fracture is more commonly seen in children as an isolated injury.

In contradistinction, fractures of the intercondylar eminence in adults are frequently the results of high-energy injuries often caused by motor vehicle accidents. In this context they can be associated with other fractures or major ligamentous disruption, or both, about the knee (see Fig. 7–23). In fractures of the medial tibial plateau, a portion or all of the intercondylar eminence is often destroyed. There may be other systemic injuries and associated fractures characteristic of multitrauma. In these instances, the priority for treatment is secondary to stabilization of long-bone fractures and major weight-bearing intra-articular fractures. Often the displacement is not significant enough in these cases to warrant operative treatment except in conjunction with an associated injury pattern.

Clinical Evaluation

A significant hemarthrosis is usually present. The knee is held in flexion and is swollen and tender to palpation. Attempted movement is painful; however, careful examination can usually be performed without too much difficulty and, in the isolated injury, often reveals no associated instability patterns. As noted earlier, this injury in the adult often accompanies other fractures or systemic trauma and may be associated with severe ligamentous injury or knee dislocation. In the latter instance, an arteriogram should be obtained in order to rule out intimal arterial injury despite the presence of peripheral pulsations.

Routine radiographs are often sufficient to make the diagnosis; the lateral view is the most revealing. CT evaluation is helpful for accurately assessing the extent of the fracture or associated fractures of the tibial plateau. MRI evaluation shows the associated soft tissue injury quite well, but it is more often indicated in the isolated injury or at the time of reconstruction in the previously multitraumatized patient. Tomograms also help delineate the extent of the lesion, and in this regard, the lateral views are the most useful. These studies need not be conducted for undisplaced fractures or for fractures obviously displaced enough to require operative treatment.

Classification

Intercondylar eminence fractures were first classified by Meyers and McKeever.[20] The following is a modification of this classification, which accounts for the rare fracture of the posterior intercondylar region and adjacent posterior tibia (type 4) to include the origin of the posterior cruciate ligament (Fig. 7–29). This fragment may be sizable and should be replaced through a posterior or posteromedial incision when significantly displaced (Fig. 7–30).

Treatment

In Meyers and McKeever's series, more than 50 per cent of these injuries occurred in children; about 80 per cent were classified as type I or II injuries responding to closed treatment and cast immobilization.[20] Therefore, in these fractures the joint should be aspirated if a tense hemarthrosis is present, and the patient is placed in a knee immobilizer that can be converted to a cylinder or a long leg cast when swelling has receded. Recommended positioning is 10° to 20° of flexion. Immobilization is continued for 6 to 8 weeks. Prognosis is good for isolated injuries occurring in children but is less favorable in adults for the reasons noted earlier.

Type III injuries—that is, significantly displaced fractures—should be treated by operative reduction and stabilization. Many of these fractures lend themselves well to arthroscopically assisted reduction and stabilization through techniques similar to those for meniscal repair. Absorbable sutures such as Vicryl can be passed through the fragment and secured to the adjacent meniscal insertions unless involved with the fragment. K-wire fixation[39] or pull-out techniques have also been successful; however, the growth plate should be avoided in the treatment of children with this lesion. Once the fragment is reduced and appropriately immobilized, no significant dynamic forces are sufficient to cause displacement. Elaborate fixation systems are not necessary.

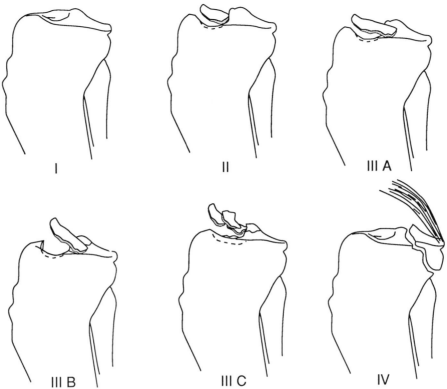

FIGURE 7–29. Classification of intercondylar eminence fractures.

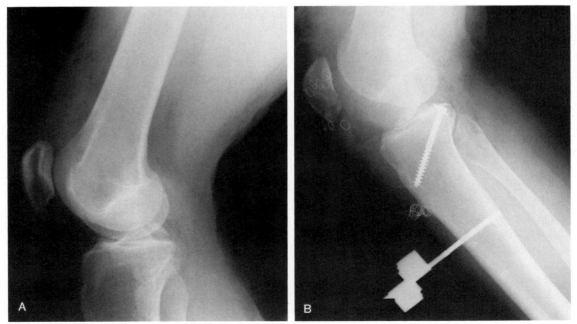

FIGURE 7–30. *(A)* Displaced intra-articular fracture posterior intercondylar eminence. Associated open tibial fracture treated with external fixator. *(B)* Lateral radiograph of the knee after open reduction and internal fixation. Fragment included the entire origin of the posterior cruciate ligament.

Postoperative Care and Prognosis

After operative repair, immobilization in a cylinder cast as in undisplaced fractures is undertaken. Healing is quite rapid through the cancellous bed of the fragment. Prognosis is very good after operative treatment of isolated injuries. If there are associated fractures or other major ligamentous injuries, the prognosis is significantly less favorable and is often more dependent on the treatment and resolution of the associated pathologic process. On occasion, un-united fragments may become symptomatic or form loose bodies, which require excision.

REFERENCES

1. Apley AG: Fractures of the lateral tibial condyle treated by skeletal traction and early mobilization: a review of sixty cases with special reference to the long-term results. J Bone Joint Surg 38B(3):699–708, 1956.
2. Blokker CP, Rorabeck CH, Bourne RB: Tibial plateau fractures: an analysis of the results of treatment in 60 patients. Clin Orthop. 162:193–199, 1984.
3. Brown A, D'Arcy JC: Internal fixation for supracondylar fractures of the femur in the elderly patient. J Bone Joint Surg 53B(3):420–424, 1971.
4. Chapman MW, Madison M (eds): Operative Orthopaedics, vol. 1. Philadelphia: JB Lippincott, 1988.
5. Chiron HS, Tremoulet J, Casey P, Muller M: Fractures of the distal third of the femur treated by internal fixation. Clin. Orthop 100:160–170, 1974.
6. Connolly JF, Dehne E, LaFollette B: Closed reduction and early cast-brace ambulation in the treatment of femoral fractures. J Bone Joint Surg 55A:1581–1599, 1973.
7. DePalma AF, Flynn JJ: Joint changes following experimental partial and total patellectomy. J Bone Joint Surg 40A(2):395–413, 1958.
8. Dovy H, Heerfordt J: Tibial condyle fractures: a Follow-up of 200 cases. Acta Chir Scand 137:521–531, 1971.
9. Drennan DB, Locher FG, Maylahn DJ: Fractures of the tibial plateau: treatment by closed reduction and spica cast. J Bone Joint Surg 61A(7):989–995, 1979.
10. Duthie HL, Hutchinson JR: The results of partial and total excision of the patella. J Bone Joint Surg 40B(1):75–81, 1958.
11. Gausewitz S, Hoh M: The significance of early motion in the treatment of tibial plateau fractures. Clin Orthop 202:135–138, 1986.
12. Geckeler EO, Quaranta AV: Patellectomy for degenerative arthritis of the knee: late results. J Bone Joint Surg 44A(6):1109–1114, 1962.
13. Giles JB, DeLee JC, Heckman JD, Keever JE: Supracondylar-intracondylar fractures of the femur treated with a supracondylar plate and lag screw. J Bone Joint Surg 64A:864–870, 1982.
14. Hohl M, Luck JV: Fractures of the tibial condyle: a clinical and experimental study. J Bone Joint Surg 38A(5):1001–1018, 1956.
15. Jensen D, Rude C, Duus B, Bjerg-Nielsen A: Tibial plateau fractures: a comparison of conservative and surgical treatment. J Bone Joint Surg 72B(1):49–52, 1990.
16. Kaufer H: Mechanical function of the patella. J Bone Joint Surg 53A(8):1551–1560, 1971.
17. Kaufer H: Patellar biomechanics. Clin Orthop 144:51–54, 1979.
18. Lansinger O, Bergman B, Korner L, Andersson GBJ: Tibial condylar fractures: a twenty-year follow-up. J Bone Joint Surg 68A(1):13–19, 1986.
19. Lieb FJ, Perry J: Quadriceps function. J Bone Joint Surg 50A(8):1535–1548, 1968.
20. Meyers MH, McKeever FM: Fracture of the intercondylar eminence of the tibia. J Bone Joint Surg 41A(2):209, 1959.
21. Mize RD, Bucholz RW, Grogan DP: Surgical treatment of displaced, comminuted fractures of the distal end of the femur. J Bone Joint Surg 64A:871–879, 1982.
22. Mooney V, Nickel VL, Harvey JP Jr, Snelson R: Cast-brace treatment for fractures of the distal part of the femur: a prospective controlled study of one hundred and fifty patients. J Bone Joint Surg 52A:1563–1578, 1970.
23. Muller ME, Allgower M, Willenegger H: The Manual of Internal Fixation, 2nd ed. New York: Springer-Verlag, 1979.
24. Neer CS, Grantham SA, Shelton ML: Supracondylar fracture of the adult femur: a study of one hundred and ten cases. J Bone Joint Surg 49A:591–613, 1967.
25. Olerud S: Operative treatment of supracondylar-condylar fractures of the femur: technique and results in fifteen cases. J Bone Joint Surg 54A:1015–1032, 1972.

26. Pettine KA: Supracondylar fractures of the femur: long-term follow-up of closed versus non-rigid internal fixation. Contemp Ortho 21:253–261, 1990.
27. Roberts JM: Fractures of the condyles of the tibia: an anatomical and clinical end-results study of one hundred cases. J Bone Joint Surg 50A(8):1515–1521, 1968.
28. Rockwood CA, Green DP (eds): Fractures, vols 1, 2. Philadelphia, J.B. Lippincott, 1975.
29. Saltzman CL, Goulet JA, McClellan RT, et al: Results of treatment of displaced patellar fractures by partial patellectomy. J Bone Joint Surg 72A:1279–1285, 1990.
30. Sanders R, Regazzoni P, Ruedi T: Treatment of supracondylar-intracondylar fractures of the femur using the dynamic condylar screw. J Orthop Trauma, 3:214–222, 1989.
31. Scapinelli R: Blood supply of the human patella: its relation to ischaemic necrosis after fracture. J Bone Joint Surg 49B(3):563–570, 1967.
32. Schatzker J, McBroom R, Bruce D: The tibial plateau fracture: the Toronto experience 1968–1975. Clin Orthop 136:94–104, 1979.
33. Shybut GT, Spiegel PG: Tibial plateau fractures. Clin Orthop 138:12–16, 1979.
34. Spiegel PG: Distal tibial intra-articular fractures. Clin Orthop 138:17, 1979.
35. Stewart MJ, Sisk TD, Wallace SL Jr: Fracture of the distal third of the femur: a comparison of methods of treatment. J Bone Joint Surg 48A:784–807, 1966.
36. Swanson TV, Marder RA, Duwelius PJ, Sharkey NA: Patellofemoral contact pressures: effects of partial patellectomy and patellar tendon reattachment. In press.
37. Weber JJ, Janecki CJ, McLeod P, et al: Efficacy of various forms of fixation of transverse fractures of the patella. J Bone Joint Surg 62A:215–220, 1980.
38. West FE: End results of patellectomy. J Bone Joint Surg 44A(6):1089–1108, 1962.
39. Zaricznyj B: Avulsion fracture of the tibial eminence: treatment by open reduction and pinning. J Bone Joint Surg 59A(8):1111–1114, 1977.
40. Zickel RE, Fietti VG Jr, Lawsing JF III, Cockran GV: A new intramedullary fixation device for the distal third of the femur. Clin Orthop 125:185–191, 1977.

CHAPTER 8

Tumors and

Their

Treatment

Dempsey S. Springfield, M.D.

William W. Tomford, M.D.

■

Musculoskeletal tumors about the knee are not common in the general population, nor are they common in comparison with traumatic abnormalities of the knee. This fact is both good and bad. It is good that musculoskeletal tumors are uncommon, but it is bad that they are so uncommon that they are often forgotten and missed by the busy physician. Only once or twice a year does a practicing orthopaedist see a patient with a musculoskeletal tumor about the knee, most of which are benign lesions, and maybe only once or twice during a career does an orthopaedist see a patient with a malignant musculoskeletal tumor about the knee. This means that orthopaedists must constantly remind themselves of the possibility of an underlying tumor as the cause of a patient's symptoms, that radiographs of the knee of almost every patient with knee symptoms should be obtained, and that the radiographs must be examined carefully in order to rule out an underlying lesion. Too often a lesion, especially a giant cell tumor of bone, is obvious in retrospect but had been missed on initial inspection. The patella has been reported as the site of almost all musculoskeletal tumors, but it is often overlooked.[12, 26]

The distal femur and proximal tibia are common sites for a variety of musculoskeletal tumors, and physicians who specialize in knee disorders see patients with musculoskeletal tumors.[19] Many patients with a musculoskeletal tumor present with an unrelated complaint, such as a sprained ligament or painful joint, and a bone lesion is an incidental finding seen on the radiograph. It is unusual for asymptomatic lesions to be of clinical significance, and for most of these, only observation is needed. Benign lesions are common and only if they change over time should a biopsy be performed.

The symptom of a clinically significant bone tumor, one that is growing and requires treatment, is most often pain; occasionally, there is an associated mass. The pain of a tumor is a dull ache, which is often worse at night, and the pain may or may not be aggravated by activity. Acute, severe pain is an indication of a pathologic fracture or infection and is not likely to be caused directly by the tumor. Patients with lesions that are immediately adjacent to the subchondral plate or the articular cartilage may manifest findings typical of internal derangement of the knee: giving way, "locking," and a feeling of instability. Most patients have had symptoms for a month or more, and they report that although the symptoms may wax and wane, they are generally progressive. Systemic symptoms from a musculoskeletal tumor are rare. An occasional patient with Ewing's sarcoma or with a very large malignant fibrous histiocytoma or osteosarcoma has a low-grade fever or loss of energy, but most patients look and feel healthy.

No physical findings are particular for musculoskeletal tumors. It is important that the examiner ask the patient about any history of a tumor and find out whether radiographs have been taken. The presence of a joint effusion should be noted, and atrophy of the thigh or calf muscles should be measured. A joint effusion is a common finding in patients with a benign chondroblastoma, as it is in patients with malignant tumors that either are directly in contact with the synovium or have broken into the joint. Ewing's sarcoma is the only musculoskeletal neoplasia that commonly produces local inflammation. None of the others are associated with an inflammatory reaction.

All radiographs should be examined for the presence of a neoplastic lesion of bone, of soft tissue, or of the joint. Usually a diagnosis can be made from the appearance of the lesion on the plain radiograph. The exact locations, what the lesion does to the host bone, how the host bone reacts, and whether the tumor has calcified cartilage or bone in it are all important characteristics. Some lesions of bone are produced by intra-articular lesions, and this possibility should be considered when the lesion is seen to communicate with the joint.

CATEGORIES OF BONE TUMORS

Before the examiner decides how extensive an evaluation is needed for a lesion, it is best to have a differential diagnosis or at least to be able to categorize the lesion as inactive/benign, active/benign, or aggressive/malignant. Such categorization is helpful for selecting the methods and the extent of an evaluation. Every lesion can be placed into one of these three categories on the basis of the presenting complaints, the physical findings, and the appearance on plain radiographs. Once the lesion has been categorized, the appropriate evaluation can be conducted and a specific diagnosis made.

INACTIVE/BENIGN. The specific tumors in this category are nonossifying fibromas, fibrous cortical defects, healing unicameral bone cysts, enchondromas, and osteochondromas. The patient usually has no pain, the lesion having been found when a radiograph was taken for another reason. Some osteochondromas are found by the patient or the patient's parent and manifest as painless masses. There are no abnormal physical findings in patients with inactive/benign tumors except that most osteochondromas can be palpated. These lesions have a typical radiographic appearance, and a specific diagnosis can be made with only the radiograph. There should be no evidence of periosteal or endosteal reaction, no cortical erosion, and a well-defined margin between the lesion and the surrounding bone, often outlined with a thin rim of bone. If the diagnosis is made from the plain radiograph, there is no reason for any further testing, but periodic follow-up is recommended (Fig. 8–1).

If a specific diagnosis is not made and there is a question about the activity of the lesion, a technetium bone scan should be done. Most lesions, even inactive/benign lesions, have increased uptake on the bone scan, but when the lesion appears to be inactive/benign on the plain radiographs and there is no increased uptake on the bone scan, further evaluation is unnecessary. If there is an intense uptake on the bone scan, the lesion is active, and further evaluation should be conducted in order to determine whether treatment is necessary. Surgical treatment is not needed for inactive/benign lesions. On occasion, a patient or a patient's parent wants histologic proof of the diagnosis or requests that a large enchondroma or osteochondroma be removed.

If biopsy is performed for a benign lesion, it is probably best to remove the entire lesion rather than to remove only a small portion of it. The lesion can be removed without an incisional biopsy if a wide margin can be obtained (excisional biopsy) or after a frozen section confirms that it is benign. An excision gives the pathologist the opportunity to review the entire specimen instead of just a small portion, the bone can then heal, and there is no persistent appearance of a lesion on subsequent radiographs.

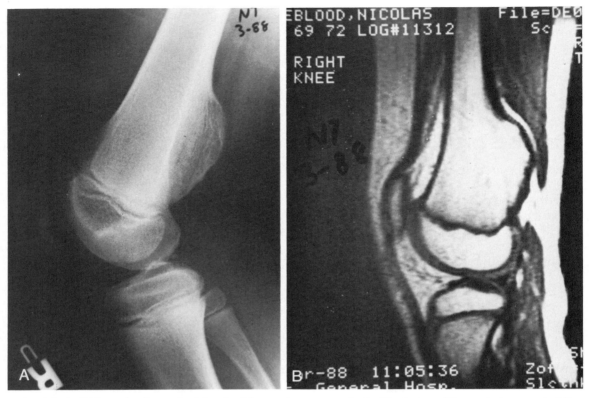

FIGURE 8–1. *(A)* Lateral radiograph of the distal femur of a young patient with a lesion of the posterior aspect of the distal femur. A definitive diagnosis can be made from the radiographic appearance. This is an osteochondroma (also called an osteocartilaginous exostosis), a typical inactive/benign lesion that does not require surgical treatment. Although parosteal osteosarcoma is commonly found in the posterior distal femur, this lesion has the typical and diagnostic characteristics of an osteochondroma: the cortex of the lesion is an extension of the cortex of the femur, and the lesion and the femur have medullary canals that communicate. Parosteal osteosarcomas attach onto the cortex. *(B)* Sagittal view of the magnetic resonance image (MRI) of the lesion shown in part *A*. The relationship between the lesion's medullary canal and cortex and the femur's medullary canal and cortex is seen better on the MRI than on the plain radiograph. This lesion is a classic sessile exostosis. The MRI was not necessary for making a diagnosis.

ACTIVE/BENIGN. The common tumors in this category are giant cell tumors of bone (the most common), aneurysmal bone cysts, active unicameral bone cysts, and chondroblastomas. Patients with one of these lesions complain of pain, often have a limp, and may or may not have a joint effusion and restricted motion. Many children less than 10 years of age with an active unicameral bone cyst and many young adults (20 to 35 years of age) with a giant cell tumor are not seen until they sustain a pathologic fracture, although usually they admit to having had an ache or mild pain before the fracture.

The radiographic appearance of each active/benign lesion is specific, and a diagnosis can be made with some confidence from the plain radiograph (Fig. 8–2). Active/benign lesions are most often treated with an intralesional curettage but occasionally require resection. Patients with such lesions need to be evaluated carefully, particularly for the extent of the lesion, before a biopsy is performed. Technetium bone scans are useful as a means of screening the skeleton for other lesions. Computed tomographic (CT) scans are most informative about the relationship of the tumor to the cortex and best depict intraosseous or extraosseous bone or calcification. Usually a technetium bone scan and a CT scan are adequate for the evaluation of active/benign lesion. MRI is a sensitive tool for determining the intramedullary extent of the tumor, but it is not as sensitive as CT in depicting intralesional bone, calcifications, or subtle cortical changes and should be used only if determining intramedullary is critical. Active/benign lesions are usually treated with aggressive curettage. Recurrent lesions should be resected. The biopsy should be performed in such a way that the incision can be excised later if necessary. Whoever performs the biopsy should be prepared to administer the definitive treatment.

AGGRESSIVE/MALIGNANT. The common tumors in this category are osteosarcomas, Ewing's sarcomas, and chondrosarcomas. Patients with one of these tumors usually have complaints and physical findings similar to those of patients with active/benign tumors. The radiograph is suggestive of the seriousness of the tumor. Any patient with a bone-forming tumor of the distal femur or the proximal tibia, especially a teenage

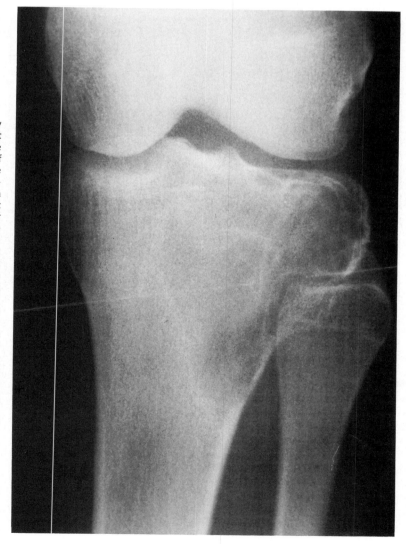

FIGURE 8–2. Anteroposterior view of the proximal tibia of a patient with a giant cell tumor of bone. The diagnosis of giant cell tumor of bone can almost always be made with certainty from a plain radiograph. This tumor is a common primary bone tumor and it is most often found in the distal femur or the proximal tibia. It involves the epiphysis and metaphysis in patients in whom the growth plates have closed. It does not have any intralesional densities and extends up to and sometimes through the subchondral plate. It is an active/benign tumor, and the recurrence rate after curettage is approximately 25 per cent, but resection is reserved for recurrent lesions or lesions that have destroyed the articular surface of the bone involved. An aggressive curettage with bone graft or packing with polymethyl methacrylate is suggested as the primary treatment.

patient, should be assumed to have an osteosarcoma (Fig. 8–3). Patients less that 30 years of age with a destructive lesion of bone, a periosteal reaction, and a soft tissue mass probably have Ewing's sarcoma. Chondrosarcomas occur in older patients and are often confused with metastatic carcinoma, but usually there are small nodules of calcification in chondrosarcoma. Metastatic carcinoma in the distal femur is unusual and is almost always accompanied by other, more proximal metastatic lesions. Metastatic carcinoma in the proximal tibia or fibula is quite uncommon.

Patients with aggressive/malignant tumors need radical surgery, often with adjuvant chemotherapy or irradiation or both. These patients need thorough evaluation both of the primary tumor and of potential sites of metastasis. The primary tumor is evaluated with CT for the same reasons as the active/benign tumor, but MRI is also useful. MRI is particularly accurate in depicting the intraosseous extent of the tumor, the extent of any soft tissue component, and intra-articular extension. Both CT and MRI are useful for determining the relationship between the neurovascular bundle and the tumor, but MRI is superior. The technetium bone scan is

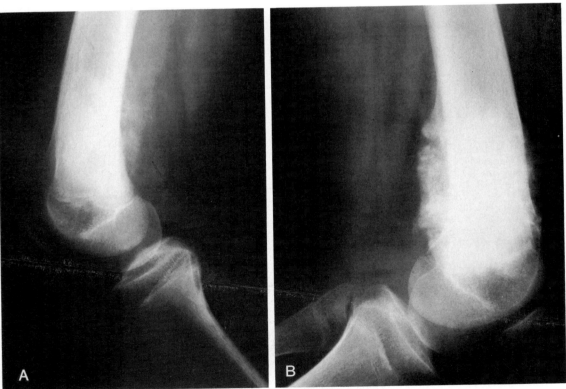

FIGURE 8–3. *(A)* Lateral radiograph of the distal femur of a patient with a classic high-grade osteosarcoma. The patient has open growth plates and is therefore young; the lesion is located in the metaphysis of the distal femur, and there is increased density and an extraosseous mass with ossification. These are the typical findings of classic osteosarcoma. Aggressive/malignant lesions have poorly defined borders, a periosteal reaction, and a permeative pattern of bone destruction. The production of bone by this tumor is the clue that this aggressive/malignant tumor is an osteosarcoma. *(B)* Lateral radiograph of the same patient's distal femur after the patient received preoperative chemotherapy. The clinical response has been excellent with decreased pain, increased motion in the knee, reduction in the size of the lesion, and increased density on the radiograph. Unfortunately, the clinical response does not correlate as well with the histologic response as expected, and only a careful histologic examination will indicate whether the response should be considered good (>90 per cent necrosis) or not. (From Springfield DS: Introduction to limb-salvage surgery for sarcomas. Orthop Clin North Am 22[1]:3, 1991.)

important as a method of screening the entire skeleton for metastasis, and a CT scan of the lungs should be taken in addition to a plain chest radiograph. Blood and urine values are of some importance in the initial evaluation of patients with a suspected aggressive/malignant tumor. The serum alkaline phosphatase, lactic dehydrogenase, erythrocyte sedimentation rate, calcium, phosphorus, blood urea nitrogen, and immunoelectrophoresis levels are the minimal studies recommended.

BIOPSY

The biopsy of a musculoskeletal tumor is not simple and should not be performed until a thorough evaluation has been completed.[20, 30] It is not performed early in the evaluation; rather, it should be the last procedure. The surgeon who performs the biopsy should be prepared to manage the lesion no matter what is found, and if the surgeon is not prepared to manage all the lesions in the prebiopsy differential diagnosis, the patient should be referred to another surgeon. It is inappropriate to perform a biopsy of a lesion in order to prove that it is serious enough to justify referring the patient to an oncology center.

If the tumor requires a wide surgical resection, the biopsy incision and all tissue exposed at the time of the biopsy must be resected with the specimen. This means that placement of the incision for the biopsy and the dissection to the tumor must be made appropriately if limb salvage is to be safe. In addition, there is a wide array of tests on fresh tumor tissue that are useful in planning treatment that cannot be conducted with tissue that has been placed in formaldehyde and methanol (Formalin) or paraffin blocks. These are the reasons why the biopsy should be performed where the patient is most likely to be treated.

Longitudinal incisions with minimal dissection of the deep tissues are best. Neurovascular bundles are avoided, and the path of the biopsy should be through overlying muscle, not between muscles. The biopsy specimen should be sharply cut from the tumor and carefully handled so that it is not crushed. The case should be discussed with the pathologist before the biopsy is performed, and a frozen section should always be taken in order to insure that diagnostic tissue has been obtained. A culture of the tissue should be performed. Hemostasis should be thorough, and the wound should be drained if there is any possibility of a postoperative hematoma. When an opening has been made in the cortex of the bone, a polymethyl methacrylate (PMMA) plug is useful as a means of reducing bleeding from the bone. In addition, if the cortex is opened the limb should be protected from stress that might produce a subsequent fracture.

SPECIFIC TUMORS

Benign

UNICAMERAL BONE CYST. Unicameral bone cysts are benign lesions commonly seen in children, but they are unusual in the distal femur, the proximal tibia, the patella, and the proximal fibula.[3, 27] Ninety per cent are found in the proximal femur and the proximal humerus. When a radiolucent lesion is seen in one of the bones around the knee, it should not be thought of first as a unicameral bone cyst. Unicameral bone cyst are found in the metaphysis (initially adjacent to the growth plate; later, usually after the patient reaches the age of 10 years, the growth plate moves away) in a central location, and there should be no periosteal reaction unless there has been a recent fracture. When there is a unicameral bone cyst in the metaphysis, the metaphysis does not remodel normally and is wider than normal; the width usually equal to but not greater than the width of the growth plate.

Unicameral bone cysts are filled with fluid (which is usually clear and yellow), and the wall is lined with synoviumlike cuboidal cells. These lesions spontaneously heal, and treatment is necessary only for those that fracture or those that are at risk for fracture. When a patient presents with a fracture through a unicameral bone cyst, it is best to treat the fracture closed and wait for the bone to unite. Although these benign cysts can heal after the bone fractures, there is no evidence that healing is more common after a fracture. Usually the cyst only appears to heal, inasmuch as it is obscured by the callus, but then it reappears as the callus remodels; therefore it is important to follow the patient's progress until the fracture has completely remodeled. If the cyst persists, an intralesional steroid injection is the best initial treatment.[3, 27, 42] It is unusual to have to operate on a unicameral bone cyst, but if it persists after repeated (probably three to six) injections, curettage and bone grafting are indicated.

ANEURYSMAL BONE CYST. Aneurysmal bone cysts have been reported in almost every bone in the skeleton, but approximately one quarter are found around the knee, mainly in the distal femur and the proximal tibia, but they also occur in the proximal fibula and the patella.[11, 35, 40] These lesions are most common in patients between the ages of 10 and 20 years. The patient usually complains of a mild pain that may be aggravated by activity. The physical findings are most commonly normal except for mild tenderness, but the radiographic abnormality is not subtle (Fig. 8–4). Aneurysmal bone cyst usually involves the medullary canal with expansion through the cortex and elevation of the periosteum. The periosteum contains the lesion and responds by producing a reactive rim of bone. The lesion occasionally arises from the cortex without involving the medullary canal but with an aneurysmal appearance to the periosteum.

Aneurysmal bone cyst can have an aggressive growth pattern and appear as an active to aggressive lesion on the radiograph; it is sometimes mistaken for a malignant lesion, but its radiographic appearance is not indicative of its clinical behavior. Although this type of cyst occasionally heals spontaneously, curettage and bone grafting are recommended. The lesion is typically a cystic cavity filled with a bloody fluid. The wall of the cavity is covered with thick, hemosiderin-stained tissue that has multinucleated giant cells, a benign fibrous stroma, benign fibroblastic appearing cells, and hemosiderin-ladened macrophages.[7] Normal mitoses and bone formation can be seen.

A note of caution: telangiectatic osteosarcoma can masquerade as an aneurysmal bone cyst. When a teenager has a lesion in the distal femur or the proximal femur, the physician must always include osteosarcoma in the differential diagnosis, even when the lesion has the appearance of an aneurysmal bone cyst. The gross appearances of the two lesions can

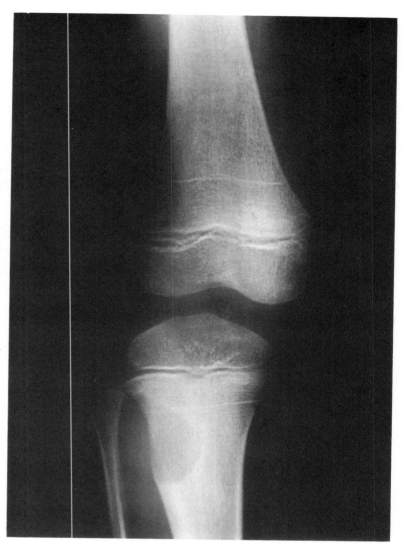

FIGURE 8–4. Anteroposterior radiograph of a 10-year-old patient complaining of pain with activity. The eccentric, metaphyseal, destructive nature of the lesion without any density suggests an active to aggressive type of lesion. It is an aneurysmal bone cyst, but in this age group the differential diagnosis also includes osteosarcoma, chondromyxofibroma, eosinophic granuloma, Ewing's sarcoma, and osteomyelitis. Usually a thin rim of periosteal bone surrounds the extraosseous component of the aneurysmal bone cyst, but it cannot be seen on this radiograph.

be identical at surgery, and only if the pathologist handles the specimen carefully will the correct diagnosis be made.

FIBROUS CORTICAL DEFECT. Fibrous cortical defects are very common; up to 40 per cent of children between the ages of 4 and 8 years have one.[9, 11] The distal femur is more commonly involved than are the other bones around the knee. The distal tibia is another common site of this lesion. Fibrous cortical defects typically are located in the cortex, are well defined by a thin reactive rim, and have a soap bubble appearance (Fig. 8–5). They are asymptomatic and heal spontaneously. Treatment is observation. Fibrous cortical defects and nonossifying fibroma are histologically identical, but nonossifying fibroma involves the medullary canal and may require curettage and bone grafting if large. Both lesions are composed of benign, spindle, fibroblastic cells arranged in a storiform pattern. Giant cells are usually present, and hemosiderin-stained cells are a typical feature.

CHONDROBLASTOMA. Chondroblastomas are most commonly found

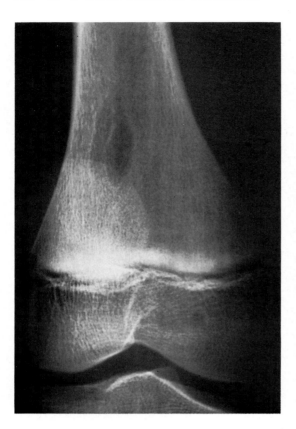

FIGURE 8–5. Anteroposterior radiograph of distal femur of a 10-year-old boy. The radiograph was taken after he hit his knee playing baseball. He had no symptoms in the knee before the injury, and the knee was normal on examination. There is a radiolucent lesion in the metaphysis with a sharp border of transition marked by a thin reactive rim of bone. It has a bubbly appearance, and there is no evidence of intralesional calcification or mineralization. This is a typical fibrous cortical defect or a nonossifying fibroma. The distinction is made on the basis of the size of the lesion (nonossifying fibromas are larger), but no measurement for differentiating the two lesions has been agreed upon.

in the proximal humerus, but approximately 35 per cent of them occur in either the distal femur or the proximal tibia. They are among the more common tumors found in the patella, but they are uncommon in the proximal fibula[2, 11, 45] (Fig. 8–6). Chondroblastoma is most common in patients with open growth plates, but up to one third of patients have completed growth when the tumor is discovered. It arises in the secondary ossification center and may extend into the metaphysis if the growth plate is closed. It is unusual for it to extend beyond the periosteum or invade into the adjacent joint. The patient usually complains of pain and has an associated joint effusion and often decreased range of motion in the adjacent joint.

The lesion may be difficult to see on the plain radiographs, and the patient may be thought to have inflammatory arthritis rather than a bone tumor. The appearance on the radiograph is of a radiolucent lesion surrounded by active bone. The lesion usually contains flecks of calcification, but these may not be seen without plain tomograms or a CT scan. There is occasionally a periosteal reaction in the metaphysis. The lesion consists predominantly of chondroblasts (cuboidal cells with a distinct nucleus, a pink cytoplasm, and a well-defined cell border) with a small amount of cartilage matrix, often with thin wisps of calcification. Multinucleated giant cells are common, but mitoses are not (Fig. 8–7). The lesion is a benign tumor that can be treated with thorough curettage. Recurrence is not uncommon (up to 25 per cent of patients), but usually

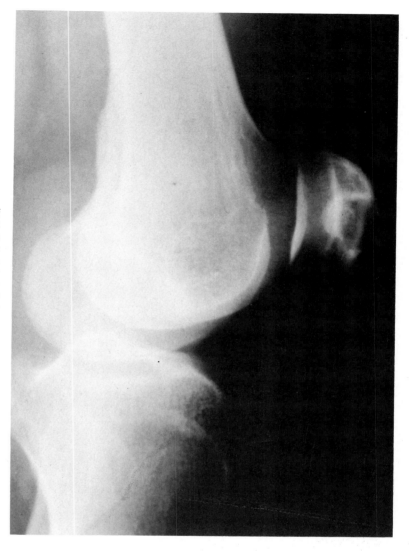

FIGURE 8–6. Lateral radiograph of a patient with a chondroblastoma of the patella. Lesions in the patella are difficult to see on plain radiographs and are often overlooked. Most chondroblastomas have calcifications within the otherwise radiolucent lesion. There is often an associated joint effusion and occasionally a periosteal reaction.

a second curettage controls the recurrence, and only very rarely is a wide resection necessary.

ENCHONDROMA. Solitary enchondromas are not common around the knee; those in the distal femur, the proximal tibia, the proximal fibula, and the patella account for only about 10 per cent of them.[11, 38] Enchondromas are most common in the hands. In children and young adults, the lesions are radiolucent, are centrally located in the metaphysis, and may prevent the normal metaphyseal remodeling, resulting in a widened metaphysis. They are asymptomatic and usually found when a radiograph is taken for another reason. They do not need treatment unless they are so large that the bone is weakened.

Enchondromas are composed of benign hyalinelike cartilage (Fig. 8–8). Enchondral ossification of those tumors seems to occur in the second or third decade of life. Enchondromas probably spontaneously heal, although there are no adequate follow-up studies to document this supposition. When they persist, they become calcified, and adults with

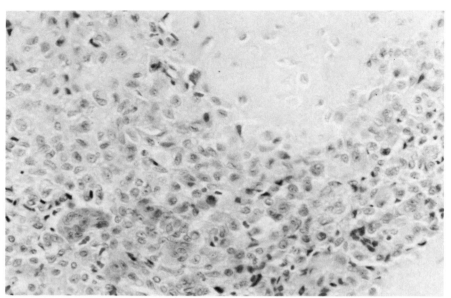

FIGURE 8–7. Typical histologic appearance (magnified 40 times) of a chondroblastoma. In the upper right portion there is a cartilage matrix; the remainder of the field is composed of the typical cuboidal chondroblasts, which are uniform in appearance. Two or three multinucleated giant cells are usually seen in chondroblastoma. (From Springfield DS: Introduction to limb salvage surgery for sarcomas. Orthop Clin North Am 22[1]:3, 1991.)

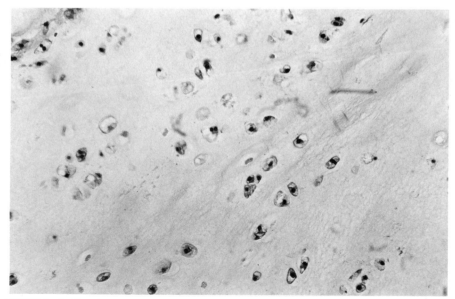

FIGURE 8–8. Histologic appearance (magnified 40 times) of benign cartilage typical of the cap of an exostosis or an enchondroma. There are a few binucleate chondrocytes, but the nuclei are small and dark; both of these features are typical of benign chondrocyte nuclei. It is difficult to differentiate low-grade malignant chondrosarcoma from active benign cartilage lesions, and the clinical manifestation is important. Patients who have no pain and whose radiographs reveal no evidence of activity (endosteal resorption or periosteal reaction) are unlikely to have a malignant cartilage tumor. A biopsy should be conducted carefully, and usually if a biopsy is performed for a benign cartilage tumor, the entire lesion should be removed.

enchondromas have intramedullary calcifications without other changes on the plain radiograph.

These lesions carry a small risk of undergoing malignant degeneration and need to be observed only once a year. When they become malignant, the patient has pain, and the appearance of the lesion on plain radiographs changes. An irregular pattern or shape of the calcification, endosteal erosion, and a periosteal reaction are all radiographic evidence of malignancy.[39] In comparison with patients who have only one enchondroma, patients with multiple enchondromas (Ollier's disease) have a higher risk of developing a malignant chondrosarcoma (approximately 15 per cent), and among patients with multiple enchondromas and hemangiomas (Maffucci's disease), there is an approximately 25 per cent incidence of developing a chondrosarcoma, but these patients also have a significant risk of developing a carcinoma at some time during their lives.

OSTEOCHONDROMA. Almost 40 per cent of solitary osteochondromas (also called osteocartilaginous exostosis) occur around the knee.[11] The lesion is usually found by a patient's parent and manifests as a painless mass. The osteochondroma grows as the patient grows but not necessarily at the same rate. It is not uncommon for the patient to complain of pain caused by repeated direct trauma or irritation of an overlying muscle, although most of these lesions are not associated with symptoms. The radiographic appearance is diagnostic (see Fig. 8–1). The cortex of the host bone blends into the stalk of the osteochondroma, which is capped with a cauliflowerlike mass with irregular calcification. The stalk may be thin (pedunculated osteochondroma) or broad (sessile osteochondroma), and the cap may be quite thick (>5 cm) in a child but should be thin (<1 cm) in an adult (Fig. 8–9). Parosteal osteosarcoma may be confused with osteochondroma.

A reliable radiographic difference between osteochondroma and par-

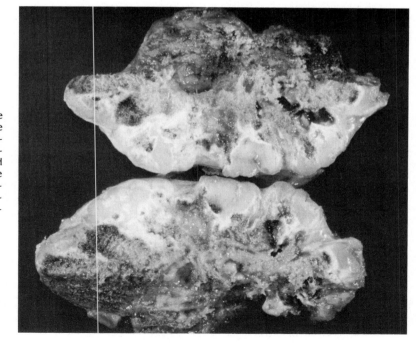

FIGURE 8–9. Gross appearance of an osteochondroma. This one has been split to show the interior. The cartilaginous cap is almost 1 cm thick in portions, and this benign lesion may be undergoing early malignant degeneration. Its broad base is characteristic of a sessile osteochondroma.

osteal osteosarcoma is the relationship of the lesion to the cortex of the host bone. As mentioned, an osteochondroma's stalk blends with the cortex of the host bone so that the medullary canal of the bone communicates with the medullary canal of the osteochondroma, but a parosteal osteosarcoma is attached to the surface of the bone (Fig. 8–10). The difference can usually be suspected on a plain radiograph, but a CT scan or MRI reveals the relationship between the lesion and host bone best and is recommended.

The indications for removal of an osteochondroma are limited in children, and recurrence is common unless the entire lesion, including the base, is removed. In adults they can be electively removed if the osteochondroma irritates local structures or if the patient chooses, but removal is required only if they are growing. An osteochondroma consist of a cartilaginous cap of hyalinelike cartilage that is undergoing enchondral ossification. The cartilage is more cellular than normal hyaline cartilage, and the ossification process is irregular. A benign osteochondroma should have a cap less than 1 cm thick. The enlarging osteochondroma with a cap more than 1 cm thick in a patient over 30 years of age should be considered a secondary chondrosarcoma and completely resected. It is impossible to know the incidence of malignant degeneration of a solitary osteochondroma, but it has been predicted to be as high as 5 per cent. Metastases from malignant degeneration of a solitary osteochondroma are

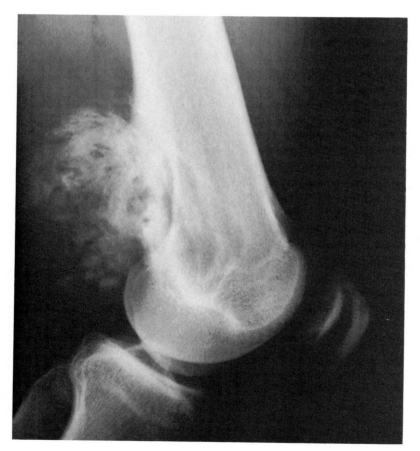

FIGURE 8–10. Lateral radiograph of the distal femur of a patient with a parosteal osteosarcoma. In contrast to the osteochondroma, the posterior cortex of the femur does not extend into the cortex of the parosteal osteosarcoma. Parosteal osteosarcoma usually does not invade the medullary canal, but this lesion had an intraosseous extension but was histologically low grade. The patient was treated with resection and osteoarticular allograft replacement, but not with chemotherapy.

extremely rare. Patients with multiple osteochondromas have a higher risk of developing a chondrosarcoma and should be so advised and examined yearly.

GIANT CELL TUMOR OF BONE. At least half of all giant cell tumors of bone occur around the knee, and they are the most common clinically significant tumor seen about the knee.[4, 11, 13, 37] The distal femur is the single most common site for a giant cell tumor of bone, and the proximal tibia is the second (Fig. 8–2). The patient is usually between 20 and 45 years of age and either complains of pain or manifests a pathologic fracture. The symptoms can suggest an internal derangement, and it is the tumor about the knee most often missed by the physician.[23]

The radiographic appearance of a giant cell tumor of bone is usually diagnostic. It involves the secondary ossification center and extends into the metaphysis. The cortex may be intact or expanded, or the tumor may have escaped the confines of bone. There is minimal reaction of the host bone to the lesion, and the lesion is entirely radiolucent. A giant cell tumor of bone is almost always immediately adjacent to the subchondral bone and often extends through the subchondral bone to the articular cartilage although it is unusual for it to breach the cartilage. Extension into a joint is usually secondary to an intra-articular fracture or by growth along the anterior cruciate ligament.

Histologic examination shows that giant cell tumors of bone consist of multinucleated giant cells, a background of benign fibrous stroma, and benign single nucleated cells whose nucleus look like the nuclei of the multinucleated giant cells (Fig. 8–11). Spontaneous necrosis is not uncommon, and normal mitoses are usually seen. The majority of giant cell tumors of bone can be managed by curettage, and primary resection is indicated only for a recurrent lesion or a very large lesion that has destroyed so much bone that reconstruction without resection is not possible. The reported incidence of local recurrence after a curettage is thought to be dependent on the aggressiveness of the curettage, but even with the most aggressive curettage, approximately 20 per cent of these tumors recur. Sometimes a second curettage is possible, and if it is technically possible, it should be done. When it is not possible to repeat the curettage, a resection is indicated.

Although it has not been proved, some authors believe that packing the cavity with PMMA after curettage reduces the incidence of local recurrence in comparison with packing with bone graft. Marcove and others advised repeated freeze/thaw cycles to control giant cell tumor of bone, but the complication rate is high, and if cryosurgery is ever appropriate, it should be performed only by surgeons who are well versed in this technique.[22, 32, 34] The author recommends a wide exposure of the lesion with a large window in the bone. The entire rim of reactive bone surrounding the lesion should be removed, and the author uses a high-speed burr to complete the curettage. After such extended curettage, the lesion is carefully hand packed with PMMA.

Up to 5 per cent of patients with benign giant cell tumors of bone develop pulmonary metastases. Most of these patients are treated successfully with resection of the pulmonary nodule. Patients with giant cell tumors of bone should have routine follow-up chest radiographs in addition to a radiograph of the original tumor site.

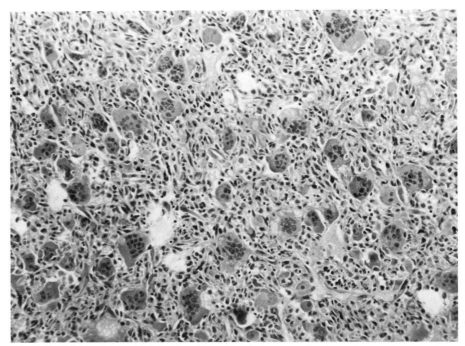

FIGURE 8–11. Typical histologic appearance (magnified 40 times) of a benign giant cell tumor of bone. It is composed of multinucleated giant cells with nuclei that are identical or similar in appearance to those in the background stromal cells. This field does not have any necrotic areas, but they are seen in benign giant cell tumor of bone. Normal but increased numbers of mitoses are also usually present.

Malignant

OSTEOSARCOMA. Osteosarcomas are malignant spindle cell tumors in which bone is produced by the malignant cells. They should be classified into at least three categories: classic, juxtacortical, and other. The other category includes low-grade interosseous, radiation induced osteosarcoma associated with Paget's disease and osteosarcoma of the jaw. The other category types are uncommon and are not discussed further. Classic osteosarcoma is common around the knee, and approximately half of all osteosarcomas occur in the distal femur, the proximal tibia, or the proximal fibula.[11] One third of all osteosarcomas occur in the distal femur alone (Fig. 8–3A).

Classic osteosarcoma is a disease of teenagers and young adults with a peak incidence between 15 and 25 years of age. Patients usually manifest an enlarging mass and minimal to mild pain. Half of the patients have an elevated serum alkaline phosphatase level. The radiographic appearance may vary greatly, but usually the diagnosis can be made from a plain radiograph. The majority of osteosarcomas are in the metaphysis, and most often there is a combination of destruction of the bone and formation of tumor bone. Almost all classic osteosarcomas extend beyond the confines of the cortex.

The histologic subtypes depend on whether the tumor is predominantly fibrous (fibroblastic), cartilaginous (chondroblastic), or osseous (osteoblastic) or is a vascular cyst (telangiectatic) but all have malignant spindle cells producing bone. Anaplasia and abnormal mitoses are present (Fig. 8–12). Adjuvant chemotherapy and surgical resection are the recommended treatment. Preoperative chemotherapy is increasingly used, and limb salvage surgery has become the norm; fewer than half of all patients require an amputation (Fig. 8–3B). The methods of reconstruction are numerous and include arthrodesis, osteoarticular allograft replacement, endoprosthetic replacement, and, for lesions in the distal femur in a young patient, rotationplasty.[21, 25, 42]

CHONDROSARCOMA. Chondrosarcoma is a malignant tumor of cartilage origin and may be either primary or secondary.[31] Primary chondrosarcomas arise within the bone without an associated abnormality, whereas secondary chondrosarcomas are malignancies that are associated with a pre-existing benign cartilage lesion (either an enchondroma or an exostosis). The bones of the knee are not common sites of chondrosarcoma although they are occasionally involved, and most chondrosarcomas in this area are of the secondary type. Patients with exostosis, either solitary or multiple, usually notice enlargement of a palpable lesion about the knee as the first indication that a secondary chondrosarcoma has developed. Those lesions that enlarge while the patient is young (less than 30 years of age) are not likely to be malignant, but when an exostosis grows after the age of 30 years, it should be assumed to have undergone malignant degeneration.

(Although there is some controversy concerning the diagnosis of secondary chondrosarcoma associated with an exostosis, most authors

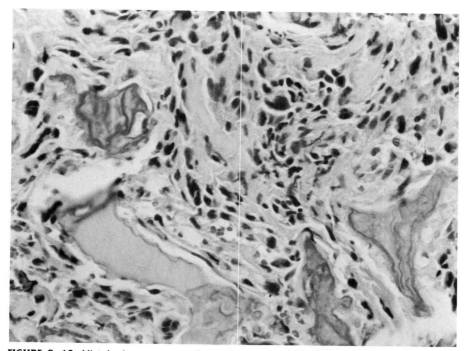

FIGURE 8–12. Histologic appearance (magnified 40 times) of a high-grade osteosarcoma. The features necessary for the diagnosis are malignant spindle cells, which are making bone. As in this field, there is usually significant variation in the size and shape of the cells and their nuclei. Mitoses are common, and bizarrely shaped mitoses can usually be found. Spontaneous necrosis is usually present.

use the thickness of the cartilaginous cap as the principle measure of the activity of the lesion. Lesions with a cartilaginous cap of less than 0.5 cm in thickness are classified as benign, and those with a cap more than 1 cm thick are classified as malignant even when the cytologic details are not diagnostic of a malignancy.)

Patients with multiple hereditary exostosis have a higher risk of developing a malignancy than do those with only one lesion. Patients with a secondary chondrosarcoma with an associated enchondroma complain of pain as the first indication of a malignancy. This pain is usually a dull ache that is unremitting and not associated with activity. The symmetric regular calcification seen on radiographs of a benign enchondroma is altered when the lesion becomes malignant. The calcification becomes irregular, the endosteal surface is eroded, and often there is a periosteal reaction. Chondrosarcomas may vary from being cytologically benign (Fig. 8–7) to being high-grade, poorly differentiated spindle cell tumors, but most are of an intermediate histologic grade (Fig. 8–13). Chondrosarcomas are treated with wide surgical resection, and adjuvant chemotherapy is not routinely used.

Synovial Tumors

PIGMENTED VILLONODULAR SYNOVITIS. Pigmented villonodular synovitis is a benign condition of the synovial lining; it is not common and can be confused with other causes of chronic synovitis.[1, 17, 18, 46] The nature of the lesion is unknown, although it behaves as a locally aggressive

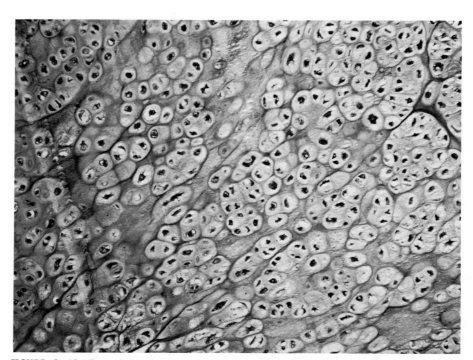

FIGURE 8–13. Typical histologic appearance (magnified 40 times) of a medium-grade chondrosarcoma. There is an increased cell-to-matrix ratio; almost every chondrocyte has more than one nucleus, which are large and irregular. Mitoses are present.

benign condition. The knee and the hip are the two most commonly affected joints. The patient complains of persistent swelling, but no pain, in the knee. The diagnosis can be made from an arthrogram. The joint fluid aspirated at the time of the arthrogram is dark brown, and the irregular villous appearance of the synovial lining is seen on the arthrogram. On occasion, these lesions erode into the bone, producing smooth irregularities in the bone. Synovectomy is the treatment of choice, although there is early evidence that the recurrence rate can be decreased by using postoperative intra-articular yttrium or dysprosium.[48]

SYNOVIAL CHONDROMATOSIS. Synovial chondromatosis is a disorder of the intermediate layer of the synovium.[11, 36] Hyaline cartilage is produced in this layer and extruded into the joint. The knee is the most commonly affected joint. The patient complains of locking and giving way of the knee and has an effusion on examination, and multiple small calcified lesions in the joint are seen on the plain radiograph. Removal of the loose bodies and a synovectomy are the treatments of choice.[10]

Soft Tissue Tumors

SOFT TISSUE SARCOMA. Soft tissue sarcoma often arises in the soft tissues around the knee, and they should be suspected whenever a patient manifests a soft tissue mass, especially one that is deep to the fascia (Fig. 8–14). Subcutaneous lesions are most often benign lipomas, but malignant fibrohistiocytomas occur often enough in the subcutaneous tissue to warrant inclusion in the differential diagnosis. Most of the deeply situated soft tissue tumors are malignant and they should be assumed to be so until proven otherwise (Fig. 8–15). A CT scan or MRI is usually specific for a lipoma or ganglion, and if these tests do not reveal that the lesion is one of these, malignant soft tissue tumor should be the first disease in the list of differential diagnoses.

Limb salvage surgery for even the largest soft tissue sarcoma is now routine with the use of irradiation in combination with surgery. Treatment is dependent on the anatomic extent and location, not the histologic type, of the tumor. It is unusual for a patient to have an amputation for a soft tissue tumor unless the tumor has been neglected or the method of the biopsy makes the risk of irradiation and surgery unreasonable. It is important that the surgeon who is to be responsible for the care of the patient be allowed to perform the biopsy. The common histologic types of soft tissue sarcoma about the knee are synovial cell sarcoma (not an intra-articular tumor), liposarcoma (common in the popliteal fossa), and malignant fibrous histiocytoma.

RECONSTRUCTIVE TECHNIQUES

Osteoarticular Allograft Reconstruction

The transplantation of large bones has provided a biologic material with which to reconstruct extremities. Before its routine use, which began with the work of Frank Parrish in 1972, biologic reconstruction was limited because only autogenous bone was available.[41] Only reconstruction with the iliac crest, the ribs, the fibula, or a partial cortex of the femur or the

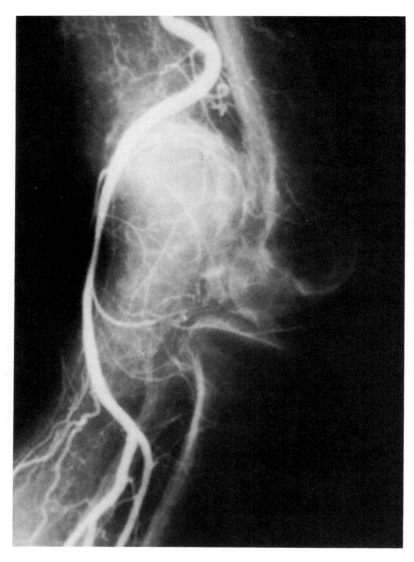

FIGURE 8–14. Lateral view of an angiogram of a patient with a popliteal mass. The popliteal artery is displaced by a vascular mass, and because it lies directly on the pseudocapsule of the tumor, it is considered involved; if a wide resection is required to control the tumor, the artery would have to be resected with the tumor. This mass proved to be pigmented villonodular synovitis, but almost all solid tumors in the popliteal fossa are malignant lesions and should be assumed to be so until proved otherwise.

tibia could be performed. Nonbiologic materials were and are used to replace resected or damaged bone and articular surfaces, but these materials have a limited life expectancy and are not optimal for young patients. Before the use of allografts, most of the biologic reconstructions performed after an articular cartilage resection with autogenous bone resulted in an arthrodesis. Only the articular surface of the distal radius (with the proximal fibula) and a hemicondyle of the tibia (with half of the patella) could be replaced with autogenous cartilage.[5, 16] Allografts can include articular surfaces, and any joint surface can now be replaced with an osteoarticular allograft. Osteoarticular replacement of the distal femur or the proximal tibia with an allograft is now considered an excellent method of reconstruction (Figs. 8–16, 8–17).

The bones with their articular surfaces are harvested from fresh cadavers under sterile conditions in an operating room, usually immediately after any organs available for transplantation have been removed.[47] These bones are cultured on numerous occasions, wrapped in sterile

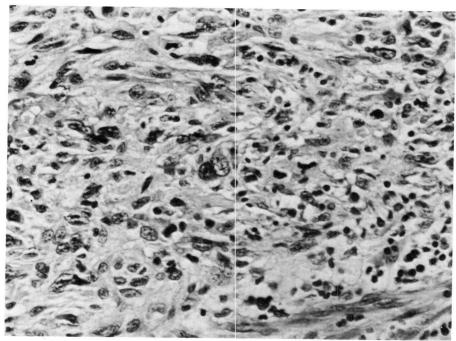

FIGURE 8–15. Histologic appearance (magnified 40 times) of the single most common soft tissue sarcoma in adults: a malignant fibrous histocytoma. This tumor has a number of subclassifications, but the diagnostic features are large irregular histocytic cells with large granular nuclei and a storiform or "whirlwind" pattern. Mitoses are common, and necrosis is almost always seen.

FIGURE 8–16. Anteroposterior radiograph of the distal femur of a patient who has had an osteoarticular allograft reconstruction after a resection of the distal femur. The operation was done two years prior and the patient has excellent function. The allograft has healed to the host bone, there has been no resorption, and the joint continues to appear normal. These patients have some instability in the knee and are asked to restrict their activities (no running or twisting activities) but otherwise lead a normal life.

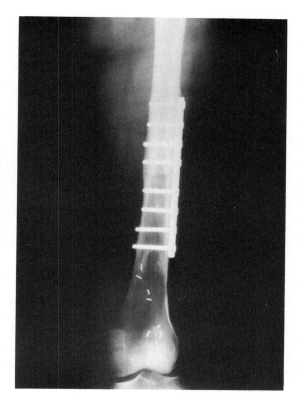

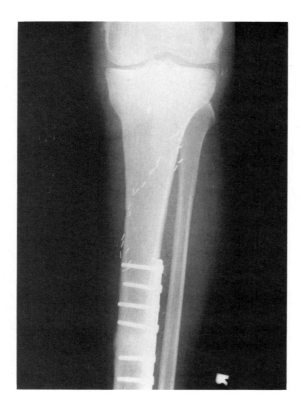

FIGURE 8–17. Anteroposterior radiograph of the proximal tibia of a patient who has had a reconstruction with an osteoarticular allograft after a resection of the proximal tibia. This radiograph was taken 4 years after the operation and there is some loss of articular cartilage on the medial side of the joint but the patient was without symptoms and walking without difficulty.

drapes and plastic, and stored at −70°C. The articular cartilage is treated with dimethylsulfoxide to help preserve the chondrocytes. The specimens are radiographed, and when a transplant is needed, the bone closest in size to the resected bone is chosen. The size articular surface of the transplant should be as close as possible to that of the resected articular surface, but if an exact match is not possible, it is better that the replacement femur is slightly smaller and the replacement tibia is slightly larger than the resected bones.

The bone and the articular cartilage are thawed in the operating room and fixed to the host bone with plates, and the ligaments are attached to the host ligaments with nonabsorbable suture. After operation, the joint is immobilized in a cast for 6 to 10 weeks; then the patient is allowed to slowly regain motion in the joint. The controlling muscles are rehabilitated with a gentle program while the allograft bone continues to heal to the host bone. Only touchdown weight bearing is allowed until there is radiographic evidence of union, and this requires 7 to 9 months. If there is no evidence of union 1 year after surgery, autogenous iliac crest bone graft is added to the site of junction. Once the junction is healed, the patient can increase weight bearing to the full extent as quickly as tolerated.[29]

The specific operative technique for an osteoarticular allograft reconstruction of either the distal femur or the proximal tibia is similar. Once the bone to be replaced has been resected and the allograft cut to the same length as the resected bone, the reconstruction can begin. Either the allograft can be fixed to the host bone first or the ligaments can be repaired first. The authors prefer to first select a plate and fix it to the allograft, being sure that it fits the host but not fix it to the host bone until the ligaments about the knee have been repaired.

After the plate has been fixed to the allograft, the posterior capsule and the collateral ligament are repaired with interrupted, nonabsorbable suture. It seems best to place all the suture first and tie them afterwards. The posterior capsule should not be too tight, and the joint should be allowed to come to full extension or just short of full extension. The collateral ligaments should be as tight as possible. If the cruciate ligaments are touching, a suture should be used to approximate them, although in most patients, the cruciate ligaments are not functioning at follow-up. After the posterior capsule and collateral ligaments have been repaired, the patella is relocated, and the remainder of the joint capsule is closed. When the proximal tibia is being replaced, the patella ligament must be repaired and the length of the patella ligament must be maintained. Before the proximal tibia is resected, the length of the patella ligament should be measured so that the reconstructed ligament can be adjusted to be equal in length to the original patella ligament.

The patient is expected to be able to walk without external aids soon after the bones have healed. They all have modest instability in all directions, the anteroposterior motion being the most abnormal. Despite this, the joint functions well for nonathletic activities. In general, patients with osteoarticular reconstructions are asked not to participate in running or jumping activities, but they are allowed to play golf, swim, and bicycle. An occasional patient prefers to wear a brace, and some patients are more active than they are advised to be. It is not uncommon for the joint to have radiographic signs of mild degeneration with thinning of the articular surface and osteophytes (host side of the joint only) and for the patient to have a minimal effusion, but symptoms are rare. If extensive degenerative changes in the joint develop, a standard endoprosthesis can be used to replace the articular surfaces. The authors use a constrained endoprosthetic knee for replacing the degenerated allograft joint (Fig. 8–18).

Endoprosthetic Reconstruction

Reconstructions of a major joint with an endoprosthesis after resection of a major portion of the bone have been performed long enough that the results can be predicted.[7, 24, 33, 43, 44] It was originally thought that the results of these mega-endoprosthetic reconstructions would be worse than those of the more standard joint reconstructions, but, surprisingly, the patients have done extremely well. One, and probably the major, reason is that patients who have a mega-endoprosthetic reconstruction have a tendency to protect their extremities and to limit their activities more than do arthritic patients, particularly young healthy patients with osteonecrosis or posttraumatic arthritis who have conventional joint replacements. The patients who must undergo major resection tend to take care of their endoprostheses, and as a result, the endoprostheses last longer than originally predicted, and the long-term results have been good. Despite this, there begins to be a significant incidence of breakage and loosening after 10 years.

The original endoprostheses were custom-made devices manufactured for each patient to the specifications of the surgeon on the basis of

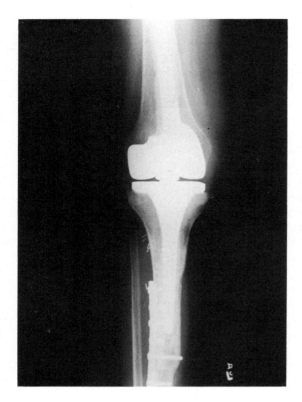

FIGURE 8–18. Anteroposterior radiograph of a patient with an allograft endoprosthetic reconstruction after a resection of the proximal tibia. The total joint was used because the patient was over 60 years of age and had early degenerative arthritis of the femoral condyles, and the allograft was used to provide an attachment for the patellar tendon. This patient has 95° of flexion and full active extension. Another advantage of the allograft is that the reconstruction can be tailored during the operation to replace the bone resected.

the predicted length of the resection and the size of the patient's joint (Fig. 8–19). The majority of the early replacements were for the proximal femur with a custom-made total hip and proximal femur. Later, distal femoral and proximal tibial resections were reconstructed with endoprostheses. Endoprosthetic replacements for the proximal tibia have been less successful than those for the other location because of the difficulty of reconstructing the patellar tendon. A variety of methods have been tried to improve the attachment of the patellar tendon to the tibial construct, and both the medial gastrocnemius flap and the fibular osteotomy work, although even with these, active extension is not normal.[24, 28] Custom-made endoprostheses continue to be used for the reconstructions, but modular endoprostheses are now available and are increasingly being used for the replacements. The advantage of the modular endoprosthesis is the ability to modify the resection and reconstruction during the operation as necessary, whereas with a custom-made device, this option is not available.

The operative technique depends on the site of the reconstruction but is not significantly different from that of the reconstruction of an arthritic knee. The major difference is that after a major resection of a tumor, the entire distal femur or the proximal tibia is gone, and the collateral ligaments are transected. The endoprosthetic knee must be intrinsically stable. The most popular model is a rotating hinge joint that allows free rotation but no varus-valgus or anterior-posterior motion. Once the resection has been completed, the nontumor side of the joint (the proximal tibia for a distal femoral lesion or the distal femur for a proximal tibial lesion) is prepared for the appropriate component of the

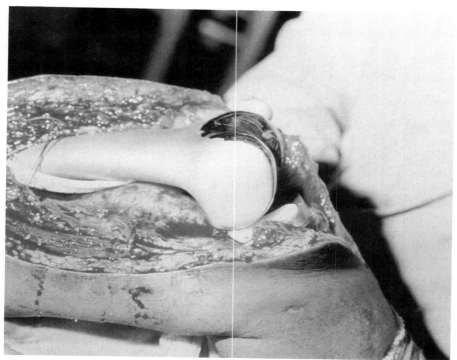

FIGURE 8–19. Intraoperative photograph of a custom-made endoprosthesis used to replace the distal femur after resection of an osteosarcoma. Endoprosthetic replacements are attractive because the patient recovers quickly and can resume most activities within a few weeks. The endoprostheses have a limited life expectancy, and when a young patient survives a malignancy, this reconstruction needs revision. The endoprosthetic reconstructions are best for older patients who must undergo osteoarticular resection.

endoprosthesis, as is done in a standard total knee endoprosthesis for the type of device chosen. On the resected side of the joint, the remaining bone is only a diaphysis, and this is prepared for the stem of the endoprosthesis by being reamed to the appropriate size.

Endoprostheses used to be fixed to the host bone with PMMA, but more recently, bone ingrowth fixation has been used, and in some endoprostheses, a combination of bone ingrowth and PMMA fixation is being used.[8] There is no consensus regarding the need for resurfacing the patellar when an endoprosthetic knee is used. When the patella is normal, there is probably no need for resurfacing the patella, but if there are abnormalities in the patella cartilage, it should be resurfaced in a standard manner.

The postoperative management of a patient who has undergone mega-endoprosthetic reconstruction is similar to the postoperative management of a patient who has undergone routine total knee replacement. The surgical wound for the former patient is larger, and it is best to delay movement for 3 or 4 days, although earlier motion from 0° to 35° is probably safe. Once the wound has begun to heal, increased motion can be allowed, and quadriceps and hamstring muscle–strengthening exercises can be undertaken. Partial weight bearing is allowed immediately if the endoprosthesis was fixed with PMMA, and full weight bearing is allowed when the quadriceps muscle is strong. Often a portion of the quadriceps muscle is resected with the distal femoral lesion, and soft tissue recon-struction is performed in order to replace the resected muscle. If this is the case, the postoperative course must be tailored to accommodate the healing of the soft tissue reconstruction.

Arthrodesis

Arthrodesis of the knee after a resection has been and continues to be an excellent method of reconstruction.[6, 14, 15] The disadvantages are obvious, and the loss of knee flexion does make sitting, especially in a confined space, difficult; however, the advantage of having a strong, painless, permanent lower extremity reconstruction with which all activities can be performed is attractive to many patients. The major indication for an arthrodesis is the reconstruction of an extremity after an extra-articular resection. Trying to keep knee motion after the extensor mechanism has been resected is difficult at best, and the function is limited. Some patients prefer the limited knee motion and accept the extensor weakness and limitation of activities required for arthroplasty reconstruction after an extra-articular resection, but they should understand the expected limited function before making a decision.

A secondary indication for an arthrodesis is complete resection of the quadriceps muscle with the femur. The patients can undergo reconstruc-tion with an allograft or an endoprosthetic device for the bone and hamstring muscle transfers for the extensor mechanism, but the best results are flexion of less than 90° and weak extension; patients who want to be physically active prefer an arthrodesis.

A final relative indication for an arthrodesis is for a young patient who wants to be, or must be, very physically active. It is unreasonable to expect a reconstructive arthroplasty to last a significant length of time in a young, active, 200-pound patient if that person continues an active life style. The arthrodesed knee is strong and permanent. There have been occasional patients in whom a knee arthrodesis was converted to an articulating endoprosthesis, but the results have not been encouraging, and this revision is not recommended.

After resection of the joint because of a tumor, the arthrodesis can be performed with autogenous or allograft bone. The fibula and a portion of the cortex of the femur or the tibia (the one not resected) or both fibulas can be used as sources of autogenous bone (Fig. 8–20).[14] When allograft arthrodesis is selected as the reconstruction, a tibia or a femoral allograft is used to replace the resected bone and joint (Fig. 8–21). The bone grafts can be held in place with either an intramedullary rod or plates. The advantage of intramedullary rods is that they permanently add to the strength of the reconstruction; their disadvantage is that their introduction exposes the entire intramedullary canal to the operative field and to potential contamination with tumor cells. Plate fixation reduces the ex-posure of tissues to potential tumor contamination, but their contribution to the strength of the reconstruction is limited. The authors prefer intramedullary rod fixation. The reconstructed limb should be approxi-mately 1 cm shorter than the normal limb in order to improve the patient's gait.

After the resection has been completed and the pathologist has reviewed the resected specimen to ensure that the margins of the resection

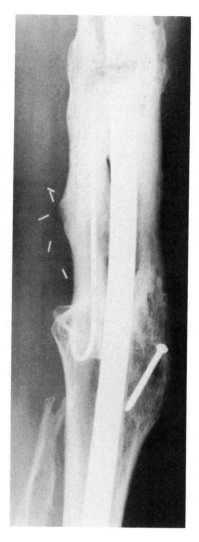

FIGURE 8–20. Lateral radiograph of the distal femur and proximal tibia of a patient who had an arthrodesis of the knee after a resection of the distal femur. The bone graft for this arthrodesis is autogenous. The anterior graft is from the anterior cortex of the tibia and the posterior graft (with the K-wire) is the ipsilateral fibula. This graft has healed and hypertrophied, and the patient is fully active without restrictions. The radiograph was taken more than 5 years after the operation.

are adequate, the arthrodesis can be performed. When autogenous bone graft is to be used, the ipsilateral fibula is harvested. The length of fibula needed is 2 to 3 cm longer than the defect to be replaced. Once the fibula has been harvested, the intramedullary canal of the femur and the tibia are reamed to accept the intramedullary rod. The authors use a fluted intramedullary rod, the proximal two thirds of which is curved and the distal third of which is straight (Kirschner Medical Corporation, New England Surgical Specialties, Inc.). The rod is passed in a retrograde fashion up the femur until it extends from the distal end of the femur 1 cm more than the length of the resection. Then the fibula is positioned posterior to the rod, in the medullary canal of the femur proximally and in the medullary canal of the tibia distally. The tibia is positioned properly (the correct rotation should be ensured), and the intramedullary rod is driven antegrade into the distal tibia. The anterior cortex of the femur or the tibia, whichever is present, is then harvested and placed anterior to the intramedullary rod. The patient is postoperatively placed in a brace and walks with crutches (toe-touch weight bearing only) until the grafts

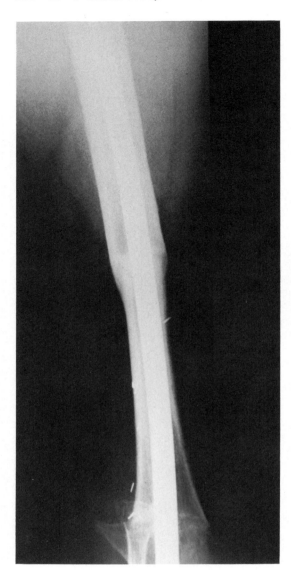

FIGURE 8–21. Lateral radiograph of the distal femur of a patient who underwent an allograft arthrodesis after an extra-articular resection of the knee joint. The allograft was threaded over a long intramedullary rod. Sixteen months after the surgery, the allograft had healed to the host bone at both ends. The patient is fully active, and his activities have not been restricted.

are well healed, usually in about 1 year. It takes approximately 2 years for the bone grafts to revascularize and regain their strength, and the patients should limit their activities during those 2 years. Once the grafts have united to the host bone and revascularized, full activities are allowed.

The major advantage of using an allograft for the reconstruction is that bone does not need to be harvested from the host. Thus the length of time required for the operation is reduced, as is the magnitude of the dissection. The allograft is cut to a length of 1 cm less than the defect created by the resection. When an intramedullary rod is to be used, the allograft must be reamed until it slips easily over the curved section of the rod. Once this has been done, the femur and the tibia are reamed, and the rod is passed in a retrograde fashion up the femur until it extends 1 cm longer than the length of the allograft. The allograft is slipped on the rod, and the rod is driven into the tibia in a forward fashion. Pressure is exerted against the foot in order to keep the junctions between the femur, the allograft, and the tibia closed during the positioning of the intramedullary rod in the tibia. The intramedullary rod is to be permenant, and it can be driven completely into the femur just below the top of the greater trochanter. The patient is postoperatively allowed to ambulate with partial weight bearing on crutches until the allograft is healed to the host bone. Then full weight bearing is allowed.

When plates are used to fix the allograft to the host bone, two plates are usually used. If possible, a single long plate is used to span the length of the allograft with screws in the femur, the allograft, and the tibia. Two additional plates are used to increase the strength of the reconstruction. None of these plates are routinely removed. The patient is postoperatively allowed to ambulate, toe touching with two crutches, until the allograft is healed to the host bone; then full weight bearing is allowed.

Rotationplasty

An unusual method of reconstruction after a resection of the distal femur is a rotationplasty.[21, 25] It is most useful for the reconstruction of a child's limb when the distal femoral epiphysis must be resected with the tumor. The resultant limb length inequality makes the other types of limb salvage reconstruction impractical unless the child is almost fully grown. Other advantages of this reconstruction are that it includes the knee joint (i.e., is an extra-articular resection), distal thigh muscles are not needed for a functional limb, and the amount of normal tissue that can be resected is greater than with other types of limb-salvaging operations. These are all oncologic advantages and decrease the risk of a local recurrence.

The limb is short, and the patient must wear a prosthesis, but the patient has an end-bearing limb and phantom sensation does not exist. The description sounds worse than cosmetic appearance of the limb actually is, and with a prosthetic limb, the patient looks normal (Fig. 8–22). Even when the prosthetic limb is not worn, most patients learn to hold the foot in maximal plantar flexion, which diminishes the effect of a "backwards" foot.

The resection and the reconstruction are straightforward. Only if the vessels are to be resected with the tumor is there any significant potential for a major difficulty. Only the nerve has to be saved because everything else between the proximal resection margin and distal margin can be sacrificed. Two elliptical incisions are made around the limb, one in the proximal thigh and the other in the proximal tibia just distal to the tibial tubercle. The angle of obliquity of the two incisions should be different in order to equalize the circumference of the incisions. The proximal incision should be more transverse than the distal incision. A posterior longitudinal incision joins these two circumferential incisions so that the sciatic nerve can be dissected out and protected. If the femoral artery and vein are to be saved, they are also dissected out and protected. If they are to be resected with the tumor, they are isolated in the proximal thigh and in the proximal leg but not ligated until just before the specimen is removed. Once the vessels have been identified, the section of the limb between the two circumferential incisions is removed by transection of all the muscles and bone.

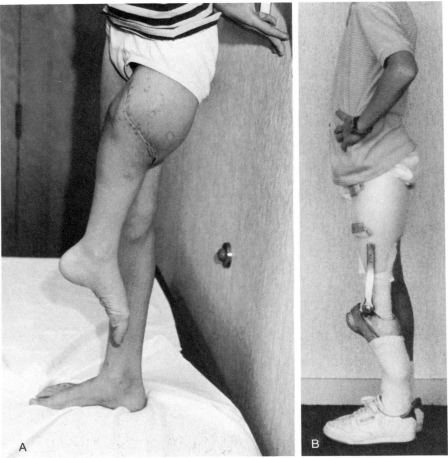
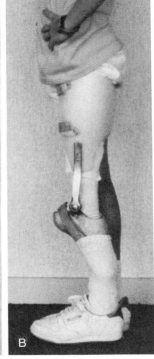

FIGURE 8–22. *(A)* Photograph of a young man who 3 weeks earlier underwent a rotationplasty reconstruction after a resection of the distal femur. He was already able to think in terms of knee extension and get the ankle to plantar flex. He even calls his old ankle a knee. *(B)* Same young man a few months later in his prosthesis. The old ankle needs to be braced to block subtalar motion to stabilize the varus and valgus motion. The prosthesis is an end-bearing prosthesis, and the patient can run and jump. He plays both football and basketball for his school.

The reconstruction consists of *externally* rotating the lower portion of the limb 180°. The axis of the ankle should be in the anteroposterior plane, and the length of the extremity should be adjusted so that the ankle of the child, when fully grown, is opposite the contralateral knee. (The expected difference in growth between the unaffected limb and the operated limb is calculated as the difference in growth between the normal distal femur and the normal distal tibia for the age of the patient. The difference is not as much as might be thought, and most of the femoral shaft needs to be removed so that the ankle is at the correct position.) The femur and the tibia are held together with a compression plate. If the vessels were resected, they are anastomosed now. The nerve and the vessels, if they were not resected, are carefully coiled in the soft tissues of the thigh. The posterior muscles (hamstrings) are sutured to the anterior muscle fascia of the leg, and the anterior muscles (quadriceps) are sutured to the posterior muscles (gastrocnemius) of the leg. The skin is closed in a routine fashion.

The leg is placed in a compressive dressing in the operating room, and this dressing is left on for the next 5 to 7 days. Non–weight-bearing ambulation, with the aid of two crutches, should begin as soon as the patient is comfortable. When the initial dressing is removed, the patient should begin exercising the ankle in order to improve the amount of plantar flexion and to get use to the reversed ankle. The patient will walk better if the ankle can be plantar flexed to at least 160°, which most children can achieve with little difficulty. The first prosthesis should be made within the first 2 or 3 weeks so that the patient can begin to get experience with using the reversed ankle motion for extension and flexion of the prosthetic knee. The prosthesis has an end-bearing socket and a hinge for the knee joint for stabilizing the subtalar motion, which is not needed at the knee. The authors have thought of performing a subtalar arthrodesis in order to eliminate the subtalar motion, but this has not yet been done. Partial weight bearing is allowed until there is radiographic evidence of union of the femur to the tibia. This usually is seen within 3 months. The authors' experience is that the patient has little difficulty learning to use the reversed ankle as a knee, and the appearance is an emotional problem more for the patient's parents than for the patient.

SUMMARY

The distal femur and the proximal tibia are two of the most common sites for bone tumor, and all physicians who evaluate patients with complaints about the knee must remember to consider a tumor as the cause of the symptoms. Often the symptoms simulate an internal derangement, and the unsuspecting physician can easily miss a tumor about the knee. The patella and the proximal fibula are also sites of tumors. When a tumor is discovered, the patient should be thoroughly evaluated. The anatomic extent and activity of the lesion should be evaluated. For lesions that have a risk of being malignant, a search for metastatic foci should be completed. Only after a thorough evaluation should a biopsy be performed, and it should be performed with care to ensure that future surgical options are not eliminated. The surgical reconstruction options available are numerous, and the patient and the surgeon must select the one most appropriate for the situation.

(Work related to allograft has been supported in part through National Institutes of Health Grant AR 21896.)

REFERENCES

1. Bentley G, McAuliffe T: Pigmented villonodular synovitis. Ann Rheum Dis 49:210–211, 1990.
2. Bloem JL, Mudler JD: Chondroblastoma: a clinical and radiological study of 104 cases. Skeletal Radiol 14:1–9, 1985.
3. Bovill DF, Skinner HB: Unicameral bone cysts: a comparison of treatment options. Orthop Rev 18:420–427, 1989.
4. Campanacci M, Baldini N, Boriani S, Sudanese A: Giant cell tumor of bone. J Bone Joint Surg 69:106–114, 1987.
5. Campanacci M, Cervellati C, Donati U: Autogenous patella as replacement for a resected femoral or tibial condyle: a report on 19 cases. J Bone Joint Surg 67B:557–563, 1985.
6. Campanacci M, Costa P: Total resection of the distal femur or proximal tibia for bone tumors: autogenous bone grafts and arthrodesis in twenty-six cases. J Bone Joint Surg 61B:455–463, 1979.

7. Capanna R, Guerra A, Ruggieri P, et al: The Kotz modular prosthesis in massive osteoarticular resections for bone tumors: preliminary results in 27 cases. Ital J Orthop Traumatol 11:271–281, 1985.
8. Chao EY: A composite fixation principle for modular segmental defect replacement (SDR) prosthesis. Orthop Clin North Am 20:439–453, 1989.
9. Clark BE, Xipell JM, Thomas DP: Benign fibrous histiocytoma of bone. Am J Surg Pathol 9:806–815, 1985.
10. Coolican MR, Dandy DJ: Arthroscopic management of synovial chondromatosis of the knee: findings and results in 18 cases. J Bone Joint Surg 71B:498–500, 1989.
11. Coster E, Van Tiggelen R, Shahabpour M, et al: Osteoblastoma of the patella: case report and review of the literature. Clin Orthop 243:216–219, 1989.
12. Dahlin DC: Bone Tumors, 3rd ed. Springfield, IL: Charles C Thomas, 1978.
13. Eckardt JJ, Grogan TJ: Giant cell tumor of bone. Clin Orthop 204:45–58, 1986.
14. Enneking WF: Musculoskeletal Tumor Surgery. New York: Churchill Livingston, 1983.
15. Enneking WF, Shirley PD: Resection arthrodesis for malignant and potentially malignant lesions about the knee using an intermedullary rod and local bone grafts. J Bone Joint Surg 59A:223–236, 1977.
16. Fineschi G, Schiavone-Panni A: Free patellar graft for the reconstruction of juxtaarticular defects in the treatment of giant-cell tumors. Clin Orthop 256:197–204, 1990.
17. Flandry F, McCann SB, Hughston JC, Kurtz DM: Roentgenographic findings in pigmented villonodular synovitis of the knee. Clin Orthop 247:208–219, 1989.
18. Franssen MJ, Boerbooms AM, Karthaus RP, et al: Treatment of pigmented villonodular synovitis of the knee with yttrium-90 silicate: prospective evaluations by arthroscopy, histology, and 99mTc pertechnetate uptake measurements. Ann Rheum Dis 48:1007–1013, 1989.
19. Gebhardt MC, Ready JE, Mankin HJ: Tumors about the knee in children. Clin Orthop 255:86–110, 1990.
20. Heare TC, Enneking WF, Heare MM: Staging techniques and biopsy of bone tumors. Orthop Clin North Am 20:273–285, 1989.
21. Jacobs PA: Limb salvage and rotationplasty for osteosarcoma in children. Clin Orthop 188:217–222, 1984.
22. Jacobs PA, Clemency RE Jr: The closed cryosurgical treatment of giant cell tumor. Clin Orthop 192:149–158, 1985.
23. Joyce MJ, Mankin HJ: Caveat arthroscopos: extra-articular lesions of bone simulating intra-articular patholog of the knee. J Bone Joint Surg 65A:289–292, 1983.
24. Kotz R, Ritschl P, Trachtenbrodt J: A modular femur-tibia reconstruction system. Orthopaedics 9:1639–1652, 1986.
25. Krajbich JI, Caroll NC: Van Nes rotationplasty with segmental limb resection. Clin Orthop 256:7–13, 1990.
26. Kransdorf MJ, Moser RP, Vinh TN, et al: Primary tumors of the patella: a review of 42 cases. Skeletal Radiol 18:365–371, 1989.
27. Makley JT, Joyce MJ: Unicameral bone cyst (simple bone cyst). Orthop Clin North Am 20:407–415, 1989.
28. Malawer MM, McHale KA: Limb-sparing surgery for high-grade malignant tumors of the proximal tibia: surgical technique and a method of extensor mechanism reconstruction. Clin Orthop 239:231–248, 1989.
29. Mankin HJ, Gebhardt MC, Tomford WW: The use of frozen cadaveric allografts in the management of patients with bone tumors of the extremities. Orth Clin North Am 18:275–289, 1987.
30. Mankin HJ, Lange TA, Spanier, SS: The hazards of biopsy in patients with malignant primary bone and soft tissue tumors. J Bone Joint Surg 64:1121–1127, 1982.
31. Marcove RC: Chondrosarcoma: diagnosis and treatment. Orthop Clin North Am 8:811–820, 1977.
32. Marcove RC: A 17-year review of cryosurgery in the treatment of bone tumors. Clin Orthop 163:231–234, 1982.
33. Marcove RC, Rosen G: En bloc resections for osteogenic sarcoma. Cancer 45:3040–3044, 1978.
34. Marcove RC, Weis LD, Vaghaiwalla MR, et al: Cryosurgery in the treatment of giant cell tumors of bone: a report of 52 consecutive cases. Cancer 41:957–969, 1978.
35. Martinez V, Sissons HA: Aneurysmal bone cyst: a review of 123 cases including primary lesions and those secondary to other bone pathology. Cancer 61:2291–2304, 1988.
36. Maurice H, Crone M, Watt I: Synovial chondromatosis. J Bone Joint Surg 70B:807–811, 1988.
37. McDonald DJ, Sim FH, McLeod RA, Dahlin DC: Giant cell tumor of bone. J Bone Joint Surg 68A:235–242, 1986.
38. Milgram JW: The origins of osteochondromas and enchondromas. A histopathologic study. Clin Orthop 174:264–284, 1983.
39. Mirra JM, Gold R, Downs J, Eckardt JJ: A new histologic approach to the differentiation

of enchondroma and chondrosarcoma of the bones: a clinicopathologic analysis of 51 cases. Clin Orthop 201:214–237, 1985.

40. Morton KS: Aneurysmal bone cyst: a review of 26 cases. Can J Surg 29:110–115, 1986.
41. Parrish FF: Allograft replacement of all or part of the end of a tumor: report of twenty-one cases. J Bone Joint Surg 55A:1–22, 1973.
42. Schwartz HS, Frassica FJ, Sim FH: Rotationplasty: an option for limb salvage in childhood osteosarcoma. Orthopaedics 12:257–263, 1989.
43. Sim FH, Beauchamp CP, Chao EY: Reconstruction of musculoskeletal defects about the knee for tumor. Clin Orthop 221:188–201, 1987.
44. Sim FH, Ivins JC, Taylor WF, et al: Limb-sparing surgery of osteosarcoma: Mayo Clinic experience. Cancer Treatment Symposia 3:139–154, 1985.
45. Springfield DS, Capanna R, Gherlinzoni F, et al: Chondroblastoma: a review of seventy cases. J Bone Joint Surg 67A:748–755, 1985.
46. Steinbach LS, Neumann CH, Stoller DW, et al: MRI of the knee in diffuse pigmented villonodular synovitis. Clin Imaging 13:305–316, 1989.
47. Tomford WW, Doppelt SH, Mankin HJ, et al: 1983 bone bank procedure. Clin Orthop 174:15–21, 1983.
48. Tsahakis PJ, Shortkroi S, Boyd AD, et al: Personal communications, Boston, MA, November 1991.

CHAPTER 9

Osteochondral Allografts for Reconstruction of Articular Defects

JOHN C. GARRETT, M.D.

■

Osteochondral mini-grafts can be used to reconstruct large articular defects resulting from trauma, arthritis, and osteochondritis dissecans. Grafts are transplanted fresh in order to preserve chondrocyte viability and minimize histologic degeneration. Rejection is minimal, which thus negates the need for tissue typing and immunosuppression. Grafts are most useful when there is a single focal defect, the ideal case being osteochondritis dissecans and cases of malunion after tibial plateau fracture (Fig. 9–1).

Large craters in the articular surface occur as the result of trauma or osteochondritis dissecans. When lesions occur in young patients, are less than 2 cm in diameter (4 cm in cross-sectional area), and have firm rims of articular cartilage, abrasion arthroplasty or Pridie spongialization may result in reasonable filling with fibrous tissue, although the resultant surfaces may be concave in comparison with a femoral condyle, which is normally convex.[3] The lamina splendans and collagen arcades of normal articular cartilage are absent; instead, a carpet of fibrous tissue or fibro-cartilage with type I rather than the type II collagen of hyaline cartilage, often rough or fissured on microscopic examination, is present from subchondral bone to the surface. Once covered with fibrous tissue, these lesions remain clinically "silent," at least initially.

In comparison with normal articular cartilage, the fibrous tissue may prove fragile, and accelerated arthritic changes may result, and so it is difficult to accept grafting these cases even as ones of qualified success. However, trouble abounds with lesions larger than 2 cm in diameter (4 cm^2 in cross sectional area), especially those on markedly convex surfaces, those with poor surrounding rims of articular cartilage, those in older

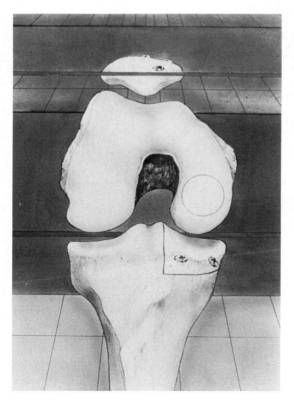

FIGURE 9–1. Osteochondral allografts: Femoral condyle, tibial plateau, and patella.

patients, or those in patients who have failed to produce adequate fibrous tissue after one or more attempts at abrasion arthroplasty. Pain, buckling, and swelling are common, and arthritis with joint space narrowing occurs in an accelerated fashion.

An alternative treatment before significant abrasion of the meniscus and contralateral articular surface occurs[1, 7] is to patch with an osteochondral graft.[5, 6, 11] Although some surgeons advocate use of heterotopic autogenous grafts from the knee,[17] these leave a secondary defect that in turn is symptomatic. In addition, they are improperly matched in terms of thickness, compliance, and surface contour. No prosthesis that mimics the characteristics of articular cartilage is currently available. Metallic implants are too hard and result in accelerated wear. Plastic implants are too soft and generate debris. In the distant future, transplantation of periosteum or populations of chondrocytes directly into the defect may offer an alternative, but whether these will reestablish the normal microscopic architecture of articular cartilage is uncertain.

The current established alternative is an osteochondral allograft. This type of graft has been used to replace defects left after resection for benign and low-grade malignant tumors (Fig. 9–2).[12, 14, 15] When a distal femur or a proximal tibia is excised en bloc, a massive allograft is implanted. Such extensive transplantation procedures are beset with a multitude of problems: sizing, balancing of collateral ligaments, and cruciate ligament reconstruction. Fracture and collapse are common postoperatively. Nevertheless, it has been demonstrated that articular cartilage survives, and when smaller grafts are used, many of these technical and postoperative problems can be circumvented. Since 1970, Alan Gross has made extensive use of these smaller, so-called mini grafts, paving the way for their use in reconstructive surgery.[16]

MECHANICS FOR OSTEOCHONDRAL ALLOGRAFTS

Osteochondral allografts are used to reconstruct articular segments lost as the result of trauma or osteochondritis dissecans. They have a lesser role in treatment of degenerative disease. The ideal candidate is a patient with a single focal defect but an otherwise healthy knee. Osteochondritis dissecans in a young person represents the ideal case. A solitary defect is present; the surrounding cartilage is sound and has a normal life span, and the menisci and the ligaments are intact. Unfortunately, most cases of trauma are far from ideal for osteochondral allografts. In many patients, more than one articular surface is damaged, menisci are lost, ligaments are disrupted, and significant arthrofibrosis is present. Nevertheless, articular grafts may improve such knees. In contrast is the development of focal changes as the result of degenerative disease or cartilage delamination. The typical patient is middle-aged. The surrounding articular cartilage is prone to progressive delamination or degeneration. In spite of a successful osteochondral allograft, the remainder of the knee may deteriorate, negating an initial success.

IMMUNOLOGY

Many scientists believe that articular cartilage, like heart valves and the cornea, is "immunologically privileged."[4, 8, 9, 10] Humoral and cell-directed

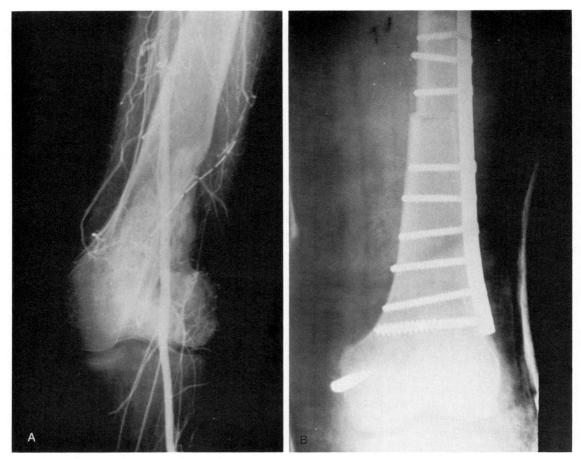

FIGURE 9–2. Of historic interest: classical large osteochondral graft for treatment of benign tumors. *(A)* Eighteen-year-old female with recurrent giant cell tumor of the femur. *(B)* Replacement with cryopreserved osteochondral allograft. (Courtesy of Henry J. Mankin, Massachusetts General Hospital, Boston, Massachusetts.)

antibodies are produced, but the rejection process is weak, presumably because antibodies are filtered out by the ground substance and fail to reach their target, the chondrocyte. Thus tissue typing is irrelevant, and immunologic suppression is unnecessary. A contrary view is held by a minority of physicians who believe that divergence in genetic matching adversely affects the fate of osteochondral allografts. Similarly, transplantation of bone is associated with an immunologic response. Fresh specimens are more reactive than frozen or denatured specimens, but the reaction is slight and thought to be clinically insignificant. The fact that thousands of allografts of bones are used each year argues against an overwhelming problem in this regard.

FRESH VERSUS FROZEN GRAFTS

Articular grafts are most effective when transplanted fresh. Viable chondrocytes are required for replenishing the ground substance within the graft and for maintaining the microscopic architecture of healthy articular surface (Fig. 9–3). If kept in tissue culture medium at 4°C, articular graft

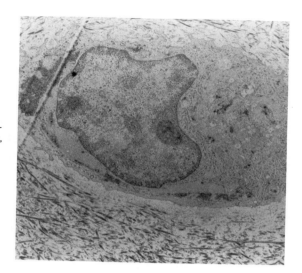

FIGURE 9–3. Chondrocyte with surrounding matrix of collagen and ground substance. (Courtesy of Charles Weiss, Miami, Florida.)

chondrocytes remain viable for 7 days; a significant decline in viability occurs thereafter. Frozen grafts demonstrate deterioration with fissuring or delamination, fibrosis, and wholesale breakdown of the surface.[16] When large segments of grafts are needed for replacement after tumor resection, such degeneration may be acceptable, but when mini grafts are used, excellence of the articular surface is required for a good result. The alternative of cryopreservation, typically with dimethyl sulfoxide, is theoretically promising but currently has a limited success rate.

TRANSPLANTATION: MICROSCOPIC ANATOMY

With transplantation, there is an implicit desire to restore normal anatomic structure in the osteochondral void. The anatomic structure of the articular cartilage has been extensively studied and noted to be complex. The horizontally directed collagen network of the lamina splendans and the microscopic rugae yield a relatively smooth surface that appears to be designed for gliding. Beneath is a series of collagen arcades, which are believed to function in load bearing. The arcades are linked to subchondral bone at the tidemark area, providing firm fixation of the articular cartilage to the underlying bony skeleton. Depending on the site, articular segments vary in thickness and compliance as well as in orientation of their surface grooves. Degeneration occurs with age; the water content changes, and fissuring develops. Thus transplantation with young, viable cartilage grafts is preferable to that with older grafts.

THE OSTEOCHONDRAL UNIT

Because transplantation of a cartilaginous cap alone does not result in bonding to the skeleton, cartilage is transplanted with an underlying plate of bone as an osteochondral unit (see Fig. 9–9). The underlying bone of the osteochondral unit is used initially as the attachment vehicle and is soon replaced by creeping substitution. Additional bone is necessary anyway for filling the void left after traumatic loss or, as in the case of osteochondritis dissecans, after resection of sclerotic bone and fibrous tissue beneath the osteochondral fragment.

MATCHING

Three factors are important in matching donors with recipients: age, size, and articular site. As with transplantation of other tissues, knee tissue from a young donor is preferred over that from an older donor. Significant surface defects in articular cartilage often occur by the fifth or sixth decade. In an attempt to match surface contour and provide adequate graft material, donors must be matched according to size. Discrepancies of less than 5 per cent are considered reasonable. Finally, isotopic transplantation with articular cartilage of similar height compliance and contour is appealing; however, subtle problems abound, especially in osteochondritis dissecans, in which the defective condyle often assumes a mushroom shape. On occasion, a donor graft or a heterotopic site that is larger than the recipient's site may be the best compromise for a graft.

SCREENING

Donors are screened in a multifactorial process according to the guidelines of the American Association of Tissue Banks.[2] The process begins with a careful social history in order to rule out groups at high risk for HIV infection, including intravenous drug users, prostitutes, runaways, and homosexual persons. It continues with a medical history in order to rule out donors with systemic disease including infection, neoplasia, and degenerative disease. Blood is screened for syphilis, types B and C hepatitis, and human immunodeficiency virus–related disease; the screening includes antigen and antibody testing. Donor tissues are cultured for bacterial and fungal infection. Finally, autopsy with lymph node evaluation is performed.

HARVESTING

Harvesting is performed under sterile operating room conditions immediately after the kidneys, the heart, and the lungs have been removed and life-support systems terminated. Knees are often excised en bloc from midfemur to midtibia, and ligaments and the capsule are included. Contrariwise, they may be divided immediately to accommodate multiple transplant needs, including femoral condyles, menisci, the tibial plateau, and ligaments. Specimens are preserved in sterile tissue culture solution at 4°C until transplantation occurs. Reasonable chondrocyte viability can be preserved for 7 days.

TRANSPLANT REGISTRY

As is the case with soft organ transplants, a number of patients at any given center typically await knee tissue transplantation. Requirements may differ according to age, size, and specific deficits. For instance, articular segments may be required alone or in conjunction with menisci and ligaments. Once the donor tissue has been identified and properly matched, the recipient is brought to the transplant site for the procedure. Because of modern air transportation, this can usually be achieved within a day or two. Transplantation can be performed during normal operating room hours when the usual complement of personnel are available.

OPERATIVE PROCEDURE

TIBIAL PLATEAU

Transplantation of the tibial plateau and the adjoining meniscus is commonly performed for malunion that follows fracture. The ideal case is an isolated tibial plateau fracture. Damage to the femoral condyles or to the contralateral tibial plateau or rupture of the cruciate or collateral ligaments may compromise an otherwise good result. The most amenable cases are those with 1 cm or less of depression. More depression or devitalization of large segments of the proximal tibia as a result of previous surgery may undermine the base of support or necessitate extremely thick grafts; both of these factors potentiate collapse.

The lateral tibial plateau is most commonly involved and may be approached through a lateral parapatellar incision. Osteotomy of the tibial tubercle allows for medial reflection of the patella and yields excellent exposure. External tibial guides used in total knee replacement are useful for resection of the tibia, which is cut parallel to the normal articular surface. The medial extent of the resection is the lateral margin of the anterior cruciate ligament. The donor material with menisci, including the anterior and posterior meniscotibial attachments, is cut according to size to fit with the knee both in extension and in flexion. Fixation is achieved with the use of multiple, obliquely oriented 4.0-mm AO cancellous screws driven through the corners of the graft into the proximal tibial metaphysis. Three or four screws typically are used in order to afford solid fixation and enable early range of motion (Fig. 9–4). The tibial tubercle is reattached with 6.5-mm AO cancellous screws, and closure is accomplished in a standard fashion.

FEMORAL CONDYLES

In osteochondritis dissecans, defects of the femoral condyles are typically round. Defects of the medial femoral condyle are 2.0 to 2.5 cm in diameter, but those of the lateral condyle are up to 3.0 cm in diameter and sometimes even larger. The standard replacement of the lesions up to 3.0 cm in diameter involves use of a set of instruments designed by the Concept Corporation (Fig. 9–5) that are similar to Cloward tools in appearance and function. For lesions wider in diameter, especially in the case of the giant lesions of osteochondritis dissecans of the far posterior aspect of the lateral femoral condyle, full-width segments of a condyle may be required.

With standard lesions the aim is to drill a cylindrical hole into the condyle removing all fibrous tissue and sclerotic bone in order to leave a healthy base. The defect is replaced with a plug of articular cartilage of similar dimensions. The orientation of the axis of the cylindrical hole is

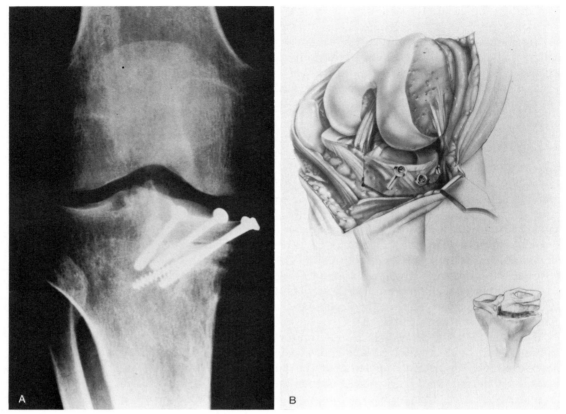

FIGURE 9–4. *(A)* Treatment of malunion after tibial plateau fracture with osteochondral allograft and attached meniscus. The meniscus is transplanted en bloc with meniscotibial ligaments and the attached tibial plateau. The height of the tibial plateau graft is dependent on the amount of depression of the tibial plateau fracture. *(B)* Fixation is achieved with insertion of multiple 4.0-mm AO cancellous screws inserted obliquely through the tibial plateau just below the joint line.

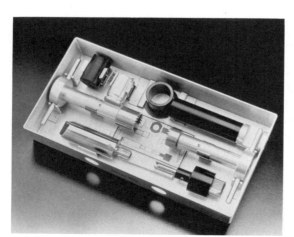

FIGURE 9–5. Instruments designed by the Concept Corporation for use with osteochondral transplantation for defects from 1.0 to 3.0 cm in diameter.

matched with that of the donor plug (Fig. 9–6A). This is achieved with a cylindrical guide, placed over the defect (Fig. 9–6B). A guide wire is driven down through the guide, into the center of the defect (Figs. 9–6C, 9–6D). A hand-powered device is used to sharply cut through the articular cartilage without creating undue torque, which might disrupt the bond between surrounding articular cartilage and underlying bone (Fig. 9–7). The bony base is then augered with a Cloward-type device until normal trabeculae and punctate hemorrhage, which are indicative of viable bone, appear. This results in a defect 4- to 5-mm deep.

The defect is matched with the corresponding portion of the donor femoral condyle (Fig. 9–8A). Templates made of dental wax are of benefit for locating the exact site for transplantation (Fig. 9–8B). In other cases, the disparity between the size or the contour of the femoral condyles or distortion of the recipient femoral condyle by osteochondritis dissecans may necessitate the use of a more distant site. A segment of the donor tissue, including the specific portion to be used in the transplant, is removed and steadied within a jig (Figs. 9–9A to 9–9C). In this manner, proper orientation to the articular surface can be established with the use of a second cylindrical guide. The jig firmly grips the donor material, resisting the torque of power drills. First the articular surface is cut with a hand-twisted instrument in order to minimize shear between the articular cartilage and the underlying bone. Then the bone is cut with a device similar to a Cloward plug cutter. The result is a cylindrical specimen of articular cartilage and underlying bone (Fig. 9–9D).

The defect is measured according to depth and care taken to match the donor plug with this void (Fig. 9–10A). The plug typically is inserted several times in order to evaluate the fit. If proud, the bone of the plug can be shaved with an oscillating saw. If excess bone has been removed, height can be regained by packing bone shavings beneath the graft. The graft is affixed with Herbert screws. There is invariably a 1- or 2-mm difference between one segment of the graft and the surrounding femoral condyle. This difference can be minimized with the compressive effect of the Herbert screws, which effectively warp a thin graft and depress an otherwise proud edge. Herbert screws are countersunk sufficiently to enable early range of motion without compromising later removal (Fig. 9–10B). When necessary, meniscal and anterior cruciate ligament reconstruction is performed concomitantly.

After surgery, a continuous passive motion machine is used to enhance motion and facilitate nutrition of the articular graft. With small grafts, weight bearing probably can be initiated immediately. With those 3 cm or more in diameter, weight bearing is restricted for 6 weeks, after which roentgenographs typically reveal healing in the surrounding femoral condyle. Eight to ten weeks after transplantation, the Herbert screws are removed, and the articular graft is inspected for viability. In the case of transplantation of the tibial plateau, screws rarely must be removed, but weight bearing is restricted longer in order to enable these grafts to heal and be incorporated so as to minimize the chance of fracture or collapse during the revascularization process. Four to six months typically suffices. Vigorous athletic activity is restricted for 6 months after a femoral condylar graft and for 12 months after a tibial plateau graft. The intensity of subsequent activity depends on the size of the graft. No strict criteria are available, but sports such as tennis and softball are permitted, whereas

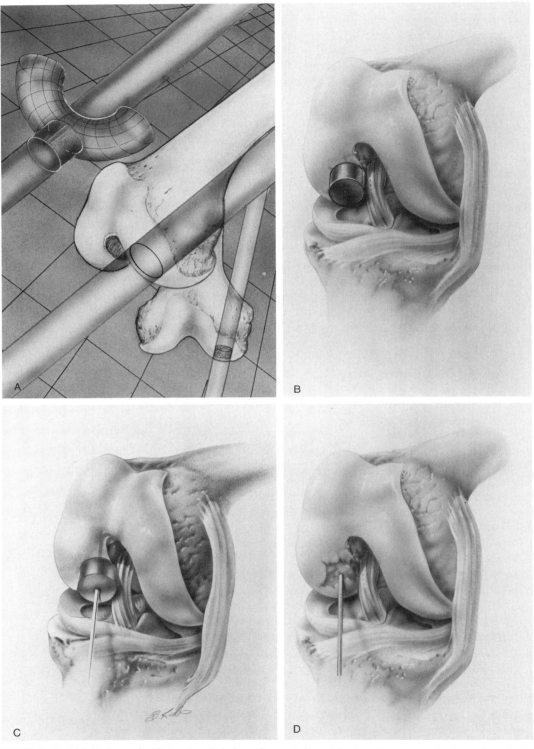

FIGURE 9–6. *(A)* Articular grafts. Osteochondral allografts are designed for insertion perpendicular to the articular surface. *(B)* Cylindrical guide. *(C, D)* Cylindrical guide with K-wire placed over the defect to facilitate orientation of the K-wire perpendicular to the surface of the defect.

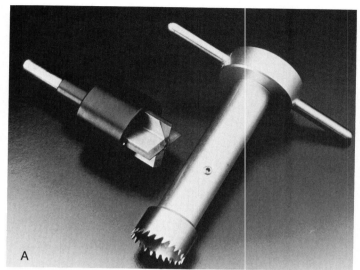

A

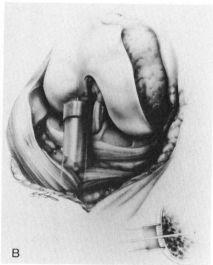

B

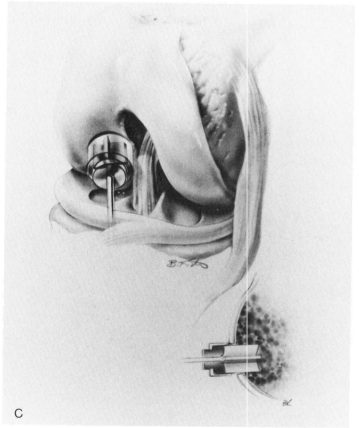

C

FIGURE 9–7. Devices used to cut the articular cartilage. Right-hand–powered device used to minimize torsion and sheer forces that might otherwise delaminate the articular cartilage from the underlying bone. (A) Cannulated plug cutting device used to cut the subchondral bone. (B) Hand-driven device used to cut the articular cartilage. (C) Power-driven device used to cut the articular cartilage.

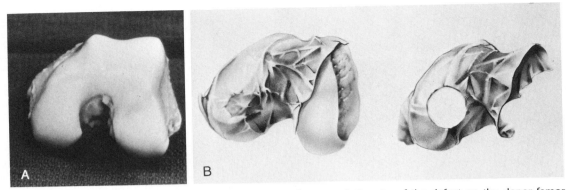

FIGURE 9–8. *(A)* Donor femur. *(B)* Template used for transfer to mark the site of the defect on the donor femoral condyle.

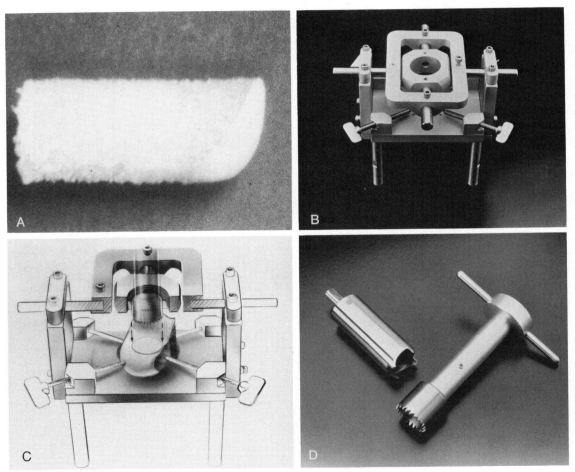

FIGURE 9–9. *(A)* Osteochondral unit with articular cartilage and underlying cancellous bone, which is used as an attachment vehicle. *(B)* Jig used to hold the donor femoral condyle and direct the cutting devices. *(C)* Jig holding donor femoral condyle. *(D) Left:* Plug cutting device used with power to cut the subchondral bone. *Right:* Hand-driver device used to minimize torsion and sheer forces on the articular cartilage, which otherwise might cause delamination from the underlying bone.

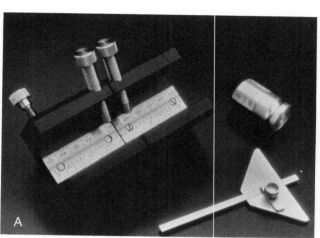
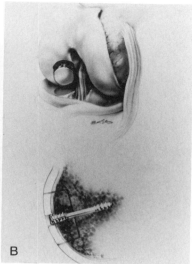

FIGURE 9–10. *(A)* Instruments for measuring depth of condylar defect and height of osteochondral graft. *(B)* After the osteochondral graft has been properly cut according to depth, it is inserted and fixed with multiple Herbert screws, which are countersunk below the articular surface.

long-distance running and basketball are typically discouraged (Figs. 9–11 to 9–15).

FACTORS AFFECTING SUCCESS OF AN OSTEOCHONDRAL ALLOGRAFT

The fit and the congruence of a graft transplanted into a condyle are easy to appreciate visually but difficult to quantify precisely. Ablating surrounding articular irregularities and creating flush margins minimizes abrasive wear, cutting, plowing, and filing. Restoring normal congruence of the femoral condyle with material of similar stiffness optimizes weight-bearing characteristics, and realigning the microscopic rugae of the graft with those of the femoral condyle enhances gliding characteristics. Grafts undoubtedly work best in knees with a meniscus and a normal opposing articular surface. When necessary, menisci can be transplanted concomitantly with osteochondral allografts.

Degenerative changes of the opposing articular surface and fibrotic degeneration elsewhere within the knee compromise overall function irrespective of their effect on the graft itself and are to be avoided. Malalignment, which might adversely affect the graft, should be corrected with osteotomy (Fig. 9–16). Small grafts, especially those buried within a femoral condyle, are probably protected by the surrounding rims of the femoral condyle. If collapse begins, the majority of the force is subsequently applied to the surrounding condyle, and therefore collapse is minimized and angulation does not develop. In contrast, collapse of graft that does not have a surrounding protective collar, as in the case of a tibial plateau, may lead to angulatory deformity, which by itself increases forces on the graft, thereby accelerating collapse.

Osteochondral allografts are currently being used in the United States

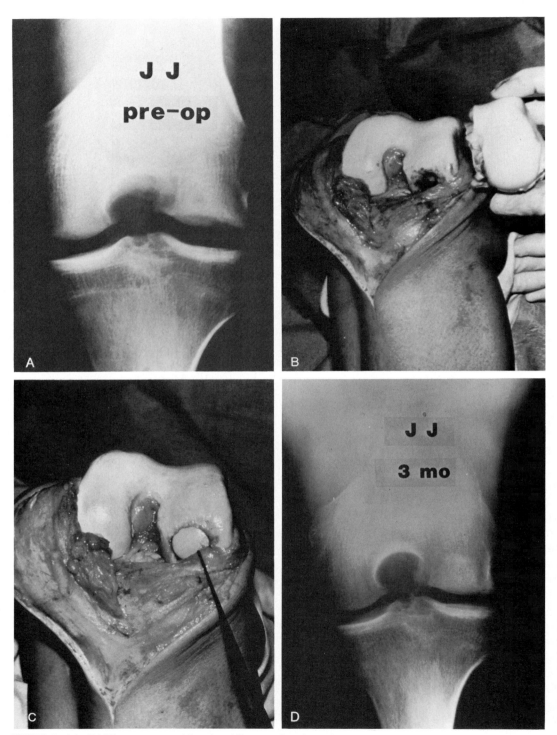

FIGURE 9–11. *(A)* Nineteen-year-old male with osteochondritis dissecans of the lateral femoral condyle. The patient had undergone multiple arthroscopic procedures for removal of loose bodies and was left with a 2-cm defect. *(B)* Defect noted at the time of surgery. Note adjacent osteochondral allograft, which came from an 18-year-old donor matched according to skeletal size. *(C)* Osteochondral allograft inserted. *(D)* Radiographs taken 3 months after surgery.

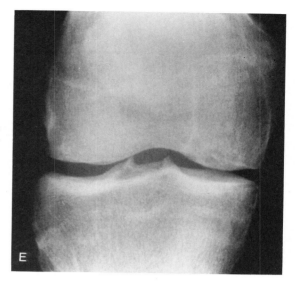

FIGURE 9–11. *Continued. (E)* Radiographs taken 7 years after osteochondral allograft. Arthroscopy revealed an intact graft.

and abroad for a variety of lesions. The overall success rate with fresh small-fragment grafts regardless of the diagnosis has been 77 per cent at 2 to 10 years, as reported by Meyers and associates.[13] Gross and colleagues reported similar success with transplant of the tibial plateau.[6] Collapse of more than 3 mm in diameter was noted in only two of 12 patients who were followed longer than 2 years; when rated according to pain and function, 10 of the 12 grafts were noted to be improved. In general, monopolar grafts (tibial or femoral grafts alone) were more successful than bipolar grafts (tibial and femoral grafts combined). In the author's

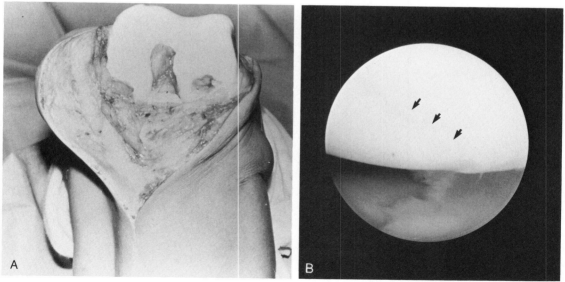

FIGURE 9–12. *(A)* Thirty-seven-year-old male with osteochondritis dissecans of the lateral femoral condyle. A 2.5-cm chondral defect remained after three operations, extraction of loose bodies, and abrasion arthroplasty. *(B)* Photograph taken 2 years after osteochondral allograft of lateral femoral condyle. Note flush margins of the graft (outlined by *arrows*).

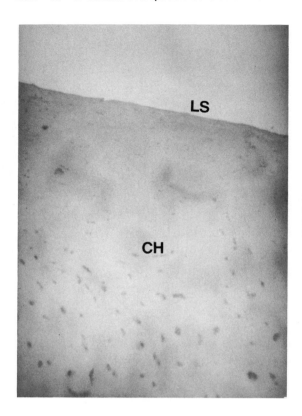

FIGURE 9–13. Biopsy 5 years after 2.5-cm osteochondral allograft of the medial femoral condyle in a 21-year-old male. Note normal lamina splendans and viable chondrocytes.

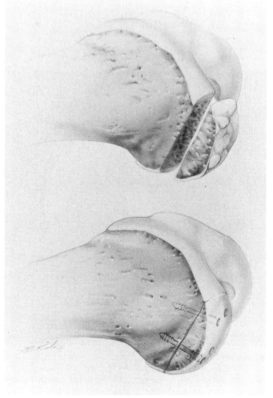

FIGURE 9–14. Alternative technique for a gigantic osteochondral defect of the far posterior aspect of the lateral femoral condyle. The entire condyle was replaced with a crescent-shaped graft fixed with Herbert screws.

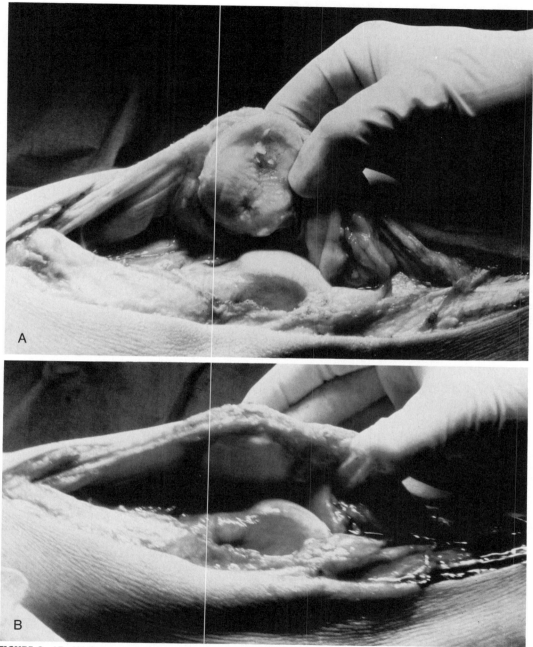

FIGURE 9–15. (A) Osteochondral resurfacing of the patella in a 39-year-old male with severe chondromalacia of the patella but a normal trochlea. (B) Photograph taken after osteochondral allograft of the entire undersurface of the patella.

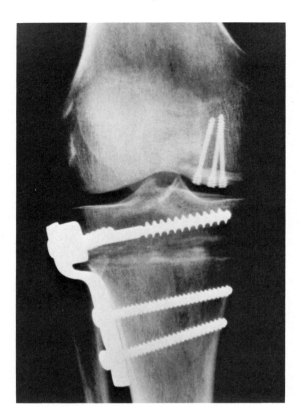

FIGURE 9–16. Osteochondral graft to medial femoral condyle combined with tibial osteotomy to correct varus deformity.

experience, specifically with osteochondritis dissecans, there has been only one case of a failure out of 40 transplants that were followed for 1 to 6 years. This remains the ideal indication for transplant. Treatment of patients for unicompartmental arthritis has been of limited success. Transplantation of populations of chondrocytes alone may prove to be a useful compromise when fresh grafts of proper size and shape are not available.

In the future, cryopreservatives may ensure that an ample supply of transplants is constantly available, obviating the long delays that currently are required in order to locate a proper donor.

REFERENCES

1. Almård LE, Wikstad I: Late results of surgery for osteochondritis dissecans of the knee joint. Acta Chir Scand 127:588–596, 1964.
2. American Association of Tissue Banks: Guidelines for the banking of musculoskeletal tissue. Am Assoc Tissue Banks Newsletter 3:2, 1979.
3. Casscells SW: Lesions of the articular cartilage. *In* Arthroscopy: Diagnostic and Surgical Practice, pp. 29–36. Philadelphia: Lea and Febiger, 1984.
4. Elves MW: Newer knowledge of the immunology of bone and cartilage. Clin Orthop 120:232–249, 1979.
5. Garrett JC: Treatment of osteochondral defects of the distal femur with fresh osteochondral allografts: a preliminary report. Arthroscopy 2:222–226, 1986.
6. Gross AE, McKee NH, Pritzker KPH, Langer F: Reconstruction of skeletal deficits at the knee: A comprehensive osteochondral transplant program. Clin Orthop 174:96–106, 1983.
7. Hughston JC, Hergenroeder PT, Courtnay BG: Osteochondritis dissecans of the femoral condyles. J Bone Joint Surg 66A:1340–1348, 1984.

8. Langer F, Czitrom A, Pritzker KP, et al: The immunogenicity of fresh and frozen allogeneic bone. J Bone Joint Surg 57A:216–220, 1975.
9. Langer F, Gross AE: Immunogenicity of allograft articular cartilage. J Bone Joint Surg 56A:297–304, 1974.
10. Langer F, Gross AE, West M, Urovitz EP: The immunogenicity of allograft knee joint transplants. Clin Orthop 132:155–162, 1978.
11. Locht R, Gross A, Langer F: Late osteochondral allograft resurfacing for tibial plateau fractures. J Bone Joint Surg 66A:328–335, 1984.
12. Mankin HJ, Doppelt S, Tomford WW: Clinical experience with allograft implantation: The first ten years. Clin Orthop 174:69–86, 1983.
13. Meyers MH, Akeson W, Convery FR: Resurfacing of the knee with fresh osteochondral allograft. J Bone Joint Surg 71A:704–713, 1989.
14. Ottolenghi CE: Massive osteo and osteo-articular bone grafts: technic and results of 62 cases. Clin Orthop 87:156–164, 1972.
15. Parrish FF: Allograft replacement of all or part of the end of a long bone following excision of a tumor. J Bone Joint Surg 55A:1–22, 1973.
16. Tomford WW, Henry WB, Trahan CA, Mankin HJ: The fate of allograft articular cartilage: fresh and frozen. Transactions of the 30th Annual Meeting of the Orthopaedic Research Society, February 6–9, 1984, p. 217. Chicago: Orthopaedic Research Society, 1984.
17. Yamashita F, Sakakida K, Suzu F, Takai S: The transplantation of an autogeneic osteochondral fragment for osteochondritis dissecans of the knee. Clin Orthop 201:43–50, 1985.

CHAPTER 10

Infectious and Inflammatory Processes of the Knee

J. ANDY SULLIVAN, M.D.

■

This chapter deals with the inflammatory and infectious problems of the knee. The most common conditions affecting the knee are described, and references are given for a more detailed review.[7, 15] The various disorders are discussed along with the means of making the diagnosis, the differential diagnosis that must be considered, and an overview of treatment.

Inflammation about the knee has a different clinical spectrum in the child than in the adult. Some of the same disease processes occur; however, the manifestations and clinical history are at times dissimilar, and the processes that must be included in the differential diagnosis are somewhat different. Although there are similarities between the child and the adult, it is best to consider them independently.

INFECTIOUS ARTHRITIS

Septic Arthritis in Childhood

Synovium is an extremely vascular tissue. The cells composing the synovium produce synovial fluid, which is essentially a transudate of serum. Thus the joint provides a closed space and nutrition, which constitute an ideal medium for a bacterial infection.

Once a bacterial infection establishes itself, deleterious effects on the articular cartilage occur. The white blood cells that enter the joint in an attempt to contain the infection release enzymes that have a degradative effect on cartilage matrix and collagen. In addition, some bacteria also produce proteases that can destroy articular cartilage. Early diagnosis and prompt treatment are the keys to adequate treatment and the prevention of long-term morbidity.

In most instances, the means by which the bacteria reach the joint are unknown. A few cases of infection do result from penetration of the joint by a foreign body. Most infections are probably borne by blood, and the reasons for their seeding in the joint are unknown.[9] In children the source of the infection can be otitis media, upper respiratory tract infection, or skin infection.

HISTORY. Children with septic arthritis of the knee usually have a history of pain, limp, and refusal to walk. It is not unusual for the child to have been seen by another physician and to be already receiving some type of antibiotic therapy for another infection. There may be a history of fever, general malaise and systemic signs of infection.

PHYSICAL EXAMINATION. Clinical examination usually reveals very limited motion that is exceedingly painful. The knee is held in flexion and may have a tense effusion. Careful examination should reveal that the effusion and the pain are in the knee joint itself. It must be established that the swelling is actually a knee effusion and not a prepatellar bursitis. The examiner must also carefully look for point tenderness in the distal femoral and proximal tibial metaphyses, which indicates acute osteomyelitis. In the remainder of the clinical examination, involvement of other joints should be ruled out. Other sources of infection should be sought, and in the young child, the examiner must carefully seek signs of meningeal irritation.

DIAGNOSTIC TESTS. Initial laboratory should include plain radiographs, a complete blood cell count, and a measuring of sedimentation rate. The sedimentation rate becomes elevated several days after onset of the infection and increases during the early course of the disease until the process begins to be contained, either by the host or by antibiotic treatment. Although the white blood cell count and the sedimentation rate are important, they can be variable, particularly in the young child and the neonate.[9, 10] The sedimentation rate is more often elevated but may also be unreliable in the neonate and is of no value in patients with sickle cell disease.

Plain radiographs should be obtained. Although they may show only soft tissue swelling, they may be of value in the differential diagnosis of a sympathetic effusion from acute, epiphyseal, or subacute osteomyelitis. They can also be diagnostic in cases of tumor or the presence of a foreign body.

Scintigraphy with technetium 99m (^{99m}Tc) phosphate is rarely indicated and not often needed for making the diagnosis of septic arthritis of the knee. It may be beneficial in cases in which the diagnosis of septic arthritis is in question or in arriving at other diagnoses such as osteomyelitis, either acute or subacute. In review of nuclear scanning in orthopaedic infections, Sullivan and colleagues found a 77 per cent accuracy rate, with three false-positive and five false-negative results.[27] Sundberg and associates found that only 13 per cent of children with proved septic arthritis had correct "blind" scan interpretation.[28] When compared with clinical findings, the scan still did not identify septic arthritis in 30 per cent of the patients and incorrectly identified septic arthritis in 32 per cent of children with no evidence of the disease.

Aspiration of a joint remains the simplest, least expensive, and most direct means of making a diagnosis of septic arthritis. It should be performed with careful sterile technique, with gloves, and with proper preparation and draping of the skin. Aspiration of the knee in cases of an effusion is usually a relatively simple procedure. Specimens should be sent for cell count, culture, and gram stain for all appropriate organisms.

Some authors have warned that any scanning with technetium should be performed before an attempt at aspiration because aspiration affects the scan. Canale and co-workers performed ^{99m}Tc bone scanning in 15 dogs.[3] The hip joint was aspirated, the distal femoral metaphysis was drilled and aspirated, and the tibial periosteum was scraped with a needle. Bone scans were obtained 5 hours to 10 days later. There was no evidence that there was any increased focal technetium uptake of any hip joint as a result of these procedures. The effect of cortical drilling did not become obvious for at least 2 days. It seems reasonable to perform aspiration of both the joint and the bone first. If the findings of both are negative, the examiner could consider proceeding with radioactive scanning in order to look for osteomyelitis or tumor.

In addition to culture, a complete cell count and a differential leukocyte count should be performed. The white blood cell count in septic arthritis is the highest that is seen in the inflammatory conditions. Polymorphonuclear cells may constitute more than 75 per cent of the white blood cells.

The cultures in septic arthritis are positive in approximately 60 to 70 per cent of cases. Immunoelectrophoresis and latex agglutination methods can be used to identify *Haemophilus influenzae*, *Pneumococcus* species, *Meningococcus* species, and group B *Streptococcus* species.[22] It is also important to obtain blood cultures, which increase the chances of identifying an organism. About half the patients with septic arthritis have a positive blood culture.

In certain instances, the organism in septic arthritis may be related to other infections. *Haemophilus influenzae* type B is a frequent cause of otitis media, which may be accompanied by septic arthritis. In one series of 23 patients with *H. influenzae* type B septic arthritis, concurrent *H. influenzae* type B meningitis was present in 30 per cent of patients and concurrent osteomyelitis in 22 per cent.[20] Patients with sickle cell disease may have *Salmonella* infection. Patients with open skin lesions, particularly those who have recently had chicken pox, may be susceptible to streptococcal infections. Gonococcal infections can be present in newborns and in sexually active teenagers.[10, 18]

DIFFERENTIAL DIAGNOSIS. The differential diagnosis of septic arthritis includes other infections such as acute osteomyelitis, subacute osteomyelitis, and epiphyseal osteomyelitis. The most frequent locations of acute osteomyelitis are the distal femur and the proximal tibia. Subacute osteomyelitis in these locations is also common. Subacute osteomyelitis is a more insidious disease process and usually can be diagnosed from the clinical history, the physical examination, and presence of a lesion on radiographs. Acute osteomyelitis manifests with metaphyseal tenderness and fever. It can also be accompanied by a sympathetic joint fluid effusion, which may be sterile.

Juvenile rheumatoid arthritis (JRA) and acute rheumatic fever are among the other inflammatory conditions that must be considered in the differential diagnosis. They are discussed later in this chapter.

TREATMENT. Of primary importance in the management of septic arthritis is the identification of the infecting organism. As stated earlier, all appropriate fluids, including joint fluid, blood, and that from any other possible source, such as a wound, should be cultured before antibiotics are taken. Once these cultures have been obtained and the clinical diagnosis of septic arthritis is established, appropriate antibiotic therapy should be begun. The physician must make an educated guess of the most likely organism on the basis of the age of the patient and the clinical presentation.

Staphylococcus aureus still remains the most common cause of septic arthritis in children, and an antibiotic such as nafcillin should be chosen to combat this organism.[10, 18, 21] Children under the age of 3 to 4 years also may have *H. influenzae* type B infections of the knee, and an antibiotic must be chosen to combat this organism as well.[20] Because some *H. influenzae* type B infections are resistant to ampicillin, chloramphenicol is usually chosen until cultures are obtained in these young children.[10] The specific antibiotics and their dosage is subject to frequent change. More extensive reviews are available.[6, 7, 10, 16, 18, 21] The treating physician must either be knowledgeable in these matters or seek appropriate consultation.

The author's preferred method of treatment is to admit all such patients to the hospital and perform aspiration. Once all cultures are obtained, consultation is obtained from either a pediatrician or a pediatric infectious disease specialist in order to help manage the antibiotic therapy. As with any infection, the goals are administration of an appropriate antibiotic and relief of pressure by the drainage of pus, which may contain deleterious enzymes. In the past, the routine was to perform arthrotomy of the knee and leave it open to heal by secondary intention or perform delayed primary closure after 4 to 5 days if the infection is contained.

Herndon and colleagues reviewed 45 children who underwent initial nonoperative treatment of septic arthritis in joints other than the hip.[8] Only joints in which symptoms had been present less than 6 days and without associated osteomyelitis were included. Of 49 joints, 34 were successfully managed by aspiration and antibiotics, whereas the remaining joints were successfully managed by surgical drainage after a lack of response to nonoperative treatment. All children had a satisfactory result after an average follow-up interval of more than 3 years.

A major criticism of such treatment is that multiple aspirations are painful and may cause further damage to the joint. Another criticism is that it was possible to manage only 34 of 49 patients in this manner. In this study, 32 of the 34 joints treated nonoperatively were managed by a single diagnostic aspiration. Even the patients who ultimately underwent surgery had a satisfactory result, so that their treatment or outcome was not affected by the delay in surgery. Other critics have quoted an animal study that showed more thinning of the cartilage in animals treated with aspiration than in those treated with arthrotomy.[5]

Only five of the patients had infections with S. aureus. The smallness of this number is probably related to the fact that we did not include patients with coexistent osteomyelitis or with symptoms for more than 5 days, both of which are common with S. aureus infections.

The conclusion was that a single aspiration followed by treatment with appropriate antibiotics is effective for the majority of children with acute pyogenic arthritis in the absence of osteomyelitis. In this study, the treatment was started within 6 days of the onset of symptoms. Rapid diagnosis and early treatment are more important than the method of drainage. Not all joints respond to drainage, and not all joints require open drainage.

Arthroscopic lavage is another alternative to arthrotomy in the management of septic arthritis. In one study, 20 patients treated by arthroscopic lavage were compared with five patients treated by arthrotomy.[24] Both groups were doing well at follow-up. The advantages of arthroscopic treatment were said to be low morbidity, minimal scarring, and much earlier functional recovery. Skyhar and Mubarak believed that the advantages over needle aspiration included complete joint visualization, thorough lavage, and easy drain placement that allowed suction-irrigation over several days. In this study, a general anesthetic was used, although it was stated that the procedure could be performed with local anesthesia and sedation in a cooperative patient. In another study, Stanitski and associates evaluated arthroscopic evacuation, irrigation, and debridement of septic knees in children and found that this treatment was effective in the management of 16 patients.[26] Ninety-four per cent (15) had S. aureus infections. Two patients were immunosuppressed, and both had S. aureus and Pseudomonas aeruginosa infections. Twenty-five per cent (four) of the patients had a foreign body in the joint (needles in three patients and a nail in one) that was removed arthroscopically. Stanitski and associates did not use any type of postoperative suction-irrigation. At 3-year follow-up, there was no evidence of persistent or recurrent infection and no radiographic evidence of joint destruction.

The duration of antibiotic treatment and the mode of administration have changed in recent years. Most of the infections in septic arthritis are treatable by antibiotics that may be administered orally. Compliance by the patient must be obtained, and a sufficient concentration of the antibiotic in the serum must be reached in order to eradicate the infection. The author's general plan has been to place patients on a regimen of intravenous antibiotics initially and, after the first few days, make a transition to oral antibiotics. Serum concentrations are monitored, and once compliance is ensured, the patient may be discharged. These patients are usually treated for 3 weeks. Patients are followed routinely after treatment for 1 to 2 years with clinical and radiographic examinations.

Infectious Arthritis in the Adult

The clinical manifestation in the adult is often pain in one or more joints that is accompanied by fever, limp, and loss of motion.

DIAGNOSTIC TESTS. The most common organisms found in adults with septic arthritis are *Gonococcus, Staphylococcus, Streptococcus,* and *Pneumococcus.* Gonococcal arthritis is currently the most common in young adults. *Staphylococcus* infection is more common in the older population. Gram-negative organisms as well as anaerobic organisms are less common but must be carefully sought. A variety of organisms can be seen in intravenous drug abusers. Because there is often an underlying illness, other foci of infection must be sought. The adult patient is also more likely to have systemic illness and to be taking medications that suppress the immune system. Patients who have received systemic steroids or are taking intravenous drugs may be infected with a variety of gram-negative and other unusual organisms. Systemic illnesses in which patients are on immunosuppressive therapy may also be associated with unusual organisms. In addition, patients with meningitis, brucellosis, or gram-negative infections may develop bacterial seeding of the joint.

Gonococcal arthritis tends to involve one or a few joints and may be accompanied by tendinitis as well. The hips and other large joints are the most commonly involved, but the knee is the joint most commonly affected by gonorrheal arthritis. The disease usually manifests with pain, swelling, and a limp. The response may be indolent, and the systemic response may be less pronounced than in other types of infectious arthritis. It is often confused with rheumatoid arthritis. Gonococcal arthritis occurs more commonly in females than in males. The joint aspirate, the blood cultures, and the cervical and urethral swabs should be examined carefully. Penicillin is the treatment of choice. Another diagnosis considered in the differential diagnosis must be Reiter's syndrome, in which there is urethral discharge and an aseptic effusion.

Adult patients with septic arthritis of the knee present with pain, limp, limited range of motion, and swelling of joint. Laboratory tests obtained should include a complete blood cell count with differential leukocyte count and sedimentation rate measurement. The joint fluid should be aspirated for cell count, gram stain, and culture. Radiographs ordinarily are normal unless the diagnosis is made at a delayed time.

TREATMENT. Treatment involves decompressing the joint and removing the harmful bacteria and debris. The joint should be rested either with traction, splinting, or casting. If the infection is detected early, multiple aspirations and perhaps lavage of the knee joint may be effective. In some instances, however, these procedures are not as effective in decompressing the joint. If there is any question, the patient should be taken to the operating room for open irrigation and debridement or for arthroscopic debridement.

In the past, it was customary to leave the joint open. As discussed in the section on septic arthritis in children, other options now include arthroscopic lavage with or without the institution of closed suction irrigation. A multicenter study of 46 cases of septic arthritis, predominantly in adults, indicated that arthroscopy is a useful means of managing this disease.[29] This series was not representative of the usual case in that the average interval from onset to treatment was 35 days. The article claimed a 78 per cent cure rate. Sixty-five per cent of the patients with an identifiable organism had *S. aureus*. It was stated that in order to be effective, the lavage must be abundant and at very strong pressure, but there was no evidence in the article to support this.

Seventy-eight patients with septic arthritis who were seen over a 10-year period at the Mayo Clinic were reviewed by Kelly and collaborators.[12] The knee, the hip, and the shoulder were the joints most commonly involved. Many patients had predisposing factors such as other sources of infection, administration of corticosteroids, or diabetes. In comparison with other series, the patients in this series were more elderly. The most common differential diagnoses were osteoarthritis, rheumatoid arthritis, or nonspecific synovitis. The erythrocyte sedimentation rate was fairly consistently elevated, whereas the white blood cell count was elevated in only 20 of 78 patients. The most common organism was, overwhelmingly, *S. aureus*. Surgical treatment was most often used, but in this series the patients with infected knees had advanced pathologic changes with irreparable damage and destruction of bone and cartilage. Many of these patients subsequently underwent arthrodesis.

In the patients whose knees were involved, joint function at follow-up was grim. Only five had flexion of 90° or more. Thirteen had undergone successful operative arthrodesis, and six had fibrous ankylosis or limited motion. Casting in hopes of spontaneous arthrodesis did not work. Kelly and collaborators cautioned that adequate treatment depended on early suspicion of infection, identification of the organism, and prompt institution of an antibacterial regimen. They believed that any patient with a pain in the joint, anemia, and an elevated sedimentation rate should undergo a careful and persistent attempt to culture an organism from the synovial fluid. Although most of the patients studied had *Staphylococcus* infections, anaerobic organisms must be sought as well.

The choice of antibiotics depends on the isolation and identification of the appropriate bacteria. Parenteral antibiotics are used initially. The duration of action is variable, depending on the clinical response and whether there are other underlying illnesses. There is no need to inject the antibiotics in the joint fluid because antibiotics achieve satisfactory levels after systemic administration.[17]

DISEASES WITH AN IMMUNE JOINT REACTION FROM REMOTE INFECTION

Acute Rheumatic Fever

Rheumatic fever is an inflammatory disorder of the joints, the heart, the skin, and the central nervous system.[14] It occurs as a complication of a group A *Streptococcus* upper respiratory infection. The incidence has declined in developed countries to the point that it is very rare, but the disease must be considered in the differential diagnosis of inflammatory conditions of the knee.

The pathogenesis is unknown. The peak incidence is in the 5- to 15-year age group. The joint involvement is a characteristic migratory polyarthritis in which the knee is frequently involved. There is joint swelling without pannus formation. The joint symptoms disappear in 3 to 4 weeks without any permanent residual effects. The diagnosis is based on the Jones criteria.[14] The major criteria are carditis, polyarthritis, chorea, erythema marginatum, and subcutaneous nodules. The minor criteria are fever; arthralgia; previous episodes of rheumatic fever or rheumatic heart disease; acute-phase elevation of the sedimentation rate, C-reactive protein levels, white blood cell count, and antistreptolysin-O levels; and a prolonged PR interval on the electrocardiogram. Confirmation of the diagnosis with high probability requires two major criteria or one major and two minor criteria. The treatment of the arthritic portion of the condition is rest and anti-inflammatory drugs. The treatment of the remainder of the condition is conducted by the primary care physician or another specialist and depends on the extent and the systems involved.

Lyme Disease

This disease is caused by a spirochete. Several thorough reviews are available.[4, 15] It often manifests in an insidious manner similar to that of the rheumatic diseases. The knee is frequently involved, and such involvement must be considered in a patient whose knee is swollen and hot, especially if the patient is in an endemic area.

The organism is a tick-borne spirochete, *Borrelia burgdorferi.* Although the disease can be harbored by a variety of ticks and hosts, it is most frequently harbored by the tick *Ixodes dammini,* which is found on whitetail deer. The disease was originally described in a group of children from Lyme, Connecticut. It has since been reported from more than half of the United States but is considered endemic in the northeast, the upper midwest, and the northwest.

The disease has three stages. The first occurs within the first few days or weeks after the tick bite and consists of a skin lesion (erythema chronicum migrans). A red macule or papule appears, usually near the bite. This lesion gradually expands and may clear in the center. Other, more remote skin lesions may appear. The second stage begins weeks to months after the bite and consists of flu-like symptoms of malaise, fever, fatigue, arthralgias, and myalgias. These symptoms may be intermittent. In some patients, serious neurologic problems such as meningitis, encephalitis, and peripheral neuritis develop. Other patients develop serious cardiac disease such as first-degree atrioventricular blockage or myocarditis. The third stage may develop months to years after onset. These patients develop arthritis in the joints. They may be subject to recurrent attacks of arthralgia and flu-like symptoms. The joints are swollen, warm, and tender.

The joint fluid reveals an elevated white blood cell count with a predominance of polymorphonuclear cells. Definitive culture of the infecting organism is rare. The patients develop an immune reaction that enables diagnosis of the disorder. Elevation of immunoglobulin M (IgM) levels in response to *B. burgdorferi* develops in the first 3 to 6 weeks of the disease and of immunoglobulin G (IgG) in the first few months. Results of Venereal Disease Research Laboratory test results are negative. Arthroscopy or biopsy of the synovium or examination of the joint may reveal changes similar to those of rheumatoid arthritis.

The organism is sensitive to a variety of antibiotics, including tetracycline, penicillin, and erythromycin. The drug chosen, the route of administration, and the duration of action depend on the age of the patient and the stage of the disease. Early in the disease course, oral medication is used; later stages require parenteral antibiotics and longer duration of action. Tetracycline is avoided in children if at all possible. Cephalosporins may be required in penicillin-sensitive patients.

INFLAMMATORY ARTHROPATHY

The most frequent types of arthritis that must be considered in the differential diagnosis of suppurative arthritis are the inflammatory disorders, of which rheumatoid arthritis is the best example. In adults, the crystalline arthropathies must also be considered.

Juvenile Rheumatoid Arthritis

JRA has three clinical manifestations. The most common is the polyarticular type (50 per cent of JRA patients), in which three or more joints are involved. This type is more common in females than in males. Rheumatoid factor is rarely positive in any JRA patients, but it is positive in 15 per cent of patients with the polyarticular variety. Pauciarticular JRA (30 per cent of patients) is a variety in which three or fewer joints are involved. This type is also more common in females. Patients who develop pauciarticular JRA at a young age must be observed at frequent intervals by an ophthalmologist for the development of iridocyclitis.[15] Some patients who initially appear to have monarticular involvement may develop multiple joint involvement. Monarticular JRA can also be accompanied by iridocyclitis.[2]

The incidences in males and females are equal in the systemic variety, which occurs in 20 per cent of patients. In systemic JRA, there can be fever, rash, an elevated white blood cell count, and hepatosplenomegaly.

The etiology of rheumatoid arthritis is unknown. Patients with adult rheumatoid arthritis and other rheumatic diseases may have a genetic predisposition. Developments in testing for human leukocyte antigens have led to blood tests that are useful in the diagnosis of rheumatoid arthritis. Class II antigens are known to be associated with rheumatoid arthritis, juvenile arthritis, and systemic lupus erythematosus. Sixty to eighty per cent of adult patients with rheumatoid arthritis may be diagnosable with a serologic type of antigen.

In JRA, the diagnosis is based on a clinical manifestation of pain in one or more joints. Loss of motion occurs but is less severe than that seen in septic arthritis. The knee is one of the most frequently involved joints. When the knee is involved, there are usually loss of extension and a limp. Radiographs ordinarily are normal in the early phase of the disease, with normal-appearing bone and a normal joint space. Joint fluid should be aspirated for cell count, culture, and microscopic examination.

The prognosis for children with rheumatoid arthritis is much better than that for adults. The majority of children eventually experience lasting remission and are able to lead a normal life. In other children, the disease is more severe and leads to lifelong disability. Growth disturbance, effects from the medications required, and joint destruction can be devastating (Fig. 10–1).

Once the diagnosis is made, the first line of treatment in children and adults is medical, with nonsteroidal anti-inflammatory drugs (NSAIDs). The variety of medications to choose from is much wider for adults, inasmuch as many of the agents have not been proved safe in children, for whom aspirin remains the initial drug of choice.

The role of synovectomy remains unclear, and the procedure is of questionable benefit. The knee is the most accessible joint, and the procedure can be performed arthroscopically. The usual indication is for a joint that is unresponsive to systemic therapy, preferably in the early stages of the disease before destruction of the articular cartilage. The most usual reasons given for surgery are for relieving pain, increasing the range of motion, and curtailing the effusion and swelling.

Jacobsen and colleagues reviewed 41 synovectomies in 30 children with JRA. At follow-up after an average of 7 years, few if any benefits in range of motion and pain were found.[11] Radiographic deterioration had increased. In some patients, the range of motion and the functional capability became more limited. In a review on knee synovectomy in adults, Parides obtained similar results.[19] The one area in which there was a possible improvement was pain relief. The range of motion was more limited, and articular cartilaginous destruction had not been prevented. Both of these series consisted mainly of open synovectomies. In another study, open synovectomy was compared with arthroscopic synovectomy.[23] The postoperative course and the early rehabilitation produced better short-term results in the group treated arthroscopically, but the long-term results were no better.

Adult Rheumatoid Arthritis

This disease occurs more commonly in females than in males, and the frequency is highest among persons in the mid-30s and 40s. The disease may manifest with systemic symptoms such as generalized weakness, lassitude, and loss of weight. The arthritis may involve either a single joint or multiple joints. The onset may be insidious. Synovial fluid in rheumatoid arthritis contains an elevated white blood cell count, 70 to 80 per cent of which is polymorphonuclear leukocytes. The total white blood

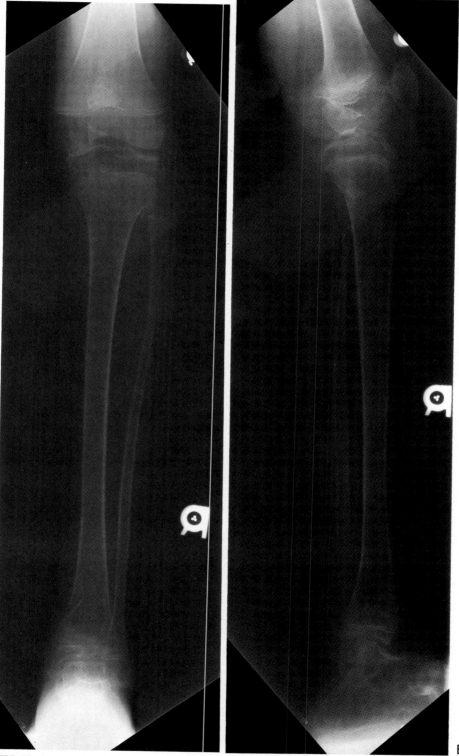

FIGURE 10-1. Anteroposterior *(A)* and lateral *(B)* views of the tibia in a patient with long-standing, polyarticular juvenile rheumatoid arthritis. Note the irregularity of the joint surfaces of the knee and ankle joints and of the epiphyses. There is also a cortical irregularity of the distal tibia, which represents a torus fracture.

cell count is usually 3000 to 7000 per milliliter. There may be a higher concentration of protein than in normal joint fluid, and the viscosity of the fluid is less than normal. Proteolytic enzymes may be isolated.

At arthroscopy or surgery of the knee, a pannus, an extension of the synovium over the articular cartilage, may be identified. The pannus occurs in the chronic inflammatory stage of the disease, contains white blood cells and macrophages, and causes erosion of the underlying cartilage.

Early in the disease course, radiographs may be normal or may show swelling of soft tissue; however, with time, joint space narrowing and erosion of articular cartilage ensue. Osteoporoses, loss of joint space, erosion, and joint subluxation occur later in the disease course (Fig. 10–2).

In the knee, the classic manifestation is pain and swelling in the joint with loss of motion and lack of full extension. The articular surface eventually collapses, and the menisci are destroyed, which causes ligamentous laxity. The synovium may be palpable and boggy, and there may be an effusion. A popliteal (Baker's) cyst may be present.

Medical management involves anti-inflammatory agents. Aspirin has been one of the main drugs in the past, but newer NSAIDs with fewer

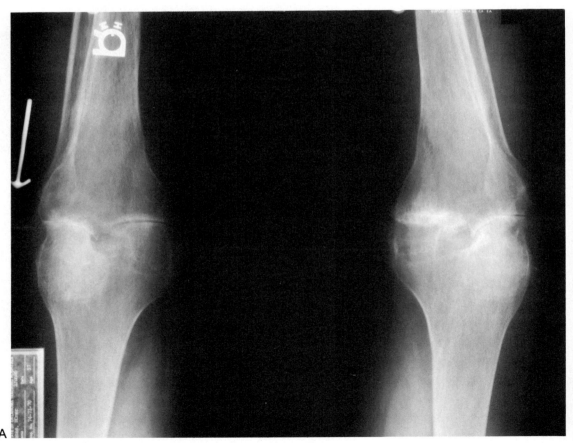

A

FIGURE 10–2. *(A)* Standing anteroposterior radiograph of a 57-year-old patient with rheumatoid arthritis. Note the total loss of joint space, the subchondral sclerosis, and the osteopenia.

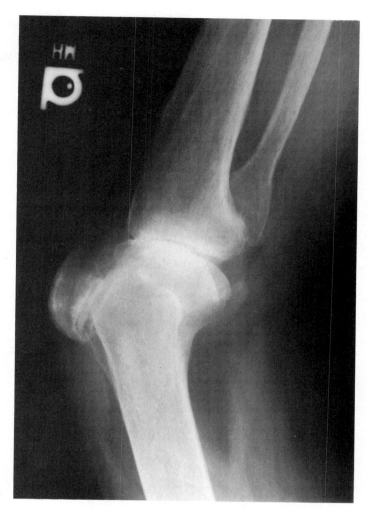

FIGURE 10–2. *Continued. (B)* Lateral radiograph of the left knee.

B

side effects are probably used more often now. A variety of other agents, including the antimalarial drug chloroquine, gold, penicillamine, and methotrexate, have been used. Oral steroids alleviate the anti-inflammatory effects, but because of the side effects, they are reserved for extremely nonresponsive cases.

Surgical options include synovectomy, debridement, and total joint replacement. Total joint replacement is frequently indicated in the advanced stages, in which there are no treatment options other than arthrodesis.

Synovectomy has been discussed earlier. Radiation synovectomy has been recommended. A variety of radioactive agents have been used. In the knee, a yttrium 90, gold 198 and dysprosium 165 have been used. The last agent has been injected in the knee when bound to ferric hydroxyapatite macroaggregates in order to prevent its spread to other parts of the body.[25] This procedure has been shown to be effective and to yield minimal leakage to other body tissues. The results are best if the bone and cartilage changes are minimal. Radioactive synovectomy is still investigational and available only in limited locations in the United States.

Although results of early studies are promising, the long-term risks, including radiation leakage to surrounding tissues, are uncertain.[13]

CRYSTALLINE ARTHROPATHY

In these disorders, abnormal crystals form in the synovium and in the synovial fluid. An inflammatory response causes the breakdown of white blood cells with release of degradative enzymes in the synovial fluid. The crystals are composed of monosodium urate, calcium pyrophosphate, calcium hydroxyapatite, or cholesterol.

Gout is probably the most common and most widely known of these disorders. It is more common in males than in females (by a ratio of 10 to 1). It classically occurs in the first metatarsophalangeal joint (podagra). There may be a history of obesity, excessive alcohol consumption, or hypertension. There is often a family history of the disease. A small percentage of patients with gout have hyperuricemia secondary to chronic intake of medication or to other diseases such as the myeloproliferative disorders. Monosodium urate or serum uric acid levels are elevated, and monosodium urate crystals are found in the synovial fluid. The diagnosis is made by aspiration of a joint and findings on polarized microscopy of needlelike birefringent crystals. Other useful findings include an elevated white blood cell count, an elevated platelet count, an elevated sedimen-

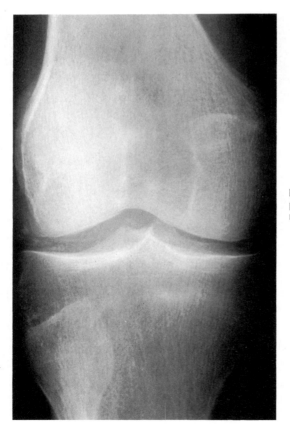

FIGURE 10–3. Anteroposterior radiograph of the knee of a patient with chondrocalcinosis. Note the calcification in the menisci.

tation rate, and an elevated level of C-reactive protein. Other joints may be involved, and tenosynovitis may be present.

The treatment of an acute attack includes NSAIDs. Aspirin has been the traditional medication but is being displaced by newer drugs that produce fewer side effects. Almost all the newer drugs, however, produce gastrointestinal side effects. Colchicine was also frequently used to control an acute attack; the response to the medication was considered diagnostic, but a similar response can be seen in chondrocalcinosis.

Adrenocorticotropic hormone (40 IU given intramuscularly) has been used in one-time doses for management of acute attacks.[1] Its benefits include fewer side effects, particularly gastrointestinal, than those of the NSAIDs. A wide variety of NSAIDs can be used, including naproxen, indomethacin, and phenylbutazone. The various risks and benefits of these drugs must be weighed in the choice of a specific agent. Allopurinol can also be used to lower the serum uric acid concentration. The management of chronic gout involves identifying any precipitating cause such as obesity. The patients must be categorized as overproducers or undersecretors and must be managed accordingly.

Chondrocalcinosis is a disorder that may manifest in a manner similar to that of gout and, indeed, is known as pseudogout. In this disease process, the crystals are calcium pyrophosphate and are deposited in the articular cartilage, the synovium, and the menisci. Deposition in the cartilage in this disease can lead to a pathognomonic radiographic appearance that can occur even in asymptomatic patients. The diagnosis can usually be made either from the radiograph or from biopsy specimens of synovium or articular cartilage (Fig. 10–3).

This disease may be present in a wide variety of metabolic abnormalities, including hyperparathyroidism, hypothyroidism, hypomagnesemia, and hemachromatosis. The hereditary form is acquired through autosomal dominance, but it may also occur as spontaneous genetic mutation. The crystals themselves are not necessarily pathognomonic, inasmuch as crystals are found in some patients with rheumatoid arthritis, osteoarthritis, and gout. Treatment is very similar to that of gout.

REFERENCES

1. Axelrod D, Preston S: Comparison of parenteral adrenocorticotrophic hormone with oral indomethacin in the treatment of acute gout. Arthritis Rheum 31:803–805, 1988.
2. Blockey NJ, Gibson AA, Goel KM: Monarticular juvenile rheumatoid arthritis. J Bone Joint Surg 62B:368–371, 1980.
3. Canale ST, Harkness RM, Thomas PA, Masse JD: Does aspiration of bones and joints affect results of later bone scanning? J Pediatr Orthop 5:23–26, 1985.
4. Davidson RS: Orthopedic complications of Lyme disease in children. Biomed Pharmacother 43:405–408, 1989.
5. Goldstein WM, Gleason TF, Barmada R: A comparison between arthrotomy and irrigation and multiple aspirations in the treatment of pyogenic arthritis. Orthopaedics 6:1309–1314, 1983.
6. Greene Edwards K: Bone and joint infections in children. Orthop Clin North Am 18:555–576, 1987.
7. Gustilo RB, Gruninger RP, Tsukayama DT (eds): Orthopaedic Infection: Diagnosis and Treatment. Philadelphia: WB Saunders, 1989.
8. Herndon WA, Knauer S, Sullivan JA, Gross RH: Management of septic arthritis in children. J Pediatr Orthop 6:576–578, 1986.
9. Heydemann JS, Morrissy RT: Bone and joint sepsis in childhood: problems in diagnosis. Orthop Trans 10:504, 1986.

10. Jackson MA, Nelson JD: Etiology and medical management of acute suppurative bone and joint infections in pediatric patients. J Pediatr Orthop 2:313–323, 1982.
11. Jacobsen ST, Levinson JE, Crawford AH: Late results of synovectomy in juvenile rheumatoid arthritis. J Bone Joint Surg 67A:8–15, 1985.
12. Kelly PJ, Martin WJ, Coventry MB: Bacterial (suppurative) arthritis in the adult. J Bone Joint Surg 52A:1595–1602, 1970.
13. Lee P: The efficacy and safety of radiosynovectomy [editorial]. J Rheumatol 9:165–168, 1982.
14. Markowitz M, Gordis L: Diagnosis. *In* Rheumatic Fever, 2nd ed, pp. 103–117. Philadelphia, WB Saunders, 1972.
15. McCarty DJ: Arthritis and Allied Conditions: A Textbook of Rheumatology, 10th ed. Philadelphia: Lea and Febiger, 1985.
16. Nade S: Acute septic arthritis in infancy and childhood. J Bone Joint Surg 65B:234–241, 1983.
17. Nelson JD: Antibiotic concentrations and septic joint effusions. N Engl J Med 284:349–353, 1971.
18. Nelson JD, Koontz WC: Septic arthritis in infants and children: a review of 117 cases. Pediatrics 38:966–971, 1966.
19. Parides LH: Synovectomy for rheumatoid arthritis of the knee. J Bone Joint Surg 57A:95–100, 1975.
20. Rotbart HA, Glode MP: *Haemophilus influenzae* type B septic arthritis in children: report of 23 cases. Pediatrics 75:254–259, 1985.
21. Scoles PV, Aronoff SC: Antimicrobial therapy of childhood skeletal infections. J Bone Joint Surg 66A:1487–1492, 1984.
22. Shackleford P, Campbell J, Feigin RD: Countercurrent immunoelectrophoresis in the evaluation of childhood infections. J Pediatr 85:478–481, 1974.
23. Shibata T, Shiraoka K, Takubo N: Comparison between arthroscopic and open synovectomy for the knee in rheumatoid arthritis. Arch Orthop Trauma Surg 105:257–262, 1986.
24. Skyhar MJ, Mubarak SJ: Arthroscopic treatment of septic knees in children. J Pediatr Orthop 7:647–651, 1987.
25. Sledge CB, Zuckerman JD, Shortkoff S, et al: Synovectomy of the rheumatoid knee using intra-articular injection of dysprosium-165-ferric hydroxide macroaggregates. J Bone Joint Surg 69A:970–975, 1987.
26. Stanitski CL, Harvell JC, Fu FH: Arthroscopy in acute septic knees: management in pediatric patients. Clin Orthop 241:209–212, 1989.
27. Sullivan JA, Vasileff T, Leonard JC: Nuclear scanning in bone and joint infection. J Pediatr Orthop 1:73–79, 1981.
28. Sundberg SB, Savage JP, Foster BK: Technetium phosphate bone scan in the diagnosis of septic arthritis in childhood. J Pediatr Orthop 9:579–585, 1989.
29. Thiery JA: Arthroscopic drainage in septic arthritides of the knee: A multi-center study. Arthroscopy 5:65–69, 1989.

CHAPTER 11

Arthritis and

Arthroplasty

PAUL J. TSAHAKIS, M.D.

GREGORY W. BRICK, M.D.

THOMAS S. THORNHILL, M.D.

■

OSTEOARTHRITIS

The destruction of the articular surface occurs through a variety of inflammatory and noninflammatory mechanisms. These arthritic disorders can conveniently be stratified into inflammatory and noninflammatory arthritis. The prototype of inflammatory arthritis is rheumatoid arthritis, in which the primary abnormality is in the synovial tissue, in which an aberrant immune system causes cellular interactions that lead to the production of cytokines, cartilage-degrading enzymes, and direct cellular injury, which in turn lead to the destruction of the articular matrix. Medical therapy for inflammatory arthritis is directed toward preventing or blocking these cell-to-cell interactions. Synovectomy (either surgical or via radiation), if performed early in the course of the disease, may delay the eventual destruction of the cartilage.[90, 96] When resurfacing is necessary, all of the articular cartilage must be replaced in order to prevent continued synovial cartilage interaction, which leads to further pain and inflammation. Unicompartmental arthroplasty or bicompartmental arthroplasty without patellar resurfacing has no role in the surgical treatment of the patient with rheumatoid arthritis.

The prototype of noninflammatory cartilage destruction is osteoarthritis. The prevalence of this disease increases with age, affects nearly 10 per cent of the population over 60 years of age, and is second only to cardiovascular disease in producing functional disability.[73] In contrast to rheumatoid arthritis, which affects three times as many women as men, osteoarthritis has no gender specificity.

Osteoarthritis can involve the axial and appendicular skeleton, affecting weight-bearing and non–weight-bearing joints. It is classified as a primary idiopathic form, or one in which a cause cannot be identified, or as secondary forms, in which predisposing conditions are known. Examples of secondary osteoarthritis are congenital factors, such as congenital dislocation of the hip and epiphyseal dysplasia, and posttraumatic forms, such as those that occur after a fracture or a ligamentous injury.

Although the exact etiologic mechanism of osteoarthritis remains unknown, most cases are thought to be caused by one of two mechanisms. The first involves conditions that lead to abnormally increased loading of normal cartilage. These excessive forces may result from juxta-articular malalignment secondary to congenital or acquired conditions and cause focal articular degeneration. Brandt[9] theorized that the sequence of events begins with cartilage surface fibrillation, followed by increased hydration of the matrix and decreased proteoglycan content. Ultimately, cartilage wear with eventual exposure of the subchondral bone occurs. When coupled with age-related loss of resiliency of the subchondral bone plate,[77] the mechanical degradation of the cartilage is magnified.

The second mechanism causing osteoarthritis may involve conditions in which abnormal cartilage is unable to accommodate normal loads. These conditions include hemochromatosis,[98] chondrocalcinosis,[33] ochronosis,[81] and hemophilia.[60] In hemochromatosis and chondrocalcinosis, cartilage destruction occurs by replacement of free water with either iron or calcium pyrophosphate. The dessicated cartilage is then unable to accommodate normal loads. The origin of cartilage destruction in hemophilia appears multifactorial. Although the exact mechanism is unclear, repeated hemarthroses may lead to free radical formation from the intra-articular degradation of hemoglobin and may induce a synovial proliferative response that may degrade cartilage by mechanisms similar to inflammatory arthritis. Ochronosis arises from a hereditary deficiency of homogentisic acid oxidase that results in the accumulation and deposition of homogentisic acid in connective tissue. Such deposition in articular cartilage causes the cartilage to become friable and eventually to be destroyed under normal loads.

ARTHROSCOPIC DEBRIDEMENT

In 1941, Magnuson[59] first introduced the concept of open debridement of the arthritic knee joint. He believed that progressive degenerative changes could be slowed by radical removal of all mechanical irritants. In 1959, Pridie introduced the concept of drilling full-thickness cartilage defects in gonarthrosis in order to stimulate cartilage formation.[74] Both of these procedures were performed through arthrotomy exposure, and rehabilitation was both painful and lengthy.

By the mid-1970s, arthroscopic access to the knee was emerging as an alternative to procedures previously performed via arthrotomy. Jackson noted that arthroscopic irrigation of an arthritic knee allowed the patient some relief of symptoms.[41] Sprague reported an 84 per cent favorable response to arthroscopic debridement in 68 knees followed for an average of 13.6 months.[93] There were, however, no consistent parameters that could be used to predict which patients would improve after the procedure. Jackson and associates[42] reported improved results in 68 per cent of patients with gonarthrosis at average follow-up of 3.3 years after debridement of condylar and meniscal tissue. Timoney and colleagues[99] reviewed the results of arthroscopic debridement in 111 knees after an average follow-up interval of 50 months. Overall, there were 50 good, 20 fair, and 41 poor results. Moreover, 74 per cent of patients judged the procedure to be of some benefit.

In an attempt to determine the extent and the duration of symptomatic relief from arthroscopic debridement on older patients with gonarthrosis, Baumgaertner and co-workers[5] reported on 49 knees in patients more than 50 years of age. Surgery was ineffectual in 39 per cent of patients; another 9 per cent experienced temporary relief, but the surgery was judged a failure after less than 3 years. Good to excellent results were reported in 52 per cent of patients, but the result was maintained in only 40 per cent after an average 33-month follow-up interval.

In an effort to help elucidate the indications for arthroscopic debridement, Salisbury and collaborators[80] demonstrated that varus malalignment of the knee was associated with poor results after arthroscopic debridement, and they recommended performing the procedure only in normally aligned knees. Other authors have also confirmed the detrimental effect of malalignment on arthroscopic debridement.[5]

Johnson was the first to introduce arthroscopic abrasion arthroplasty as a treatment for the arthritic knee.[45] In this procedure, eburnated bone is removed, and intracortical blood vessels are exposed. Johnson believed that the depth of the debridement must remain within the intracortical layer of bone and that exposure of cancellous bone is associated with poor results. A hematoma forms over the abraded area and ultimately differentiates into fibrocartilage.[23] In 1986, Johnson reported 74 good results with this procedure on 96 knees after a minimum of two years. Fifteen knees were worse at follow-up, and 7 knees were unchanged.[45] Mankin demonstrated that this fibrocartilage has poor wear characteristics in comparison with normal hyaline cartilage, and therefore long-term results are not predictable.[61, 62]

Friedman and associates[23] retrospectively compared the results of arthroscopic abrasion arthroplasty with arthroscopic debridement alone. They noted improvement in 60 per cent of patients who underwent abrasion arthroplasty, as opposed to only 32 per cent of patients who underwent debridement. Follow-up, however, averaged only 1 year, and 83 per cent of patients who had undergone abrasion still experienced pain.

Bert and Maschka also compared the two procedures in the treatment of unicompartmental gonarthrosis and reported their 5-year results.[7] Good to excellent results were reported in 66 per cent of patients who underwent debridement alone, as opposed to 51 per cent who underwent abrasion arthroplasty. Moreover, the observation at follow-up that radiographic joint space widening was not correlated with an improved result is consistent with Mankin's earlier reports.[61, 62] Of importance is that the results of both of these procedures were totally unpredictable.

In summary, it appears that for approximately 50 to 70 per cent of patients, arthroscopic debridement results in improvement that lasts for a variable period of several months to 5 years. The ideal candidate for this procedure is a patient with moderate radiographic change and whose symptoms are mainly those of internal derangement (locking, buckling, effusion) secondary to a degenerative meniscal tear and moderate cartilage wear. Debridement of the meniscal tear often leads to satisfactory results.[57] This procedure has a limited role in the treatment of gonarthrosis. In younger patients, however, it can be considered as a palliative alternative to more extensive procedures such as osteotomy or knee replacement. The minimal sacrifice of tissue makes the procedure appealing in that future reconstructive procedures are not jeopardized. It appears that repeated attempts to induce functional cartilage regeneration through abrasion arthroplasty have been unsuccessful. The results are unpredictable and appear to be inferior to those of debridement alone.

OSTEOTOMY

Rationale for Osteotomy

Although first described by Volkmann[100] in 1875, osteotomy was initially thought to be a dangerous procedure in light of the complications associated with tibial fractures (especially arterial injuries). Tibial osteotomy was first used in the treatment of degenerative arthritis of the knee in the early 1950s. It was first reported by Gariepy[24] and Jackson & Waugh[43] as being a safe and effective method of treatment for osteoarthritis of the knee. The effect of osteotomy in the treatment of unicompartmental arthritis may be purely mechanical[29] and associated with redistribution of the load to a less involved compartment.[64] An alternative theory about the effectiveness of osteotomy is related to the alteration in circulation and the possible lowering of intraosseous venous pressure.[2] The medial joint space may appear widened on follow-up radiographs after osteotomy and may be associated with cartilage regeneration.[63, 64] Coventry reported autopsy and biopsy findings that demonstrated an improvement in the articular cartilage after osteotomy.[16]

Varus Deformity

Varus deformity in association with medial compartmentaı osteoarthritis is the most common clinical situation experienced. With increasing varus deformity, there is associated stretching of the fibular collateral ligament, the popliteal tendon, and other lateral structures, thereby creating instability. When the varus deformity is more than 15°, the instability is usually combined with lateral subluxation of the tibia and significant medial bone loss. In this clinical situation, described by Kettelkamp and colleagues[51] as the "teeter" effect, osteotomy is contraindicated because it is usually associated with poor results. Maquet,[63] however, reported findings with tibial osteotomy in 41 patients with a varus deformity of more than 15° and subluxation on weight-bearing radiographs; results were excellent in 32 patients. He reported spontaneous tightening of the lax lateral structures, particularly if slightover correction was produced.

Valgus Deformity

With increasing valgus deformity, increasing loss of lateral femoral condylar bone stock usually occurs (cf. loss of tibial bone stock associated with varus deformity). Obliquity of the joint is associated with this bone stock loss. It is recommended that if the joint line is more than 10° from the horizontal or if a valgus deformity of more than 12° is present, a femoral osteotomy should be performed in order to produce a more horizontal joint line and thereby prevent continued stress on the lateral compartment and associated tibial subluxation. This recommendation does not apply to previous lateral tibial plateau fractures, in which loss of bone stock occurs on the tibial side and obliquity of the joint is not encountered. In this instance, a varus tibial osteotomy may be the appropriate method of treatment. Coventry[15] reported successful results in patients undergoing varus tibial osteotomy and a joint obliquity of 10° or less. Removal of a medial wedge is associated with relative lengthening of the medial collateral ligament.

Techniques of varus osteotomy include a lateral approach and removal of a medially based wedge. A 95° AO condylar blade plate may be used for fixation. An alternative technique may be used with a medial approach for removal of a medially based wedge. Through this approach, it is necessary to use an AO/ASIF 90° osteotomy blade plate. The disadvantages of a medial approach include possible injury to the superficial femoral vessels and a tender medial scar.

Healy and collaborators[31] reported the results of 23 distal femoral osteotomies, for valgus deformity, in 21 patients at an average follow-up of 4 years. Results were good or excellent in 14 of 15 patients treated for osteoarthritis. Osteotomy was not recommended in patients with rheumatoid arthritis or poor preoperative motion. These results are not long term and may deteriorate with time.

Selection of Patients

Patients who are active and whose symptoms are referable to the affected compartment should be selected. If symptoms appear to be in the radiographically noninvolved compartment, a bone scan may demonstrate changes in this compartment. Patients experiencing mechanical symptoms should undergo a preoperative arthroscopy in order to rule out a meniscal tear or a loose body as the cause of the symptoms. There should be a flexion contracture of less than 15° and a minimum of 90° of knee flexion.[36] The patient ideally should be less than 60 years of age; poor results of osteotomies have been reported in patients more than 60 yrs of age.[47] This is possibly because of more widespread cartilage damage in this age group or because previously unloaded cartilage in the more normal compartment is less resilient. Deficiency of the anterior cruciate ligament does not appear to preclude a good result.[32]

Patellofemoral arthritis is not thought to be a contraindication to osteotomy. Patellofemoral symptoms that manifest preoperatively may continue postoperatively, and the patient should be warned of this. It is possible for these symptoms to improve after valgus realignment because of a change in patellar tracking. Anterior displacement of the tibial tubercle at the time of tibial osteotomy may also improve patellofemoral symptoms.

Theoretically, preoperative arthroscopy would be appealing for assessing the involvement of the lateral compartment and patellofemoral joint, thereby aiding in selection of patients. Keene and Dyreby,[48] however, reported that arthroscopic assessment of the uninvolved compartment was of little value for predicting the clinical results of high tibial osteotomy.

Assessment of the Femorotibial Axis

Maquet[64] recommended the use of radiographs with patients standing that include the hip, the knee, and the ankle in order to calculate the mechanical axis. He recommended a correction to 2° to 4° of mechanical valgus angulation. There is some difference of opinion in the literature, however, as to the ideal postoperative angle. Most authors recommend slight overcorrection to valgus angulation. Bauer and co-workers[4] recommended 3° to 16° of valgus angulation, Coventry[14] favored 10° to 13°, Kettelkamp and colleagues[51] preferred 5°, and MacIntosh and Welsh[58] advocated 5° to 7°. Although excessive valgus angulation may be cosmetically unacceptable, it may not prejudice function.

For correcting a valgus deformity, Coventry[15] recommended correction to 0° of anatomical tibiofemoral alignment in order to prevent recurrence of the valgus deformity and to decrease the load on the lateral tibiofemoral compartment.

In the normally aligned knee, approximately 60 per cent of the forces are experienced through the medial compartment and 40 per cent are experienced through the lateral compartment.[50] Morrison[70] confirmed that loading in the normal knee is predominantly medial. Static analysis does not predict dynamic forces experienced during gait. During stance, horizontal medially directed forces (the adduction moment) act to increase the forces in the medial compartment. Static measurements are correlated with dynamic measurements only when the femorotibial angle is 5° or more of varus angulation. Gait analysis after tibial osteomy has confirmed that even when the static load is in the lateral compartment, half of the patients who undergo the procedure experience more loading in the medial compartment.[44]

Bauer and co-workers[4] recommended that once the angle of correction has been calculated, a lateral based wedge of 1 mm for each degree of correction required should be removed. This calculation produces satisfactory results in women. In men, however, removal of a wedge of 10 mm produces approximately 8° of correction. Slocum and associates[91] recommended the construction of a template with the angle of correction required and the use of a scale for the different thicknesses of the tibial osteotomy. They reported an average error of 1.6° and a range of 0° to 6° with this method. Myrnerts[71] described the use of the SAAB jig as an aid in high tibial osteotomy. Other jigs for calculating the size of the wedge to be removed are now commercially available.

Osteotomy Techniques

A variety of osteotomy techniques have been described. Jackson and Waugh,[43] who initially reported on osteotomies below the tibial tubercle, subsequently altered their technique to a supratubercular osteotomy. The large surface area of cancellous bone proximal to the tibial tubercle enables more rapid healing of the osteotomy, and the correction is closer to the site of deformity. Also, contraction of the quadriceps muscle allows compression of the osteotomy surfaces. If the fibular remains intact, it acts as a tether, preventing adequate correction. Initially, it was recommended that an osteotomy be performed on the fibular shaft.[43, 101] This may be ineffective inasmuch as the tethering effect of the fibula is not fully relieved as long as the intraosseous membrane remains intact. Gariepy[24] and Coventry[14] recommended excision of the fibular head, removal of the fibular collateral ligament, and reattachment of the fibular head. Most authors now recommend division or excision of the superior tibiofibular joint without detachment of the fibular collateral ligament or of the biceps tendon.

Methods of fixation of the tibial osteotomy include cast immobilization, stepped staples, and a modified blade plate or screws. The use of external fixation is not recommended because of a high incidence of pin tract infections and peroneal nerve palsy associated with its use.[58] If in the long term a high tibial osteotomy fails, a previous pin tract infection may preclude total knee arthroplasty.

The use of continuous passive motion in the early postoperative period assists in the avoidance of loss of motion in the knee and enables early rehabilitation.

Results

The early results of high tibial osteotomy have been correlated with the degree of correction obtained. Although patients are encouraged to resume normal activity, most patients are initially unable to resume jumping or sports activities that require sudden rapid changes in direction. They may be able to run on a limited basis.[32] In a long-term follow-up study, Holden and colleagues[32] reported that 13 of 15 patients with excellent results were able to resume swimming, bicycling, hiking, tennis, golf, hunting, and softball. Four patients ran three times a week, and three skied frequently. Two patients were unable to take part in recreational activity for other reasons. Holden and colleagues also reported on 51 osteotomies in 45 patients, aged 50 or less, with an average follow-up of 10 years. Seventy per cent of the patients were regarded as having achieved good or excellent results, and 30 per cent, fair or poor results. In this series, there was no correlation between the degree of arthritis observed radiographically and the long-term result. There was a possible correlation of improved result with increased angle of correction. The most important factor predicting long-term outcome was the preoperative level of disease; patients with higher preoperative knee scores experienced better long-term results.

In a further long-term follow-up of 83 patients undergoing 95 osteotomies, Insall and collaborators[36] reported that 97 per cent of the results were satisfactory at 2 years, 85 per cent were satisfactory at 5 years, and 63 per cent were satisfactory at 8.9 years; 23 per cent of the patients underwent total knee arthroplasty for failure. Insall and collaborators reported marginally better results when 10° to 14° of valgus angulation was obtained. They also reported gradual deterioration of acceptable results with longer follow-up. In a review of 81 knees at a 5.7-year follow-up, 75 per cent were regarded as having achieved acceptable results and 50 per cent as having achieved good results. Of 65 patients followed to 11.9 years, 43 per cent demonstrated good results.

Prodromos and co-workers[75] reported pre- and postoperative gait analysis in 21 patients undergoing osteotomy. All patients demonstrating a low preoperative adduction moment experienced good clinical results, whereas 50 per cent of those patients with a high preoperative adduction moment developed a recurrent deformity and subsequent poor clinical results. This outcome suggests that although a patient may fulfill the clinical criteria for osteotomy and may undergo satisfactory correction, a poor result may be experienced when a high preoperative adduction moment exists.

Complications

Although osteotomy may be technically demanding, the complications reported in the literature are relatively low. Insall and collaborators,[36] in a series of 95 osteotomies, reported one intraoperative cardiac arrest and one fatal pulmonary embolism. There was one instance of nonunion related to the use of a power saw rather than an osteotome for the osteotomy. Loss of correction occurred in one patient. There were no wound infections, peroneal nerve palsies, or intraoperative fractures. Ivarsson and associates,[40] in a series of 99 osteotomies, reported a 9 per cent rate of superficial wound infections, one instance of peroneal nerve palsy, and two deep vein thromboses. Holden and colleagues,[32] in a series of 51 osteotomies, reported one instance of peroneal nerve palsy, two pulmonary emboli, and one loss of correction with no skin problems or wound infections.

Preoperative planning is essential before an osteotomy about the knee is performed. The surgeon must determine the preoperative deformity and the desired angle of correction. In general, varus knee deformities are corrected on the tibial side and valgus knee deformities are corrected on the femoral side. This is because most valgus abnormalities are caused predominately by excessive distal femoral valgus angulation. Because genu varum is more common in the osteoarthritic knee, most osteotomies are performed on the tibial side.

In a varus knee deformity, the surgeon must determine the optimal postoperative alignment and the angle of correction. In general, the authors prefer a proximal, lateral based wedge for corrections of less than 14°. For greater corrections, an oblique metaphyseal osteotomy or a barrel vault osteotomy is preferred.

Internal fixation is routinely used to maintain the angle of correction and enable early joint motion.

Authors' Preferred Technique

A 36-inch radiograph is obtained with the patient standing and includes the hip, the knee, and the ankle joint. The patient is instructed to stand on both feet but to put most of the weight on the affected limb. Care is taken to keep the tibia and femur in neutral rotation. A line is drawn from the center of the femoral head to the center of the talus. This determines the center of effort and is invariably to the medial side. The surgeon then determines where the center of effort should cross the knee joint postoperatively. This crossing is generally at some point between the lateral tibial spine and the lateral edge of the tibial surface. A more laterally aligned center of effort is chosen in people with extensive medial destruction (i.e., eburnated bone) or lateral laxity and in female patients who have more preoperative physical valgus angulation.

A line is drawn from the center of the femoral head through the ideal postoperative center of effort to a point lateral to the talus. This line marks the postoperative position of the talus in relation to the knee joint. A line is then drawn from the center of the tibia at the joint line to the center of the talus, and a second line is drawn from the center of the tibia to the ideal talor position. Perpendicular lines from these lines are constructed at the proximal tibia to form a laterally based wedge whose apex is at the medial cortex. This method is used to determine the size of wedge required to bring the center of effort to the desired position (Fig. 11–1). Unfortunately, variabilities in bone quality, the possibility of opening medially, and differences in compression across the osteotomy can significantly influence the angular correction. For this reason, the tibial osteotomy is checked with fluoroscopy during surgery in order to confirm the desired correction.

The preferred technique for construction of a laterally based proximal tibial wedge to correct a varus knee deformity requiring less than 14° of correction is described as follows. The patient is prepared and draped on an operative table adapted for intraoperative fluoroscopy. A trochanteric roll is placed under the hip in order to bring the femur to a neutral position. A pneumatic tourniquet is placed on the thigh. A transverse incision is made approximately 2 cm distal and parallel to the joint line.

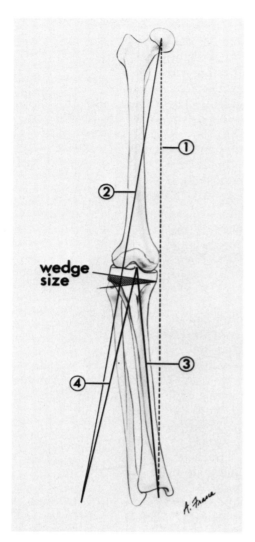

wedge size

FIGURE 11–1. Wedge determination. A three-foot standing radiograph that includes the hip, knee, and ankle joint is obtained. A line is drawn from the center of the femoral head to the center of the talus. This determines the center of effort and is invariably to the medial side in varus knees. The surgeon then determines where the center of effort should cross the knee joint postoperatively. This is generally at some point between the lateral tibial spine and the lateral edge of the tibial surface. A line is drawn from the center of the femoral head through the ideal postoperative center of effort to a point lateral to the talus. This marks the postoperative position of the talus in relation to the knee joint. A line is then drawn from the center of the tibia at the joint line to the center of the talus, and a second line is drawn from the center of the tibia to the ideal talar position. Perpendiculars from these lines are constructed at the proximal tibia in order to form a laterally based wedge whose apex is at the medial cortex. This will determine the size of wedge required to bring the center of effort to the desired position. Intraoperative fluoroscopy is used to confirm the desired correction.

It begins at the fibular head and ends near the midline (Fig. 11–2). The subcutaneous tissues are divided in order to expose the lateral capsule, the iliotibial band, and the anterolateral musculature. A flap that begins just lateral to the infrapatellar tendon and is approximately 1 cm below and parallel to the joint line is created. It divides a portion of the iliotibial band from Gerdy's tubercle and continues back to the position of the anterior third of the fibular head.

The dissection is carried distally 90° to this line and crosses the anterior third of the fibular head. Care is taken to avoid the insertion of the biceps femoris muscle and lateral collateral ligament. The flap is reflected to expose the tibiofibular joint and the lateral surface of the tibia (Fig. 11–3). The tibiofibular joint is excised with the use of an osteotome, a rongeur, and a curette (Fig. 11–4). A retractor is placed in this space and around the back of the tibial surface in order to protect the peroneal nerve. A second retractor is placed in the infrapatellar bursa in order to protect the infrapatellar tendon. A small Steinmann pin is drilled across

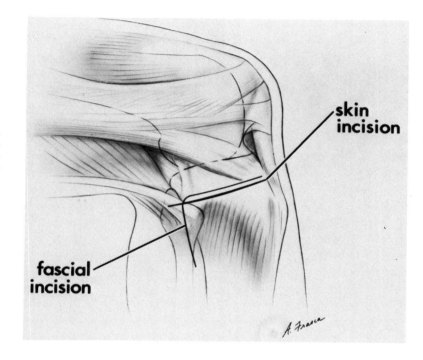

FIGURE 11–2. Exposure. A transverse incision is made approximately 2 cm distal and parallel to the joint line. It begins at the fibular head and ends near the midline. The subcutaneous tissues are divided to expose the lateral capsule, the iliotibial band, and the anterolateral musculature.

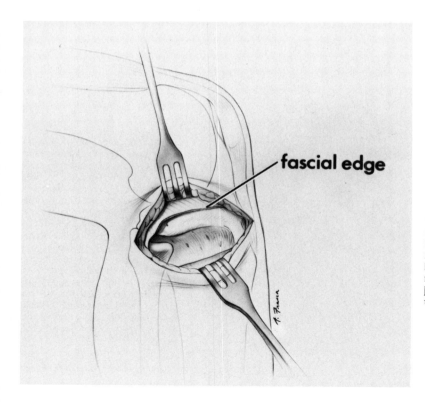

FIGURE 11–3. Exposure (continued). A flap that begins just lateral to the infrapatellar tendon and is approximately 1 cm distal and parallel to the joint line is created. It divides a portion of the iliotibial band from Gerdy's tubercle and continues back to the position of the anterior third of the fibular head. The dissection is carried distally 90° to this line and crosses the anterior third of the fibular head. Care is taken to avoid the insertion of the biceps femoris muscle and the lateral collateral ligament. This flap is now reflected to expose the tibiofibular joint and the lateral surface of the tibia.

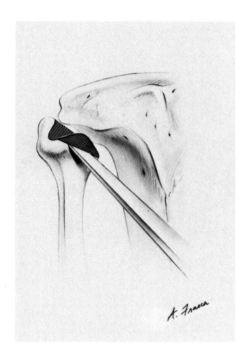

FIGURE 11–4. Tibiofibular joint resection. The tibiofibular joint is resected with the use of an osteotome and a rongeur.

the tibia approximately 1 cm distal to the joint. It is centered in the anteroposterior dimension so as to cross the widest part of the tibial surface, which measures about 8 cm in the mediolateral dimension at that level. This track is used for the proximal limb of the staple (Fig. 11–5).

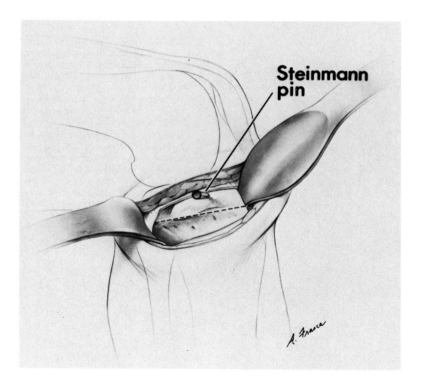

FIGURE 11–5. Retractor placement. A retractor is placed in the excised tibiofibular joint interval and around the back of the tibia to protect the peroneal nerve. A second retractor is placed in the infrapatellar bursa to protect the infrapatellar tendon. Under fluoroscopic control, a small Steinmann pin is now drilled across the tibia approximately 1 cm distal to the femorotibial joint. It is centered in the anteroposterior dimension to cross the widest part of the tibial surface (usually 8 cm). This track will ultimately be used for the proximal limb of the staple.

Fluoroscopy is used to confirm that the pin is parallel to the joint and approximately 1 cm distal to the surface. The pin is driven about 1 cm beyond the medial cortex so that it may be palpated beneath the skin and serve as a guideline to direct the osteotomy. The osteotomy is made 1 cm distal and parallel to this pin with the use of an oscillating saw. The base of the preferred wedge, as determined by the preoperative radiographs, is scribed on the lateral shaft of the tibia with the electric cautery. An oscillating saw is used to complete the wedge.

The surgeon has several options at this point. A variety of guides for ensuring that the cuts meet at the apex are commercially available. The osteotomy may be cut under fluoroscopic control, but this requires that the leg be in extension and provides less protection to the posterior vasculature. The authors prefer to make the distal limb of the wedge incomplete and to remove a trapezoidal wedge of bone so as to enable the rest of the osteotomy to be made under direct visualization, the apex being completed with an osteotome (Fig. 11–6). The medial cortex is then perforated with a K-wire but not completely disrupted.

The osteotomy is closed, and bone apposition is confirmed fluoroscopically. A metal wire (usually the electrocautery cord) is run from the center of the femoral head (determined by a preoperative marker) to the center of the talus. When the osteotomy is closed, the center of effort is determined and compared with the ideal position. The osteotomy cuts and the compression can be adjusted at this time. The guide wire is removed, and the proximal limb of a step staple is inserted in its tract (Fig. 11–7). As the distal limb of the staple approaches the lateral cortex,

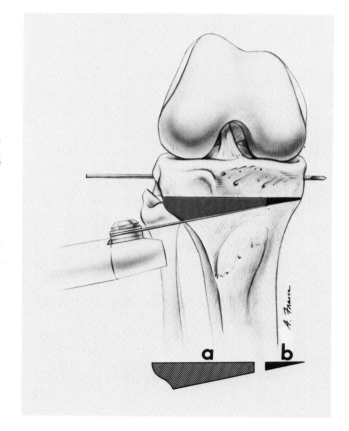

FIGURE 11–6. Wedge resection. An osteotomy is made 1 cm distal to and parallel to this pin with the use of an oscillating saw. The base of the preferred wedge as determined by the pre-operative radiograph is scribed on the lateral shaft of the tibia by the electric cautery. An oscillating saw is used to complete the wedge. At this point, the authors prefer to make the distal limb of the wedge incomplete and remove a trapezoid wedge of bone, allowing the rest of the osteotomy to be made under direct visualization, the apex being completed with the use of an osteotome. The medial cortex is perforated with a K-wire but not completely disrupted. The osteotomy is closed, and closure is confirmed fluoroscopically.

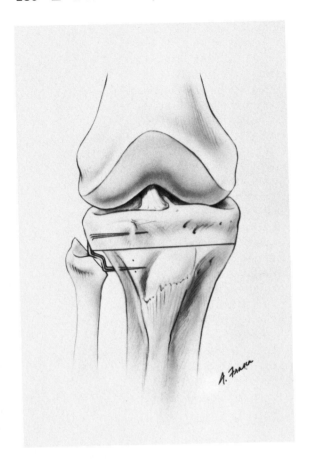

FIGURE 11–7. Fixation. The guide wire is removed, and the proximal limb of a step-cut staple is inserted in its tract. As the distal limb of the staple approaches the lateral cortex, a 7/64-inch drill is used to make a hole in the cortex just distal to the staple. This allows slight further compression across the osteotomy.

a 7/64-inch drill is used to make a hole in the cortex just distal to the staple. This enables slight further compression across the osteotomy site. The center of effort is again confirmed radiographically (Fig. 11–8), and the knee is carried through a range of motion. If the osteotomy is unstable, a second staple may be required.

The tourniquet is deflated, and hemostasis is achieved. The soft tissue flap is now resutured anatomically or is advanced in order to correct lateral instability. A drain is left in place for 24 hours.

Continuous passive motion is part of postoperative management until 90° of flexion is obtained. The patient may then be discharged in a hinged cast brace or a solid cast, depending on the stability of the osteotomy, the extent of lateral laxity, and the extent of compliance by the patient. The patient's limb is protected until the osteotomy has healed.

McKEEVER HEMIARTHROPLASTY

Symptomatic unicompartmental gonarthrosis in young, active patients may result from intra-articular fractures about the knee,[54] from osteochondritis dissecans, or after total meniscectomy.[20] The surgical treatment options for these patients are limited. If the patient is not a candidate for an arthroscopic procedure, and if high tibial osteotomy has failed or is

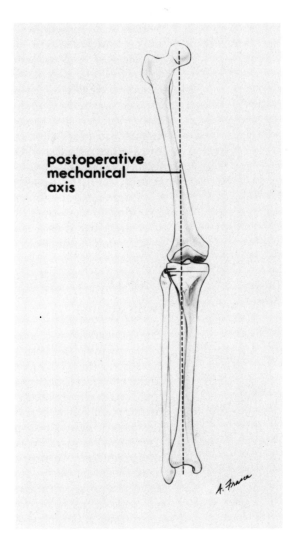

postoperative mechanical axis

FIGURE 11–8. Postoperative alignment. The center of effort is again confirmed fluoroscopically, and the knee carried through a range of motion. If the osteotomy is unstable, a second staple may be required.

contraindicated because of limited range of motion or instability, an interpositional hemiarthroplasty is an attractive alternative. Because the rates of loosening and wear of cemented prosthetic components increase with time and activity level,[38] cemented arthroplasties should be avoided in this group of patients.

McKeever[67] introduced a noncemented hemiarthroplasty for the tibial plateau in the late 1950s. It consists of a metallic plate with a slightly concave surface, and it is fixed into the tibia with a cruciate stem. Mirror-image components allow medial or lateral application. Plates ranging in thickness from 2 to 15 mm are available to help correct any varus/valgus malalignment.

Fixation and stability of the prosthesis is achieved through a fibrocartilaginous interface that is formed beneath the implant as a result of repeated compressive loads. Because cement is not required, there is no potential for formation of acrylic debris with increased wear.

Minimal amounts of bone are resected in this procedure. This is important for future arthroplasties, which are probably inevitable in these patients. In the series of McKeever hemiarthroplasties reported by Scott and co-authors,[84] 14 per cent of knees required revision because of inadequate relief of pain. In each case, the hemiarthroplasty was easily converted to a unicompartmental or a bicompartmental knee arthroplasty. Good to excellent results were achieved by 70 per cent of patients with an average follow-up interval of 8 years. In this series, patients with a poor preoperative range of motion showed improvement after surgery, which included debridement of impinging osteophytes and release of intra-articular adhesions. Obesity, which is at least a theoretical concern in any knee prosthetic arthroplasty, did not seem to adversely affect the results. Similar results have been reported by other authors.[18]

Hemiarthroplasty of the knee, although rarely indicated, should be included in the list of options for the surgical treatment of noninflammatory arthritis. It is a conservative procedure and can be converted to a unicompartmental or a total knee arthroplasty when indicated.

UNICOMPARTMENTAL KNEE ARTHROPLASTY

Indications

The indications for unicompartmental knee arthroplasty have evolved as improvements in selection of patients, in surgical techniques, and in prosthetic designs have been made. Comparisons of unicompartmental replacement with other treatment options, including arthroscopic debridement, high tibial osteotomy, and total knee arthroplasty, have also helped to establish the indications for this procedure.

The principal indication for unicompartmental replacement is unicompartmental gonarthrosis in patients with low activity demands whose symptoms are refractory to conservative measures. The patient should be near the ideal body weight, because obesity has been implicated in the failure of this procedure.[3] Only noninflammatory types of arthritis such as osteoarthritis, posttraumatic arthritis, and osteonecrosis should be considered for this procedure. Inflammatory arthritides such as rheumatoid arthritis represent panarticular processes secondary to diffuse synovial involvement and are not suitable for unicompartmental procedures.

Conditions that alter the ability of articular cartilage to accommodate normal loads are relative contraindications to unicompartmental arthroplasty because the remaining cartilage would still be at risk for degeneration. These conditions include chondrocalcinosis,[33] hemochromatosis,[98] hemophilia,[60] and ochronosis.[81]

The decision to perform an osteotomy or a unicompartmental arthroplasty is based on preoperative parameters. Although high tibial osteotomy remains the treatment of choice in young, active patients, comparisons of the long-term outcomes of the two procedures in older patients reveal superior results with unicompartmental arthroplasty.[66] Moreover, rehabilitation is faster with unicompartmental replacement because patients are frequently placed in a cast after high tibial osteotomy. Of interest, successful outcomes have been reported with unicompartmental arthroplasties after a failed high tibial osteotomy.

The final decision of whether to proceed with unicompartmental replacement or total knee arthroplasty occurs at the time of operation. Extensive degenerative changes must be limited to the compartment that is to be replaced. Areas of frank ulceration involving more than 10 per cent of the weight-bearing surface of the tibiofemoral articulation should be treated with a bi- or tricompartmental replacement.[85] An erosion is frequently seen on the non–weight-bearing surface of the medial aspect of the lateral femoral condyle; this erosion results from intercondylar impingement of tibial spine osteophytes. These can be removed and do not preclude unicompartmental replacement. Peripheral osteophytes in an otherwise normal-appearing compartment may also be removed and a unicompartmental replacement performed.[65] Although asymptomatic chondromalacia patellae does not preclude unicompartmental replacement,[85] the patellofemoral joint must not demonstrate any exposed subchondral bone, especially on the trochlear side.

Most authors agree that both cruciate ligaments must be intact in order for unicompartmental replacement to be successful. Moller and associates[69] demonstrated in a cadaver study that sectioning the anterior cruciate ligament caused the articulation between the prosthetic tibial and the femoral components to move posteriorly; they concluded that deficiency of the anterior cruciate ligament precludes unicompartmental knee arthroplasty. Goodfellow and colleagues[25] noted a higher incidence of failure in anterior cruciate ligament–deficient knees.

A deformity of up to 15° in the frontal plane and a flexion deformity of less than 20° can usually be corrected after soft tissue release and debridement of osteophytes.[65] If these maneuvers do not result in the correction of the deformity, bi- or tricompartmental replacement should be performed.

Authors' Preferred Technique

The surgical exposure is performed through a midline longitudinal skin incision commencing over the midshaft of the femur 10 cm above the patella, crossing the junction of the middle and medial third of the patella to 6 to 8 cm below the patella and 15 mm medial to the tibial tubercle (Fig. 11–9A). The quadriceps tendon is exposed and the vastus medialis identified. An arthrotomy is performed at the proximal medial pole of the patella, protecting the vastus medialis (Fig. 11–9B). The incision is continued proximally in the quadriceps tendon at the junction of the medial and middle third, extending to the articularis genu muscle. The incision is continued distally through the medial capsule and the infrapatellar fat pad.

If a medial unicompartmental arthroplasty is to be undertaken, the remaining anterior horn of the medial meniscus may be incised and the proximal medial tibia exposed. If a lateral unicompartmental replacement is being performed, the anterior horn of the medial meniscus should be protected by incising the infrapatellar fat pad more laterally or by using a lateral parapatellar approach.

The patella is everted, and the knee is flexed. A knee retractor is placed within the joint so as to protect the medial collateral ligament. The remainder of the medial meniscus is excised. The joint is then inspected in order to assess the need for a uni-, bi-, or tricompartmental replacement. Once a unicompartmental replacement is chosen, a sponge is placed over the patellofemoral joint and the lateral compartment in order to prevent

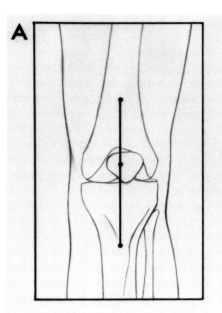
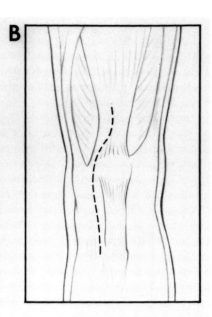

FIGURE 11–9. (*A*) A longitudinal skin incision is centered over the junction of the medial and middle thirds of the patella and is overlying the midshaft of the femur proximally and the medial aspect of the tibial tubercle distally. (*B*) Medial parapatellar arthrotomy follows; care should be taken to avoid the fibers of the vastus medialis musculature. (From Tsahakis PA, Sledge CB: The unicompartmental knee arthroplasty. *In* Chapman MW [ed]: Operative Orthopaedics, 2nd ed. Philadelphia: JB Lippincott, in press.)

debris from contaminating these compartments and to prevent dessication of the cartilage surface.

With the knee held in full extension, the leading edge of the anterior tibia is marked with methylene blue on the femoral condyle (Fig. 11–10*A*). This edge represents the most anterior extent of contact between the tibial and femoral articular surfaces. The sizing jig (Fig. 11–10*B*) is then used to estimate the size of the femoral component to be inserted. The foot is placed under the femoral condyle, and the leading edge of the guide is placed on the methylene blue mark.

To obtain adequate seating of the posterior condylar cutting guide, it may be necessary to contour the distal femur with a burr (Fig. 11–11). This enables the distal condylar cutting guide to accurately match the profile of the femoral condyle and prevents unwanted flexion of the femoral component.

Care is taken to orient the condylar cutting guide so as to avoid excessive internal or external rotation (Fig. 11–12*A*). In the lateral plane, the handle of the cutting guide is placed at 90°. Each pin track is predrilled before insertion of the pin. Drilling the pins and inserting them sequentially avoids possible toggling or loss of position of the guide (Fig. 11–12*B*). A narrow bladed saw is then used to perform the posterior condylar cut, protecting both the collateral ligament and the cruciate ligaments (Fig. 11–13). The femoral component drill guide is placed on the distal femur, and an osteotome is used to confirm that the mechanical axis of 5° to 7° is obtained (Fig. 11–14). Once the holes have been completed, the trial femoral component is seated, and care is taken to ensure that there is adequate prosthesis bone contact. There should be a smooth transition

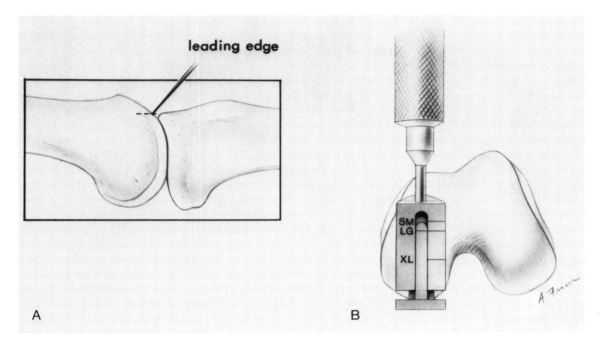

FIGURE 11–10. (*A*) The anterior extent of the tibiofemoral contact is identified by placing the knee in extension and marking the contact of the tibia with the femoral articular surface. (*B*) Sizing of the femoral condyle is performed with the knee in 90° of flexion and aligning the femoral sizing guide with the previously marked leading edge. (From Tsahakis PA, Sledge CB: The unicompartmental knee arthroplasty. *In* Chapman MW [ed]: Operative Orthopaedics, 2nd ed. Philadelphia: JB Lippincott, in press.)

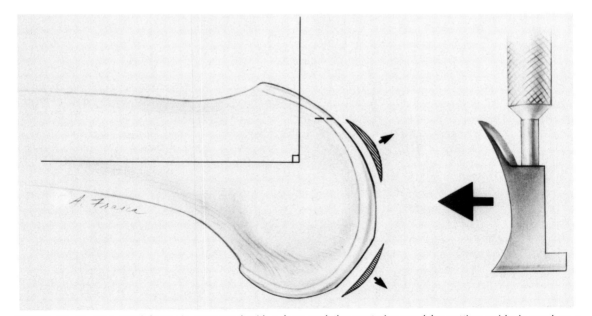

FIGURE 11–11. The distal femur is contoured with a burr, and the posterior condylar cutting guide is used as a template. (From Tsahakis PA, Sledge CB: The unicompartmental knee arthroplasty. *In* Chapman MW [ed]: Operative Orthopaedics, 2nd ed. Philadelphia: JB Lippincott, in press.)

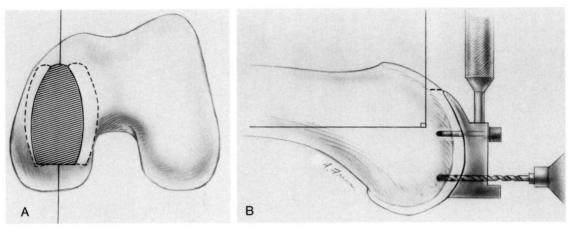

FIGURE 11–12. (*A*) The posterior condylar cutting guide is oriented in the anteroposterior plane to avoid malrotation of the femoral component. (*B*) In the sagittal plane, the posterior condylar cutting guide is aligned at 90° in relation to the long axis of the femur. Predrilling the pin sites prevents toggling of the guide when the pins are tapped through eburnated bone. (From Tsahakis PA, Sledge CB: The unicompartmental knee arthroplasty. *In* Chapman MW [ed]: Operative Orthopaedics, 2nd ed. Philadelphia: JB Lippincott, in press.)

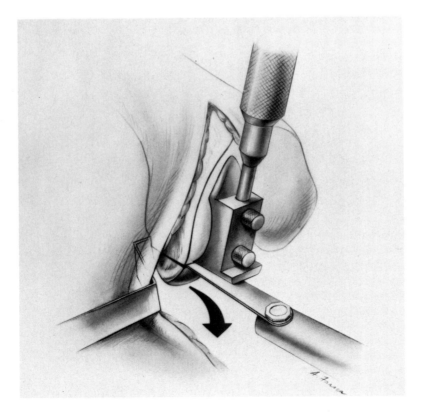

FIGURE 11–13. The posterior condylar resection is executed with an oscillating saw. (From Tsahakis PA, Sledge CB: The unicompartmental knee arthroplasty. *In* Chapman MW [ed]: Operative Orthopaedics, 2nd ed. Philadelphia: JB Lippincott, in press.)

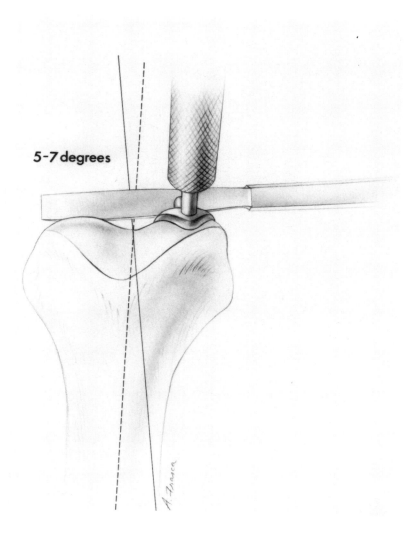

5-7 degrees

FIGURE 11–14. The femoral component drill guide is oriented on the distal femur so that a mechanical axis of 5° to 7° is achieved. This angle can be confirmed intraoperatively by placing an osteotome across the proposed location of the drill guide and observing its intersection with the anatomic axis on the femur. (From Tsahakis PA, Sledge CB: The unicompartmental knee arthroplasty. *In* Chapman MW [ed]: Operative Orthopaedics, 2nd ed. Philadelphia: JB Lippincott, in press.)

between the articular cartilage of the unresurfaced femur and the femoral component.

An osteotome may again be used to determine the mechanical axis of the femur (Fig. 11–15). The knee is placed in full extension, and a line is drawn on the tibial plateau 2 mm lateral (or medial) to the edge of the femoral component. The knee is then flexed, and the line is continued posteriorly. This line marks the lateral (or medial) limit of the tibial resection and assists in ensuring rotational congruity (Fig. 11–16). The tibial alignment guide may then be placed on the femur. With the knee in extension and held in normal alignment, the proposed tibial resection is marked (Fig. 11–17A). The guide is then removed, the knee is flexed, and a tibial resection guide is placed against the tibia. This guide should closely approximate the line previously constructed with the tibial alignment guide (Fig. 11–17B). The tibial resection is completed with approximately a 3° posterior slope. This slope matches the normal tibial slope and prevents impingement in flexion.

A trial reduction is performed with the femoral and tibial components in situ. The correct rotational alignment of the tibial component is

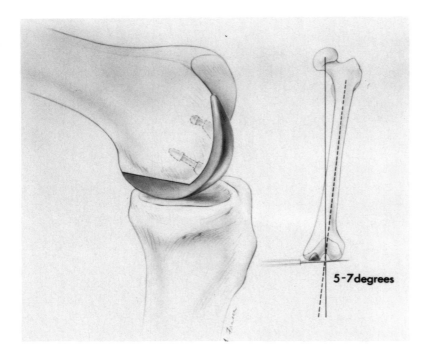

5-7degrees

FIGURE 11–15. The appropriate-sized trial femoral component is inserted, and adequate prosthesis-bone contact is confirmed. The leading edge of the femoral component should provide a smooth transition of the remaining distal femoral cartilage anteriorly. The orientation of the trial femoral component in the anteroposterior plane can once more be checked by again placing an osteotome across the distal femur and determining the mechanical axis. (From Tsahakis PA, Sledge CB: The unicompartmental knee arthroplasty. *In* Chapman MW [ed]: Operative Orthopaedics, 2nd ed. Philadelphia: JB Lippincott, in press.)

established (Fig. 11–18). The fixation holes for the tibial component are then marked and completed with a burr.

A final trial reduction is performed with the real components in situ; there must be no impingement of the tibial spines in extension or rocking of the tibial or femoral components with flexion and extension. The patella is relocated for the trial reduction; again, there should be no impingement of the patella articular cartilage on the femoral component.

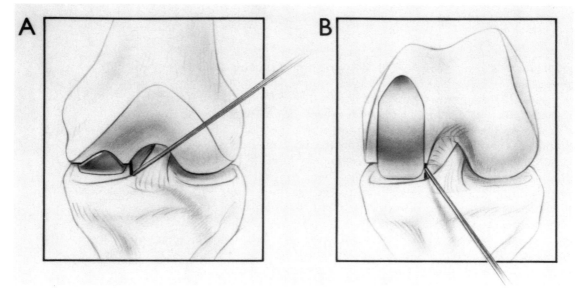

FIGURE 11–16. (*A*) With the trial component in place, the knee is placed in full extension, and a line is begun on the tibial plateau with methylene blue 2 mm lateral to the edge of the component. (*B*) The knee is then flexed to 90° and the line is completed. (From Tsahakis PA, Sledge CB: The unicompartmental knee arthroplasty. *In* Chapman MW [ed]: Operative Orthopaedics, 2nd ed. Philadelphia: JB Lippincott, in press.)

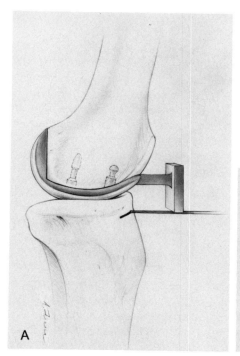

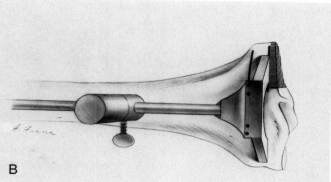

FIGURE 11–17. (A) With the use of the tibial alignment guide, a horizontal line is drawn on the anterior aspect of the proximal tibia while a valgus force is applied to the fully extended knee. (B) With a tibial resection guide aligned with the previously drawn line, a minimal tibial resection is accomplished with an oscillating saw. (From Tsahakis PA, Sledge CB: The unicompartmental knee arthroplasty. *In* Chapman MW [ed]: Operative Orthopaedics, 2nd ed. Philadelphia: JB Lippincott, in press.)

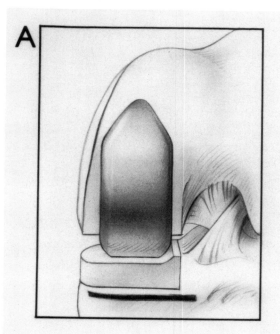

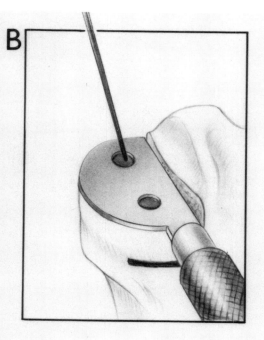

FIGURE 11–18. (A) The axis of rotation of the tibial component is established by inserting trial components and observing the knee through its range of motion. Particular attention is paid to the congruency and stability of the components. (B) Once the position of the tibial components is confirmed, the trial components are removed, and the position of the tibial fixation lugs is marked. The fixation holes can be created with a burr. (From Tsahakis PA, Sledge CB: The unicompartmental knee arthroplasty. *In* Chapman MW [ed]: Operative Orthopaedics, 2nd ed. Philadelphia: JB Lippincott, in press.)

The components are removed and thoroughly cleaned, the bone surfaces are thoroughly water picked and dried, and the components are cemented (Fig. 11–19). The tibial component is placed first. The knee is held in extension until the cement has hardened. Any additional cement that has extruded is removed with a ¼-inch osteotome. Care is taken to ensure that no cement remains posteriorly on either the tibial plateau or the femoral component.

The knee is once more thoroughly irrigated to remove all debris, the tourniquet is deflated, hemostasis is obtained, and the wound is closed in layers over two intra-articular closed suction drains.

TOTAL KNEE ARTHROPLASTY

Historical Perspective

In 1940, Campbell[12] reported the successful use of a metallic interposition femoral mold. Shortly thereafter, M. N. Smith-Petersen, at the Massachusetts General Hospital, developed a similar arthroplasty that was initially used to treat rheumatoid arthritis patients with ankylosed knees. Subsequently, in 1953, a femoral stem was added.[46] MacIntosh[57a] and, shortly thereafter, McKeever[67] reported the use of a hemiarthroplasty that served as an interposition on the tibial side.

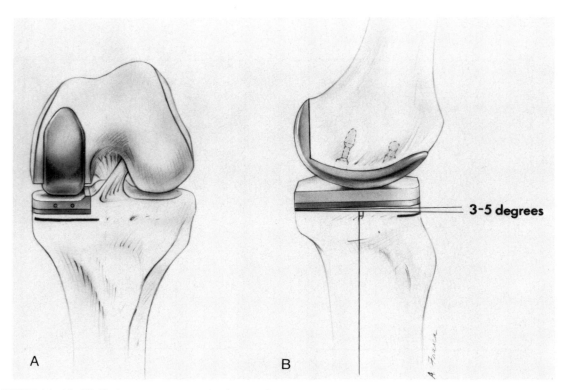

FIGURE 11–19. (A) The components are simultaneously cemented in place. After curing and removal of any excess cement, the knee is again placed through its range of motion, and any impingement with the patella or tibial spines and prosthetic components is observed. Proper soft tissue tension and prosthetic congruency are confirmed. (B) In the sagittal plane, the tibial component should be sloped posteriorly 3° to 5° in order to avoid prosthetic impingement in flexion. (From Tsahakis PA, Sledge CB: The unicompartmental knee arthroplasty. *In* Chapman MW [ed]: Operative Orthopaedics, 2nd ed. Philadelphia: JB Lippincott, in press.)

A second line of development began when B. Walldius introduced the first hinged prosthesis in 1951. Other hinges such as Shier's[87] hinge and the Guepar hinge were developed. These metal hinged prostheses corrected severe deformities while providing at least 90° of painless knee motion. Their excessive constraint, however, and the metal-on-metal design led to frequent loosening and a high rate of infection.[72] Less constrained hinges, the Spherocentric hinge and the Kinematic rotating hinge, were developed. These designs, however, still entailed unacceptably high failure rates.[72]

Gunston and MacKenzie[26, 27] heralded the era of modern knee replacements by introducing an unlinked prosthesis with metallic femoral runners that articulated with polyethylene troughs on the tibial side. In order to secure the components to the underlying bone, acrylic cement was used for the first time. This polycentric knee replacement was the first cemented surface replacement, and its design was based on the changing arc of radius of the femoral condyles with flexion. The collateral and cruciate ligaments were retained in this design in order to enhance joint stability.

Two schools of thought then developed with regard to prosthetic design and the posterior cruciate ligament. The cruciate-sparing design, with the duocondylar prosthesis as a prototype, was developed in the early 1970s. It did not allow patellofemoral replacement. Residual patellofemoral symptoms in 20 per cent of patients[89] led to the development of the duopatellar replacement, which did provide for resurfacing the patella. Further improvements in all of the prosthetic components led to the RBBH (Robert Breck Brigham Hospital) knee. These changes included a deepened trochlear groove aligned in 7° of valgus angulation in order to improve patellar tracking. A one-piece central stemmed polyethylene tibial component was ultimately added to buffer varus-valgus forces and compression-distraction forces in the sagittal plane. In an effort to decrease tibial component loosening, metal backing was added in 1980 on the premise that loads would be more uniformly transferred to the proximal tibia. Several current metal-to-metal plastic designs allow for cruciate retention in an unconstrained device.

The cruciate-sacrificing design was introduced by Freeman and Swanson, and results with this prosthesis were reported in 1973.[21] The most successful cruciate-sacrificing prosthesis, the total condylar knee prosthesis, was designed in 1973 and is still available in its original form. It comprised a dome-shaped polyethylene patellar component with a central, rectangular fixation lug. Limited flexion to only 90° led to the development of the cruciate-substituting design, in which an intercondylar eminence articulates with the femoral component in flexion, enabling femoral rollback to occur.[37]

Posterior Cruciate Ligament

One of the most enduring and controversial subjects in total knee arthroplasty has concerned retention or excision of the posterior cruciate ligament. A brief review of the role of this ligament in normal knee kinematics is useful for understanding this debate. As the strongest ligament in the knee,[49] the posterior cruciate ligament serves many purposes. As a stabilizer, it absorbs anterior and posterior shearing forces, ultimately preventing posterior subluxation of the tibia on the femur. The posterior cruciate ligament is responsible for the combination of rolling and gliding of the femoral condyles in relation to the tibia during flexion, which enable the tibiofemoral contact point to move posteriorly. Through this mechanism, physiologic flexion occurs. Also, the movement posteriorly of the tibiofemoral contact point enhances the efficiency of the quadriceps mechanism by producing a longer lever arm.

All of these functions of the posterior cruciate ligament are useful in total knee arthroplasty. Certainly, one of the biggest problems in cemented total knee arthroplasty has been loosening of the tibial component and polyethylene wear. Sledge and Ewald[88] demonstrated that the bone-cement interface is at risk from shear forces. Through resection of the posterior cruciate ligament, stresses that are otherwise dissipated through this natural stabilizer are borne by a necessarily more constrained prosthesis, leading to increased stress at the critical bone-cement interface and at the metal-polyethylene articulation. Ultimately, these forces could allow premature loosening, although both cruciate retention and cruciate resection designs have similar loosening rates at 5- to 9-year follow-up.[35, 103]

One of the purposes of total knee arthroplasty is to improve function. In the knee, this is accomplished by providing a stable joint with as near normal a range of motion as can be achieved. Andriacchi and co-authors evaluated gait patterns after total knee arthroplasty and demonstrated improved stability on stairs, especially during descent, with prostheses that retained the posterior cruciate ligament, as opposed to prostheses in which the ligament was sacrificed.[1] Also, because the posterior cruciate ligament allows more physiologic motion to occur, its retention should enhance function and lead to greater satisfaction on the part of the patient after total knee arthroplasty.

Advocates for posterior cruciate sacrifice/substitution designs point out that resection of the posterior cruciate ligament enables a technically less demanding arthroplasty to be accomplished. It obviates the need to balance the posterior cruciate ligament in flexion and extension.

In summary, it appears beneficial to preserve the posterior cruciate ligament in patients without severe deformity because function is enhanced. Longer follow-up periods are necessary for determining any differences in rates of loosening that results from increased stresses at the bone-cement interface with cruciate resection designs.

Indications

The indications for total knee arthroplasty in patients with osteoarthritis are (1) disabling pain that is unresponsive to nonsteroidal anti-inflammatory drugs and (2) marked functional impairment. Older patients with a sedentary lifestyle and whose recreational activities involve low-impact sports such as golf, biking, or swimming should be selected. There should be clinical and radiographic evidence of tricompartmental degenerative changes, and the patient should not be a candidate for a simpler procedure such as arthroscopic debridement or osteotomy.

Active pyogenic sepsis is an absolute contraindication to total knee arthroplasty. The procedure can, however, be safely performed in patients who were previously treated for sepsis and those who have suffered a previous bout of tuberculosis after systemic chemotherapy, debridement, and aspiration of the joint with negative findings.[52]

Although obesity poses theoretical concerns regarding potentially increased rates of wear and loosening, Stern and Insall[95] reported no difference in overall knee scores between obese and nonobese patients. They did, however, note an increased rate of patellofemoral symptoms in obese patients.

Neuropathic arthropathy may mimic osteoarthritis in some patients. It has traditionally been considered a contraindication to total knee arthroplasty secondary to high failure rates. Recent reports, however, have documented success in this setting with unconstrained prostheses if appropriate surgical technique is followed.[92]

Preoperative Evaluation

RADIOGRAPHS

Radiographs that should be obtained for a patient being considered for total knee arthroplasty include standing anteroposterior, lateral, and skyline views. Assessment of the joint space, general bone quality, bone stock, and periarticular deformity can be made on these views and help guide surgical planning. Also, a 36-inch radiograph of the patient standing should be obtained in order to determine mechanical axis and to evaluate any deformity in the femur, the tibia, or both.[53]

RESULTS OF INGROWTH VERSUS CEMENTED FIXATION

Total knee arthroplasty has undergone many advances since 1970 in terms of implant design and prophylaxis for sepsis and thromboembolic disease. One remaining controversial and unsolved problem involves prosthetic component fixation. Whereas the most frequent cause of failure in early knee arthroplasties was prosthetic loosening,[39] several more recent reports of cemented implants have shown a low incidence of failure through this mechanism at follow-up for up to nine years.[35, 103]

Excellent results have been reported with both cemented posterior cruciate ligament–sparing and ligament–sacrificing prostheses at 5- to 9-year follow-up.[35, 103] Both prosthetic designs have low rates of loosening and complications. The main difference has been a slightly higher arc of flexion with the ligament–sparing design. Wright and co-workers[103] reported an average flexion arc of 109° with the kinematic prosthesis. In fact, among 65 per cent of patients, average flexion arc was 110° to 135°.

These encouraging results have increased the confidence of surgeons who perform total knee arthroplasties, and as a result, the lower age limit for this procedure continues to fall. The long-term follow-up experience with total hip replacement and recognized problems with acrylic cement debris, however, have caused investigators to question the routine use of cement in prosthetic fixation and to evaluate uncemented implants as an alternative form of fixation.

Cementless implants consist of porous coatings applied to solid metal components. Optimal pore size for ingrowth is between 50 and 100 μm.[8] The metals most commonly used are cobalt-chromium-molybdenum alloy and titanium alloy. Fixation occurs through ingrowth of bony and fibrous tissue.

Two requirements relating to surgical technique have been identified for ingrowth of bone into the porous coating of cementless implants.[28] The first is that the porous coating on the prosthetic component must be in intimate contact with the bone. Significantly less bony ingrowth has been observed in animal studies if this contact is not achieved.[30] The second consideration regards movement at the bone-prosthesis interface. Motion at this interface has been shown to inhibit bone ingrowth.[11] Methods of limiting this movement include impacting the prosthesis onto the bony surface or rigidly fixing the prosthesis through the use of screws or pegs.

Several authors have reviewed the outcome of cementless fixation in total knee arthroplasties with short and medium-length follow-up. Rorabeck and collaborators[78] prospectively reviewed the short-term results of cemented and cementless total knee arthroplasties and noted a higher rate of reoperation and a poorer clinical outcome among patients undergoing the cementless procedure.

Rosenberg and associates[79] compared the results of cemented and cementless fixation at 3- to 6-year follow-up. In contrast to Rorabeck and collaborators' report, they observed similar results between the two groups. In fact, the results of the cementless procedure improved with longer follow-up, which Rosenberg and associates thought reflected the biologic nature of this type of fixation.

Dodd and associates[17] recently reported on 18 patients with an average follow-up interval of 5 years who underwent staged bilateral total knee arthroplasties with the porous coated anatomic prosthesis. Each patient was treated with a cemented prosthesis on one side and an uncemented prosthesis on the contralateral side. Similar functional and clinical results were noted in both groups.

Wright and co-workers[104] reported the results of a posterior cruciate ligament–sparing prosthesis with an uncemented femoral component after an average follow-up interval of 2.8 years. Good to excellent results were noted in 93 per cent of patients. Moreover, there was no evidence of component loosening. These results compare favorably with those of cemented femoral fixation at similar follow-up intervals.

An alternative cementless prosthesis designed by Ewald and colleagues[19] involves press fit fixation without provision for bony ingrowth. It is theorized that a new supportive subchondral bone plate forms secondary to multiple microtrabecular fractures from cyclical loading between the proximal tibia and the smooth metal surface of the prosthesis.

Rackemann and associates examined the results of this prosthesis after average follow-up of 43 months in 17 patients whose average age was 52 years.[76] The diagnoses included revision arthroplasties and post-sepsis reconstructions failed. Pain relief was complete in 16 of 17 patients, and range of motion averaged 99° of flexion. Ambulation was unrestricted in the majority of patients, who were relatively young and active, and prosthetic loosening and migration was not observed. This form of cementless knee arthroplasty should be considered as an alternative to other forms of fixation in young, active patients who are not candidates for lesser procedures.

Authors' Preferred Technique

Patients undergoing total knee arthroplasty should be prepared and draped so that the entire leg is visualized. A pneumatic tourniquet is placed on the upper thigh. A standard midline incision is made, and the capsule is opened in a medial parapatellar fashion; the arthrotomy is carried proximally to the articularis genu and distally along the medial side of the infrapatellar tendon (Fig. 11–20). The patella is then everted, the patellofemoral ligament is sacrificed, and an initial joint inspection is performed (Fig. 11–21). A preliminary balancing of soft tissue is performed on the basis of the patient's preoperative deformity. In a varus knee, a preliminary medial release is performed. In a valgus knee, a preliminary lateral release is performed. In a tight valgus knee or a knee with difficult exposure, a lateral retinacular release for patellar tracking may be performed as a preliminary portion of the soft tissue balancing. Final adjustment of the soft tissues in total knee arthroplasty is performed once the trial components have been inserted. Tensioning is performed through the use of the trial components with appropriate thicknesses of tibial inserts.

Before performing the bone cuts, it is essential to obtain adequate exposure. In most cases, the tibia can be subluxed anterior to the femur in four steps. The first is to release the patellofemoral ligament; such release loosens the lateral side (Fig. 11–22). In addition, it is important to expose the anterolateral surface of the tibia, which may require removal of a portion of the iliotibial band from Gerdy's tubercle. A portion of the fat pad may be removed if necessary for obtaining full visualization of the surface. The second step is to take a curved osteotome and sharply reflect the posterior oblique ligament from the posteromedial corner of the knee (Fig. 11–23). The dissection is carried around to the semimembranosus tendon. The third step is to remove the entire anterior cruciate ligament. Finally, it is important to release the posteromedial and posterolateral meniscal attachments from the back of the tibia (Fig. 11–24). At this point, the tibia can be generally subluxed anterior to the femur.

The sequence of bone cuts is not critical as long as proper alignment is restored. Alignment can be considered as correction of the coronal,

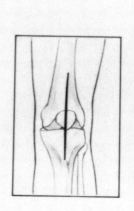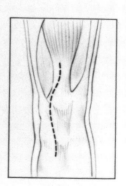

FIGURE 11–20. The approach. A longitudinal skin incision is centered over the junction of the middle and medial thirds of the patella and is overlying the midshaft of the femur proximally and the medial aspect of the tibial tubercle distally. Then a medial parapatellar arthrotomy, extending proximally to the articularis genu and distally along the medial side of the infrapatellar tendon, is made.

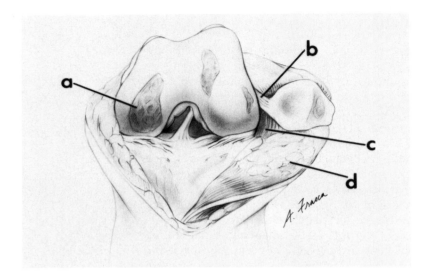

FIGURE 11–21. Preliminary exposure in an osteoarthritic knee: eburnated bone (a), patellofemoral ligament (b), iliotibial band (c), and infrapatellar fat pad (d).

sagittal, and transverse or rotational axis. The coronal and sagittal axes are determined by the proximal tibia and distal femoral cuts. These cuts determine the varus/valgus alignment, femoral flexion, and tibial posterior slope. They should be made independent of one another and according to bony landmarks. Correct alignment of the transverse or rotational axis is more difficult. Femoral rotation is determined by the femoral anterior, posterior, and chamfer cuts. Rotation of the tibia is the alignment of the tibial component in relation to the tibial tubercle. Patellar alignment is a function of the patellar resection coupled with quadriceps soft tissue balancing.

The proximal tibial cut can be made by means of an intramedullary or extramedullary system. The authors prefer an extramedullary system on the tibia because the bony landmarks are readily palpable and the

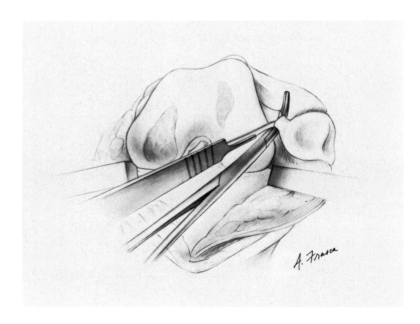

FIGURE 11–22. The exposure is increased until the tibia can be subluxed anterior to the femur. This is usually accomplished in four steps, the first of which is to release the patellofemoral ligament.

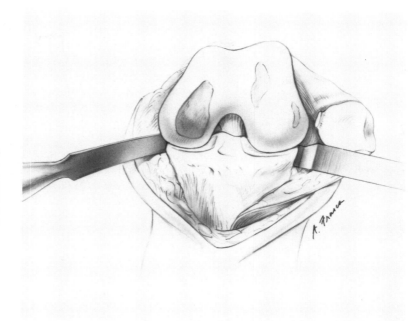

FIGURE 11–23. The second step of the exposure is to sharply reflect the posterior oblique ligament from the posteromedial corner of the knee with a curved osteotome. The third step is to excise the entire anterior cruciate ligament.

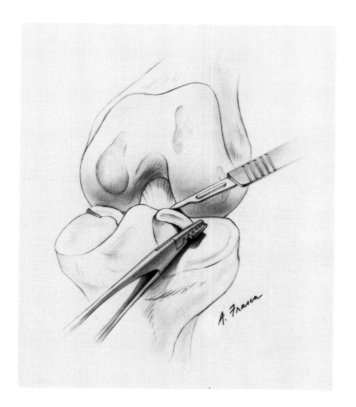

FIGURE 11–24. The final step of the exposure involves the excision of the posteromedial and posterolateral meniscal attachments. At this point, the tibia can be generally subluxed anterior to the femur.

posterior slope can be adjusted independently. Intramedullary tibial cuts require making a hole in the proximal tibia that is not generally in the same position as the lugs or the central peg for tibial fixation. Intramedullary tibial alignment is accurate for varus knees, but in certain valgus knees with exaggerated tibial bows, the intramedullary rod cannot be placed in a proper position. Intramedullary tibial fixation is helpful in cases of severe obesity or peripheral edema that would mask the normal bony landmarks.

The first step in extramedullary fixation of the tibia is to determine the approximate position of the anterior aspect of the tibial component in relationship with the tibial tubercle. This point is generally midway between the medial and lateral edges of the tibial plateau, in the center of the piece of the tibial spines, and at the junction of the middle third and lateral two thirds of the infrapatellar tendon (Fig. 11–25). This mark is made for three specific reasons. First, it is a guide for placing the tibial resection jig along the anterior face of the proximal tibia. Second, it prevents placement of the jig in relative internal rotation to the tibia. If the jig is placed in internal rotation and if posterior slope is built into the cut, an abnormal valgus resection could result. The third reason for marking the front of the tibia is to serve as a guide for final tibial component rotation. There is a tendency to internally rotate the tibial prosthesis on the tibia as the patellar tendon and fat pad can block lateral exposure. An internally rotated tibial component increases the quadriceps angle and makes patellar tracking more difficult. Moreover, if the posterior cruciate ligament is retained, an internally rotated tibial component ne-

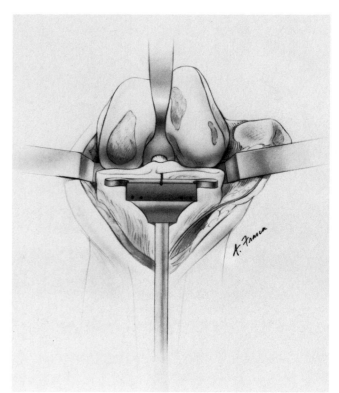

FIGURE 11–25. Tibial resection. The approximate midpoint of the tibial plateau is marked with methylene blue. This point is generally midway between the medial and lateral edges of the tibial plateau, in the center of the tibial spines and at the junction of the middle third and the lateral two thirds of the infrapatellar tendon. This point aids in placing the tibial resection guide along the anterior face of the proximal tibia. Retractors are placed to protect the medial and lateral collateral ligaments and to keep the tibia anteriorly subluxed.

cessitates internal rotation of the femoral component for congruity and may again predispose the knee to patellar problems.

Once the tibial alignment jig is applied proximally, it must be adjusted distally in the coronal plane in order to establish varus/valgus alignment. Centering the alignment guide between the malleolae results in a more varus tibial cut as the lateral malleolus causes the intermalleolar center to be about 3 to 5 mm lateral to the center of the talus. The distal portion of the tibial alignment guide should therefore be subluxed medially in order to center it over the talus (Fig. 11–26). The cutaneous landmarks for the center of the talus include the sulcus just lateral to the tibialis anterior tendon and the point just distal to the sharp anterior crest of the tibia and parallel to the second ray (if there is no midfoot or hindfoot abnormality).

Once the tibial alignment guide is placed, the level of resection is determined, and the resection is executed with an oscillating saw (Fig. 11–27). As a general rule, the surgeon should remove the same amount of bone as will be replaced by the prosthesis in order to prevent artificial raising or lowering of the joint line. In cases of bone defects, the size of the defect can generally be determined from the preoperative radiograph. This technique involves drawing a line perpendicular to the mechanical axis of the tibia that goes along the joint side of the normal plateau. A

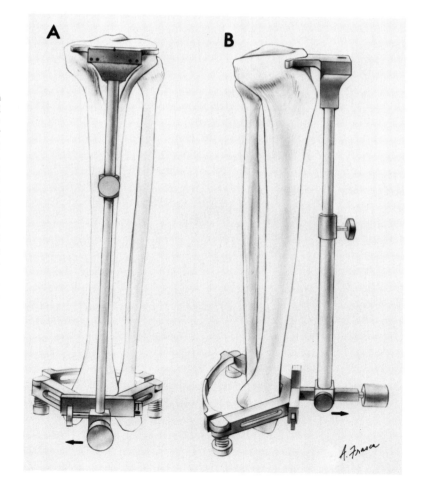

FIGURE 11–26. Tibial resection (continued). (*A*) Once the tibial alignment guide is applied proximally, it must be adjusted distally in the coronal plane in order to establish varus/valgus alignment. The distal portion of the guide is subluxed medially in order to center it over the talus. The cutaneous landmarks for the center of the talus include the sulcus just lateral to the tibialis anterior tendon and the point just distal to the sharp anterior crest of the tibia and parallel to the second ray. The level of resection is determined in such a way that the amount of bone removed equals that replaced by the prosthesis. This avoids raising or lowering the joint line. (*B*) In the sagittal plane, the guide is adjusted to reproduce the patient's anatomy. This usually results in 0° to 5° of posterior slope.

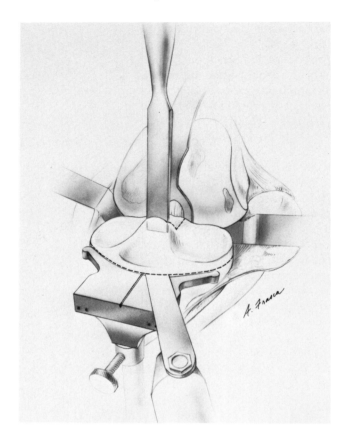

FIGURE 11–27. Tibial resection (continued). After the precutting of a bone block anterior to the posterior cruciate ligament, the proximal tibia is resected with an oscillating saw. A half-inch osteotome protects the posterior cruciate ligament.

line vertical to this line at the largest area of defect, when corrected for radiographic magnification, is a measure of the total defect present. If an 8-mm portion is to be removed from the normal condyle, the residual defect will be the size of the original defect minus 8 mm. It is the authors' opinion that the patient's posterior slope should be reproduced if there is no severe posterior erosion. The amount of posterior slope is a function of the patient's anatomy, the prosthetic design, the preoperative range of motion and the integrity of the soft tissue.

The proximal tibial cut has been used to determine the coronal and sagittal planes for the tibial component. The next cut should be on the

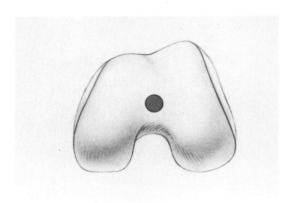

FIGURE 11–28. Distal femoral resection. The authors recommend an intramedullary guide for the distal femoral resection. This cut determines both the coronal and sagittal plane alignment. The medullary canal is entered just anterior to the femoral attachment of the posterior cruciate ligament with a $5/16$-inch drill.

distal femur and is used to determine both its coronal and sagittal planes. It is easiest to make this with an intramedullary device at 5°, 7°, or 9° of valgus angulation, depending on the preoperative determination of the difference between the anatomic and mechanical axes of the femur. It is important to remove any remaining cartilage and any osteophytes that project distally as their presence may result in underresection of the distal femur. The femoral medullary canal is entered just anterior to the femoral attachment of the posterior cruciate ligament (Fig. 11–28). In general, 8 mm is removed from the most prominant condyle in order to be replaced with an 8-mm prosthesis and to maintain the femoral joint line (Figs. 11–29, 11–30).

The next cuts on the anterior and posterior femur determine the femoral rotation. In the absence of any posteromedial or posterolateral bone deficiency, a standard guide can key off the femoral posterior condyles in order to ensure a neutral rotation (Fig. 11–31). There are several instances in which slight external rotation of the femur is desirable. The most likely is a varus knee that has undergone more lateral than medial plateau resection in order to return the tibial cut to a neutral alignment. This, coupled with tighter medial soft tissues, leaves a posteromedial gap that is smaller than the posterolateral gap. Some of this difference can be corrected by release of medial soft tissue, but it is also helpful to externally rotate the femoral component. This rotation also faces the trochlear flange somewhat laterally to track better with the patella.

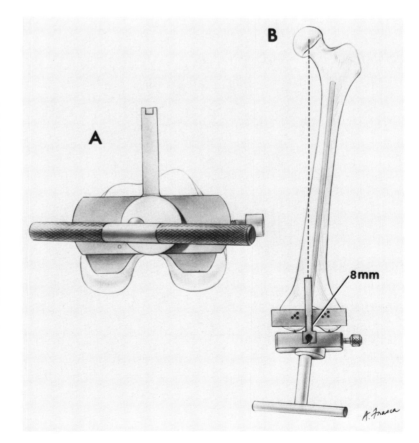

FIGURE 11–29. Distal femoral resection (continued). (*A*) The intramedullary guide is set at 5°, 7°, or 9° of valgus angulation, depending on the preoperative determination of the difference between the anatomic and mechanical axes of the femur. The rotation alignment of the guide is adjusted with reference to the posterior femoral condyles. If one condyle is deficient, the medial and lateral epicondyles can be used for rotational alignment. This initial rotation is further adjusted at the time of the anteroposterior femoral resection. (*B*) Typically, 8 mm are removed from the most prominent condyle and are replaced with 8 mm of prosthesis in order to maintain the femoral joint line.

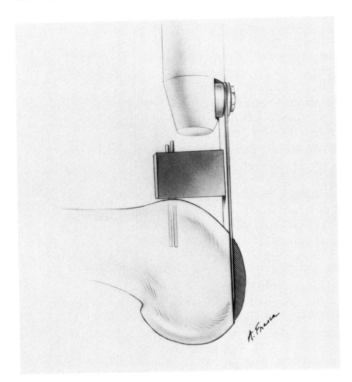

FIGURE 11–30. Distal femoral resection (continued). This distal femoral resection is executed with an oscillating saw. The resected surface must be carefully checked to ensure that it is perfectly flat.

FIGURE 11–31. Anteroposterior femoral resection. (*A*) The appropriate-sized femoral drill guide is positioned against the resected distal femur. A stylus keyed off the anterior femoral cortex may be used to confirm the proposed size. (*B*) Femoral rotational alignment is determined by aligning the drill guide skids with the posterior condyles. The guide should be perpendicular to the mechanical axis of the tibia at 90° of knee flexion. The femoral drill guide may be used to place the femoral component in 3° of external rotation. This is particularly useful in a varus knee in which an asymmetric tibial resection (lateral plateau greater than medial plateau) is required for neutral tibial alignment. This also aids in patellar tracking.

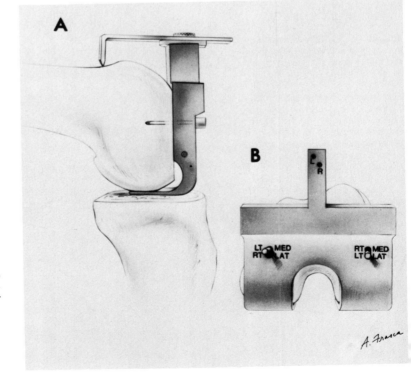

Moreover, slight external rotation of the femoral component allows a commensurate external rotation of the tibial component on the tibia. This external rotation of the tibial component brings it more underneath the tibial tubercle, thereby decreasing the quadriceps angle and facilitating patellar tracking.

Once the femoral cuts have been made (Figs. 11–32, 11–33), a trial femoral component is seated (Fig. 11–34) and matched with a trial tibial component with an appropriate insert. The size of the tibial component is based on the amount that most fully caps but does not overhang the tibia (Fig. 11–35). The key to femoral sizing is bringing the anterior flange of the component flush with the anterior cortex of the femur. Care must be taken not to overresect anteriorly and to avoid notching, which would weaken the bone, and not to underresect and raise the flange of the prosthetic femur, which artificially tightens the quadriceps.

With the trial components in place, the leg is extended and the tibial tray is rotated in order to ensure proper congruity with the femur. This tibial rotational alignment is marked and is the final determination of the rotational orientation of the tibial component (Fig. 11–36). The proper thickness of tibial insert is chosen in order to obtain soft tissue stability without excessive tightness. The leg should come into extension, but not hyperextension. The collateral ligaments should be tight, but not overly tight. There may be 1 mm of play with the leg in full extension and 5° of flexion. The knee should be flexed with the patella in the trochlea; there should be no tendency for the femur to sublux to the posterior part of the tibial component, and the tibial tray without a fixation stem should not lift off anteriorly. Such subluxation or lift-off generally indicates excessive tightness of the posterior cruciate ligament, the posterior structures, or both. In this case, further posterior release and a posterior cruciate resection is indicated. With the trial tibial tray as a template, a series of punches are used to prepare the proximal tibia for the keel of the tibial component (Fig. 11–37).

The final cut is on the patella; before the cut is made, it is important to remove the soft tissues about the patella and to define the chondro-osseous junction. The cut should go from the chondro-osseous junction on the medial side to the same junction on the lateral side. This means removing more bone on the medial half than on the lateral half. The anterior and superior margins are determined by the quadriceps tendon insertion and the infrapatellar tendon, respectively. The patella should be

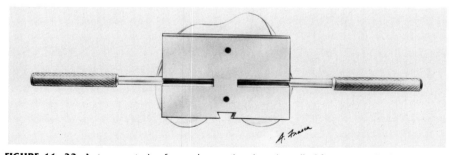

FIGURE 11–32. Anteroposterior femoral resection (continued). After removal of the femoral drill guide, the corresponding anteroposterior cutting block is applied to the distal femur; the previously tapped holes are used as templates for placement.

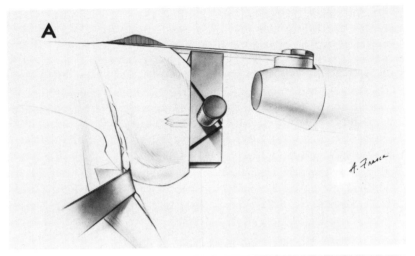

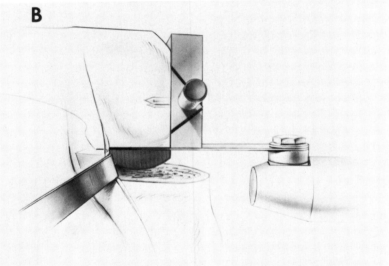

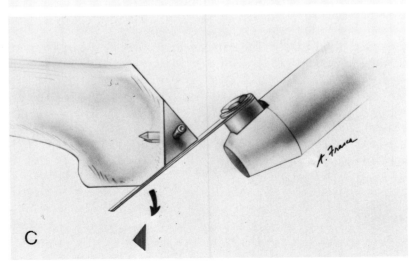

FIGURE 11–33. Anteroposterior femoral resection. (*A, B*) The anterior and posterior femoral cuts are executed with an oscillating saw. Retractors are positioned in order to protect the collateral ligaments. (*C*) The correspondingly sized chamfer guide is applied to the distal femur, and the femoral cuts are completed.

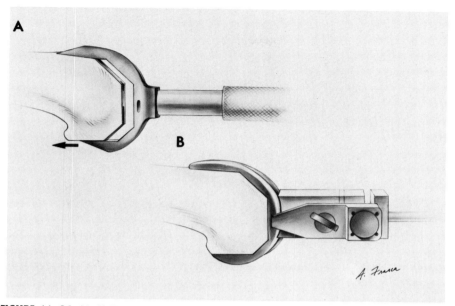

FIGURE 11–34. (*A, B*) Femoral trial reduction. A trial femoral component is fully seated. The prosthesis bone interfaces are critically inspected for an intimate fit, and neutral sagittal plane alignment is confirmed.

FIGURE 11–35. Tibial trial reduction. A trial tibial component that most fully caps the proximal tibia without any component overhang is chosen.

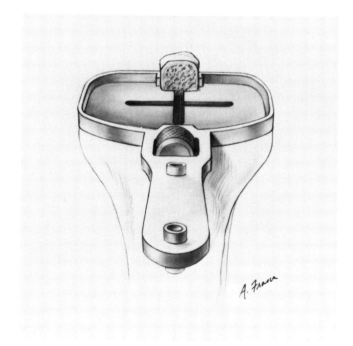

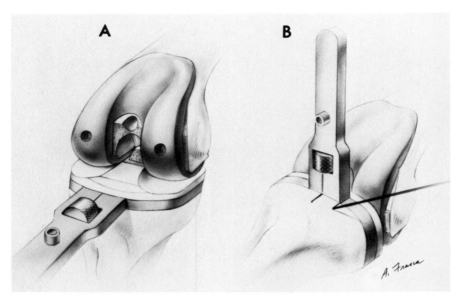

FIGURE 11–36. Femorotibial trial reduction. (A) The trial femoral and tibial components are now placed with an appropriate-sized tibial insert. The proper thickness of the insert allows the knee to come into full extension but not hyperextension. The collateral ligaments should be tight, but not overly tight. There may be 1 mm of play with the leg in full extension as well as in 5° of flexion. (B) With the leg in extension, the tibial tray is rotated in order to ensure proper congruity with the femoral component. This is marked and will be the final determination of the tibial component's rotational alignment.

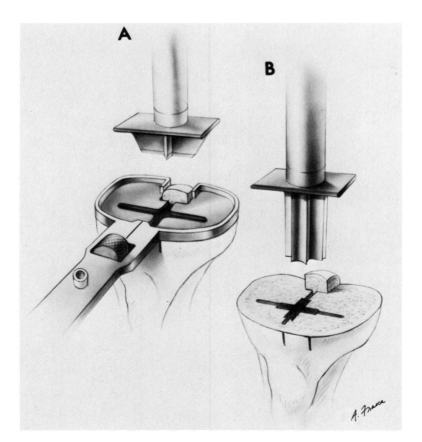

FIGURE 11–37. Tibial keel preparation. (A, B) With the trial tibial tray as a template, a series of punches are used to prepare the proximal tibia for the keel of the tibial component.

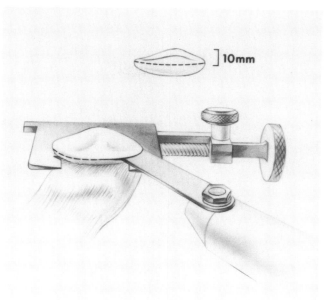

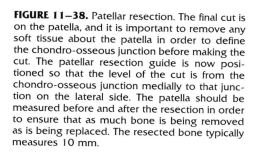

FIGURE 11–38. Patellar resection. The final cut is on the patella, and it is important to remove any soft tissue about the patella in order to define the chondro-osseous junction before making the cut. The patellar resection guide is now positioned so that the level of the cut is from the chondro-osseous junction medially to that junction on the lateral side. The patella should be measured before and after the resection in order to ensure that as much bone is being removed as is being replaced. The resected bone typically measures 10 mm.

measured before and after resection in order to ensure that as much bone is being removed as is being replaced (Fig. 11–38).

The patellar drill guide is aligned, and holes are prepared for the patellar component (Fig. 11–39). The patellar trial is positioned, and the patella is returned to its proper trochlear orientation. The knee is then flexed, and with the medial capsule opened, the patella should stay in the trochlear groove. Moreover, with the knee flexed at 90°, the medial portion of the polyethylene patella button should be in contact with the medial femoral flange (Fig. 11–40). If the patella tends to sublux laterally at this point, or if there is no medial contact, a lateral retinacular release is performed. Before the release, the superolateral geniculate vessels are identified. They form the base of a triangle between the vastus lateralis

FIGURE 11–39. Patellar resection (continued). The patellar drill guide is aligned so that two drill holes are placed in the medial patellar facet and one hole in the lateral patellar facet.

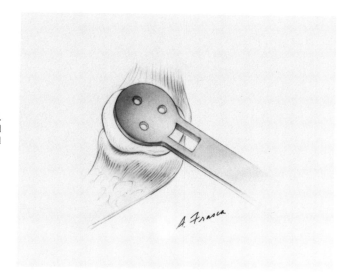

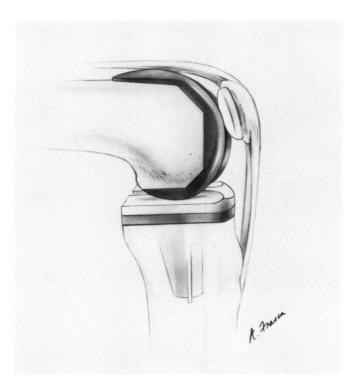

FIGURE 11–40. Trial patellar reduction. The patellar trial is now positioned and the patella reduced in the trochlear groove. The knee is then observed through a full range of motion. With the knee flexed at 90°, the medial portion of the polyethylene patellar button should be in contact with the medial femoral flange. If the patella tends to sublux laterally, a lateral retinacular release should be performed.

muscle and the lateral shaft of the femur. The release is performed from inside out and begins several centimeters posterior to the patellar button. It can be carried distally to the tibia and proximally along the lateral intermuscular septum.

The prostheses are then inserted according to standard techniques of cemented or uncemented designs. The authors advocate the use of a cemented all-polyethylene patellar component. A patellar clamp is used to maintain pressurization at the prosthesis-cement interface during curing of the methyl methacrylate (Fig. 11–41).

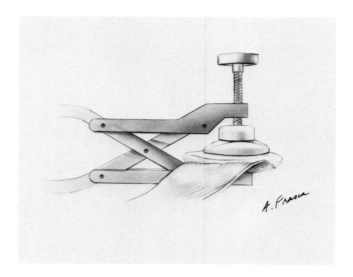

FIGURE 11–41. Implanting the components. The components are then implanted according to standard techniques of cemented or cementless designs. The authors advocate the use of a cemented all-polyethylene patellar component. A patellar clamp is used to maintain pressurization at the prosthesis-cement interface during curing of the methyl methacrylate.

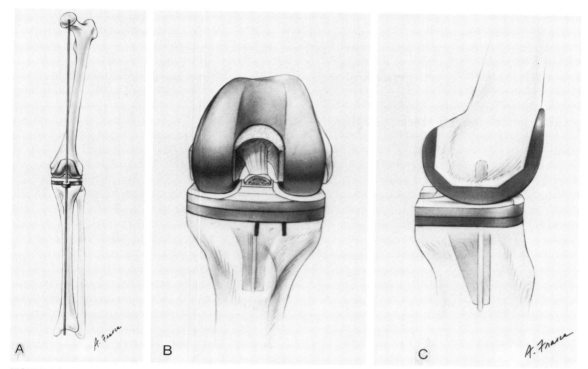

FIGURE 11–42. Final inspection. (A, B, C) After placement of the components, a final inspection is carried out so as to confirm congruent femorotibial orientation, acceptable prosthetic alignment, and proper soft tissue tension. After capsular closure, the knee is flexed to ensure adequate patellar tracking.

The tourniquet is deflated, and hemostasis is achieved. A final inspection is carried out to confirm congruent femorotibial orientation as well as proper soft tissue tension (Fig. 11–42). Capsular closure is in two standard layers, and the knee is flexed after capsular closure so as to make certain that the patella tracks and the closure is secure and to note the final amount of flexion.

PATELLOFEMORAL RESURFACING

Patellofemoral complications account for up to 50 per cent of the complications that follow total knee replacement. Complications experienced include patellofemoral discomfort in the unresurfaced patella, patella instability, fracture, osteonecrosis, wear, and loosening. Changes in design of patellar components, combined with changes in cementing and surgical techniques, may in the future reduce patellofemoral complications. There are, however, no reports in the literature that confirm reduced complications associated with these changes.

Biomechanics

The patellofemoral joint is subjected to between one and one and half times body weight while walking on level ground and up to seven times body weight in squatting and climbing stairs.[34] The patella is also subjected to bending moments that tend to deform the peripheral margins of a prosthetic patellar component. Stresses in the patella are also altered by the thickness of the patella/prosthesis composite. If the resurfaced patella is thicker than the original patella, stresses within the bony patella are increased, and flexion in a total knee replacement may be limited.

Prosthetic Design

There are a number of reports of failure of metal-backed patellar components.[6, 56] This failure does not appear to be design or manufacturer specific. Failure has occurred with excessive wear and fracture of the polyethylene as well as dissociation of the polyethylene from the metal backing. It is recommended that if patellar resurfacing is undertaken, an all-plastic patellar component should be used. Central fixation lugs are subjected to higher stresses than are peripheral fixation lugs.[13] Lugs oriented in a transverse direction are subjected to 50 per cent less stress than are lugs oriented in a longitudinal or proximal/distal direction.[13] Most patellar components are now oval in shape for better capping of the patella. This change in design is supported by retrieval studies that have demonstrated that circular dome–shaped prostheses tend to deform into a more elliptical shape.

Indications for Patellofemoral Resurfacing

Most investigators agree that in rheumatoid arthritis, the patella should be resurfaced. Thomas and collaborators[97] reported residual patellofemoral pain in 10 rheumatoid arthritis patients who did not undergo patellar resurfacing at the time of total knee replacement. Laboratory studies and clinical observation have suggested that residual cartilage in a rheumatoid arthritic knee after total knee arthroplasty may interact with the active rheumatoid synovium, causing the inflammatory process to continue.[94] It is therefore recommended that all patellae in patients with rheumatoid arthritis be resurfaced.

Resurfacing of the osteoarthritic patella is more controversial. Brick and Scott[10] compared 82 osteoarthritic knees with unresurfaced patellae and 156 osteoarthritic knees with resurfaced patellae and reported a higher incidence of significant patellofemoral pain in the unresurfaced patellae. The reoperation rate was similar in both groups (2.4 and 2.5 per cent). With improved prosthetic design and cementing techniques, the incidence of loosening and patellar fracture may be reduced. With improved femoral component design, however, and the associated improved tracking of unresurfaced patellae, the incidence of patellofemoral pain may also be reduced. The authors' current practice is to resurface all patellae in osteoarthritic knees. In a small percentage of patients, bone stock is insufficient for resurfacing the patella (approximately 3 per cent of patients with rheumatoid arthritis).

Surgical Technique

A preoperative axial tangential patellar radiograph demonstrates subluxation or dislocation, abnormal anatomy, and any erosions or cysts that may be present. A medial arthrotomy combined with a complete lateral meniscectomy disrupts all blood supply to the patella with the exception of the supply from the superior lateral genicular artery. Consequently, when a lateral retinacular release is required, care should be taken to preserve this vessel.[102]

In order to obtain satisfactory exposure and adequate patellar eversion, the patellofemoral ligament should be routinely sectioned. Before the patellar cut is made, a caliper may be used to measure the patellar thickness. Once the trial patellar component has been inserted, the thickness of the patella/prosthetic composite can be measured so as to ensure that it corresponds with pre-resection patellar thickness.

A common error made in resurfacing the patella involves resection of too little medial patellar bone stock, causing the bone cut to be asymmetric. Once the patella is resurfaced, the patella should track on trial reduction without subluxing or tilting in the absence of a restraining thumb.[82] If the patella tends to sublux laterally, a lateral retinacular release should be performed; care should be taken to preserve the superior lateral geniculate artery.[68]

Complications

SUBLUXATION AND DISLOCATION. The combination of subluxation and dislocation is the most common complication and is related to abnormal tracking of the patellar component. In 90 per cent of cases, the subluxation occurs in flexion. In 10 per cent, however, it occurs in extension, and relocation of the patella occurs in flexion. Causes of subluxation include dynamic or static imbalance of soft tissue, component malposition, capsular dehiscence, patella alta, and postoperative hemarthrosis. Dislocation in extension is more commonly related to overactivity of the vastus lateralis, excessive valgus of the femoral component, or an uncorrected valgus deformity.

FRACTURE. Stress fractures of the patella have been reported in 1 and 21 per cent of patients.[86] These fractures are more likely to occur when a large central patella fixation lug has been used and when the patella blood supply has been compromised. Patellar fracture was reported by Insall and associates as an incidental finding.[37] Eight of 10 fractures were diagnosed at routine follow-up evaluation. Other presentations included a history of minor trauma or giving way associated with an increased quadriceps force. A patient who has minimal discomfort and no significant extensor lag may be treated with closed management. Indications for surgical treatment include fracture displacement of more than 2 cm, a significant extensor lag that causes instability, or a loose, displaced prosthesis. Open reduction and internal fixation may be attempted. It is often not possible to resurface the patella, and it may be more appropriate to undertake a partial patellectomy with repair of the quadriceps tendon or ligamentum patellae. Patellectomy should be considered for comminuted fractures and when fixation has failed.

LOOSENING. A loose patellar component may be asymptomatic and may not require revision surgery. Factors that predispose to loosening include osteonecrosis, osteoporosis subluxation, and component malposition. In a series of 16 loose patellar components at the author's institution,[10] 12 patients required revision surgery. In two knees, the displaced patella component had caused significant abrasion of the ligamentum patellae or quadriceps tendon. If on radiographs a displaced component appears to lie within either of these structures, a revision may be indicated in order to prevent attritional wear and rupture of either structure.

PATELLOFEMORAL PAIN. This may occur in both resurfaced and unresurfaced patellae. Significantly improved pain relief in osteoarthritic knees with patellar resurfacing was reported by Freeman and colleagues[22] and Leval and co-workers.[55] There was no correlation between patellar erosion seen on radiographs and patellofemoral pain in the unresurfaced patellae.[39] Insall and collaborators[39] reported patellofemoral pain and decreased clinical knee scores in six of 33 knees that did not undergo patellar resurfacing. At the authors' institution, in a series of 82 osteoarthritic knees without patellar resurfacing, 11 per cent of patients experienced significant patellofemoral pain, in comparison with 5.3 per cent of osteoarthritic knees with patellar resurfacing.

SOFT TISSUE IMPINGEMENT. Insall and collaborators[39] reported entrapment of a fibrous synovial meniscus that may regenerate in relation to the prosthetic patella and cause mechanical symptoms.

OSTEONECROSIS. Osteonecrosis of the patella may follow vascular[68, 83] injury, which predisposes the prosthesis to loosening and the patella to stress fracture. When possible, the lateral superior genicular artery should be saved during total knee arthroplasty in order to reduce the incidence of this complication.

PATELLAR LIGAMENT AVULSION. Although this is an uncommon complication, it presents a difficult surgical problem. Of four patients at the authors' institution who have sustained this complication during the years 1980 to 1990, three underwent multiple revision procedures. Three knees treated with patellar ligament reconstruction subsequently developed deep joint infections. The arthroplasties in all four knees were clinical failures.

WEAR. Wear of metal-backed patellar components has presented a major problem with metal synovitis.[6, 56] Although wear with polyethylene components may occur and require revision, the incidence of problems associated with wear in an all-polyethylene component appears to be much reduced.

REFERENCES

1. Andriacchi TP, Galante JO, Fermier RW: The influence of total knee replacement design on walking and stair-climbing. J Bone Joint Surg 64A:1328, 1982.
2. Arnoldi CC, Lemperg RR, Linderholm H: Intra-osseous hypertension and pain in the knee. J Bone Joint Surg 57B:360, 1975.
3. Bae DK, Guhl JF, Keane SP: Unicompartmental knee arthroplasty for single compartment disease: clinical experience with an average 4-year follow-up study. Clin Orthop 176:233, 1983.
4. Bauer GC, Insall JN, Koshino T: Tibial osteotomy in gonarthrosis (osteo-arthritis of the knee). J Bone Joint Surg 51A:1545–1563, 1969.
5. Baumgaertner MR, Cannon WD Jr, Vittori JM, et al: Arthroscopic debridement of the arthritic knee. Clin Orthop 253:197, 1990.
6. Bayley JC, Scott RD, Ewall FC, Holmes GB: Failure of the metal-backed patellar component after total knee replacement. J Bone Joint Surg 70A:668, 1988.
7. Bert JM, Maschka K: The arthroscopic treatment of unicompartmental gonarthrosis: a five year follow-up of abrasion arthroplasty plus arthroscopic debridement and arthroscopic debridement alone. Arthroscopy 5:25, 1989.

8. Bobyn JD, Pilliar RM, Cameron HU, Weatherly GC: The optimum pore size for the fixation of porous-surfaced metal implants by the ingrowth of bone. Clin Orthop 150:263, 1980.
9. Brandt KD: Pathogenesis of osteoarthritis (OA). *In* Kelley WN, Harris ED Jr, Ruddy S, Sledge CB (eds): Textbook of Rheumatology, pp. 1457–1470. Philadelphia: WB Saunders, 1985.
10. Brick GW, Scott, RD: The patello-femoral component of total knee arthroplasty. Clin Orthop 231:163, 1988.
11. Cameron HU, Pilliar RM, MacNab I: The effect of movement on the bonding of porous metal to bone. J Biomed Mater Res 7:301, 1973.
12. Campbell WC: Inter-position of Vitallium plates in arthroplasties of the knee: preliminary report. Am J Surg 47:639, 1940.
13. Cheal EJ, Hayes WC, Harry JD, et al: Influence of component orientation on peg failure of patellar surface replacements. *Presented at* the 32nd annual meeting of the Orthopaedic Research Society, New Orleans, February 1986.
14. Coventry MB: Osteotomy about the knee for degenerative and rheumatoid arthritis, indications, operative technique, and results. J Bone Joint Surg 55A:23, 1973.
15. Coventry MB: Proximal tibial varus osteotomy for osteoarthritis of the lateral compartment of the knee. J Bone Joint Surg 69A:32, 1987.
16. Coventry MB, Bowman PW: Long-term results of upper tibial osteotomy for degenerative arthritis of the knee. Acta Orthop 48:139, 1982.
17. Dodd CAF, Hungerford DS, Krakow KA: Total knee arthroplasty fixation: comparison of the early results of paired cemented versus uncemented porous coated anatomic knee prostheses. Clin Orthop 260:66–70, 1990.
18. Emerson RH, Potter T: The use of the McKeever metallic hemi-arthroplasty for unicompartmental arthritis. J Bone Joint Surg 67A:208, 1985.
19. Ewald FC, Walker PS, Poss R, et al: Uncemented, press-fit total knee replacement. *In* Rand JA, Dorr LD (eds): Total Arthroplasty of the Knee: Proceedings of the Knee Society—1985 & 1986, p. 173. Rockville, MD: Aspen, 1986.
20. Fairbanks TJ: Knee joint changes after meniscectomy. J Bone Joint Surg 30B:664, 1948.
21. Freeman MAR, Swanson SAV: Total prosthetic replacement of the knee. J Bone Joint Surg 54B:170, 1972.
22. Freeman MAR, Swanson SAV, Todd RC: Total replacement of the knee using Freeman-Swanson knee prosthesis. Clin Orthop 94:153–170, 1973.
23. Friedman JJ, Berasi CC, Fox JM, et al: Preliminary results with abrasion arthroplasty in the osteoarthritic knee. Clin Orthop 182:200, 1984.
24. Gariepy R: Genu varum treated by high tibial osteotomy. *In* Proceedings of the Joint Meeting of the Orthopaedic Associations of the English Speaking World. J Bone Joint Surg 46B:783, 1964.
25. Goodfellow JW, Kershaw CJ, Benson MK, O'Connor JJ: The Oxford Knee for unicompartmental osteoarthritis: the first 103 cases. J Bone Joint Surg 70B:692–701, 1988.
26. Gunston FH: Polycentric knee arthroplasty: prosthetic simulation of normal knee movement. J Bone Joint Surg 53B:272, 1971.
27. Gunston FH, MacKenzie RI: Complications of polycentric knee arthroplasty. Clin Orthop 120:11, 1976.
28. Haddad RJ, Cook SD, Thomas KA: Current concepts review: biological fixation of porous-coated implants. J Bone Joint Surg 69A:1459, 1987.
29. Harms WR, Kostuik JP: High tibial osteotomy for osteoarthritis of the knee. J Bone Joint Surg 52A:330, 1970.
30. Harris WH, Jasty M: Bone ingrowth into porous coated canine acetabular replacements: the effect of pore size, apposition and dislocation. *In* The Hip: Proceedings of the Thirteenth Open Scientific Meeting of the Hip Society, pp. 214–234. St. Louis: CV Mosby, 1985.
31. Healy WL, Anglen JO, Wasilewski SA, Krackow KA: Distal femoral osteotomy. J Bone Joint Surg 70A:107, 1988.
32. Holden DL, James SL, Larson RL, Slocum DB: Proximal tibial osteotomy in patients who are fifty years old or less. J Bone Joint Surg 70A:977, 1988.
33. Howell DS: Diseases due to the deposition of calcium pyrophosphate and hydroxyapatite. *In* Kelley WN, Harris E Jr, Ruddy S, Sledge CB (eds): Textbook of Rheumatology, pp. 1438–1454. Philadelphia: WB Saunders, 1985.
34. Huberti HH, Hayes WC: Patello-femoral contact pressures. J Bone Joint Surg 66A:715, 1984.
35. Insall JN, Hood RW, Flawn CB, Sullivan DJ: The total condylar knee prosthesis in gonarthrosis: a five- to nine-year follow-up of the first one hundred consecutive replacements. J Bone Joint Surg 65A:619, 1983.
36. Insall JN, Joseph DM, Msika C: High tibial osteotomy for varus gonarthrosis. J Bone Joint Surg 66A:1040, 1984.
37. Insall JN, Lachiewicz PF, Burstein AH: The posterior stabilized condylar prosthesis: a modification of the total condylar design. Two to four year clinical experience. J Bone Joint Surg 64A:1317, 1982.

38. Insall JN, Ranawat CS, Aglietti P, et al: A comparison of four models of total knee replacement prostheses. J Bone Joint Surg 58A:745, 1976.
39. Insall JN, Scott WN, Ranawat CS: The total condylar knee prostheses: a report of two hundred and twenty cases. J Bone Joint Surg 61A:173, 1979.
40. Ivarsson I, Myrnerts R, Gillquist J: High tibial osteotomy for medial osteoarthritis of the knee: a 5 to 7 and an 11 year follow-up. J Bone Joint Surg 72B:238–244, 1990.
41. Jackson RW: The role of arthroscopy in the management of the arthritic knee. Clin Orthop 101:28, 1974.
42. Jackson RW, Silver R, Marans H: The arthroscopic treatment of degenerative joint disease. Arthroscopy 2:114, 1986.
43. Jackson JP, Waugh W: Tibial osteotomy for osteoarthritis of the knee. J Bone Joint Surg 43B:746, 1961.
44. Johnson F, Leitl S, Waugh W: The distribution of load across the knee. J Bone Joint Surg 62B:346, 1980.
45. Johnson LL: Arthroscopic abrasion arthroplasty: historical and pathologic perspective. Present status. Arthroscopy 2:54, 1986.
46. Jones WN, Aufranc OE, Kermond WL: Mold arthroplasty of the knee. J Bone Joint Surg 49A:1022, 1967.
47. Joseph D, Insall J, Msika C: High tibial osteotomy: a long-term clinical review. *Presented at* the annual meeting of the American Academy of Orthopaedic Surgeons, Anaheim, CA, 1983.
48. Keene JS, Dyreby JR Jr: High tibial osteotomy in the treatment of osteoarthritis of the knee: the role of pre-operative arthroscopy. J Bone Joint Surg 65A:36, 1983.
49. Kennedy JC: Tension studies of human knee ligaments. J Bone Joint Surg 58A:350, 1976.
50. Kettelkamp DB, Chao EY: A method for quantitative analysis of medial and lateral compressive forces at the knee during standing. Clin Orthop 83:202–213, 1972.
51. Kettelkamp DB, Wegner DR, Chao EYS, et al: Results of proximal tibial osteotomy: the effects of tibio-femoral angle, stance-phase, flexion-extension and medial-plateau force. J Bone Joint Surg 58A:952, 1976.
52. Kim YH: Total knee arthroplasty for tuberculous arthritis. J Bone Joint Surg 70A:1322, 1988.
53. Krushell R, Deland J, Miegel RE, et al: A comparison of the mechanical and anatomic axes in arthritic knees. *In* Rand JA, Dorr LD (eds): Total Arthroplasty of the Knee: Proceedings of the Knee Society—1985 & 1986. Rockville, MD: Aspen, 1987.
54. Lansinger O, Bergman B, Korner L, et al: Tibial condylar fractures. J Bone Joint Surg 68A:13, 1968.
55. Leval JP, McCloud HC, Freeman MAR: Why not resurface the patella? J Bone Joint Surg 65B:448, 1983.
56. Lombardi AV, Engh JA, Volz RG, et al: Fracture/dislocation of the polyethylene in metal-backed patellar components in total knee arthroplasty. J Bone Joint Surg 70A:675, 1988.
57. Lotke PA, Lefkoe RT, Ecker M: Late results following medial meniscectomy in an older population. J Bone Joint Surg 63A:115, 1981.
57a. MacIntosh DL: Hemiarthroplasty of the knee using a space occupying prosthesis for painful varus and valgus deformities. J Bone Joint Surg 40A:1431, 1958.
58. MacIntosh DL, Welsh RP: Joint débridement—a complement to high tibial osteotomy in the treatment of degenerative arthritis of the knee. J Bone Joint Surg 50A:1094–1097, 1977.
59. Magnuson PB: Technique of debridement of the knee joint for arthritis. Surg Clin North Am 26:249, 1946.
60. Mainardi CL, Levin PH: Hemophilia and arthritis. *In* Kelley WN, Harris ED Jr, Ruddy S, Sledge CB (eds): Textbook of Rheumatology, pp. 1605–1613. Philadelphia: WB Saunders, 1985.
61. Mankin HJ: The reaction of articular cartilage to injury and osteoarthritis, Part I. N Engl J Med 219:1285, 1974.
62. Mankin HJ: The reaction of articular cartilage to injury and osteoarthritis, Part II. N Engl J Med 291:1335, 1974.
63. Maquet P: Valgus osteotomy for osteoarthritis of the knee. Clin Orthop 120:143, 1976.
64. Maquet P: The biomechanics of the knee and surgical possibilities of healing osteoarthritic knee joints. Clin Orthop 146:102, 1980.
65. Marmor L: Selection of patients for unicompartmental knee replacement. Tech Orthop 5:3, 1990.
66. Marmor L: Unicompartmental knee arthroplasty: 10- to 13-year follow-up study. Clin Orthop 226:14, 1987.
67. McKeever DC: Tibial plateau prosthesis. Clin Orthop 18:86, 1960.
68. Merkow RL, Soudry M, Insall JN: Patellar dislocation following total knee replacement. J Bone Joint Surg 67A:1321–1327, 1985.

69. Moller JT, Weeth RE, Keller JO: Unicompartmental arthroplasty of the knee: cadaver study of tibial component placement. Acta Orthop Scand 56:115, 1985.

70. Morrison JB: Bioengineering analysis for force actions transmitted by the knee joint. Biomed Eng 3:164, 1968.

71. Myrnerts R: The SAAB jig: an aid in high tibial osteotomy. Acta Orthop Scand 49:85–88, 1978.

72. Oglesby JW, Wilson FC: The evolution of knee arthroplasty: results with three generations of prostheses. Clin Orthop 186:96, 1984.

73. Peyron JG: Osteoarthritis: the epidemiologic viewpoint. Clin Orthop 213:13, 1986.

74. Pridie KH: A method of resurfacing osteoarthritis knee joints. J Bone Joint Surg 41B:618, 1959.

75. Prodromos CC, Andriacchi TP, Galante JO: A relationship between gait and clinical changes following high tibial osteotomy. J Bone Joint Surg 67A:1188, 1985.

76. Rackemann S, Mintzer CM, Walker PS, Ewald FC: Uncemented press-fit total knee arthroplasty. Arthroplasty 5:307, 1990.

77. Radin EL, Rose RM: Role of subchondral bone in the initiation and progression of cartilage damage. Clin Orthop 213:34, 1986.

78. Rorabeck CH, Bourne RB, Nott L: The cemented Kinematic-II and the non-cemented porous coated anatomic prosthesis for total knee replacement: a prospective evaluation. J Bone Joint Surg 70A:483, 1988.

79. Rosenberg AG, Barden RM, Galante JO: Cemented and ingrowth fixation of the Miller-Galante prosthesis. Clin Orthop 260:71, 1990.

80. Salisbury RB, Nottage WM, Gardner V: The effect of alignment on results in arthroscopic debridement of the degenerative knee. Clin Orthop 198:268, 1985.

81. Schumacher HR Jr: Secondary osteoarthritis. *In* Moskowitz RW, Howell DS, Goldberg VM, Mankin HJ (eds): Osteoarthritis, Diagnosis, and Management, pp. 235–264. Philadelphia: WB Saunders, 1984.

82. Scott RD: Prosthetic replacement of the patello-femoral joint. Orthop Clin North Am 10:129, 1979.

83. Scott RD: Duopatellar total knee replacement: The Brigham experience. Orthop Clin North Am 13:89, 1982.

84. Scott RD, Joyce MJ, Ewald FC, et al: McKeever metallic hemi-arthroplasty of the knee in unicompartmental degenerative arthritis: long-term clinical follow-up and current indications. J Bone Joint Surg 67A:203, 1985.

85. Scott RD, Santore RF: Unicondylar unicompartmental replacement for osteoarthritis of the knee. J Bone Joint Surg 63:536, 1981.

86. Scott RD, Turoff N, Ewald FC: Stress fracture of patella following duopatellar total knee arthroplasty with patellar resurfacing. Clin Orthop 170:147–151, 1982.

87. Shiers LGP: Arthroplasty of the knee: preliminary report of a new method. J Bone Joint Surg 36B:553, 1954.

88. Sledge CB, Ewald FC: Total knee arthroplasty experience at the Robert Breck Brigham Hospital. Clin Orthop 145:78, 1979.

89. Sledge CB, Stern P, Thomas WH: Two-year followup of the duocondylar total knee replacement. Orthop Trans 2:193, 1978.

90. Sledge CB, Zuckerman JD, Shortkroff S, et al: Synovectomy of the rheumatoid knee using intra-articular injection of dysprosium-165-ferric hydroxide macroaggregate. J Bone Joint Surg 69A:970, 1987.

91. Slocum DB, Larson RL, James SL, Grenier R: High tibial osteotomy. Clin Orthop 104:239, 1974.

92. Soudry M, Binazzi R, Johanson NA, et al: Total knee arthroplasty in Charcot and Charcot-like joints. Clin Orthop 208:199, 1986.

93. Sprague NF III: Arthroscopic debridement for degenerative knee joint disease. Clin Orthop 160:118, 1981.

94. Steinberg J, Sledge CB, Noble J, Stirrat CR: A tissue culture model of cartilage breakdown in rheumatoid arthritis: quantitative aspects of proteoglycan release. J Biochem 180:403, 1979.

95. Stern SH, Insall JN: Total knee arthroplasty in obese patients. J Bone Joint Surg 72A:1400, 1990.

96. Taylor AR, Harbison JS, Pepler C: Synovectomy of the knee in rheumatoid arthritis: results of surgery. Ann Rheum Dis 31:159, 1972.

97. Thomas WH, Ewald FC, Poss R, Sledge CB: Duopatellar total knee arthroplasty. Orthop Trans 4:329, 1980.

98. Thornhill TS, Scott RD: Unicompartment total knee arthroplasty. Orthop Clin North Am 20:245, 1989.

99. Timoney JM, Kneisl JS, Barrack RL, et al: Arthroscopy in the osteoarthritis knee: long-term follow-up. Orthop Rev 19:371, 1990.

100. Volkmann R: Osteotomy for knee joint deformity. Edinburgh Med J [translated from Berl Klin Wochenschr, p. 794, 1875].

101. Wardle EN: Osteotomy of the tibia and fibula. Surg Gynecol Obstet 115:61, 1962.
102. Welzner SM, Bezreh JS, Scott RD, et al: Bone scanning and assessment of patella viability following knee replacement. Clin Orthop 199:125, 1985.
103. Wright J, Ewald FC, Walker PS, et al: Total knee arthroplasty with the kinematic prosthesis. Results after five to nine years: A follow-up note. J Bone Joint Surg 72A:1003, 1990.
104. Wright RJ, Lima J, Scott RD, Thornhill TS: Two- to four-year results of posterior cruciate–sparing condylar total knee arthroplasty with an uncemented femoral component. Clin Orthop 260:80, 1990.

CHAPTER 12

Extra-Articular

and Overuse

Problems

WILLIAM A. GRANA, M.D.

■

A variety of connective tissue problems about the knee do not affect the internal structures of the joint or do not fit easily into any differential diagnostic or anatomic classification. Nonetheless, these entities cause pain and common problems in day-to-day life as well as in sports, such as reduced performance on the athletic field or time loss on the job. These disease processes usually result in localized pain, and if the affected anatomic structure is recognized, diagnosis is usually readily apparent. The purpose of this chapter is to describe those disease processes, their causes, and recognition and management.

CONSIDERATION OF OVERUSE PROBLEMS

As human performance levels have increased, overuse problems have become more and more frequent. The rewards for early diagnosis of these overuse problems are an earlier recovery and earlier return to the previous level of performance. However, when the condition is not recognized, when warning symptoms are ignored, or when treatment is not acted on, complete recovery may be much slower. The earliest recognition of overuse problems was recorded in the 19th century by M. D. Breithaupt, a military surgeon, who described the painful, swollen feet of soldiers after long marches. Later, in the early 20th century, A. W. Sterchow was able to identify metatarsal stress fractures on radiographs, and these fractures were called "march fractures." Since that time, it has been recognized that these overuse problems occur not only in the bone but in the soft tissues as well.[3, 13]

The interest in aerobic activities has increased dramatically with the accumulation of evidence that aerobic exercise improves cardiovascular fitness and promotes weight loss. Activities in which large muscle groups are used and a minimal exercise intensity of 50 per cent of maximal oxygen consumption for 20 to 30 minutes is required are termed aerobic. The dominant source of energy for aerobic exercise is fat, whereas more intense anaerobic exercise involves mainly the use of carbohydrates. For this reason, aerobic exercise is preferred for promoting general fitness and weight loss because it burns fat. Aerobic exercise includes distance running, bicycling, swimming, cross-country skiing, and rowing.[17]

Overuse problems usually involve some form of impact loading or repetitive stress. Certain aerobic exercises such as running seem to be associated with these problems more than others. The principle is that forces that normally would not produce an acute injury are applied repetitively to produce microinjury, which subsequently becomes symptomatic as a result of the inflammatory response elicited. If the duration or the intensity of this activity reaches threshold level for the person, microinjury occurs and adversely affects a variety of structures about the joint, particularly a weight-bearing joint such as the knee. Structures that are affected include articular cartilage, the meniscus, tendons, and the bone.[13]

With regard to articular cartilage, joints are normally capable of handling stresses with impact loading activity without any detrimental effects. The normal joint is able to dissipate the energy produced from weight-bearing and impact-loading activity through its frictionless articulation and muscular support. This is accomplished through a well-conditioned muscular system about the knee as well as the lubricating mechanisms in the normal shock-absorbing capacity of the articular cartilage and the meniscus.[1, 7] In boundary lubrication, molecules of synovial fluid adhere momentarily to the free borders or the boundary of the opposing articular surfaces, and motion occurs between the molecules of synovial fluid. This boundary lubrication works under low-velocity normal loads. As repetition increases the loading, weeping lubrication provided by transudation of water from the articular cartilage becomes the main mechanism for limiting friction and providing smooth articulation. The molecules of water roll between the opposing surfaces of the joint. This is an efficient type of lubrication under high-loading conditions. Changes in the mechanism of lubrication, such as those seen in osteoarthritis with increases in friction between the joint surfaces and those seen in weight-bearing or impact-loading activities, hasten cartilage breakdown.[7, 17, 19] Therefore, in patients who have pre-existing problems, it is important to recognize this process and to limit impact-loading activities.

In addition, repetitive impact loading in the patient with osteoarthritis causes trabecular microfracture in the subchondral bone. The result is hypertrophy of the subchondral bone and stiffening in response to impact loading. This stiffening results in increased stress placed across the articular surface, which can lead to additional cartilage breakdown and subsequent joint degeneration. The response of the articular cartilage is to produce mucopolysaccharides and increase the number of cells in the articular cartilage. However, in the presence of repetitive loading, there is a significant loss of mucopolysaccharides and, as a result, a decrease in the effectiveness of the articular surface as a weight-bearing structure. This leads to further breakdown of the mechanical integrity of the articular cartilage. Load with function increases, and there is more loss of articular cartilage. Osteophytes form at the periphery as the joint attempts to distribute the load over a larger surface area; however, the osteophytes that form are not capable of handling the forces transmitted across the joint, and the result is additional deformity and destruction with advancing osteoarthritis.[15, 19]

Therefore, if the physician recognizes that there are pre-existing abnormalities in a weight-bearing joint such as the knee, the patient who wishes to participate in aerobic exercise should choose activities that do not place repetitive impact-loading forces on the joint. Activities such as swimming, bicycling, and rowing are better for such a patient than is running.

The meniscus is thought to transmit approximately 50 per cent of the load in normal walking. In running, these loads are clearly increased. In the absence of menisci, the articular surface of the knee is exposed to more concentrated and increased stress, which thus leads to articular cartilage breakdown. This process is well documented by the substantial increased evidence of compartmental deterioration after meniscectomy. Retention of the outer rim of the meniscus or regrowth of the rim after total meniscectomies spares the articular cartilage from osteoarthritic damage. This result emphasizes the benefits of partial meniscectomy in alleviating stress in the compartment of the knee and the importance of the meniscus in impact-loading activity.[12, 19]

The structure of the meniscus is different from that of articular cartilage. Although it is made up of collagen and proteoglycan, the

proteoglycan content of the meniscus is one-tenth that of articular cartilage. In addition, the permeability of the meniscus is extremely low, and
this may be the dominant factor that determines its ability to act in
response to compressive load. Tensile behavior of the meniscus appears
to be controlled by the collagen. Structural organization of the surface
layer provides a coating for the more coarse, fibrous material of the
interior, which is oriented in a circumferential direction. This strengthens
the meniscus with regard to circumferential loads but weakens it in a
radial direction while providing a smooth, nearly frictionless articulating
surface.[18] With repetitive stress, disruption of this fibril bundle arrangement can occur, and the result is a degenerative tear of the meniscus.
These horizontal cleavage, flap, or complex types of tears occur with
increasing age.[19] In degenerative tears, there typically is no history of
specific injury, and the tear involves either or both of the menisci with
frequently associated degenerative articular cartilage change as well. In
general, the meniscus has little ability to respond to such injury, particularly when the injury is in the inner two thirds, and therefore partial
meniscectomy is usually the treatment of such overuse change.[12]

Overuse problems can also affect the muscle-tendon unit. Repetitive
stress of the muscle can produce exhaustive injury, which results in
localized myonecrosis with complex degenerative sequelae that occur after
strenuous exercise. However, because optimal conditions for regeneration
are usually present after this type of injury, normal function usually
returns except in the most severe instances.[8]

Contraction-induced injury is also seen after eccentric exercise and
results in a strain type of injury. A strain of a muscle-tendon unit results
in varying degrees of partial injury.[8, 16] Don H. O'Donoghue graded these
injuries as I, II, and III, depending on the severity of the injury. Grade I
involves bleeding into the tendon or the muscle without any actual tearing.
Grade II involves partial tearing of the tendon or the muscle. Grade III
involves a complete rupture of the tendon or the muscle within its
substance; a variant of a Grade III strain is an avulsion of the tendon from
the bone with or without a piece of bone. Partial or complete rupture of
the muscle is much less common than microfailure within the tendon
itself. Such failure is most common in the midsubstance of the tendon at
high rates of loading. Injury at the insertion site is less common.[8] Bony
avulsions with minimal displacement (3 to 5 mm) usually heal well. With
more extensive displacement, repair is necessary.

More often tension that is produced by muscles and transmitted
through the muscle to the tendon results in injury at the myotendinous
junction. Repetitive stress also results in muscle soreness, which occurs
24 to 72 hours after intense exercise.[8] This pain is an aching, generalized
kind of discomfort that is distinguishable from the pain associated with
fatigue, which results in cramping and painful spasm. Fatigue pain is a
reversible type of injury that is more likely to occur after eccentric exercise.
Strain injury is also much more likely to occur with eccentric loading at
the myotendinous junction. The tendon avulses from the muscle with a
short length of muscle fiber still attached. Incomplete tears (grades I and
II) are more common and usually heal with decreased ability to produce
tension for about 1 week after the injury.[16]

If the force applied to the tendon is insufficient for producing
immediate bleeding or disruption of the tendon, it can still produce injury

through microtears of the tendon with resulting inflammation. This is the entity recognized as tendinitis, which produces localized pain with resisted motion that is controlled by the particular muscle group involved. Localized inflammation results in pain and swelling, and if a bursa is involved, bursitis usually occurs as well.

If muscular strength develops more rapidly than bony remodeling can occur, there is a temporary imbalance and an increase in mechanical loading of the bone. Muscles normally act to dampen the peak stresses in bone by eccentric contraction during loading. Stress fracture, in its early stages, is a stress reaction. If the load is appropriately decreased, healing in the form of hypertrophy of the bone occurs with resolution of the symptoms. If the stress continues unaltered, a stress fracture occurs. Microstructural damage to the bone occurs with subthreshold fracture loads as a result of fatigue failure. If this damage occurs over a period of weeks, bone formation may take place and maintain the structural integrity of the bone. On the other hand, osteoclastic removal of the stressed bone may actually accelerate the microstructural damage. Accumulative microdamage to the bone may then progress to a symptomatic stress fracture.[3, 4, 21]

These injuries are more likely to occur in bone of decreased density or in a lamellar bone with a lower percentage of osteons than normal. About the knee, stress fractures occur most commonly in the proximal tibia and the patella. These fractures are discussed later in this chapter.[3, 14, 21]

COMMON PROBLEMS

Bursitis

PES ANSERINUS BURSITIS. This problem occurs commonly in runners, soccer players, or persons involved in other sports in which side-to-side movement or cutting is common activity. The manifestation is of pain with valgus stress or rotation of the tibia in the area of the pes anserinus tendons. The pain is occasionally associated with a mass or a painful snapping of the pes anserinus tendons. Usually the onset is insidious, and the problem becomes worse with physical activity over a period of 7 to 21 days (Fig. 12–1).

The diagnosis is made on the basis of the localized tenderness over the pes anserinus tendons. There is often a mass, fullness, or focal swelling in this area. This problem is often associated with an exostosis, and therefore the patient may be aware of a small mass in this area before the development of symptoms. There is tenderness to palpation over the pes anserinus tendons and over the palpable mass, as well as tenderness with resisted internal rotation and flexion of the knee. Valgus stress may reproduce the symptoms.

Radiographs may show an exostosis in the metaphyseal area, which predisposes the area to the development of pes anserinus bursitis and causes the snapping of the tendon over the bony mass.

Nonoperative management of this problem consists of local application of ice, restriction of activity, and nonsteroidal anti-inflammatory drugs (NSAIDs). A topical steroid injection, with care to avoid the

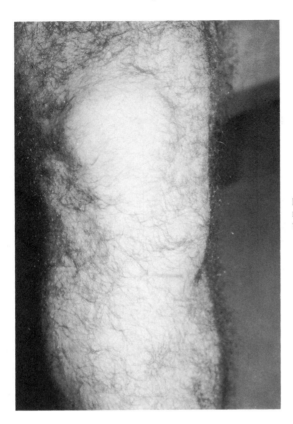

FIGURE 12–1. Pes anserinus bursitis manifests as a painful mass beneath the pes tendons. Such a mass with localized tenderness to palpation is depicted here.

tendons, may also be of use in reducing the inflammation. Finally, a period of immobilization of up to 2 weeks may help to reduce the symptoms as well.

According to the author's experience, if a mature exostosis is present and the symptoms are disabling, either the exostosis must be resected in order to remove the inciting cause of the irritation or the patient must markedly restrict activity. The operative management consists of excision of the bursa and any bony exostosis that is present. The indication for this is chronic pain that limits activity for a sustained period of time, usually 6 to 8 weeks.

The operative technique begins with an incision over the superior margin of the pes anserinus tendons. These usually are palpable at the anteromedial aspect of the knee. The incision is oblique along the course of the tendons. The tendons are retracted distally in order to expose and excise the bursa, or, if an exostosis is present, the tendons are retracted proximally and distally in order to expose the base of the exostosis. The exostosis is usually present between the sartorius and gracilis tendons. The bursa is excised sharply with a knife or scissors, and the exostosis is excised with an osteotome. Usually the pes anserinus tendons do not require any repair.

The patient is managed postoperatively in a knee immobilizer and extension or a slight flexion for 10 days and then begins a regimen of active range-of-motion exercises by taking the splint off twice a day and continuing straight-leg resistive exercise. In 3 weeks, use of the brace is discontinued. The patient continues a progressive resistive-exercise program until full strength and motion are regained.

SEMIMEMBRANOSUS BURSITIS. This problem usually occurs in runners or is associated with a degree of hamstring tendinitis after running and cutting activities. There may be local swelling over the posteromedial corner of the knee.

The diagnosis is made on the basis of localized tenderness to palpation over the posteromedial corner of the knee below the joint line with local swelling in this area. There is usually no effusion in the knee. There is tenderness with resisted flexion and occasionally with valgus stress.

The nonoperative treatment, as with pes anserinus bursitis, is initially restriction of activity, application of ice, NSAIDs, or a topical steroid injection. Again, immobilization may be of value for a 2- to 3-week period.

The indication for operative intervention is usually the development of a large mass caused by enlargement of the semimembranosus bursa. This results in unremitting pain and swelling, which limit activity.

The operative technique is a straight longitudinal incision over the posteromedial corner in order to identify the semimembranosus tendon deep to the pes anserinus tendons. The tendon is dissected proximally and anteriorly, and the bursa is resected from its medial aspect. Postoperative management is similar to that for pes anserinus bursitis.

PREPATELLAR BURSITIS. This problem is a result of direct trauma caused by a fall on the knee. The injury occurs most commonly in wrestling and football and results in an acute hemorrhagic prepatellar bursitis. Alternatively, an indirect injury associated with repetitive stress on the quadriceps or patellar tendon results in tendinitis, which may produce a sympathetic local effusion in the prepatellar bursa.[9]

The diagnosis is made on the basis of the appearance of a mass with localized tenderness in the prepatellar area. There is accumulation of fluid that is usually ballotable and may be aspirated.

Nonoperative treatment is aspiration, compression, and a period of immobilization. Application of ice and an NSAID may be of benefit. Avoidance of further irritation either by decreasing bent-knee activity or by avoiding direct trauma is the best way of preventing recurrence.

The indications for operative treatment are as follows. If the patient's problem persists for 6 to 8 weeks and limits activity, excision of prepatellar bursa should be considered. This decision must involve both the patient and the physician, and the patient must be convinced that ameliorating the disability outweighs any risk of the surgery.

The surgical technique is a straight incision in the midline, exposing the prepatellar bursa, and completely excising it, particularly in the medial and lateral recesses. Care must be taken to avoid buttonholing the skin in the medial and lateral extent of the wound. Postoperative management includes compression dressing and immobilization in a knee immobilizer for 3 weeks. Range-of-motion exercises begin at about 10 days to 2 weeks, and the patient progresses through a resistive-exercise program in order to strengthen the quadriceps and hamstring muscles as motion returns.

INFRAPATELLAR BURSITIS. Infrapatellar bursitis is often associated with chronic tendinitis of the patellar tendon. The management of this problem is an integral part of the management of the patellar tendinitis and is discussed in the next section.

Tendinitis

PATELLAR OR QUADRICEPS TENDINITIS. Patellar or quadriceps tendinitis frequently occurs in sports with the deceleration activity of jumping, such as basketball and volleyball. Manifestation is the insidious onset of pain localized to the tendon during activity and the resolution of symptoms when the activity is stopped. It is when the pain persists after activity that the patient usually comes to the physician with complaints of disability, such as decreased function. The diagnosis is based on localized tenderness over the tendon, and in the case of the patellar tendon, there may be a localized infrapatellar bursitis associated with the tendinitis as well. The nonoperative management of these problems include local application of ice, oral NSAIDs, and restriction of activity. After local pain decreases, eccentric quadriceps muscle–strengthening exercises may be of value. The author has not used steroid injections for these particular problems because there is significant risk of rupture of these tendons about a weight-bearing joint.

Radiographs are helpful in the evaluation and diagnosis of this problem because calcification occurs in either the quadriceps muscle or the patellar tendon and may indicate the presence of a more chronic problem that is difficult to treat nonoperatively without complete cessation of the inciting physical activity, and therefore an operative approach to the problem will be required. Ultrasonography and magnetic resonance imaging (MRI) may be used for an evaluation of these tendon problems in order to determine the presence of degenerative change within the tendon. If such change is present, a more aggressive approach or a much longer period of restricted activity (about 3 to 6 months) may be indicated.

Operative intervention has been reserved for patients who have prolonged chronic symptoms as well as localized evidence of degeneration of the tendon or, in the case of the patellar tendon, the development of an infrapatellar bony spur. The operative technique includes a straight longitudinal incision over the tendon in the area of discomfort. In the case of the patellar tendon, a local excision of the infrapatellar bursa is made, and exploration in the line of the tendon fibers with excision of any degenerated tendon is undertaken. Any patellar spurs are removed with a rongeur, multiple small holes are drilled in the tip of the patella, and careful closure of the tendon is performed.

Postoperative management is a 3-week period of immobilization, and at 10 days, active range-of-motion exercises are begun. Resistive straight-leg raising exercises begin at the time of surgery and at 3 weeks progress to short-arc and then long-arc quadriceps muscle–strengthening exercise.[9]

ILIOTIBIAL BAND TENDINITIS. In runners, painful, disabling inflammation of the iliotibial band may occur, particularly in the area in which the band crosses over the femoral condyle. The diagnosis is based on localized tenderness, and the symptoms are reproduced by having the patient run on a treadmill until the pain occurs. The problem is often associated with varus alignment of the knee and excessive supination of the hindfoot. Sudden changes in intensity and duration of the runner's activity are also often associated with this problem (Fig. 12–2).[11, 13]

The management of this problem is, almost without exception, nonoperative. The patient is treated with NSAIDs, perhaps through a local injection in the medial portion of the iliotibial band, and the patient begins

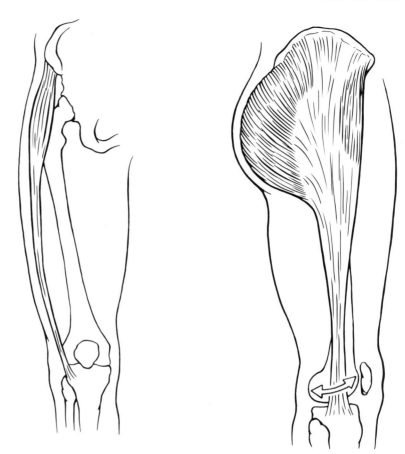

FIGURE 12–2. Iliotibial band tendinitis results from the repetitive back-and-forth motion of the iliotibial band with running.

a program of stretching as well as of strengthening of the hip adductors. An orthosis may be useful for balancing the supination of the hindfoot, correcting valgus deformity–producing heel wedge, or slightly changing the weight-bearing line at the knee. In general, appropriate exercise and a decrease in activity over a 4- to 6-week period leads to a resolution of the symptoms.

Operative management is infrequently needed but should include a simple incision over the iliotibial band at the level of its insertion to the intermuscular septum and a simple release of the posterior 2 cm by transverse incision. The patient then resumes a stretching program for strengthening of the abductor as well as the quadriceps and hamstring muscles.

Muscle Tendon Strain Injury

Indirect muscle injuries are a result of excessive force, usually from an eccentric contraction rather than from direct trauma. These injuries are frequent, and several common types occur about the knee, including quadriceps, hamstring, and gastrocnemius muscle strains. In this section, these partial injuries, including quadriceps tendon rupture and patellar tendon rupture are described.

QUADRICEPS STRAIN. The manifestation is usually of localized pain in the anterior central aspect of the quadriceps muscle, commonly after an acute injury in jumping sports such as basketball or volleyball. The diagnosis is based on the presence of localized pain over the muscle and increased discomfort with flexion of the knee or resisted active extension of the knee. There may be a palpable defect over the quadriceps muscle; this usually occurs in the rectus portion of the muscle (Fig. 12–3).[10]

Management is essentially nonoperative. Gait is supported as necessary. Gentle active range-of-motion exercise is started through the pain-free range. It is useful to measure thigh circumference in order to follow the change in swelling that occurs with treatment. Local application of ice and NSAIDs is started. Three to five days after injury, ultrasonography may be useful for preventing the formation of local scarring.

As the decrease in pain allows, short-arc and then full-arc exercises are undertaken until full range of motion and strength are achieved, at which time normal activity is resumed. Heterotopic bone occasionally may form in the muscle injured. The patient whose pain seems to be lingering should have radiographs of the thigh in order to rule out this complication of quadriceps strain.

HAMSTRING STRAIN. This strain occurs most commonly in activities that require sprinting, such as track, football, and soccer. The diagnosis is based on localized tenderness over the hamstring muscle, most often on the medial side. The pain occurs with passive extension of the knee and active flexion of the knee. Again, there may be a defect palpable. Nonoperative management proceeds in the same way as for the quadriceps strain. In this instance, the patient starts resistive exercise with prone bending and prone flexion, using a light weight (2 to 5 pounds), and then progresses to heavier weights (20 to 25 pounds) as pain subsides and range of motion allows. The patient should perform backward walking

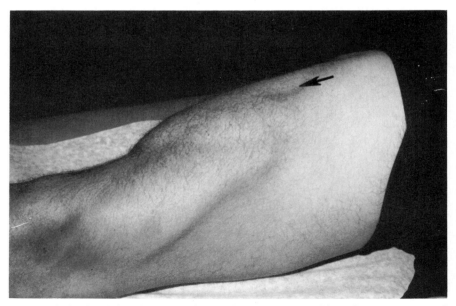

FIGURE 12–3. The defect *(arrow)* in the quadriceps is compatible with some tearing of muscle fibers in this quadriceps strain.

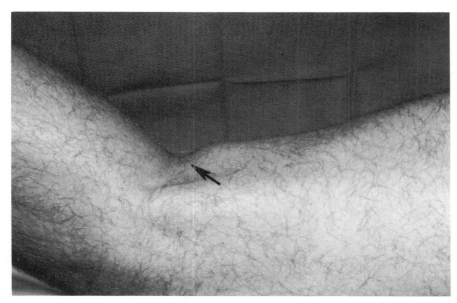

FIGURE 12–4. This hamstring strain shows a palpable and visible defect *(arrow)* with resisted flexion.

with progression to running and cutting before returning to sports. The patient is taught hamstring muscle–stretching exercises and follows a maintenance strength program once return to activity is initiated (Fig. 12–4).[10]

MEDIAL HEAD OF THE GASTROCNEMIUS. This strain occurs in racquet sports, particularly during overhead motion. It has been called tennis leg. The diagnosis is based on tenderness at the musculotendinous junction, most commonly in the medial head of the gastrocnemius muscle. The pain also occurs with passive dorsiflexion and active plantar flexion of the foot and ankle. This pain is made worse by extension of the knee. Many patients have localized discoloration and swelling in the calf, and the calf should be measured periodically in order to follow the progress of the injury as treatment is instituted (Fig. 12–5).

Nonoperative management includes use of a heel lift, local application of ice, NSAIDs, and ultrasonography 3 to 5 days after injury. Compression or wearing of support hosiery may be helpful for relieving the pain, and crutches may be useful for supporting gait. The patient then follows a stretching program until full motion and full strength are regained.

Prevention of these muscle injuries includes a warm-up or conditioning period, which has been shown to be effective to alter the biomechanical properties of the muscle tendon unit. Stretching of the tendon in this way results in the ability to develop more force and to stretch farther when the tendon is pulled to failure, in comparison with the non-preconditioned muscle tendon unit. Therefore, experimental evidence supports the use of a stretching program in order to prevent this strain type of injury.[8, 9]

Stress Fractures

The tibia is a common site of stress fracture, accounting for about 20 per cent of all stress fractures seen. Most tibial stress fractures involve the

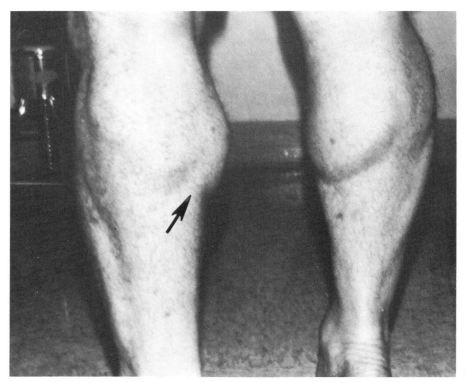

FIGURE 12–5. "Tennis leg" is a grade 2 strain of the medial gastrocnemius muscle with localized swelling *(arrow)* and tenderness.

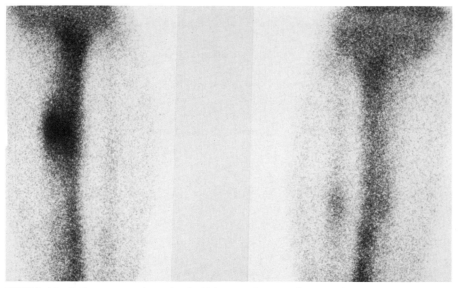

FIGURE 12–6. Bone scan of proximal tibial stress fracture that manifested with tenderness over the pes tendons.

proximal or the distal third of the bone. Those that occur in the proximal third may manifest as knee pain. Young athletes seem prone to stress fracture of the proximal third of the tibia. The patient usually presents with activity-related pain.[3, 5, 14] Point tenderness may be noted over a small, specific area in the posteromedial aspect of the proximal tibia. Pain with resisted knee or ankle motion is usually not seen, but when it does occur, it is frequently in the area of the pes anserinus tendons and bursa, and so it must be differentiated from pes anserinus bursitis. Bringing the patient's tibia over the examiner's knee and using the examiner's knee as a fulcrum often reproduces the pain.[5] The diagnosis is usually made with a plain radiograph, or a bone scintigram demonstrates the lesion at the time of presentation (Fig. 12–6). Treatment usually consists of restriction of activity for 4 to 6 weeks with alternative aerobic exercise such as swimming or bicycling, depending on the occurrence of pain. Return to normal activity, with symptoms dictating the progression of training, should be gradual.[2, 3, 5]

Patellar stress fractures may occur in young athletes and frequently involve the distal pole of the patella close to the attachment of the patellar tendon. Both transverse and longitudinal fractures have been described. Nonoperative treatment, outlined earlier, is the treatment of choice.[3]

Masses of the Joint Line and the Popliteal Area

A variety of masses occur about the knee, but three types are of concern in this chapter. The popliteal cyst arises from the posterior aspect of the knee, usually between the medial head of the gastrocnemius muscle and the semimembranosus tendon. Such a mass is usually associated with internal derangement problems such as a meniscal tear, osteoarthritis, a loose body, or some other source of effusion.[6, 20] The mass often becomes progressively larger as a result of a ball-valve effect at the entrance of the mass from the joint. It must first be determined whether the mass is indeed a popliteal cyst or some solid tumor, and usually that can be accomplished with ultrasonography or MRI. Management includes aspiration of the knee and the mass itself with local instillation of steroid into the mass, NSAIDs, and restriction of activity. If swelling is persistent, the treatment initially consists of management of the intra-articular problem and observation of the cyst. If the cyst persists, open excision should be performed.

Most popliteal cysts disappear without surgery, and those that are removed may recur. In a study of 120 such cysts, 50 were treated surgically, and of these, 21 recurred; 70 were treated nonsurgically, and 19 of these recurred.[6] The causes of popliteal cysts are mechanical and synovial. Seropositive and seronegative arthritis may be manifested as a popliteal cyst with effusion in the knee.[6, 20] Rupture of the cyst may occur, producing severe pain in the calf, and this is an early manifestation of rheumatoid arthritis. Arthrography, ultrasonography, and MRI are all diagnostic methods useful for evaluating such masses.

A second type of mass that can occur is a degenerative meniscal cyst. These occur most commonly on the lateral side of the knee and are discussed more fully in Chapter 16.

A third type of mass is a cyst that is similar to the popliteal cyst but

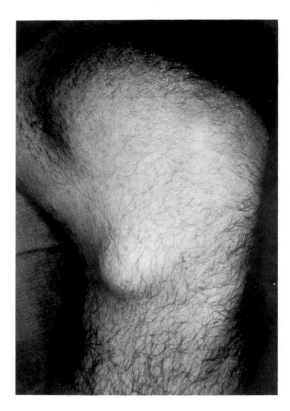

FIGURE 12–7. A semimembranosus cyst similar to a ganglion cyst. This was excised and found to be filled with a gelatinous material.

usually forms medially, anteriorly, and superiorly to the attachment to the semimembranosus tendon. This may be an extrinsic enlargement of the semimembranosus bursa (Fig. 12–7). It is often filled with a gelatinous material, much like a ganglion cyst of the wrist or the foot. This type of cyst can be managed by aspiration and local instillation of steroid. If this does not resolve the problem, local excision is the treatment of choice.

THE RUNNER AND KNEE PAIN

The number of persons who jog increases annually. It has been estimated that each year, two of three runners are affected by injury.[11] The repetitive nature of impact loading on the lower extremity has been discussed earlier in this chapter. About 30 per cent of runners' complaints are localized to the knee.[10] Many patients present after a change in the intensity or the duration of activity or in some other aspect of the training regimen or equipment. In addition, an evaluation with thorough history taking should include reports of the occurrence of static and dynamic malalignment problems, the location and duration of the symptoms, and their temporal relationship to running. Most of these problems are overuse problems, and a search for predisposing factors such as anatomic alignment variation, change in training regimen, equipment, or surface run is of value.

Most runners' problems are of three general types: patellofemoral pain, iliotibial band tendinitis, or intra-articular abnormality. Specific entities are discussed elsewhere in this book, but some general comments are in order. One third of runners with pain have iliotibial band tendinitis, and another one third have patellofemoral pain. In patients with pre-existing knee problems, intra-articular abnormalities are most common.[10] Management of these problems is mainly nonoperative, with some restriction or alteration of activity. Prevention of the symptoms should focus on limiting sudden changes in intensity and duration of workout and on building an awareness of the common problems encountered and how they relate to knee alignment and pre-existing degenerative change. The most important single preventive factor is a pre-exercise conditioning program for the hip, thigh, and calf musculature as well as a stretching program to provide preloading in the muscle tendon units about the joint.[9, 11, 13]

REFERENCES

1. Ahmed AM, Burke DL: In-vitro measurement of static pressure distribution in synovial joints: part I. Tibial surface of the knee. J Biomech Eng 105:216–225, 1983.
2. Apple DV, O'Toole J, Annia C: Professional basketball injuries. Phys Sportsmed 10:81–86, 1982.
3. Bruns BR, Yngve D: Stress reaction and stress fracture. *In* Grana WA, Lombardo JA, Sharkey BJ, Stone JA (eds): Advances in Sports Medicine and Fitness, vol 2, pp. 201–221. Chicago: Year Book Medical Publishers, 1989.
4. Demak R: The pain that won't go away. Sports Illust 27:60–71, April 1987.
5. Devas MB: Stress fractures of the tibia in athletes or "shin soreness." J Bone Joint Surg 40B:227–239, 1958.
6. Dinham JM: Popliteal cysts in children: the case against surgery. J Bone Joint Surg 57B:69–71, 1975.
7. Enneking WF: Arthritis. *In* Enneking WF (ed): Clinical Musculoskeletal Pathology, pp. 331–354. Gainesville, FL: Storer, 1984.
8. Garrett WE Jr, Almekinders LC, Seaber AV: Biomechanics of muscle tears in stretching injuries. Trans Orthop Res Soc 9:384, 1984.
9. Grana WA: Disorders of the knee. *In* Grana WA, Kalenak A (eds): Clinical Sports Medicine, pp. 451–455. Philadelphia: WB Saunders, 1991.
10. Grana WA, Coniglione TC: Knee disorders in runners. Phys Sportsmed 13(5):127–133, 1985.
11. Grana WA, Goodhart CW: Evaluation and management of knee pain in the runner. Techniques Orthop 5(3):23–29, 1990.
12. Hamberg P, Gillquist J, Lysholm J: A comparison between arthroscopic meniscectomy and modified open meniscectomy: a prospective randomized study with emphasis on postoperative rehabilitation. J Bone Joint Surg 66B:189–192, 1984.
13. Hanks GA, Kalenak A: Running injuries. *In* Grana WA, Kalenak A (eds): Clinical Sports Medicine, pp. 458–465. Philadelphia: WB Saunders, 1991.
14. Kimball PR, Savastano AA: Fatigue fractures of the proximal tibia. Clin Orthop 70:170–173, 1970.
15. Kurosawa H, Fukubayashi T, Nakajima H: Load-bearing mode of the knee joint: physical behavior of the knee joint with or without menisci. Clin Orthop 149:283–290, 1980.
16. McMaster PE: Tendon and muscle ruptures: clinical and experimental studies on the causes and location of subcutaneous ruptures. J Bone Joint Surg 15:705–722, 1933.
17. Pascale MS, Grana WA: Does running cause osteoarthritis?. Phys Sportsmed 17(3):156–166, 1989.
18. Radin EL, de Lamotte F, Maquet P: Role of the menisci in the distribution of stress in the knee. Clin Orthop 185:290–294, 1984.
19. Radin EL, Paul IL, Rose RM: Role of mechanical factors in pathogenesis of primary osteoarthritis. Lancet 1:519–522, 1972.
20. Soslow AR: Popliteal cysts in a pediatric patient. Ann Emerg Med 16:588–591, 1987.
21. Stanitski CL, McMaster JH, Scranton PE: On the nature of stress fractures. Am J Sports Med 6:391–396, 1978.

PART III

Orthopaedic

Sports

Traumatology

■

CHAPTER 13

Arthroscopy

JOHN F. MEYERS, M.D.

■

DEVELOPMENT OF ARTHROSCOPY

The modern era of arthroscopy began in the 1950s in Japan when Masaki Watanabe developed the Watanabe No. 21 arthroscope. His arthroscope provided an excellent view of the knee joint. The light that illuminated the knee was provided by an incandescent bulb at the end of the arthroscope. This proved to be a problem because it was easily bent and broken. The subsequent development of fiberoptic light sources solved this problem.

Arthroscopy was brought to North America when Robert Jackson of Toronto visited Watanabe in 1964. Jackson returned to Toronto with a Watanabe No. 21 arthroscope and began diagnostic arthroscopy of the knee. The late Richard O'Connor also studied with Watanabe and began performing arthroscopic surgical procedures in the early 1970s. Initial surgical procedures were performed with the use of an operative arthroscope, which consisted of a double-barreled sheath. The arthroscope was inserted down one barrel of the sheath, and an operative instrument, such as a punch, was placed down the parallel barrel. The development of the techniques of triangulation have rendered the operative arthroscope obsolete.

Lanny Johnson developed the first motorized instruments for arthroscopic surgery. The initial instrument was called a chondroplastic shaver and consisted of a motorized hand piece, a suction, and a revolving blade within a sheath. This device was inserted through a cannula into the knee joint. Tissue was suctioned into a small window in the side of the sheath and cut by the revolving blade. More aggressive instruments that cut meniscal tissue and burr or abrade bone have since been developed. All of these instruments function according to the same basic principle developed by Johnson.

The 1970s was the era of development of arthroscopic surgery. Instruments and techniques were developed and refined during this time. The 1980s was the era of acceptance of arthroscopic surgery. The orthopaedic community initially regarded arthroscopic surgery with skepticism, but its acceptance by patients and the documentation of clinical results have led to widespread acceptance of the procedure. It is estimated that 90 per cent of orthopaedic surgeons now use arthroscopy in some portion of their practice.

EQUIPMENT

The manufacturers' displays at the annual meetings of the American Academy of Orthopaedic Surgeons contain an overwhelming variety of equipment available to the arthroscopic surgeon. Some instruments are essential for arthroscopic surgery, some are nice to have, and some are superfluous. Through experience, the author has developed an inventory of equipment that provides for many needs in arthroscopic knee surgery (Table 13–1). Specific brands of equipment are not recommended; a good working relationship with a detail representative, the use of loaner equipment when the surgeon's own equipment is broken, and fast turnaround time for repairs are much more important than knowing specific brands of equipment. Most manufacturers are willing to let

TABLE 13–1. Arthroscopic Equipment for Knee Surgery

No. 4.0 arthroscopes, 30° and 70°
Hand-held camera and C-mount
Light source and cable
Color television monitor
Video recorder, ½ and ¾ inch
Power cutter with blades: meniscus cutter, synovectomy blade, and burr

No. 3 knife handle
18-g 3-inch spinal needle
5.5-mm cannula with sharp and blunt trocar
4.5-mm cannula with sharp and blunt trocar
Inflow (Christmas-tree) adapter
Disposable plastic cannulae, 4.5 and 5.5 mm
Hook probe
Grasping forceps
Johnson Jaws
Two switching sticks
Basket forceps: straight, curved up, curved right, curved left, and 90° right and left
Beaver knife handle: long, Arthro-Lok blades, banana No. 6984, curved meniscectomy
Curettes (including ring)
Arthroscopic rasps
Golden retriever, 2.0 mm

Small K-wires, ³⁄₃₂ down
ACL alignment guide
Battery-operated hand-held drill
Cannulated reamers: 9 mm, 10 mm, 11 mm, and 12 mm
Davis tonsil-free needles, curved small Mayo needles

Ochsner clamp
Hemostats
Needle holder
Scissors (Mayo straight)
Retractors:
    Army/Navy retractors (two)
    Small Hohmann retractor (one)
    Gelpi retractor (one)
    Senn retractor (two)
    Soup spoon
    Small vaginal speculum
Adson thumb forceps with teeth

Electrocautery system with hook electrode

Meniscal repair cannula
Suture punch with cannula
LCR staple set
Cannulated screw set: small and large

Leg holder
Aqua Vac for floor drainage

LCR, Ligamentous and Capsular Repair system.

surgeons use their equipment on a trial basis, and surgeons should do this before purchasing the equipment.

The standard arthroscope used for knee arthroscopy is the 4.0-mm, 30° oblique arthroscope that fits down a 5.0-mm sheath. The 30° obliquity offers a field of view of 60° by rotating the arthroscope within the sheath. A 70° oblique arthroscope (Fig. 13–1) is necessary for good visualization of the posterior compartments of the knee when the arthroscope is inserted through the intercondylar notch into the posterior compartments. At least three 4.0-mm arthroscopes should be available in an operating room. The

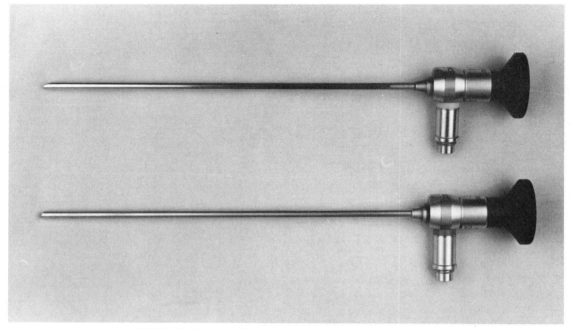

FIGURE 13–1. *Top:* 70° arthroscope; *bottom:* 30° arthroscope.

first arthroscope is for use in surgery, the second is for backup, and the third is for backup when one of the other two is out for service. One arthroscope should be kept gas-sterilized so that there is no delay in changing arthroscopes if one of the others is broken or contaminated. For the same reason, three light cords are essential. One of these should also be kept gas-sterilized.

Most of the light sources now in use for arthroscopic surgery are equipped with metal halide bulbs. These bulbs have a life of approximately 40 hours and cost between $400 and $500 to replace. Xenon bulbs have been available in the past, but in order to replace the bulb, the light source must be sent back to the factory. Xenon light sources that enable changing the bulb in the operating room are now being made. These bulbs last up to 500 hours and cost between $700 and $800. Light sources with xenon bulbs should therefore be considered when a new light source is to be bought or when a worn-out one is to be replaced. Light sources should have multiple ports that accept different types of fiberoptic light cables.

In all types of arthroscopic surgery, a camera is attached to the arthroscope. The camera should be soakable in disinfectant for use in multiple operations. The camera should have at least 450 lines of horizontal resolution. The size of the image projected on the monitor depends on the size of the arthroscope and the focal length between the camera and the lens. In general, larger images on the screen are sharper than smaller images. Many cameras have microprocessors that control the amount of light admitted to the camera on the basis of the brightness of the object in the center of the visual field; this feature makes brightness of image constant.

If laser energy is to be used in arthroscopic surgery, a camera that filters laser light should be chosen. A standard camera attaches to the eyepiece on the arthroscope by means of a C-mount adapter. A vent or a suction port on the C-mount adapter helps keep the lens from fogging. Video-dedicated arthroscopes (Fig. 13–2) do not have an eyepiece, and the arthroscope screws directly into the camera. This feature prevents moisture from getting between the eyepiece and the camera. The disadvantage of the video-dedicated arthroscope is that two camera heads are necessary for changing from a 30° to a 70° arthroscope. The regular camera and C-mount adapter are probably preferable unless the surgeon's budget allows for the purchase of multiple camera heads.

The image from the camera is displayed on a video monitor. A smaller monitor provides a sharper image of the projected signal. A 13-inch monitor with at least 450 lines of horizontal resolution provides the clearest image.

Documentation in arthroscopic surgery is important not only for educating the patient but also for medicolegal purposes. Many surgeons record their surgical cases on videotape. Three-quarter-inch video recorders are slightly more expensive than VHS recorders but provide a sharper image. Three-quarter-inch videotape can also be edited several times without appreciable loss of quality. The disadvantage of documentation on videotape is the storage space required for keeping the videotapes. If videotapes are to be used for documentation, they should probably be edited in order to save only the pertinent portions of the case. Video printers in which a thermal ink transfer process is used to make a print of the video image are now available. The newer generation of printers can produce from one to nine images per print. Microprocessor adapters can be attached to the video printer and enable storage of fifty images on one two inch floppy disk. Character generators available for the printers make titles, arrows, and other graphics on the prints. Videotapes and prints are excellent for educating patients and for documentation; how-

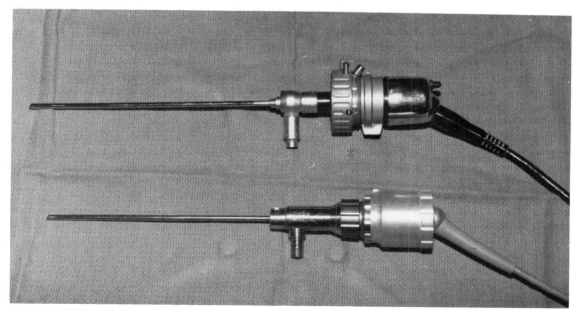

FIGURE 13–2. *Top:* C-mount camera and arthroscope; *bottom:* video-dedicated arthroscope.

ever, they lack clarity for publication in textbooks and articles. Documentation for these purposes should be made with a 35-mm camera. The techniques of arthroscopic photography are beyond the scope of this chapter but have been documented in the literature.[7, 18]

The choice of electronic equipment for arthroscopic surgery should be based on the service available from the manufacturer's representative, the availability of loaner equipment, and the surgeon's personal preference after trial usage of several types of the equipment to be purchased.

Arthroscopic knee surgery requires the use of a leg holder for stabilizing the patient's thigh and enabling the operating surgeon to open the medial and lateral compartments. Many leg holders are designed for use in conjunction with a tourniquet. Low-profile leg holders enable access to the superior portals with instruments brought in from above. Some leg holders are designed to facilitate bilateral knee arthroscopy (Fig. 13–3). The patient's pelvis should be secured with a pelvic strap when the leg holder is used. If the pelvis is not secured, the thigh can easily rotate within the confines of the leg holder.

Cannulae are used for fluid distention of the knee and facilitate easy passage of instruments through the soft tissue. The 5.5-mm cannulae are designed for inflow of fluid; 4.5-mm cannulae are used for instrument passage. Disposable plastic cannulae have a diaphragm that prevents egress of fluid when instruments are passed and an inflow port on the side.

Switching sticks are useful when arthroscopic and operative portals are changed. These sticks are long, blunt-tipped rods that are inserted

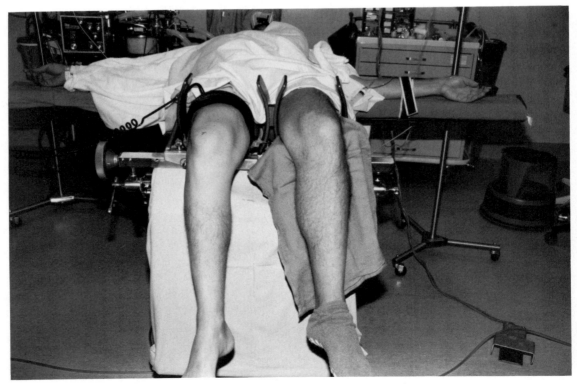

FIGURE 13–3. Leg holder, which allows bilateral knee arthroscopy.

down through the cannula. The cannula is then removed, and a different cannula can be easily inserted over the switching stick.

Hand-held instruments are necessary for exploration, cutting, and grasping. A hook probe is useful for manipulating loose bodies and palpating menisci and ligaments. The probe should fit through an operating cannula and be scored in order to facilitate measuring. Punches are used for removing meniscal tissue, synovium, and articular cartilage. A basic set of punches should include a straight punch, an upbiting punch, and left and right cutting punches (Fig. 13–4). Grasping instruments for removing loose tissue should have serrated teeth. Both a large grasping forceps and a grasping forceps that fits through an operative cannula should be available to the surgeon. Disposable knife blades (Fig. 13–5) are sharper and more effective than nondisposable knives.

Motorized instruments are powered by either electricity or gas. Electric-powered motors allow for cutting at between 600 and 4000 rpm. The gas-powered instruments cut at approximately 3000 rpm and are generally more aggressive because more torque is generated. Instruments with both hand and foot controls are available. The author has found the foot controls somewhat easier to use because the hand is free for fine manipulation of the instruments. Interchangeable blades are available in diameters between 3.5 and 5.5 mm. Blades are designed for synovial shaving, aggressive cutting of meniscal tissue, and burring of bone (Fig. 13–6). Disposable blades are probably preferable because they are always sharp.

Drill guides and cannulated reamers are used for ligament reconstruction and drilling and for bone grafting of osteochondritic lesions. The drill guide should be light-weight, sturdy, and easily manipulated. The cannulated reamers require periodic sharpening. After several years of use,

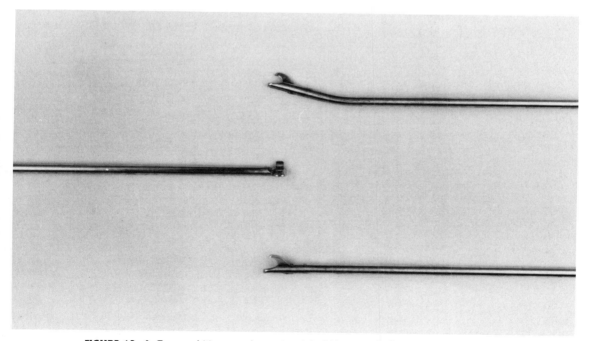

FIGURE 13–4. *Top:* up-biting punch; *center:* right-biting punch; *bottom:* straight punch.

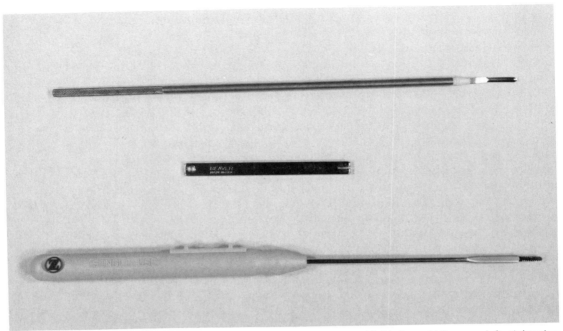

FIGURE 13–5. Disposable knife blades. *Top:* permanent handle with disposable blades; *middle:* wrench for tightening disposable blade; *bottom:* disposable knife with retractable blade.

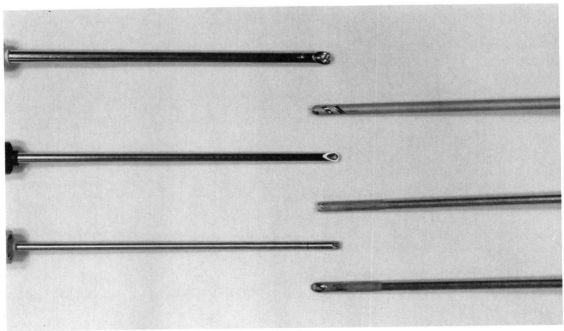

FIGURE 13–6. Disposable shaver blades. *Top to bottom:* motorized burr, air-powered synovial blade, motorized synovial blade, air-powered meniscal blade, motorized meniscal blade, air-powered burr.

these systems develop excess play and do not reproducibly insert guide wires in the intended spot. When this development occurs, they should be replaced. Power drills are necessary for use with the drill guides. The rechargeable battery-powered drills are easier to manipulate than the air-powered drills and are recommended for arthroscopic surgery.

Meniscus repair sets come in various designs. Most consist of cannulae with various curves that enable the passage of long needles (Fig. 13–7). Retractors used for protecting the posterior neurovascular structures from the needles are necessary. Several types are manufactured. A soup spoon or one limb of a pediatric vaginal speculum work quite well (Fig. 13–8).

Pumps control fluid distention of the joint and are useful in knees with degenerative arthritis and proliferative synovitis, which can block the inflow portal. One less portal than usual is necessary when a pump is used because the inflow is through the arthroscopic sheath. Tourniquets are usually not necessary when a pump is used because bleeding can be controlled by intra-articular pressure. The disadvantage of pumps includes the extra cost of the pump and tubing, additional clutter in the operating room, and the possibility of excessive soft tissue distention with fluid.

Electrocautery systems are available for cutting and coagulation. They offer no advantage over mechanical means for cutting tissue. The cautery feature is useful in controlling bleeding after lateral retinacular release and synovectomy. Most cautery systems require the use of water rather than saline or Ringer's lactate for distention.

Laser systems are now being marketed for use in arthroscopic surgery. The CO_2 laser only works in a gas medium. The Contact ND:Yag laser

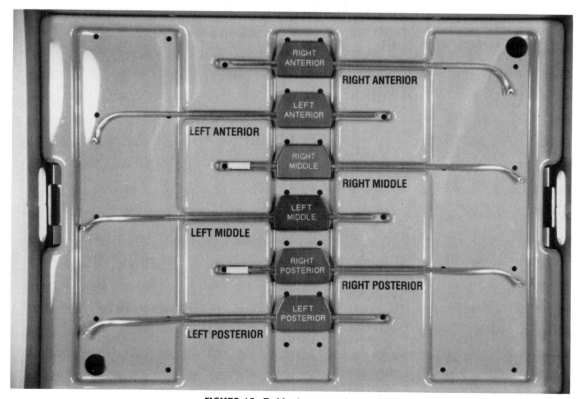

FIGURE 13–7. Meniscus repair set.

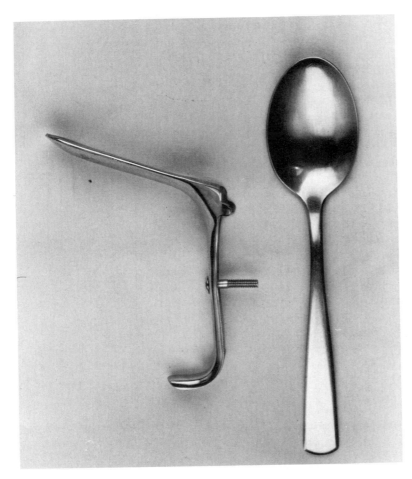

FIGURE 13–8. Vaginal speculum and soup spoon, used as retractors in meniscal repair.

works in a fluid medium and cuts only the tissue that it contacts. The laser systems offer no advantage over mechanical systems in ability to cut and remove tissue. A potential advantage of laser energy may be an ability to incite a healing response in articular cartilage and meniscal tissue. Experimental evidence of this characteristic of laser energy is inconclusive at this point.

Other instruments that may on occasion be useful include a cannulated screw set. Large cancellous screws are used for arthroscopic reduction and internal fixation of tibial plateau fractures. Smaller screws can be used for intra-articular osteochondral fractures. Suture punches are occasionally used for anterior cruciate ligament repairs. Intra-articular staples have limited application in arthroscopic knee surgery.

Arthroscopic surgery requires the use of many delicate, specialized instruments. Provisions should be made for safe and efficient storage of this equipment. Cabinets for storage of video equipment and power sources are satisfactory in a general operating room. If the operating room is used specifically for arthroscopic surgery, retractable storage shelves suspended from the ceiling are a good alternative to cabinets (Fig. 13–9).

Control of water on the floor is often a problem. Mats with attached suction can keep the floor dry. This is a much better alternative to throwing blankets onto the floor and wringing them out.

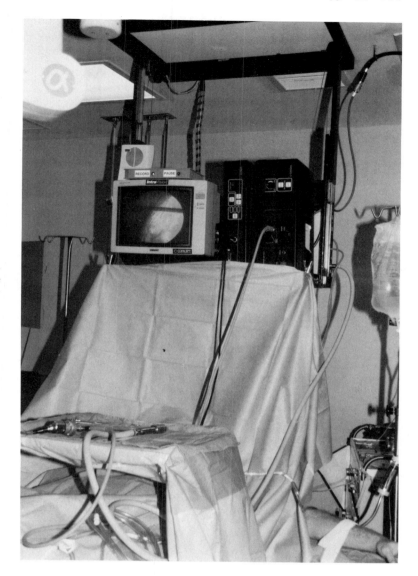

FIGURE 13–9. Arthroscopy equipment suspended from retractable storage unit in ceiling over operating table.

ANESTHESIA AND POSITIONING OF THE PATIENT

Arthroscopic knee surgery can be performed with the patient under general, epidural, spinal, or local anesthesia. General, epidural, or spinal anesthesia is usually necessary for ligament reconstructive procedures. The choice of anesthesia should be based on the preference of the anesthesiologist, the surgeon, and the patient.

The patient is placed in a supine position on the operating table with the operative knee positioned over the distal flex of the operating table. The foot of the table is flexed 90°, and a foam pad is placed behind the patient's nonoperative knee. If a tourniquet is used, it should be placed 10 to 12 cm above the superior pole of the patella with the operative knee in extension. The leg is then exsanguinated with the use of an Esmarch bandage from the toes to the tourniquet, the knee is flexed to full flexion, and the tourniquet is inflated. The leg holder is then applied, and the pelvis is secured to the operating table with a strap in order to prevent rotation of the limb.

The knee is shaved just before surgery. The author usually scrubs and paints the patient's knee with an iodophor compound. Some surgeons use only an iodophor paint.

Approximately half of arthroscopic surgeons administer prophylactic antibiotics to patients. Prophylactic antibiotics should probably always be administered to patients undergoing ligament reconstructions and meniscal repairs that require a posterior incision.

PORTALS AND TECHNIQUES OF DIAGNOSTIC ARTHROSCOPY

Establishing Portals

Multiple portals have been described for arthroscopic knee surgery.[28] Most arthroscopic surgery can be performed through five basic portals: inflow portal, anterolateral portal, anteromedial portal, posteromedial portal, and posterolateral portal (Fig. 13–10). A superolateral portal and a transpatellar tendon portal are occasionally necessary. The inflow portal is established superior to the superior pole of the patella and parallel to the medial border of the patella.

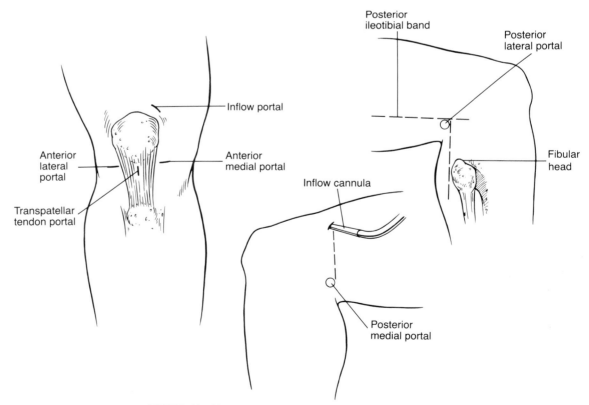

FIGURE 13–10. Basic portals for arthroscopic knee surgery.

After the knee has been inflated with lactated Ringer solution through the inflow portal, a bulge develops in the sulcus just lateral to the patellar tendon. The anterolateral portal is established in the center of this bulge. This portal is usually established one finger's breadth lateral to the superior aspect of the patellar tendon. The other portals can then be established under direct visualization by inserting a spinal needle in order to determine the proper placement of the portal. The anteromedial portal is established approximately one finger's breadth medial to the patellar tendon, but this position may be varied on the basis of intra-articular placement of the probing spinal needle.

The posterior portals are established under direct visualization by inserting the arthroscope through the intercondylar notch into the posterior compartments. The arthroscope is directed from the anterolateral portal along the medial wall of the intercondylar notch and into the posteromedial compartment (Fig. 13–11). Finger palpation posteriorly along the medial joint line reveals a soft spot just behind the posterior border of the tibia. A perpendicular line dropping from the inflow portal with the knee flexed 90° should cross the medial joint line at the approximate entry site. A spinal needle is inserted and necessary adjustments are made before the puncture wound is made.

The posterolateral puncture wound is also made under direct visualization. The arthroscope is inserted through the anteromedial portal along the lateral wall of the intercondylar notch and into the posterolateral compartment. With the knee flexed at 90°, the spinal needle should be inserted at the junction of the posterior margin of the iliotibial band and a line parallel to the posterior aspect of the head of the fibula. The needle should be angled 15° forward and 15° caudad. Minor adjustments in angulation can be made, depending on where the needle enters the posterior lateral compartment. Both posterior portals are established with the knee flexed at 90°.

The superolateral portal is sometimes used for lateral retinacular release and for observing patellar tracking. This portal can be made under direct visualization and is approximately one finger's breadth above the superior pole of the patella and parallel to the lateral border of the patella.

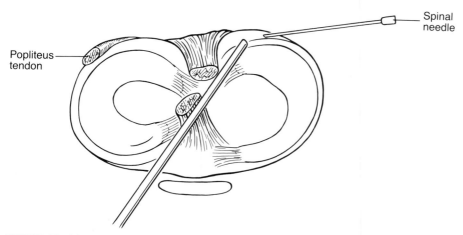

FIGURE 13–11. Arthroscope is inserted through the intercondylar notch into the posteromedial compartment. A spinal needle has been inserted into the posteromedial compartment under direct visualization.

The transpatellar tendon portal is made in the center of the patellar tendon, just distal to the inferior pole of the patella. The cut should be made parallel to the fibers of the patellar tendon. This portal is sometimes useful in cruciate ligament reconstructions.

Diagnostic Arthroscopy

A systematic method for examining the knee should be developed and used in every instance of diagnostic arthroscopy. If attention is focused immediately on the suspected pathologic process, other symptomatic conditions can be overlooked. After the inflow portal has been established and the knee has been inflated with lactated Ringer solution, the arthroscopic cannula should be inserted into the intercondylar notch with the use of the blunt obturator and with the patient's knee flexed 90°. The knee is extended, and the arthroscopic cannula is directed into the suprapatellar pouch. The arthroscope is then inserted, and the suprapatellar pouch is examined for the presence of suprapatellar plica, loose bodies, or synovial pathologic processes.

The undersurface of the patella is examined and the trochlear groove observed. The knee is flexed and extended, and patellar tracking is observed. The arthroscope is then swept down over the medial femoral condyle in order to detect the presence of a medial plica and to observe the condition of the femoral articular cartilage. A valgus stress is then placed on the knee, and the arthroscope is directed into the medial compartment. At this point, the anteromedial portal is established with the use of a spinal needle to determine proper placement of the puncture wound. A hook probe can then be inserted for palpation. The medial meniscus is examined and palpated, and the articular cartilage of the distal femur and tibial plateau is examined. The stress is removed from the knee, and the arthroscope is directed laterally over the ligamentum synovium. The anterior and posterior cruciate ligaments can then be examined with the knee flexed and extended.

Next, varus stress is placed on the knee, and the arthroscope is directed into the lateral compartment, in which the meniscus and the articular cartilage of the femur and the tibia are examined visually and with the hook probe. The arthroscope is directed along the lateral gutter and then removed from the sheath, and the blunt obturator is inserted. The arthroscope is directed into the posteromedial compartment by palpation. The 30° angle on the arthroscope makes it very difficult to direct the instrument into this compartment under direct visualization. At this point, a posteromedial portal can be established. This portal is helpful for examining the posterior cruciate ligament. It is also used for removing loose bodies posteriorly and for performing synovectomies.

The arthroscope is removed from the knee, and the arthroscopic cannula is inserted through the anteromedial portal with the knee flexed at 90°. The knee is extended, and the arthroscope is directed into the suprapatellar pouch. The pouch and the patella are again inspected. Changing portals alters viewing perspective and different areas of disease can be discovered. The hook probe can be inserted through the anterolateral portal in order to palpate the articular cartilage of the patella and the trochlear groove. The arthroscope is then swept down over the lateral femoral condyle and into the lateral compartment. The menisci and articular cartilage are again visualized. The arthroscope is next directed across the intercondylar notch for another view of the cruciate ligaments. A valgus stress is then applied, and the medial compartment is reexamined. The arthroscope should be removed from the sheath and the blunt obturator inserted. The arthroscopic sheath is then directed by palpation into the posterior lateral compartment. The arthroscope is reinserted, and a posterolateral portal may be established if necessary.

These procedures constitute a complete diagnostic arthroscopic examination and should be performed for every patient.

INDICATIONS AND TECHNIQUES FOR ARTHROSCOPIC SURGERY

Synovectomy

The development of techniques of arthroscopic synovectomy have rendered this procedure more benign than open synovectomy. Arthroscopic synovectomy decreases the postoperative morbidity and the loss of motion seen after open synovectomy. Arthroscopic techniques enable more thorough synovectomy that can easily include the posterior compartments.

Arthroscopic synovectomy is a well-accepted technique in the treatment of pigmented villonodular synovitis.[23, 28] This benign and neoplastic condition of the synovium consists of synovial proliferation and hemosiderin deposits. It can be either localized or diffuse within the knee joint. The localized conditions are easily cured by arthroscopic resection of the affected tissue. Diffuse pigmented villonodular synovitis responds well to total synovectomy, but some recurrences are to be expected. These recurrences can be treated by repeated synovectomy.

Synovial chondromatosis is a metaplastic condition of the synovium in which the synovium manufactures cartilaginous bodies, which break free within the joint and may calcify or ossify. Arthroscopic synovectomy has been advocated as a treatment for synovial chondromatosis with generally good results. Dorfmann and colleagues[6] advocated arthroscopic removal of the loose bodies without synovectomy as treatment.

Arthroscopic synovectomy for rheumatoid arthritis has been successful in both short-term and long-term studies.[16, 25, 27] For the best results, synovectomy should be performed in patients in whom effusion and synovitis have persisted after 6 months of adequate medical treatment. Synovectomy is most successful if performed early before radiographic changes are present. The removal of the diseased synovium appears to slow down or, in some cases, halt the progression of the disease.

Arthroscopic synovectomy has also been used for the treatment of recurrent hemarthrosis of the knee in hemophilia.[29] Although a significant decrease in recurrent hemarthrosis can be accomplished, the procedure does entail a high complication rate. Because of the extensive medical care required, this procedure should probably be performed in centers specializing in the treatment of hemophilia.

TECHNIQUES OF ARTHROSCOPIC SYNOVECTOMY

Arthroscopic synovectomy is one of the most technically demanding surgical procedures. The surgeon must be accomplished in the use of multiple arthroscopic portals in order to accomplish a complete synovectomy. This procedure requires a great deal of patience and a methodical approach. At least five portals must be used.

The inflow cannula is inserted through the superomedial portal. The arthroscope is inserted into the anterolateral portal, and the motorized shaver is inserted through the anteromedial portal (Fig. 13–12). The arthroscope is directed into the suprapatellar pouch, and the motorized shaver is used to resect synovium in the suprapatellar pouch, the peripatellar area, the fat pad, and the medial gutter. The arthroscope and the motorized shaver are then directed into the medial compartment, and synovium is resected from below and above the medial meniscus and from around the cruciate ligaments.

The inflow cannula remains in the superomedial portal, and the arthroscope and the operative cannula are interchanged (Fig. 13–13). Switching sticks are useful for this maneuver. The arthroscope is directed into the suprapatellar pouch, and the synovectomy in the suprapatellar pouch and along the lateral aspect of the patella is completed. Next, the lateral gutter is visualized, and synovectomy is performed. The arthroscope is then directed into the lateral compartment, and the synovial resector is used to remove synovium from above and below the lateral meniscus, around the popliteus tendon, and around the cruciate ligaments.

At this point, all the synovium has been removed from the anterior aspect of the knee joint. In order to complete the synovectomy, the posterior compartments must be visualized. The arthroscope is removed from the arthroscopic sheath, and the blunt obturator is inserted. The arthroscopic sheath is directed from the anteromedial portal through the intercondylar notch and into the posterior lateral compartment. The 70° arthroscope is inserted into the arthroscopic cannula in order to visualize the posterolateral compartment. The posterolateral portal is made under

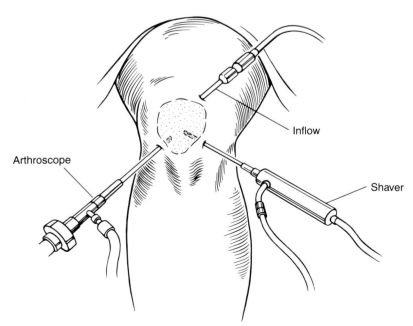

Arthroscope

Inflow

Shaver

FIGURE 13–12. Arthroscopic synovectomy, step 1. The arthroscope is in the anterolateral portal. The motorized shaver is in the anteromedial portal.

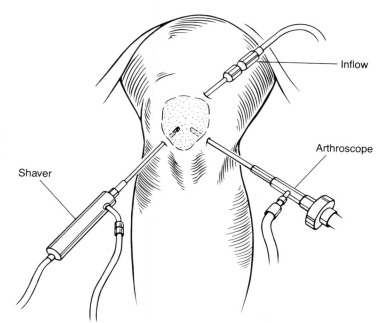

FIGURE 13–13. Arthroscopic synovectomy, step 2. The arthroscope and the motorized shaver are interchanged. The shaver enters through the anterolateral portal and the arthroscope through the anteromedial portal.

direct visualization with the use of a spinal needle to determine proper placement for the operative cannula. The motorized shaver is inserted through the posterolateral portal, and the posterolateral synovectomy is completed (Fig. 13–14). The arthroscope is then removed and inserted through the anterolateral portal into the posteromedial compartment. A posteromedial portal is established, and the synovium is removed from the posteromedial compartment. If difficulty is encountered in inserting the arthroscope into the posterior compartments, a transpatellar tendon portal may be helpful.

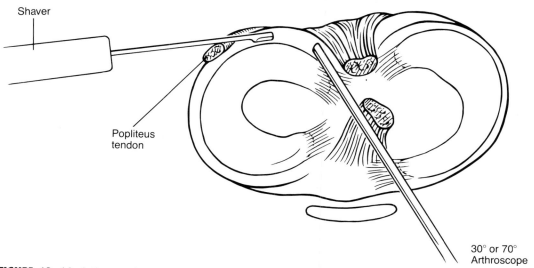

FIGURE 13–14. Arthroscopic synovectomy, step 3. The arthroscope is inserted through the intercondylar notch into the posterolateral compartment. A motorized shaver is inserted into the posterolateral compartment.

A final arthroscopic examination of the joint should be performed and any remaining abnormal synovium resected. This can usually be accomplished through the existing portals, but on occasion it is necessary to insert the shaver through a superior portal in order to complete the synovectomy.

A medium Hemovac drain is placed through the superomedial cannula before the cannula is removed. A sterile, bulky dressing is applied, and the puncture wounds are infiltrated with 0.5 per cent bupivacaine (Marcaine) with epinephrine. It is usually possible to remove the Hemovac drain before the patient is discharged from the outpatient surgical center. Range-of-motion and leg-lift exercises are started on the first postoperative day. The bulky dressing is also removed on the first postoperative day, and an elastic bandage is reapplied and worn until all swelling resolves. After 1 week, the patient is seen in the orthopaedist's office and is given ankle weights for use with leg-lift exercises. Two weeks after surgery, progressive resistive quadriceps and hamstring muscle exercises are started. Patients are referred for formal physical therapy if they have difficulty rehabilitating the knee at home.

Plica

During embryologic development, the knee joint is initially divided into three compartments by septa. The septa involute, and the knee joint becomes one large cavity. Remnants of these three septa remain in some

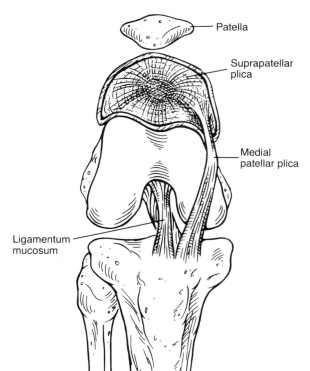

Patella

Suprapatellar plica

Medial patellar plica

Ligamentum mucosum

FIGURE 13–15. Artist's rendering of suprapatellar plica and medial patellar plica.

people and exist as synovial folds known as plica. The three plica most commonly encountered are the suprapatellar plica, the infrapatellar plica (or ligamentum mucosum) and the medial patellar plica (Fig. 13–15). The suprapatellar plica (Fig. 13–16) runs transversely across the suprapatellar pouch. It often has an opening centrally or laterally. The clinical significance of the suprapatellar plica is that loose bodies can become trapped behind it and be missed during arthroscopic examination. The infrapatellar plica runs from the intercondylar notch to the infrapatellar fat pad. Its significance in arthroscopic surgery is that it may pull the fat pad into the intercondylar notch, obscuring visualization of the cruciate ligaments. It can be easily sectioned arthroscopically in order to provide better access to the intercondylar notch.

The medial patellar plica is the synovial fold most likely to cause clinical symptoms.[19, 21] This synovial fold arises from the medial joint capsule at the level of the superior pole of the patella (Fig. 13–17). It courses distally and anteriorly across the anteromedial portion of the medial femoral condyle and inserts into the fat pad. Blunt trauma to the plica can cause hemorrhage, resulting in thickening and fibrosis of the plica. The plica then rubs across the medial femoral condyle with flexion and extension, and this rubbing causes pain. These symptoms have also occurred after overuse syndromes in microtrauma associated with athletic activity.

Patients may or may not have a history of blunt trauma to the knee. They complain of medial knee pain and, often, of snapping. Physical examination often reveals atrophy of the quadriceps muscle and a palpable band, which can be rolled beneath the examiner's finger, just medial to the patella over the medial femoral condyle. On occasion, the medial patellar plica causes symptoms of lateral joint line pain, possibly from retraction of the fat pad into the lateral joint space. Conservative treatment

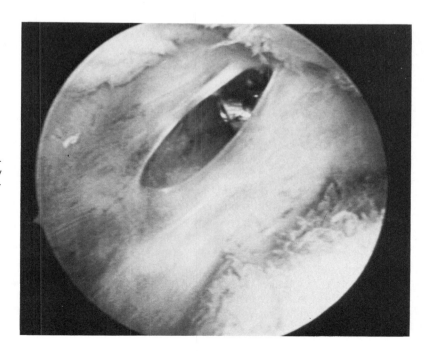

FIGURE 13–16. Arthroscopic picture of suprapatellar plica. Inflow cannula is visible through a fenestration in the suprapatellar plica.

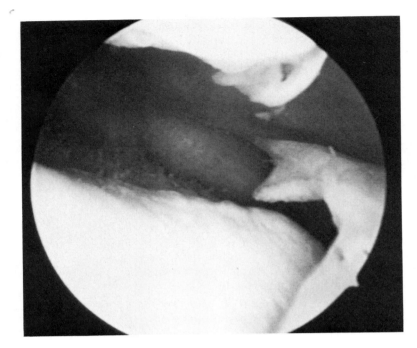

FIGURE 13–17. Arthroscopic view of medial patellar plica. *Top:* patella; *bottom left:* medial femoral condyle; *bottom right:* fibrotic medial patellar plica.

consists of rehabilitative exercises, nonsteroidal anti-inflammatory drugs, and the injection of steroid preparations into the plica.

ARTHROSCOPIC TREATMENT OF MEDIAL PATELLAR PLICA

The superomedial portal is used for inflow of lactated Ringer solution into the knee. The arthroscope is inserted through the anterolateral portal and directed into the suprapatellar pouch. The medial patellar plica can be seen originating from the medial capsule and coursing across the medial border of the medial femoral condyle. It is often difficult to sweep the arthroscope beneath the plica in order to examine the medial compartment. The knee should be hyperextended and the arthroscope brought beneath the undersurface of the plica and then directed down over the medial femoral condyle. The medial femoral condyle should be carefully examined for evidence of erosion secondary to the plica. If no erosion is seen, it is unlikely that the plica is the cause of the symptoms, and other pathologic processes should be sought.

The plica can also cause erosion on the medial facet of the patella. An anteromedial portal is established, and the arthroscope and shaver are directed into the suprapatellar pouch. A meniscectomy blade for the motorized shaver easily removes the thickened synovial fold. The fold should be completely resected back to the medial capsule and into the fat pad. The mere presence of a plica does not justify its removal; to qualify for removal, the plica should be clinically painful to palpation, and arthroscopic evidence of impingement on articular cartilage should exist.

Postoperative care is usually uncomplicated. Initial rehabilitation consists of straight-leg raising and range-of-motion exercises. When full painless range of motion has been achieved, progressive resistive quadriceps and hamstring exercises are begun.

Degenerative Arthritis

The arthroscopic treatment of degenerative arthritis remains a controversial topic. Although studies[12] have shown up to 80 per cent improvement after arthroscopic debridement of the knee, Burks[4] reached the following conclusions after a review of the literature on arthroscopic treatment of degenerative arthritis:

1. There have been few long-term reports of significant benefits from arthroscopic debridement.

2. Debridement seems to be more beneficial to older patients, probably because of a lower level of physical activity.

3. Patients with malalignment experience poorer results than do other patients.

4. Even with short-term follow-up, complete resolution of symptoms cannot be expected.

Most authors agree that arthroscopic debridement is not curative but is only a palliative procedure in the treatment of degenerative arthritis and should be considered a temporizing measure.

The following procedures have been advocated in the arthroscopic treatment of degenerative arthritis: lavage of the knee, debridement of loose articular cartilage, treatment of associated disease such as degenerative meniscal tears and loose bodies, removal of bone spurs, and abrasion arthroplasty. Arthroscopic lavage alone has been shown to provide symptomatic relief in degenerative arthritis.[4] It is theorized that lavage removes articular debris, which can cause painful synovitis. It is also theorized that the removal of enzymes and prostaglandins contributes to the improvement in symptoms.

Painful osteophytes may be easily removed from the patella and the femur. These are well visualized arthroscopically and can be removed with a burr. Tibial osteophytes are covered by the joint capsule and cannot be removed arthroscopically.

The removal of loose bodies and of unstable meniscal tissue can alleviate the mechanical symptoms of locking and catching. The removal of meniscal tissue should be extremely conservative: only mobile fragments should be removed. Meniscal tissue with minor damage, such as horizontal cleavage tears, may still transmit forces and protect articular cartilage.[11]

TECHNIQUES OF ARTHROSCOPIC DEBRIDEMENT

The three standard anterior arthroscopic portals are usually the only portals that are necessary for an arthroscopic debridement procedure. On occasion, posterior portals are required if loose bodies are trapped in the posterior compartments. If only a diagnostic arthroscopy and lavage are indicated, at least 6 L of lactated Ringer solution should be flushed through the knee. The knee should be flexed and extended and the posterior compartments palpated in order to remove any chondral debris. Loose and fragmented articular cartilage can be removed by a motorized shaver or punches. A ring curette is often useful for removal of degenerative articular cartilage. Localized areas of inflamed synovium are easily debrided with a motorized shaver.

Complete synovectomy has not proved helpful in the treatment of degenerative arthritis. Loose bodies generally reside in the suprapatellar pouch, the medial and lateral gutters, and the posterior compartments. Loose bodies occasionally slip beneath the meniscus and become trapped between the meniscotibial ligament and the tibia. Radiographic or image-intensification localization of these loose bodies may be necessary during surgery. When a loose body has been found, grasping forceps are inserted for removal. It is often necessary to enlarge the capsular incision around the forceps before removing loose bodies. Extremely large loose bodies may be morselized by a pituitary rongeur inserted through the arthroscopic portals. It is often helpful to insert a spinal needle through the capsule of the knee joint and impale the loose body, so that it is not lost while the grasping forceps is inserted.

Mobile fragments of meniscal tissue are removed by either a motorized cutter or punches. Arthroscopic knife blades are occasionally necessary, but their use has diminished with the development of better punches and better motorized cutting tools. Horizontal cleavage tears are probably best left alone in the degenerative knee. If tissue is removed, it is best to remove the inferior flap and leave the superior flap intact.

Motorized burrs can be used to remove osteophytes from the patella and the medial and lateral femoral condyles (Fig. 13–18). These spurs are often covered with articular cartilage, but a demarcation is present between the normal articular cartilage and the articular cartilage covering the spur. The spur should be resected back to this demarcation.

Johnson has advocated abrasion arthroplasty for the treatment of

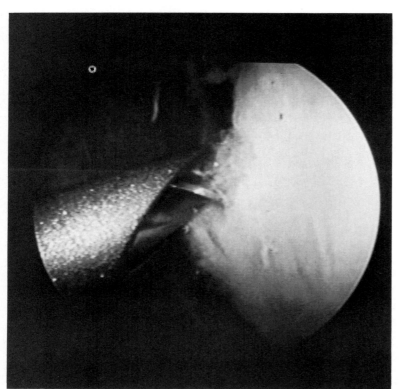

FIGURE 13–18. Motorized burr removing a spur from the lateral femoral condyle of a right knee.

grade four outer-bridge lesions of the articular cartilage.[13] The technique involves the removal of 1 to 2 mm of sclerotic bone by a motorized burr. The abrasion should not be taken down to cancellous bone. The depth of the cut can be checked by clamping the inflow tubing and applying suction to the arthroscope. If the cut is down to the proper depth, small bleeders are seen in the abraded surface. The abrasion should be carried 1 to 2 mm into the adjacent cartilage. Johnson believed that concomitant lesions of the tibia and the femur could be treated with abrasion.

Postoperative treatment consists of regaining range of motion and strengthening the quadriceps and hamstring muscles. If abrasion arthroplasty is performed, the patient should avoid weight bearing for 8 weeks. The healing response consists of formation of a blood clot over the abraded area. Over time, this clot gradually becomes adherent, and fibrocartilage covers the abraded area. Weight bearing before the end of the 8 weeks disturbs this process. However, symptoms can continue to improve for up to a year after the abrasion.

ARTHROSCOPIC TREATMENT OF SEPTIC ARTHRITIS OF THE KNEE

The knee joint may become infected in three ways: bacteria can be introduced by hematogenous spread, by direct trauma, or iatrogenically at the time of surgery. Arthroscopy has assumed a major role in the treatment of septic arthritis of the knee.

The predominant symptom in septic arthritis is extreme pain in the joint. Swelling, redness, and increased temperature are present. The patient is often febrile, and the white blood cell count and the sedimentation rate are elevated. The joint should be aspirated, and the specimen should be sent for cell count, blood sugar measurement, culture, and gram stain. The cell count is often higher than 100,000, and polymorphonuclear white cells predominate. The gram stain may or may not be revealing, but the cultures are usually positive. The patient should be admitted to the hospital and given intravenous broad-spectrum antibiotics pending the results of the culture. Arthroscopic treatment should be started as soon as possible in order to decrease the bacterial count and remove proteolytic enzymes from the knee.

The basic principles of arthroscopic treatment are copious lavage of the knee and removal of necrotic debris. A large inflow cannula should be inserted through the superomedial portal. The arthroscope sheath is inserted through the anterolateral portal and directed into the suprapatellar pouch. With the blunt obturator, the arthroscope sheath is swept through the pouch, down both gutters, and across both the medial and lateral joint surfaces to lyse adhesions. The knee is then thoroughly irrigated with 6 to 12 L of lactated Ringer solution. An arthroscopic examination is then performed in order to search for loculations and necrotic debris. A motorized shaver can be used to remove necrotic debris, but a synovectomy should not be performed. The arthroscope should be directed into the posteromedial and posterolateral compartments in order to check for loculations and necrotic tissue. If this tissue cannot adequately be irrigated from the posterior compartments, posterior operative portals should be established for complete cleansing.

Jackson[10] recommended leaving two ⅛-inch tubes in the knee inserted through the arthroscopic portals. He used a distension/irrigation technique in which the joint was progressively filled to capacity with an antibiotic solution over a 3-hour period. Over the next hour, it was drained dry by suction. A mucolytic agent and antibiotics were added to the irrigating solution. This system was kept in place for 4 to 5 days. Jackson[10] reported 100 per cent good and excellent results in 14 patients managed with this technique. He concluded that the success of the procedure resulted from the distention process, which prevented loculations and enabled the antibiotic to diffuse throughout the joint. Smith[26] reported equally good results in 30 patients treated by arthroscopic irrigation followed by the use of a Hemovac drain for 48 hours. Parenteral antibiotics were used for 48 to 72 hours postoperatively, and treatment was switched to oral antibiotics for the next month.

The author has used both of these techniques with good results. The distention/irrigation technique requires a great deal of postoperative attention. The tubes often become occluded with fibrinous exudate, and suctioning or reversal of the flow through the tubing is required for maintaining an open system. The author now uses the postoperative Hemovac technique.

Loose Bodies

There are multiple sources for loose bodies in the knee joint. In synovial chondromatosis, a metaplastic area of synovium manufactures loose bodies. In degenerative arthritis, small fragments of loose articular cartilage can break free and grow within the knee joint, being nourished by the synovial fluid. Loose bodies may be created during an acute patellar dislocation. The dislocation can cause an osteochondral fracture of the medial aspect of the patella or the lateral femoral condyle. Osteochondral fractures in other areas of the knee are less common but can certainly create loose bodies. The largest loose bodies are created when areas of osteochondritis dissecans become loose within the knee joint.

If loose bodies are identified in the knee joint, they should be removed. The diagnosis of loose bodies is usually based on history from the patient. Loose bodies usually cause mechanical symptoms, such as locking or catching in the knee joint. Many patients describe the loose body as being palpable in the suprapatellar pouch or along one of the gutters of the knee joint. The diagnosis is usually confirmed radiographically, but occasionally loose bodies do not have a bony central nidus. Magnetic resonance imaging may be helpful for localizing nonosseous loose bodies.

TECHNIQUE OF REMOVAL

Removal of loose bodies is often a simple procedure. It can also be one of the most challenging procedures in arthroscopic knee surgery. The standard arthroscopic portals are used. The arthroscope is first introduced into the anterolateral portal and directed into the suprapatellar pouch. A thorough systematic examination of the knee joint is conducted. Common hiding spots for loose bodies are in the suprapatellar pouch, specifically behind a suprapatellar plica. Loose bodies are also frequently found in the medial and lateral gutters. They can also hide in the posteromedial and posterolateral compartments. The area in which it is most difficult to find a loose body is beneath the menisci, wedged between the menisco-tibial ligament and the tibia. If the loose body is not found after a thorough inspection of the suprapatellar pouch and the anterior aspect of the knee joint, an operative cannula should be inserted through the anteromedial portal. Suction is applied to the end of the cannula while the posterior compartments are balloted through the popliteal fossa. If the loose body is not found in this manner, the arthroscope should be directed into the posterior compartments through the intercondylar notch. Removal of a loose body from the posterior compartments requires a posterior puncture for insertion of the grasping forceps.

When the loose body has been localized, it is often helpful to impale the loose body with a spinal needle inserted percutaneously. This tech-nique works especially well in the suprapatellar pouch and in the medial and lateral gutters. Several different types of grasping forceps are available (Fig. 13–19). The forceps should have serrated teeth and strong jaws. Self-locking forceps are available, but difficulty in opening them smoothly may negate their advantages. A set of small grasping forceps that fit down an operative cannula should also be available. After the loose body is securely grasped, it should be drawn up against the capsule. A No. 11 knife blade should be used to cut down on the grasping forceps and enlarge the hole in the capsule enough for removing the loose body. It is also sometimes necessary to enlarge the skin incision. Loose bodies can be lost between the capsule and the skin. The arthroscope should be focused on the loose body as it is pulled out of the capsule. If the loose body is then lost, the skin incision can be enlarged and retractors used for finding the loose body in the soft tissue.

Loose bodies are occasionally so large that they must be removed

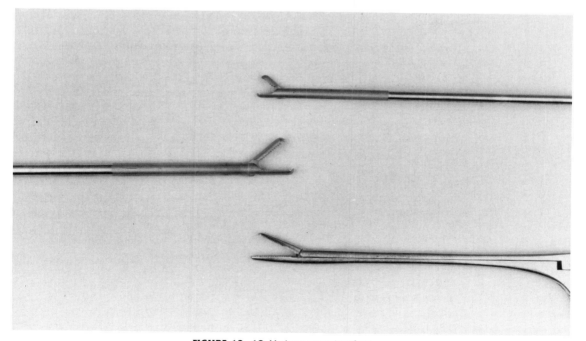

FIGURE 13–19. Various grasping forceps.

piecemeal. A pituitary rongeur is a good instrument to use for breaking the large loose bodies into smaller, removable fragments.

If after a thorough search the loose body cannot be found, then a radiograph should be taken. Intraoperative radiographs have been particularly helpful in localizing loose bodies trapped beneath the meniscus. Balloting the knee and using suction usually push these loose bodies from beneath the meniscus; however, it is occasionally necessary to perform a posterior arthrotomy and detach the meniscotibial ligament in order to remove these loose bodies. The meniscotibial ligament should then be repaired.

Arthroscopic Evaluation of the Patellofemoral Joint

The surgical treatment of patellofemoral pain remains a controversial topic. Shaving of loose patellar and trochlear groove articular cartilage, abrasion arthroplasty, lateral retinacular release, and medial imbrication are all methods for treating diseases of the patellofemoral joint arthroscopically. The indications for these procedures are described in Chapter 15. Physical examination, radiographs (including the Merchant view of the patellofemoral joint), and arthroscopic evaluation of the patellofemoral joint are all useful in determining treatment options. Patella alta and patella baja are easily documented on radiographic evaluation. Tracking of the patella, however, is more difficult to evaluate. Fulkerson and associates[8] described computed tomography as a method of evaluating patellofemoral tracking. This is an excellent test, but is not available in all radiology departments.

Johnson[14] described normal patellar tracking in anesthetized patients with the use of a tourniquet and a leg holder with the patient's knee distended. Patellar tracking should be evaluated on all arthroscopies in order to obtain a sense of normal patellar tracking. Patellofemoral tracking can often be evaluated from the anterolateral portal; however, synovium and fat occasionally obscure the patellofemoral joint as the knee is brought into flexion. A more reliable method of evaluating patellofemoral tracking is viewing the patellofemoral joint from above. The arthroscope may be inserted through the anteromedial portal and the inflow brought in through the anterolateral portal.

When the patellofemoral joint is viewed, neither surface of the patella contacts the trochlear groove in extension (Fig. 13–20). If the knee is flexed to 20° (Fig. 13–21), the lateral facet of the patella engages the lateral femoral condyle. At 45° of flexion, the patella centralizes in the trochlear groove and the medial facet of the patella touches the medial femoral condyle (Fig. 13–22). Further flexion tightens this area of contact. Failure of the patella to obtain secure contact in the trochlear groove by 60° of flexion indicates some degree of tightness in the lateral retinaculum or laxity in the medial retinaculum.

In addition to the evaluation of patellar and trochlear articular cartilage and of patellofemoral tracking, arthroscopy can be useful in the treatment of acute dislocations of the patella. The author initially performed arthroscopy on all patients who had an acute dislocation of the patella. He found that unless there was radiographic evidence of an osteochondral fracture,

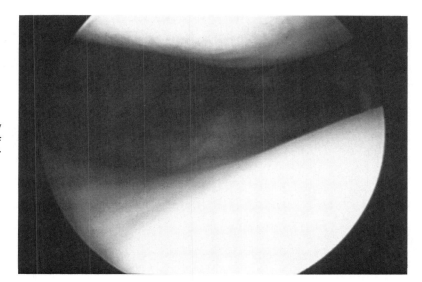

FIGURE 13–20. Arthroscopic view of left knee in extension. *Top:* patella; *bottom:* trochlear groove.

the yield of evidence from arthroscopy in these patients was fairly low. Patients without evidence of osteochondral fractures are now treated conservatively. If later mechanical symptoms develop, or if recurrent instability is a problem, arthroscopy is indicated.

When arthroscopy is indicated, the joint should be thoroughly irrigated in order to remove hematoma and facilitate visualization. Loose bodies, if found, should be removed. The medial retinaculum can often be repaired arthroscopically with the use of large curved needles passed percutaneously or with the use of meniscus repair cannulae and needles passed from inside the joint to outside the joint. After repair of the medial retinaculum, patellofemoral tracking is evaluated, and lateral release is performed if indicated.

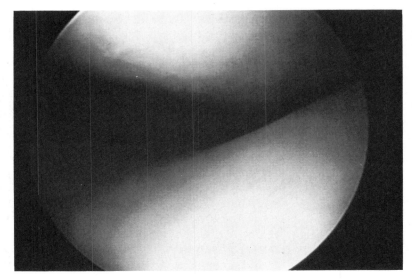

FIGURE 13–21. Arthroscopic view of left knee flexed 20°. The lateral facet of the patella has engaged the lateral femoral condyle.

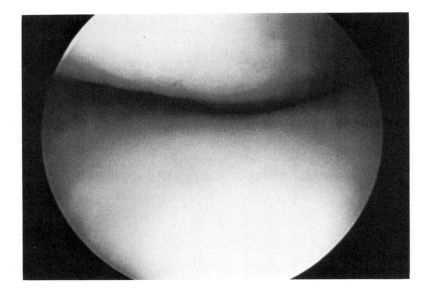

FIGURE 13–22. Arthroscopic view of left knee in 45° of flexion. The patella has centralized in the trochlear groove.

PROBLEM SOLVING IN ARTHROSCOPIC SURGERY

Arthroscopic surgery can be a frustrating experience during the learning phase. Many problems in arthroscopic surgery can be avoided or solved by careful attention to small details, knowledge of special techniques, and a systematic approach to the procedure. Just as in open surgery, clear exposure is mandatory. In arthroscopic surgery, this translates to obtaining and maintaining clear visualization of the joint. The time spent in obtaining clear visualization for the surgical procedure often exceeds the time actually spent performing the procedure.

The equipment must be of good quality and be well maintained. One person should be in charge of maintaining this equipment and inspecting it between each operation. Duplicate equipment should be available as back-up should equipment in use fail because of damage or wear.

Problems of Visualization

It is often easy to obtain a clear view in the large distended suprapatellar pouch. As the arthroscope is moved down across the femoral condyle and into the medial or lateral compartment, synovium and fat pad often obscure the view. When this happens, the arthroscope should be removed from the cannula and the blunt obturator inserted. The cannula should then be inserted deeper into the joint and withdrawn slowly. By this procedure, it is often possible to pull the synovium back along the sheath, leaving the end of the arthroscope uncovered. In cases of proliferative synovitis, it is often necessary to resect some of the synovium with a motorized shaver in order to obtain clear visualization. Another helpful technique is to section the ligamentum mucosum running from the fat pad to the top of the intercondylar notch. This allows the synovium and fat pad to fall anteriorly, enhancing the view of both the medial and lateral compartments and the intercondylar notch.

When operating on a knee with hemarthrosis, the knee should be thoroughly irrigated before arthroscopy. The inflow cannula and the arthroscope should be inserted through the standard portals. The knee is then thoroughly irrigated by means of suction applied to the arthroscopic cannula. The knee should be flexed and extended and the posterior compartments balloted in order to remove hematoma from these areas during the irrigation. Arthroscopy can begin when the fluid egress from the arthroscopic cannula is clear.

The obscuring of visualization by blood during an operative procedure is usually caused by inadequate distention of the knee. Varus and valgus stress placed on the knee in flexion often blocks the inflow cannula. Stress should be released and the inflow cannula repositioned. The fluid supply should also be checked. Fluid bags should be suspended approximately 3 m from the floor. The valve on the tubing leading to the inflow cannula should be checked. It is not uncommon for examiners, after turning the valve off when repositioning the scope or cannula, to forget to turn it back on. Sometimes switching the inflow to one of the side portals on the arthroscopic sheath facilitates visualization and clears blood from the knee. Occasionally, a fluid pump is helpful in this situation. The tourniquet line and the tourniquet should be checked for malfunction if bleeding persists.

Visualization can be distorted by bubbles in the joint. Bubbles occur, of course, because air is being sucked into the knee. This often occurs because of loose connections on equipment. Systematic checks should be made of connections between the cannula and the tubing, the cannula and the instruments, the arthroscope and the sheath, and the valves on the arthroscope. If all of these connections are tight, air is being sucked in through the puncture wounds around the instruments. The suction must then be decreased by turning down the suction source or by partially clamping the suction tubing.

The joint must be adequately illuminated for proper visualization. Light is delivered into the joint by a system of fiberoptics. A flexible fiber light cable extends from the light source to the arthroscope. A rigid fiberoptic system runs down the arthroscope to the end of the lens. The light cables consist of very small, continuous fibers of glass. With constant use, increasing numbers of these fibers break; eventually, this breakage noticeably affects the amount of light delivered into the joint. Light cables usually last for 100 to 200 operations, but the number can vary greatly, depending on how carefully the arthroscope is used. Several spare light cables should be available. The fiberoptic system in the arthroscope should last indefinitely unless the arthroscope is bent or dropped. Because such accidents do happen, spare arthroscopes should be available. Other causes of loss of the light in the joint include a dimming or failure of the light source, inadvertent unplugging of the light source, and failure in the camera system.

Damage to Articular Cartilage

Articular cartilage may be damaged because of inadequate opening of the joint space, poor selection of portals, improper use of instruments, poor choice of instruments, and gouging from the end of the arthroscope.

The use of a leg-holding device is mandatory for successful arthroscopic surgery. It allows clear exposure and adequate space for insertion of operative instruments. The leg holder allows the surgeon to be in total control of the exposure. By resting the patient's operative leg on the surgeon's hip, the surgeon controls lateral stress and flexion and extension.

Proper portal placement can be accomplished by first inserting an 18-gauge spinal needle under arthroscopic control. The needle should be manipulated in order to ensure that all aspects of the pathologic process can be reached without impinging on the articular cartilage. When the proper site has been chosen, a stab wound is made, and, again under arthroscopic control, a blunt trocar and cannula system can be inserted.

Proper selection and use of instruments is the next important step. A wide variety of motorized instruments, punches, grasping forceps, and knives should be available in the operating room. Instruments must be sharp. More damage to joints is caused by dull instruments and excessive force than by the occasional slip of a sharp instrument. The articular cartilage must not be used as a chopping block for meniscal tissue. Cutting should occur on a horizontal rather than a vertical plane. If, despite all precautions, articular cartilage is damaged, flaps should be removed because they have the potential to become loose bodies. This removal is best accomplished with a motorized shaver or a ring curette.

Broken Instruments

An instrument broken inside the joint is probably the most anxiety-producing situation in arthroscopic surgery. Thorough inspection of instruments between operations decreases the incidence of this problem. Equipment for retrieving broken instruments from the joint should always be available in the operating room. An operative cannula, forceps that fit through the cannula, and a magnetized suction device are useful. Radiographic facilities should also be available.

If an instrument should break inside the joint, the primary rule is to remain calm. The broken instrument should be removed in a stepwise fashion:

1. Stop all movement and keep the broken piece in clear view.
2. Slowly and smoothly remove the intact portion of the instrument from the joint.
3. Plan the removal of the broken piece and make sure all necessary equipment is available.
4. If a cannula was used for the instrument insertion, leave it in place and carefully insert forceps or a magnetized suction device for removal of the broken piece.
5. If a cannula was not used, use extreme care in inserting forceps through the portal so that inadvertent movement does not cause the broken piece to disappear.
6. Firmly grasp the broken piece and withdraw it under arthroscopic control. If a magnetized suction device is used, slip the cannula over the instrument and then withdraw both the cannula and the contained broken piece.

When the broken piece is lost inside the joint, it usually travels to the most dependent part of the joint. When the patient is supine, the most dependent parts are the posteromedial and posterolateral compartments of the knee. The surgeon should be familiar with insertion of the arthroscope through the intercondylar notch into the posterior compartments and the establishment of posterior portals for removal of the broken pieces.

If the broken piece cannot be found, radiographs can localize it. Broken pieces can even be removed without arthroscopic visualization by means of the image intensifier.

COMPLICATIONS IN ARTHROSCOPIC SURGERY

Operative Complications

Other than articular cartilage damage and broken instruments, few operative complications have been reported. Operative complications can arise from use of a tourniquet. The extent of tourniquet-induced nerve ischemia and paralysis is related to time used for the tourniquet and to pressure of inflation.[22] The tourniquet should be inflated to only 150 mm above the patient's systolic blood pressure. In a rare instance, in which tourniquet time reaches 1.5 hours, the tourniquet should be deflated for 10 minutes before the surgery proceeds further. Massive swelling of the calf can result from capsular leakage and infusion of fluid into the soft tissues during arthroscopic surgery. The appearance of such swelling is quite alarming, but it resolves rapidly. The author has tried to document increased compartmental pressures, but pressures have returned to normal by the time they were taken (15 minutes postoperatively). If arthroscopy is performed on a knee with known capsular damage, the procedure should be performed rapidly in order to prevent fluid leakage.

Collateral ligaments can be ruptured by excessive stress with the use of a leg holder. These isolated ligament ruptures generally heal without specific treatment and have produced no long-term sequelae in the author's experience.

Potential complications of meniscectomy and meniscus repair are damage to the posterior neurovascular structures. When meniscectomies are performed, the tip of the cutting instrument should always be in clear view in order to prevent damage to popliteal structures. When needles for arthroscopic meniscus repair are passed, small retractors should be placed between the posterior capsule and the neurovascular structures in order to prevent the needle from entering these structures. The peroneal nerve is at particular risk during lateral meniscus repair.

Lateral retinacular release involves cutting the superolateral geniculate artery. This can cause massive postoperative hemarthrosis if the vessel is not cauterized. After the lateral release, the tourniquet should be deflated, and intra-articular pressure in the knee should be decreased in order to visualize and cauterize the bleeders. One case of rupture of the quadriceps tendon after lateral release has been reported.[3] If the lateral release is performed with cutting cautery, the overlying skin can be burned and subsequently slough. Problems associated with arthroscopic synovectomy have included inadvertent resection of the meniscotibial ligament and resection of the patellar ligament.[1]

Postoperative Complications

The incidence of postoperative infections in arthroscopic surgery has been low. Infection rates of 0.04 per cent[15] and 0.07 per cent[24] have been reported. Thromboembolic disease has been less a problem in arthroscopic surgery than in open knee surgery because of the more rapid mobilization of the patient. Thrombophlebitis has been reported to occur in 0.17 per cent of arthroscopic procedures in the lower extremities.[24] Pulmonary emboli after arthroscopic surgery have been reported.[24]

Complications involving fat pad herniation and granuloma that require reoperation have been reported.[17] Minor postoperative complications such as painful scars, persistent effusions, and hemarthrosis are fairly frequent[20] but of little long-term consequence.

OTHER INDICATIONS FOR ARTHROSCOPIC KNEE SURGERY

Arthroscopy now has a major role in the treatment of injuries to the knee joint. Techniques for arthroscopic meniscectomy, arthroscopic meniscus repair, ligament reconstruction, the treatment of osteochondritis dissecans, and the treatment of disorders of the patellofemoral joint are described in other chapters. Arthroscopy of the knee not only has proved to be a valuable therapeutic modality but also is an excellent research tool. Second looks have enabled examiners to evaluate the effectiveness of this treatment and have led to changes and improvement of surgical technique and postoperative care.[19]

REFERENCES

1. Bachner EJ, Parker RD, Zaas RD: Case report: resection of the patellar ligament: a complication of arthroscopic synovectomy. Arthros 5:76–78, 1989.
2. Beguin J, Locker B, Vielpeau C, Souquieres G: Pigmented villonodular synovitis of the knee: results from 13 cases. Arthros 5:62–64, 1989.
3. Blasier RB, Cuillo JV: Case report: rupture of the quadriceps tendon after arthroscopic lateral release. Arthros 2:262–263, 1986.
4. Burks RT: Arthroscopy and degenerative arthritis of the knee: a review of the literature. Arthros 6:43–47, 1990.
5. Casscells SW: The torn or degenerated meniscus and its relationship to degeneration of the weight bearing areas of the femur and tibia. Clin Orthop 132:196–200, 1978.
6. Dorfmann H, De Bie B, Bonvarlet JP, Boyer T: Arthroscopic treatment of synovial chondromatosis of the knee. Arthros 5:48–51, 1989.
7. Ewing JW: Documentation in arthroscopy. *In* McGinty JB (ed): Operative Arthroscopy. New York: Raven Press, 1991.
8. Fulkerson J, Schutzer S, Ramsby G, Bernstein R: Computerized tomography of the patellofemoral joint before and after lateral release or realignment. Arthros 3:19–24, 1987.
9. Hardaker WT, Whipple TL, Bassett FH: Diagnosis and treatment of the plica syndrome of the knee. J Bone Joint Surg 62A:221–225, 1980.
10. Jackson RW: The septic knee—arthroscopic treatment. Arthros 1:194–197, 1985.
11. Jackson RW, Abe I: The role of arthroscopy in the management of disorders of the knee: analysis of 200 consecutive cases. J Bone Joint Surg 54B:310–322, 1972.
12. Jackson RW, Marans HJ, Silver RS: The arthroscopic treatment of degenerative arthritis of the knee. (Reports and Proceedings: Eighth combined meeting of the Orthopedic Association of the English-Speaking World, Washington, D.C.) J Bone Joint Surg 70B:332, 1988.
13. Johnson LL: Arthroscopic abrasion arthroplasty historical and pathologic perspective: present status. Arthros 2:54–69, 1986.

14. Johnson LL: Patellar tracking. *In* Johnson LL (ed): Arthroscopic Surgery: Principles and Practice, pp. 823–826. Saint Louis: CV Mosby, 1986.
15. Johnson LL, Shneider DA, Austin MD, et al: Two per cent glutaraldehyde: a disinfectant in arthroscopy and arthroscopic surgery. J Bone Joint Surg 64A:237–239, 1982.
16. Klein W, Jensen K-U: Arthroscopic synovectomy of the knee joint: indication, technique, and follow-up results. Arthros 4:63–71, 1988.
17. Lindenbaum BL: Complications of knee joint arthroscopy. Clin Arthros 160:158, 1981.
18. McGinty JB: Photography in arthroscopy. *In* Casscells WS (ed): Arthroscopy: Diagnostic and Surgical Practice, pp. 9–15. Philadelphia: Lea and Febiger, 1984.
19. Meyers JF, St. Pierre RK, Sutter JS, et al: Arthroscopic evaluation of anterior cruciate ligament reconstructions. Arthros 2:155–161, 1986.
20. Mulholland J: Symposium: arthroscopic surgery. Contemp Orthop 5(2):79–112, 1982.
21. Patel D: Arthroscopy of the plica—synovial folds and their significance. Am J Sports Med 6:217–225, 1978.
22. Rarabech C: Tourniquet-induced nerve ischemia: an experimental investigation. J Trauma 20:280–286, 1980.
23. Sim FH: Synovial proliferative disorders: role of synovectomy. Arthros 1:198–204, 1985.
24. Small NC: Complications in arthroscopy: the knee and other joints. Arthros 2:253–258, 1986.
25. Smiley P, Wasilewski SA: Arthroscopic synovectomy. Arthros 6:18–23, 1990.
26. Smith MJ: Arthroscopic treatment of the septic knee. Arthros 2:30–34, 1986.
27. Taylor AR: Synovectomy of the knee in rheumatoid arthritis: long term results [Abstract]. J Bone Joint Surg 61B:121, 1979.
28. Whipple TL, Bassett FH 3rd: Arthroscopic examination of the knee: polypuncture technique with percutaneous intra-articular manipulation. J Bone Joint Surg 60A:444–453, 1978.
29. Wiedel JD: Arthroscopic synovectomy for chronic hemophilic synovitis of the knee. Arthros 1:205–209, 1985.

CHAPTER 14

Rehabilitation

WILLIAM A. GRANA, M.D.

PRINCIPLES OF REHABILITATION

The goal of rehabilitation of the knee is to reduce symptoms after injury or surgery in order to maintain a high level of function. The purpose of this discussion is to review and emphasize the rehabilitation techniques that facilitate these goals. It is essential that the rehabilitation process produce an environment that enhances healing. Rehabilitation is focused not just on the knee but on the patient as a whole person. Physiologic health and emotional health are preserved through participation in as many normal activities of daily living as possible. The suggested progression of rehabilitation consists of the following steps: maintenance of cardiovascular fitness, achievement of full motion, prevention of muscle atrophy, renewal of the proprioceptive function of the joint, improvement of strength, power and endurance, return of agility in specific activities, and, finally, the return to participation in work or sports. The total rehabilitation encompasses all of these overlapping steps, which build on one another in order to reach the goal of return to activity.[24, 28, 42]

The physician must use a systematic approach to treating the injury. This begins by an accurate recognition of the problem and its severity in order to define a plan of management. The initial management includes modalities for diminishing inflammation, such as rest, application of ice, compression, and elevation with protected mobilization. The second phase of management is the prevention of further injury and includes the control of hemorrhage, the diminution of inflammation, limitation of muscle spasm, early passive and active motion exercises, and protection from further injury. The third phase includes continued repetitive evaluation, mobilization, strengthening of muscles, and protection from further injury. The fourth and final phase is the return to athletic activity. The return must be gradual, progressive, symptom free, and specifically related to the sport involved. During these specific phases of treatment, the athlete maintains a general cardiovascular fitness program so as to prevent deconditioning. An effort is made to compress the time frame of each stage in order to allow the athlete's return to high performance while protecting the athlete from new injury or reinjury.[23, 26, 46]

For the knee, a reasonable course of rehabilitation is based on the patient's injury problem, the severity, and the chosen management. Basic science investigation has produced a better understanding of the effects of applied stress on soft tissue and bone.[1, 3, 9] As a result of this understanding, the general trend is toward following knee injury or surgery with a more aggressive rehabilitation program that complements the use of anatomic repair or replacement of tissues through improved fixation techniques. This is especially true of rehabilitation after ligamentous injury, particularly anterior cruciate ligament (ACL) reconstruction. These principles have allowed for more rapid rehabilitation of knee problems.[4, 34, 35, 36] However, in spite of this aggressive approach, constraints are still placed on the speed of rehabilitation by the normal course of soft healing. For example, no study has shown more than a 50 per cent return of an autograft to normal ACL strength.[26, 34] Deacon and colleagues noted that grafts never return to a histologically normal appearance. They also noted that collagen fibers do not return to the large diameter expected in a normal ACL.[16] Therefore, rapid rehabilitation is built on an empirical rather than a scientific basis. Thus until there is objective documentation, a cautious approach to the return to functional activity, particularly sports, is warranted.

Four types of exercise are used to gain range of motion: passive, assisted, active, and resistive. Passive and assisted motion are used in settings in which the patient cannot negotiate an active contraction of the muscle to move the knee or in which it is not safe to do that because of the effect of active contraction on injured or reconstructed structures. However, most mobilization activity involves active motion or resisted motion in order to regain strength at the same time that mobility is achieved.[42, 46]

The second step in rehabilitation involves the improvement of muscle function. Three aspects of muscle function require attention during rehabilitation: strength, power, and endurance. Strength training maximizes the ability of the muscle to move a resisting force through a given range of motion of the joint. Power is force times distance, or the ability to move a resistance rapidly during intense exercise for short periods of time. In muscular endurance activity, less weight is used, but the duration of exercise is longer. There are three types of resistive exercise for strengthening muscles: isometric, isotonic, and isokinetic. The choice of a specific type depends on the progress of the patient during rehabilitation.[8]

Once motion and strength are obtained, a transitional step helps the patient progress from these basic neuromuscular activities to daily function or to the athletic field. This phase of rehabilitation integrates strength and endurance, range of motion, and proprioception into specific activities (Fig. 14–1). The athlete gains confidence by participating in controlled activity. Strength at slow speeds forms the basis for developing strength at higher speeds of activity. The athlete should gradually increase the resistance by adding body weight exercises such as squats and pushups as well as increasing speed of motion. Plyometrics exercises are effective for developing power, but because they are extremely demanding, they should be initiated only if the athlete tolerates them well. A variety of agility and coordination drills are useful at this point. Before specific drills are implemented, the patient progresses from jogging to full-speed running straight ahead and then to cutting in controlled drills to improve speed and activity. Close attention should be paid to the specific task or sport involved, and portions of these activities should be integrated into the rehabilitation program.[38]

Finally, the patient returns to full activity whether it is in the home, on the job, or on the athletic field. Throughout rehabilitation, a general conditioning program is maintained. With regard to the knee, this is accomplished with non–impact-loading activity such as cycling, use of a rowing machine, or water activity such as swimming or running in the water with a buoyant vest. Although these activities may not be sports specific, the work done is calculated to be at about the same caloric level as the patient's usual functional activity. This minimizes the deconditioning effects after injury and surgery.[42]

These are the specific steps of a rehabilitation program for the knee that are needed in order to achieve complete rehabilitation. Some of these specific steps and activities are discussed in more detail in the following sections. In order to have a successful rehabilitation program for the injured knee, it is important that the physician, the physical therapist, and the trainer communicate adequately with the patient. A trust must

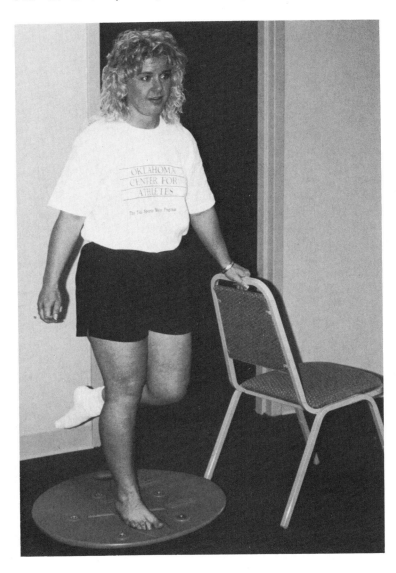

FIGURE 14–1. The use of a biomechanical ankle platform system (BAPS) board helps integrate strength, range of motion, and endurance capabilities of athletes before they begin specific sports activities.

be established between members of the medical team, and the patient must reach an understanding about the goals of the program on which the medical team has decided. Finally, together the team and the patient must establish a definitive program that the patient feels is realistic and that the patient can follow over the prescribed period of time.

THERAPEUTIC EXERCISE

Mobilization Exercise

Four types of exercise are used to gain range of motion: passive, assisted, active, and resisted. For the stretching of a muscle to restore a full range of motion, active and resistive holding/relaxing exercises are the most beneficial after soft tissue injury or surgery. In active exercise, the patient provides all stimulus for motion. The holding/relaxing exercise involves isometric contraction followed by an active move to a new range of motion.[42]

By far the most common exercise for regaining motion is active motion, in which the patient's own musculature is used. Excesses in muscle contraction that may occur must be avoided, and undue stress must not be placed on injured or reconstructed tissues. In addition, it must be recognized, as noted earlier in Chapter 3, that certain muscles are antagonists of the function of certain ligamentous structures. For example, the hamstrings are used actively after ACL injury, but not the quadriceps muscles, which produce the translation resisted by the ACL. For the same reason, the quadriceps muscle is used actively after the posterior cruciate ligament injury, but not the hamstrings. Therefore, after ACL reconstruction, active quadriceps contraction without axial load of the joint is potentially dangerous for the reconstructed tissues. When sufficient active range of motion is obtained and pain is diminished, resisted exercises can begin. The timing of this varies, depending on the specific problem, its severity, and the patient's response to that trauma (Fig. 14–2).

Proprioceptive neuromuscular facilitation (PNF) is an active-resisted mobilization and strengthening technique.[29, 48] This method of exercise

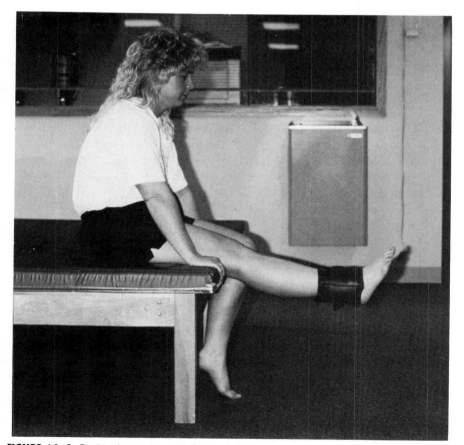

FIGURE 14–2. Resisted exercise with free weights begin when range of motion is sufficient. Progression can be from gravity resistance only to these cuff type weights to a weight bench.

produces a neuromuscular response through innervation of the stretch receptor. It was originally developed for neurologic problems, but it is also used effectively in rehabilitation of the knee. The patient can perform the exercise alone after proper instruction, but more frequently it is performed with a therapist or a partner. PNF incorporates the use of diagonal and spiral functional motor patterns in the lower extremity, which duplicate walking and kicking motions. PNF is beneficial because it accelerates coordinated sequential muscular contraction necessary for performing complex movements. It can serve as a transitional step from the active range-of-motion and resistive-weighted exercises that are performed before coordination activities begin. The resistance is typically applied against the concentric contraction, but it can also be applied eccentrically by pulling back to the starting position while the patient resists. The keys to PNF are the manual contact and correct hand placement for providing stimulation and resistance. Commands are used to facilitate the correct movement, pressure, or distraction gauged to stimulate the stretch reflex; the application of manual assistance provides stimulation of the muscle while enabling movement; and the pattern or sequence of movement proceeds in a spiral and diagonal manner. A program consists of three to five sets of 10 to 15 repetitions graded according to the strength of the patient. Initially, the manual resistance is applied, and weight can be added later.

Two methods are commonly used for passive motion in rehabilitation. They are used most frequently in conditions that are restrictive to the patient's movement or when the management of a fracture or another problem entails a period of enforced immobility. Passive motion without stretching is used most commonly after reconstruction of the knee to regain motion early while still protecting the injured, repaired, or reconstructed tissues.

Motion is beneficial for the healing of articular cartilage, ligaments, and tendons. The initial concern of the orthopaedist has traditionally been about the potential disruptive effects of motion. This concept was replaced as surgical techniques for anatomic placement with adequate fixation were developed. For example, in soft tissue reconstruction of the knee, the critical factor is anatomic placement of the graft or repaired tissue, which allows a range of motion with activities of daily living that puts minimal stress on these tissues. Motion is beneficial for the healing and the strength of the graft. It is also beneficial for regaining the normal biomechanics of the joint, for lubrication of the joint, and for re-education of the proprioceptive function of the joint.[26]

Passive motion without stretching is required in order to overcome the deleterious effects of inflammation that follow injury or surgery. The hemorrhage, swelling, spasm, and pain that follow musculoskeletal trauma significantly limit motion. The use of muscles to move a joint may increase this discomfort initially, depending on the severity of the trauma. Passive motion can be used to overcome these effects. After total knee replacement, ligamentous reconstruction, or osteochondral injury, there are swelling and spasm, which may prevent a patient from effectively performing active range-of-motion exercises. Passive range-of-motion exercises performed gently through the pain-free range enable the patient to receive the beneficial effects of motion for the joint (Fig. 14–3). With large anterior wounds, there may be concern about healing, and the

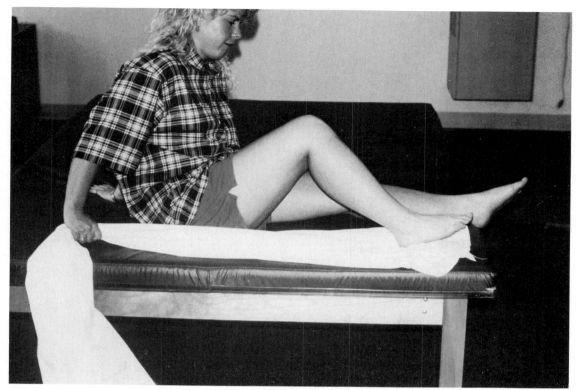

FIGURE 14–3. Passive range of motion can be performed without a continuous passive motion (CPM) device. Here the towel is used to assist a passive flexion slide without active use of the hamstrings or the quadriceps muscle.

amount of motion is therefore limited. Use of a continuous passive motion device or passive range of motion exercises with the assistance of a physical therapist or by the patient alone are effective for achieving these goals.[13, 14, 21, 22, 39]

In a limited way, stretching types of passive range-of-motion exercise are performed in order to regain motion in the later phases of a rehabilitation program after the 4- to 6-week period. The risk is that the patient loses control of protective mechanisms, and an injury may recur or worsen. Stretching may be integrated with resistive exercise and a stretching/relaxing type of activity in order to regain motion, and the stretch reflex may be used to help in this process. Isometric contraction against the manual resistance is followed by an active move to a new range of motion (Fig. 14–4). However, such passive manipulation is most efficacious when accompanied by surgical release of adhesions and by mechanical blocks with concomitant manipulation.

Strengthening Exercise

Once active range of motion is started, resistive exercises are begun through a pain-free range of motion. These exercises can take the form of manual resistance with progress to surgical tubing or an elastic band and then to free weights. Resistive exercise through weight training consists of isometric, isotonic, or isokinetic exercise to improve muscular strength,

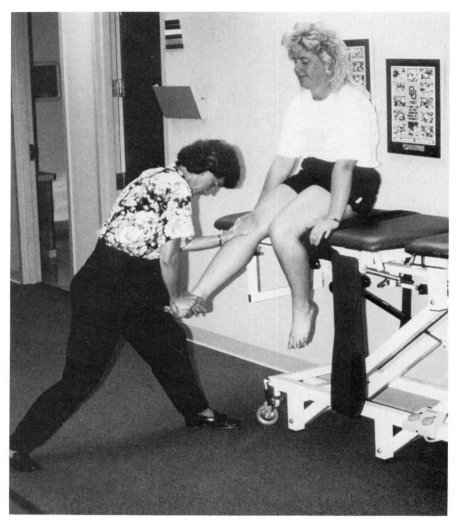

FIGURE 14–4. Contracting/relaxing exercise can be used to facilitate range of motion and at the same time provide some degree of strengthening activity as well.

power, and endurance. In conditioning or reconditioning the muscle for more complex activity after an injury or surgery, it is necessary to understand the SAID principle: that the muscle specifically *a*dapts to *i*mposed *d*emands.[2, 5, 17] Simply stated, conditioning programs must adapt the muscle to the demands that are made on it. Thus the work performed must approximate the intensity and duration of the demands of any exercise once full activity is accomplished. The patient, the therapist, and the physician must keep this in mind at all times during the rehabilitation program.

In isometric exercise, muscular force is generated without shortening of the muscle fibers. Isometric exercise is usually the first step for the athlete in a rehabilitation program. Usually in the hospital, quadriceps and hamstring exercise begins isometrically until an active range of motion is tolerated or safe (Fig. 14–5). However, isometric exercise does not carry over to functional activity. Static muscular contraction reduces maximal

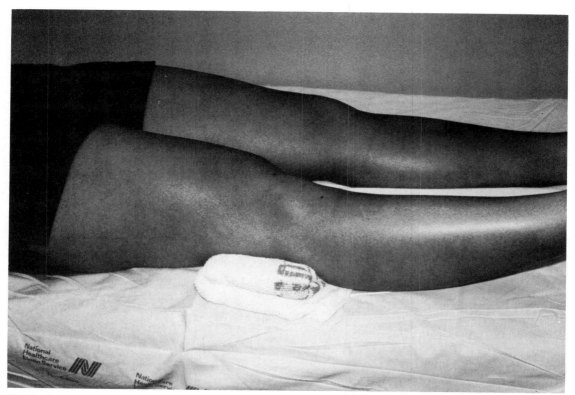

FIGURE 14–5. Isometric quadriceps sets and hamstring sets of exercises can be accomplished in the hospital immediately after reconstructive surgery. The muscle quadriceps *(foreground)* is actively contracted, whereas the thigh *(background)* is not contracted.

limb speed. On the other hand, isometric training requires no special equipment; any immovable object that provides sufficient resistance can be used. Strength gains are specific to the angle of the knee during the contraction. Therefore, there is little value in isometric weight training for fitness or general conditioning and, with regard to the SAID principle, for return to function.

Isometric exercise does have an important role in rehabilitation during the initial phase that follows injury or surgery. At this time, the patient, alone or with a therapist, uses isometric contraction to maintain muscle tone when range of motion is limited. Caution must be used for the patient who has hypertension because isometric work increases systolic and diastolic arterial blood pressure, and its use may therefore be contraindicated for such patients. The advantages are that this type of muscle contraction is usually pain free except in certain patellofemoral problems and can serve as a first step in the rehabilitation program. The patient is taught to have the muscle contract for 5 seconds per repetition and to perform three or four sets of 10 repetitions.

In isotonic weight training, a fixed resistance with a variable speed of movement is used throughout the range of motion. Most isotonic-resistive exercise for the knee is carried out from full extension to approximately 90° of flexion. There are two types of isotonic contraction: concentric and eccentric. In the concentric contraction, the muscle shortens as it develops tension in order to overcome the resistance. During an eccentric contraction, the muscle develops tension as it lengthens. For example, in order to perform an eccentric quadriceps contraction, the opposite leg is used to lift the injured knee from 90° to full extension, and then the knee is lowered to 90° while the quadriceps muscle contracts and lengthens. Eccentric contractions have become an integral part of rehabilitation. So-called closed-chain kinetic exercise involves principally eccentric contractions. It is important during isotonic exercise to control the velocity of the movement in order to prevent ballistic motion, which can increase the potential for injury (Fig. 14–6).[8]

Progressive resistive exercise is built upon isotonic weight training with gradually increasing weight. The *daily adjustment of the progressive resistive exercise* program, called the DAPRE technique, with the use of free weights is the foundation of the rehabilitation exercise program for rehabilitating muscular strength.[28] A repetition maximum is the maximal weight that can be lifted one time. Four sets of exercise are usually performed in accordance with the guidelines in Tables 14–1 and 14–2.

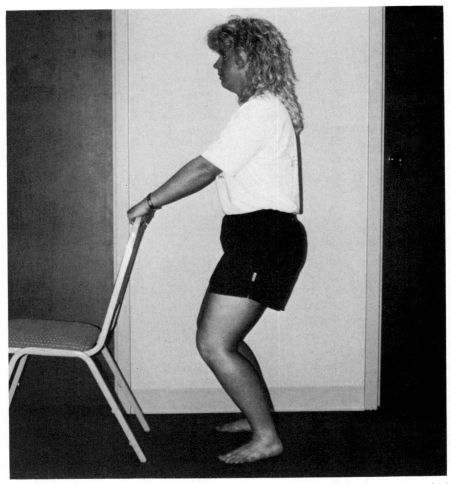

FIGURE 14–6. A quarter squat is one example of a closed-chained kinetic exercise, which involves strengthening the quadriceps and hamstring muscles while the foot remains fixed, eliminating the torque effect of the leg and foot when the foot is free.

TABLE 14–1. The DAPRE Technique

Set	Portion of Working Weight Used	No. of Repetitions
1	50 per cent	10
2	75 per cent	6
3	Full	Maximum*
4	Adjusted	Maximum†

From Knight KL: Guidelines for rehabilitation of sports Injuries. Clin Sports Med 4:413, 1985. DAPRE, daily adjustment of progressive resistive exercise.

*The number of repetitions performed during the third set is used to determine the adjusted working weight for the fourth set according to the guidelines in Table 14–2.

†The number of repetitions performed during the fourth set is used to determine the adjusted working weight for the next day according to the guidelines in Table 14–2.

This enables the patient to derive the maximal benefit from the exercise program. In a practical sense, the average woman in a quadriceps exercise program should achieve lifts of 20 to 25 pounds, and the average man, 25 to 30 pounds; patients should be able to perform three or four sets of 10 lifts at these weights. For the competitive athlete, weights are increased from 30 to 50 pounds; any occurrence of pain and swelling is a guide to appropriate weight. Once these goals are reached, or as pain and healing allow, the next step of the resistive exercise program is the use of a variable resistance machine, which is a slightly more efficient method of exercise, and then the use of an accommodating resistance, the so-called isokinetic technique. In isokinetic exercise, an accommodating resistance matches the force that the patient produces. These machines have been designed for therapeutic purposes but are also valuable for diagnostic testing. Isokinetic testing is used to measure eccentric strength as well as concentric strength (Fig. 14–7).[37]

In order to produce strength, power, and endurance, the format of the progressive resistive exercise program is adjusted. For improving muscular endurance, more repetitions are performed with less weight. In order to increase muscular or anaerobic power, shorter rest intervals and increased weight are used in accordance with the SAID principle: maximizing the patient's rehabilitation work.[8, 42]

Tables 14–3 to 14–6 provide an outline of a variety of rehabilitation programs for different types of knee problems. The patellofemoral exercise program concentrates on quadriceps strength and is used for most kinds of patellofemoral pain syndrome and chondromalacia. The nonoperative

TABLE 14–2. General Guidelines for Adjustment of Working Weight

No. of Repetitions Performed During Set	Adjustment to Working Weight For:	
	Fourth Set*	Next Day†
0 to 2	Decrease 5 to 10 pounds and perform the set over	
3 to 4	Decrease 0 to 5 pounds	Keep the same
5 to 7	Keep the same	Increase 5 to 10 pounds
8 to 12	Increase 5 to 10 pounds	Increase 5 to 15 pounds
13 or more	Increase 10 to 15 pounds	Increase 10 to 20 pounds

From Knight KL: Guidelines for rehabilitation of sports injuries. Clin Sports Med 4:414, 1985.

*The number of repetitions performed during the third set is used to determine the adjusted working weight for the fourth set according to the guidelines in Table 14–1.

†The number of repetitions performed during the fourth set is used to determine the adjusted working weight for the next day according to the guidelines in Table 14–1.

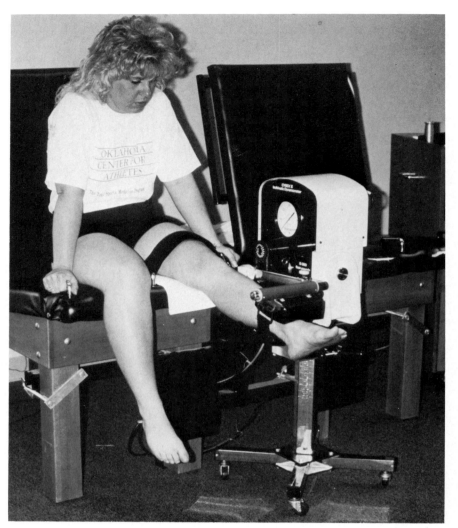

FIGURE 14–7. Isokinetic testing is used to measure eccentric strength as well as concentric strength, depending on the device used.

rehabilitation program is for ligamentous injury of grades I and II severity. The postsurgical program is followed after ACL reconstruction with or without combined meniscus injury.

Plyometric Exercise

Plyometric strengthening exercises serve as a good interface between the traditional weighted resistance exercises and coordination or agility drills. Plyometric exercises combine strength and speed to produce explosive movement. The techniques involve various types of jumping and hopping. The patient either jumps up into the air or down from a certain height onto a landing surface, which provides for an eccentric type contraction followed by a concentric contraction in which the patient takes off in a countermovement. Plyometric exercises enhance flexibility and agility;

Text continued on page 391

TABLE 14–3. Knee Rehabilitation Program: General Guidelines

Phase I

The early stage of rehabilitation focuses on prevention of muscle atrophy, reduction of swelling, and increasing or maintaining range of motion. The type of rehabilitation also must account for the specific type of injury and its subsequent precautions/restrictions. May last 24 hours to 10 days, depending on pain and swelling.

Range of Motion: Perform Four Times a Day, 40 Repetitions
Heel slides
Flexion/extension (sitting)
Patellar mobilization (5 minutes, 4 times a day)

Isometric Exercises: Perform 100 Repetitions a Day, Hold 6 Counts
Quadriceps setting
Hamstring setting
Quadriceps-hamstring co-contraction

Isotonic Exercises: Perform Two to Four Times a Day, 40 Repetitions
Straight-leg raise (supine) as tolerated, weight to 15 pounds
Straight-leg raise (sitting) as tolerated, weight to 15 pounds
Hamstring curls (prone) as tolerated, weight to 15 pounds
Hamstring curls (standing) as tolerated, weight to 15 pounds
Hip abduction as tolerated, weight to 15 pounds
Hip adduction as tolerated, weight to 15 pounds
Hip extension as tolerated, weight to 15 pounds
Hip rotation as tolerated, weight to 15 pounds
Ankle circles/pumps

Ice: Apply After Exercise (15 to 20 minutes) and as Often as Every 2 Hours Thereafter
Other: Electrical Stimulation, Other Modalities as Needed for Muscle Stimulation and Relief of Pain

Phase II

The second stage of rehabilitation concentrates on increasing strength while achieving full range of motion. Progression is based on the degree of pain, swelling, and achievement of full range of motion.

Range of Motion: Four Times a Day, 40 Repetitions
Heel slides
Flexion/extension
Quadriceps and Hamstring stretching (prolonged stretching, 20 seconds in comfortable range, 10 stretches before/ after exercise)

Isometric Exercises: 100 Repetitions a Day, Hold 6 Counts
Quadriceps sets
Hamstring sets
Quadriceps-hamstring co-contraction

Isotonic Exercises: Continue PRE Program, Using DAPRE Technique
Straight-leg raise (supine)
Straight-leg raise (sitting)
Hamstring curls (prone)
Hamstring curls (standing)
Hip abduction
Hip adduction
Hip extension
Hip rotation
Ankle pumps-circles

Ice: Continue Postexercise Application of Ice
Other: Other Modalities as Indicated

Phase III

The third stage of rehabilitation begins when full range of motion has been achieved and there is no swelling or pain with exercise.

Stretching: Pre-/Postexercise, 10 Stretches for 20 Seconds
Quadriceps stretching
Hamstring stretching

Isometric Exercises: 100 Repetitions a Day, Hold 6 Counts
Quadriceps sets
Hamstring sets
Quadriceps-hamstring co-contraction

Isotonic Exercises: Continue DAPRE Technique
Leg-extension raises (sitting)
Hamstring curls (prone)
Partial squats (100/day)
Step-ups (100/day)
Toe/heel raises
Hip abduction, adduction, extension, rotation

Table continued on following page

TABLE 14–3. Knee Rehabilitation Program: General Guidelines *Continued*

Cycling: Start With 10 Minutes, Progressing to 20 Minutes; Resistance May Progress From Light to Heavy
Proprioceptive Exercises
Balance board/BAPS program
PNF patterns (manual resistance or pulleys)
Isokinetic Exercise: Begin Isokinetic Work at Moderate Speeds (90° to 180°)
Ice: Postexercise Application, 15 to 20 Minutes

Phase IV
The strengthening program continues while gradual functional activities are begun.
Stretching: Pre-/Postexercise; 10 Stretches for 20 Seconds
Quadriceps stretching
Hamstring stretching
Isometric Exercises: 100 Repetitions a Day, Hold 6 Counts
Quadriceps sets
Hamstring sets
Quadriceps-hamstring co-contraction
Isotonic Exercises: Continue Increasing PRE per DAPRE/Derlome Method
Leg-extension raises (sitting)
Hamstring curls (prone)
Partial squats
Step-ups
Toe/heel raises
Hip abduction, adduction, extension, rotation
Cycling: Continue Progression
Proprioceptive Exercises
Balance board/BAPS program
PNF patterns (increase resistance)
Isokinetic Exercise: Progress to Full-Spectrum Rehabilitation
Agility Drills: Start at Slow Speed, Progress as Tolerated
Cariocca
Side-to-side
Backwards
Figure 8
Plyometric Exercises: Begin Basic Drills, Progress as Tolerated
Jogging: Start Jog/Walk Program; Progress as Tolerated
Ice: Postexercise; 15 to 20 Minutes

Phase V
This phase should involve primarily functional activities for return to play. Isokinetic testing should indicate no
strength deficits.
Stretching: Continue Pre-/Postexercise Stretching
Isometric Exercises: Continue as in Previous Stages
Isometric Exercises: May Be Reduced to Maintenance Phase or Increased, Depending on Strength Deficits
Isokinetic Exercises: Continue Spectrum Rehabilitation Program
Proprioceptive Exercises: Continue to Progress in Difficulty of Program
Agility Drills: Increase Speed and Difficulty
Plyometric Exercises: Increase Height and Distance
Running Program: Increase to Full-Speed Activity
Sports Specific Skills

PRE, progressive resistive exercise; DAPRE, daily adjustment of the PRE; BAPS, biomechanical ankle platform system; PNF, proprioceptive neuromuscular facilitation.

TABLE 14—4. Patellofemoral Joint Pain Home Program

Stretching

Do each stretch five times, holding 20 seconds.

Hamstrings

Sit with your knee straight and your other knee bent in with your foot touching the opposite knee. Lean toward your straight leg, keeping your back straight. Lean only until you feel a gentle stretch, then hold.

Stand facing a table or chair with your leg propped up on it. Lean toward your leg, keeping your back straight. Lean only until you feel a gentle stretch, then hold.

Iliotibial Band

Stand with the involved side toward the wall with your hand on the wall. Cross the involved leg behind other leg. Push the involved hip toward the wall, keeping your arm and leg straight. You should feel the stretch in the hip closest to the wall.

Quadriceps

Strengthening

Quadriceps sets: Lie on back with the involved leg bent 5° to 10°. Tighten the muscles on the top of your thigh. Think of straightening your knee; you should feel your kneecap move toward your head. Hold for count of 10. Relax. Do two sets of 10.

Straight-leg raises: Bend the uninvolved hip and knee so your foot is flat on a mat. Tighten the muscles on top of the involved leg and lift it 6 to 8 inches. Hold, then lower your leg slowly. This is to be done in two positions: flat on the back and propped on the elbows. Do four to six sets of 10 repetitions, weights at 2+ pounds (increase as tolerated).

Short-arc quadriceps: Sit propped up on your hands and place a rolled-up towel or a can under your involved leg so that your knee is slightly bent. Straighten the involved knee as far as you are able, and slowly lower. Do four to six sets of 10 repetitions, weights at 2+ pounds (increase as tolerated), using DAPRE technique.

Short knee dips: Stand up straight with your knees straight. Slowly bend your knees until your knees block out your toes. Remember to keep your back straight and to keep your eyes, knees, and toes in alignment. Repeat 10 times. Increase to 50 times.

Step-ups: Stand facing a step. Place the involved foot on the step. Bend your knee forward until your knee blocks out your toe. Slowly raise yourself up on the step by straightening your knee. Remember to keep your back straight and to go slowly with a smooth motion. Do not hop up the stair. Repeat five times. Increase to 30 times.

Progress to straight-ahead sprints and then to figure 8 sprints around cones 10 yards apart.

May progress in full-arc leg extensions as tolerated with the PRE program by the DAPRE technique.

This program can follow the generic protocol as outlined but with attention to patellar pain associated with flexed knee quadriceps exercise.

DAPRE, daily adjustment of progressive resistive exercise (PRE).

TABLE 14-5. Nonoperative Collateral Ligament Strengthening Program

Week 1

Any brace should be removed before exercise unless it is hinged or unless physician instructs otherwise.

Quadriceps sets: While the knee is passively extended, tighten your top thigh muscle and hold for a count of 6. Concentrate on getting a good muscle contraction. Perform 100 per day.

Hamstring sets: With your knee bent to 50°, push your heel down, tightening the back of your thigh muscles.

Straight-leg raises (brace on): Bend the uninvolved hip and knee so the foot is flat on mat. Tighten the muscles on top of the involved leg and lift it up 6 to 8 inches. Hold the position, then lower the leg slowly. This is to be done in two positions: flat on the back and propped on the elbows.

Hip abduction: Lie on the uninvolved side with your bottom leg slightly bent. Slowly raise and lower the involved leg toward the ceiling, keeping the knee bent to 45° and pointed forward.

Hip adduction: Lie on the involved side. Bend the top leg across the front or behind with the foot flat on the ground. Slowly raise and lower the involved leg, keeping the knee bent to 45°.

Hip extension: Lie on your stomach. Raise the involved leg toward ceiling, keeping the knee bent to 45°.

Patellar mobilization: While the knee is passively extended, firmly push the kneecap from side to side and up and down. Perform for 5 minutes three to four times per day.

Ice: Ice is important in reduction of joint swelling. Ice may be applied over the knee as often as 20 minutes every 2 hours. Remember to remove ice once the area becomes numb.

Week 2

Perform all exercises as in Week 1, with the addition of the following:

Range of motion (ROM) exercises: Begin ROM exercises out of the brace but within pain-free limits.

Progressive resistance exercise: Perform the straight-leg raises, using weight. Begin with 2 to 5 pounds. Increase by DAPRE technique.

Week 3

Continue previous exercises, with the addition of the following:

Progressive resistance exercise: Use DAPRE techniques.

Knee extension: Sitting, straighten the involved knee as far as possible. Hold, then slowly lower the leg to the starting position.

Knee curls: In prone position, bend the involved knee as far as possible. Hold, then slowly lower the leg to the starting position.

Isokinetic exercise: Use at high speeds only.

Weeks 4 to 6

Continue all exercises, with addition of the following:

Jog/walk program
Cutting/figure 8
Plyometric exercises
Isokinetic test of strength, power, and endurance

Criteria for Return to Play

Knee is pain free
No evidence of swelling
Full ROM
Full strength
No problems with running, jumping, or cutting

DAPRE, daily adjustment of progressive resistive exercise.

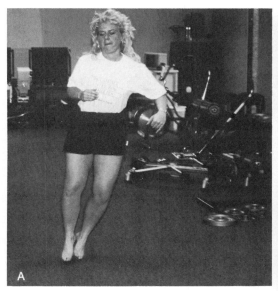
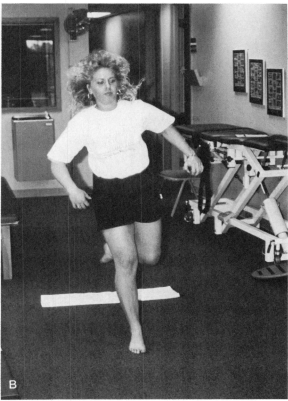

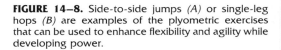

FIGURE 14–8. Side-to-side jumps *(A)* or single-leg hops *(B)* are examples of the plyometric exercises that can be used to enhance flexibility and agility while developing power.

therefore, there should be an adequate warm-up period that includes stretching. These exercises are demanding activities, and adequate rest between bouts should therefore be observed in order to allow maximal intensity during the exercise itself. Muscle strength as well as flexibility clearly must be adequate. Figures 14–8*A* and 14–8*B* illustrate some examples of these exercise activities. They must be individualized for the specific patient.[38]

ROLE OF MODALITIES (PHYSICAL AGENTS)

Heat and Cold

Both heat and cold can be used in the management of certain phases of the rehabilitation after knee injury or surgery. However, there are some specific indications for each modality. In general, the application of heat in the form of a hot pack, a whirlpool, a contrast bath, or ultrasonography is used primarily for muscular problems in order to relieve discomfort and improve extensibility of collagen. In general, heat is contraindicated in the early phases of a rehabilitation program or for specific problems related to the joint alone. Indications for heat are pain and stiffness, muscle spasm, and limited range of motion of the knee secondary to muscular contusion or contracture. Contraindications are impairment of sensation to pain or temperature and acute inflammation after trauma or neurologic impairment. The application is usually by moist towels,

TABLE 14–6. Anterior Cruciate Ligament Postoperative Rehabilitation Program

Week	Brace	Crutches	Exercises
1	Knee immobilizer with popliteal wedge Drain removed first postoperative day	Weight bearing as tolerated	1. Bent leg raises; set of 10, four sets/day in brace 2. Isometric quadriceps and hamstring sets, four sets of 10, three times a day 3. Isometric hamstring/quadriceps co-contraction in brace 4. Passive ROM with physical therapy instructions; heel slides out of brace 5. Ankle pumps
2 to 4	Functional brace 10° to 90° Brace to be worn at all times except during showering	Weight bearing as tolerated May wean off crutches by week 2 to 4	1. Bent leg raises, four sets of 10 at least two times a day; begin weights at 2 pounds, increase to 10 pounds 2. 90° to 40° leg extensions, set of 10 repetitions, up to four sets; work up to 10-pound weight on ankle 3. Ankle: Theraband and/or semiclosed chain 4. Abduction, adduction, and extension of hip with up to 10 pounds 5. Patellar mobility: 5 minutes, four times a day 6. Standing hamstring curls with up to 10 pounds 7. Closed-chain partial squats (body weight) if no meniscal repair
4 to 8	10° to full flexion Brace may be taken off for sleeping	Should be off crutches by week 5; full weight bearing	1. Increase weight to 20 pounds 2. Exercise bike in brace up to 25 minutes a day with low resistance 3. Step-ups, short knee dips 4. May swim starting at week 6 (flutter kick only) 5. Partial squats with Theraband or sport cord
8 to 16	May be out of knee brace, but full extension *not* forced; work on full flexion of the knee	Full weightbearing	1. Advance weight to 20 to 25 pounds of knee extension exercises (90° to 40°) 2. Exercise bike: increase resistance, working up to 30 minutes a day 3. Continue bent leg raises and hamstring curls

Week		Brace	Exercises
16 to 24	—	No brace required; goal is full motion, 5° to full flexion. Brace should be worn during exercises	1. Leg extension: work full arc 90° through 0°; work up to 25 pounds, multiple sets 2. Work to achieve 1:1 quadriceps/hamstring ratio 3. Continue cycling 4. Office visits every 4 weeks to check for knee stability; exercises may be advanced or decreased on the basis of examination findings
24 to 36	—	Brace should be worn during exercises	1. Continue quadriceps and hamstring strengthening up to full strength 2. Running: begin with jogging ½ mile every other day; advance to 2 miles over 1 to 2 months (modified if complete meniscectomy) 3. Cybex test performed; if involved leg has 70 per cent of quadriceps strength and 90 per cent hamstring strength of opposite leg, running program begins 4. May begin cutting and return to sports activities during weeks 32 to 36 if stability is maintained and Cybex test shows 85 per cent quadriceps strength in comparison with that in opposite leg, with a 1:1 quadriceps hamstring ratio
36 to 52	—	Custom brace to be worn for all sports activities	1. Continue muscular strengthening 2. Practice skills to sports played 3. Cybex test repeated; goal is quadriceps 90 per cent, hamstring 100 per cent strength in comparison with that in opposite leg
After 1 year	—	Custom brace should be worn during sports for 6 months (18 months after surgery)	1. Maintain exercise program two to three times a week

Progression is based on (1) muscle strength, (2) ROM (range of motion), (3) laxity, and (4) edema.

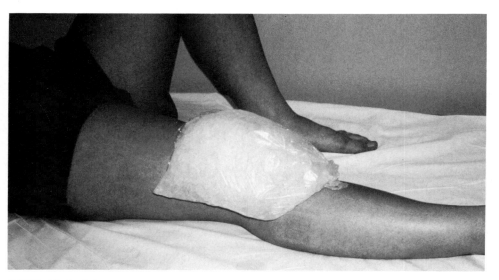

FIGURE 14–9. Cold has a much larger role than does heat in the immediate and late rehabilitation of knee problems.

Hydrocollator pads, or whirlpool baths. In specific instances after strain type injuries, as discussed earlier, ultrasonography with or without a hydrocortisone cream is useful for diminishing formation of scars and for improving flexibility of the muscles.[15]

Cold has a much larger role in acute rehabilitation after injury or surgery. The effects of cold are a decrease in metabolism, a decrease in local circulation, and a delay of inflammation. Cold also increases collagen stiffness. The best forms of cold, when available, are crushed ice in the form of ice packs and ice massages with an ice cup. An ice bath may also be useful but is usually not practical for disorders of the knee. In the initial phase after injury, cold is used for reducing pain, spasm, and extension of the hematoma. In the rehabilitation phase, it is used in connection with the contracting/relaxing type of assisted exercise in order to provide early motion by decreasing spasm and pain. Its use is contraindicated in patients who have Raynaud's disease or cold allergy and is relatively contraindicated in patients who have cardiac disease, arthritis, or anesthetic or hypesthetic skin in the area of the knee. In general, cold has a much larger role in most types of rehabilitation after knee injury or surgery (Fig. 14–9).[23]

Electricity

Electric modalities have also been used for the management of pain during rehabilitation after injury or surgery. However, the scientific basis for the use of electric devices is less certain. These devices can put out either an alternating current or a direct current like that produced by a battery. Electricity has been used in three clinical applications: to relieve pain, to increase strength, and to promote soft tissue healing. Very little scientific information is available about the value of electricity in soft tissue healing; therefore, its main applications have been for pain control and muscle strengthening.[44]

Transcutaneous electric nerve stimulation (TENS) is usually defined as the application of an electric current through the skin for the control of pain. The mechanism of that action is either release of natural opiates, called beta endorphins, as a result of the electric stimulation or flooding of the pathways to the brain that stimulate pain perception as a result of electrical stimulation. By closing this "gate" to transmission along pain fibers, the current diminishes the awareness of the painful stimuli. The problem with the scientific evaluation of the effectiveness of TENS is the result of the so-called placebo effect. In most evaluations of pain relief, investigators fail to take into account this effect, which can be responsible for up to 30 per cent of pain relief. The placebo effect is maximal when electricity is applied directly to the site of the pain, and it often decreases with time. Both of these factors are characteristics of the use of the TENS unit. Some studies have shown that patients who used a TENS unit experienced less pain and required less narcotic medication after knee surgery. However, seemingly equally good studies have shown that TENS is not effective clinically or cost effective when the same parameters are evaluated.[44] The results are not conclusive. In general, in the author's practice, TENS is used not routinely but only for patients who seem to have difficulty in rehabilitation as a result of poor pain control or for patients with causalgia of the knee (Fig. 14–10).

Electrical muscle stimulation (EMS) is the use of an electrical stimulus to cause a contraction in a muscle. EMS has been shown to be very effective in abnormal muscles; that is, muscles that have lost normal neural innervation benefit from EMS to maintain a degree of strength. Muscle stimulation can decrease strength loss that occurs as the result of immobilization, but this tends to be a short-term benefit. In addition, the stimulation does not increase the girth of the leg, and so the atrophy that is seen is often not affected. In a similar manner, EMS alone can increase the strength of a normal muscle when used in a variety of protocols.

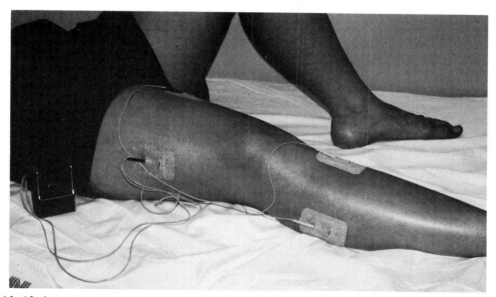

FIGURE 14–10. A transcutaneous electric nerve stimulation (TENS) unit is used for providing pain relief after surgery or injury in order to allow early range of motion safely.

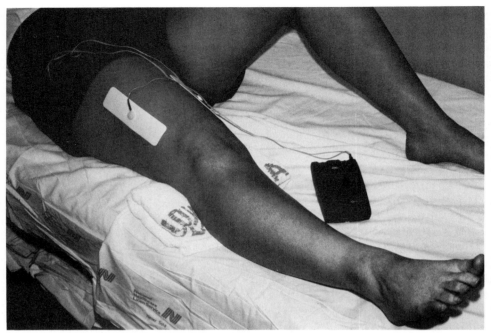

FIGURE 14–11. A muscle stimulator is used in patients who are unable to achieve voluntary contraction and for augmenting a supervised exercise program and the services of a physical therapist.

However, it has not been demonstrated that EMS, when used alone or combined with an exercise program, is any more effective in the development of strength than is a good voluntary resistive strength program. EMS is useful perhaps in the early phases of the rehabilitation program for patients who are unable to generate a voluntary contraction. Electrical stimulation, however, does not improve strength in normal muscles when voluntary muscle action is present.[44] In the author's practice, EMS is used for patients who are unable to achieve voluntary contraction and for augmenting the supervised exercise program of the physical therapist in the immediate postoperative period (Fig. 14–11).

Continuous Passive Motion Devices

The acronym CPM has become a buzz word for the cutting edge of science in the management and rehabilitation of orthopaedic problems, especially in the knee. An advertisement noted that a CPM device "blitzes post surgical pain and edema."[47] This device extends the original work on the effect of continuous passive motion on the healing of defects in articular cartilage to a variety of orthopaedic problems in which the effects of disuse are manifest. Most recently, the beneficial effects of motion on healing after reconstruction of ligaments about the knee have been emphasized.[13, 22, 43] However, there is insufficient information for defining an appropriate protocol for CPM. What motion is sufficient? How frequently is it applied? What is the duration of treatment? What is the best method of application? CPM, with the use of a device, is not to be confused with the passive motion discussed earlier in this chapter. There are few scientific data to support the use of CPM devices for reconstruction beyond the first few postoperative days (Fig. 14–12).

The scientific information that motion is useful for preventing the effects of disuse and deconditioning that accompany immobilization dates to about 1900. Around 1970, the importance of motion for the knee after fracture was emphasized and led to the use of ambulatory casts and braces as well as rigid internal fixation. Mooney and colleagues used a CPM device to avoid the effects of disuse after injury and surgery.[33] About 1980, R. B. Salter proposed that continuous passive motion did have a beneficial effect on the healing of articular cartilage defects and septic joints in the rabbit model. Subsequently, investigators believed that there was less overall morbidity, and especially less pain, with CPM. Much interest in the effects of the use of CPM devices on a variety of knee problems has developed. Clinical investigation supports the use of the CPM devices after the release of flexion contraction of the knee, after total knee replacement, after synovectomy, and for neuromuscular problems.[30, 31, 39] However, problems with compressive neuropathy and wound healing have been noted with such use.[10, 21, 27] None of these studies avoided the placebo effect discussed earlier, and it is therefore difficult to know the real benefit of a CPM device.

The question of duration and frequency of treatment remains unanswered in these clinical situations. Duration varies from a few days to weeks and from constant to less than 1 hour per day. Studies have indicated that 3 days is effective, and R. B. Salter said that the first week is the critical time for CPM. It is this area of question on which the manufacturers capitalize in recommending long-term use for CPM devices. With most of these uses, there is little understanding of the mechanics of action or the mechanics of the effect, and for some investigators, the initial enthusiasm has cooled. A CPM device is no substitute for active motion, and this principle must not be forgotten.

The detrimental effects of immobilization have been noted in the

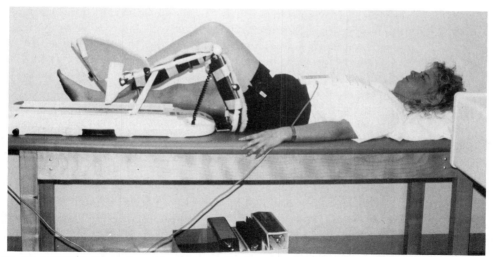

FIGURE 14–12. A CPM device such as this one is used in the management of intra-articular fracture or osteochondral injuries as well as sepsis of the knee. In a limited way, it may be useful during the hospital stay after total knee replacement or ligamentous reconstruction.

study of reconstructive surgery of the knee. This work shows that changes associated with immobilization affect the mechanical and biochemical properties of soft tissue and bone.[3] Although exercise is beneficial, it does not prevent disuse-induced mechanical changes unless it is accompanied by weight-bearing activities. The threshold of activity necessary for preventing the effects of immobilization is unknown at this time. CPM devices have not been demonstrated to improve nutrient uptake of an ACL graft, and they are potentially detrimental to graft integrity, depending on the specific techniques used.[10] The prospective clinical reviews of ACL reconstruction, in which CPM is compared with more traditional rehabilitation protocols, indicate that CPM devices did not produce any benefit over early limited active range of motion in flexion. In practice, active motion, when allowed, is more effective than passive motion or a CPM device.[4, 12, 36] Active motion with weight bearing is the most beneficial method of preventing the immobilization disease that Swiss researchers have noted after cast application. The most important time to use passive motion seems to be in the first 2 to 7 days, and whether a CPM device is used is a matter of preference, compliance, and cost.[40, 49] In addition, the studies of these devices that indicate improvement of pain tolerance have not taken into account the placebo effect. In the author's practice, a CPM device is used in the hospital after reconstruction with a stiff graft (bone–patellar tendon–bone), after total knee replacement, for intra-articular fracture, or for osteochondral defect until the patient tolerates active range of motion.

Generalized Cardiovascular Conditioning

Cardiovascular conditioning of the patient must be addressed and undertaken during the rehabilitation program for a specific knee problem. It is essential that general aerobic conditioning be started early in order to prevent deconditioning, and it is much easier to maintain the cardiovascular fitness program than it is to resume one. Conditioning assists in caloric balance and weight control during the period of relative sedentary activity. It is frequently difficult to match a conditioning program to an athlete's sport in terms of weight control. Alternative activities may be substituted with a workload that is similar to the workload involved in the patient's sport or job; thus cycling, running with a buoyant vest in a swimming pool, or rowing are activities that may be acceptable, as opposed to running or jumping.

The major objective in a conditioning program is to maintain and improve the overall level of fitness after an injury or surgery. Although factors that affect performance vary, the specificity principle, discussed with regard to muscular exercise, pertains to all forms of exercise whether aerobic or anaerobic. Factors that affect an appropriate conditioning program are the initial fitness level, the intensity of exercise, the duration of exercise, the frequency of exercise, and the type of exercise.

A maintenance conditioning program requires an evaluation of the patient's initial fitness level. This must be accomplished by some method other than running activity, such as bicycle ergometer. Once that level is established, the training exercise activity is prescribed. The patient trains at a designated target heart rate that is about 60 to 70 per cent of the maximal heart rate. This is calculated by subtracting the age from 220 and multiplying by 70 per cent; therefore, the maximal heart rate of a 40-year-old man would be 180 beats per minute and a target exercise heart rate would be about 126 beats per minute. This target exercise heart rate should be maintained for a period of 15 to 20 minutes with a total exercise time of 30 minutes, 2 to 5 days per week. This duration and this frequency enable maintenance of aerobic conditioning.

In addition, upper body exercise to maintain strength in the major muscle groups is without risk. Training benefits lapse within 2 to 3 weeks after a decrease in work load; therefore, it is important to resume a conditioning program as early as possible after the injury or surgery. As much as possible, a patient should work toward attaining a workload that corresponds to a workload that would be seen in a regular activity or in a regular job.[18]

ORTHOTIC DEVICES FOR THE KNEE

The use of braces to treat disorders of the knee began with interest in limiting motion and has progressed to stabilization of the knee with pathologic laxity while providing as much function as possible. Leather and stainless steel braces first were used early in the 1900s; today, the light-weight form-fitted braces of metal and plastic allow a great deal of movement and freedom. Use of a brace depends on the specific problem. Is the primary reason to provide restriction of motion or enforced rest, to provide relief of pathologic laxity, or to overcome some neuromuscular problem? When goal is defined, the specific brace is prescribed. An orthotist should be an integral participant on the treatment team. The simplest braces are those that restrict motion, such as a Velcro-fastened cylinder immobilizer, which is used to enforce restriction of motion when pain and swelling follow acute injury. The type of orthosis is distinctly different from a functional brace used for ACL insufficiency, which provides for the maximal motion possible. In addition, for many braces (particularly the frequently used knee sleeves), the benefit may be through the placebo effect. The brace simply makes the patient "feel better." The purpose of this section is to discuss some of the commonly used braces and their limitations as well as indications.

Prophylactic Braces

Since 1980, there has been a great deal of interest in the possibility of preventing knee injury by the use of an appropriate brace. The attention focused on the use of so-called lateral stabilizing braces, which consist of two lateral posts that are attached to the thigh and the calf and are connected by a hinge. Scientific data indicate that although these braces can reduce abduction force placed on the knee either in cutting or as a result of direct contact, many of the braces used are biomechanically inadequate and can produce potentially harmful effects on the knee. Improvements in design must be effected before these braces can be used safely and with predictable results. Much of the concern centers on proper fit and application of the brace. A poorly designed brace or a brace that is fitted improperly can fail, prematurely focusing load at the joint line, which then increases the potential for ligament or bone damage.[6, 19]

With regard to epidemiologic study of the value of such prophylactic knee braces, the information available is contradictory. The results depend on specific setting in which the brace is used, who applies the brace, who attends to its continued proper fit during athletic activity, and the compliance with use of the brace. From a variety of such studies, there is no persuasive evidence to support positive or negative recommendations about the use of these braces. In particular, for high school athletes, the use of such braces has not proved to be a cost-effective method of preventing knee injury. The best that can be said is that in a college athletic setting, the braces may offer some protection when applied properly. On the other hand, at the high school level, there does not seem to be any evidence to support the use of these braces in the prevention of knee injury.[20, 25, 41, 45]

The second kind of brace is the functional brace used for nonoperative management of ACL injury or for postoperative management after ACL reconstruction (Fig. 14–13). The scientific investigations of these braces indicate that some are more effective in controlling anterior tibial displacement than are others. However, many questions as to how these braces

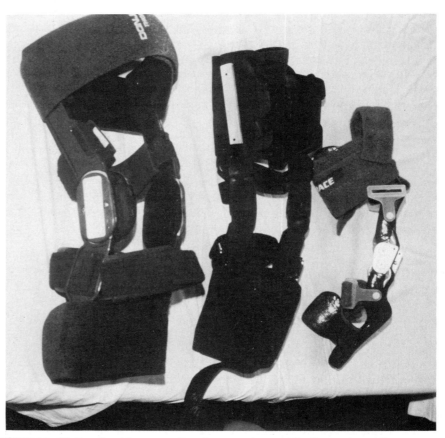

FIGURE 14–13. Functional braces such as these can be used for the postoperative management of reconstruction of the anterior cruciate ligament as well as other, more complicated ligament reconstructions.

contribute to the success of the nonoperative or postoperative treatment of ACL-deficient knees remain unanswered. It is clear that the hinge, post, and shell type of brace performs consistently better than the hinge, post, and strap type of brace in the performance of this function. Clinically, the hinge, post, and shell type of brace enables better running and cutting performance by athletes, but these braces do not seem to entirely prevent abnormal anterior tibial displacement in the absence of an ACL.[7, 11, 32]

On the basis of the information just given and what is known about the natural history of the ACL graft, it seems reasonable to recommend the use of such a brace for a period of 12 to 18 months after ACL reconstruction. In addition, for the ACL-deficient knee in nonoperative management, such a brace is useful. Also of importance is that the long-term effects of brace wear are not known, and when episodes of giving way occur, patients who wear the brace should be managed the same way that nonbrace patients would be: with restriction or modification of activity.[32]

Other Braces

One other type of brace that is frequently used potentially modifies or improves patellar motion. In most of these braces, direct pressure is used to alter the normal valgus vector of patellar tracking and can improve symptoms in patients with lateral tracking or true instability. A trial wearing is usually worthwhile. Many patients seem to experience relief from symptoms. However, this discussion is not meant to be a scientific appraisal of the function of these braces, and their entire effect may be proprioceptive rather than actual biomechanical (Fig. 14–14).

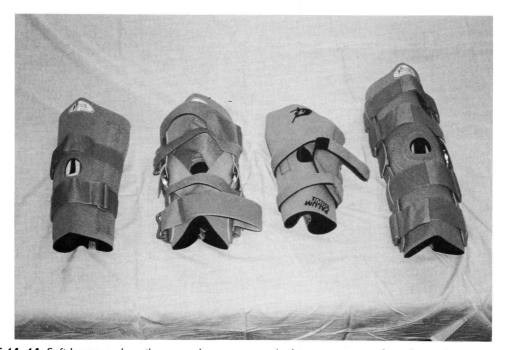

FIGURE 14–14. Soft braces such as these may have some use in the management of patellar tracking abnormalities, but they provide little true stability for the pathologically lax knee.

REFERENCES

1. Akeson W, Woo SL-Y, Amiel D, et al: The biology of ligaments. *In* Funk FJ, Hunter LY (eds): Rehabilitation of the Injured Knee, pp. 133–148. St. Louis: CV Mosby, 1984.
2. American Orthopedic Society for Sports Medicine: Strength Training Workshop, Indianapolis, 1985.
3. Amiel D, Woo SL-Y, Harwood FL, et al: The effect of immobilization on collagen turnover in connective tissue: a biochemical-biomechanical correlation. Acta Orthop Scand 53:325–332, 1982.
4. Anderson AF, Lipscomb AB: Analysis of rehabilitation techniques after anterior cruciate reconstruction. Am J Sports Med 17:154–160, 1989.
5. Atha J: Strengthening muscle. Exercise and Sports Science Reviews 9:1–73, 1981.
6. Baker BE, Van Hanswyk E, Bogosian S, et al: A biomechanical study of the static stabilizing effect of knee braces on medial stability. Am J Sports Med 15:566–570, 1987.
7. Beck C, Drez D Jr, Young J, et al: Instrumented testing of functional knee braces. Am J Sports Med 14:253–256, 1986.
8. Beckham-Burnett S: Exercise equipment and weight training for athletes. *In* Grana WA, Kalenak A (eds): Clinical Sports Medicine, pp. 264–276. Philadelphia: WB Saunders, 1991.
9. Buckley PD, Grana WA, Pascale MS: The biomechanical and physiologic basis of rehabilitation. *In* Grana WA, Kalenak A (eds): Clinical Sports Medicine, pp. 233–250. Philadelphia: WB Saunders, 1991.
10. Burks R, Daniel D, Losse G: The effect of continuous passive motion on anterior cruciate ligament reconstruction stability. Am J Sports Med 12:323–327, 1984.
11. Cook FF, Tibone JE, Redfern FC: A dynamic analysis of a functional brace for anterior cruciate ligament insufficiency. Am J Sports Med 17:519–524, 1989.
12. Cornwall MW, Leveau BF: The effect of physical activity on ligamentous strength: an overview. J Orthop Sports Phys Ther 5:275–277, 1984.
13. Coutts RD, Craig EV, Mooney V, et al: Symposium: the use of continuous passive motion in the rehabilitation of orthopaedic problems. Comtemp Orthop 16:75–111, 1988.
14. Coutts RD, Toth C, Kaita JH: The role of continuous passive motion in the rehabilitation of the total knee patient. *In* Hunderford DS, Krackow KA, Kenna RV (eds): Total Knee Arthroplasty: A Comprehensive Approach, pp. 126–132. Baltimore: Williams & Wilkins, 1984.
15. Cox JS, Andrish JT, Indelicato PA, Walsh WM: Heat Modalities. *In* Drez D Jr (ed): Therapeutic Modalities for Sports Injuries, pp. 1–23. Chicago: Year Book Medical, 1986.
16. Deacon OW, McLean I, Oakes BW: Ultra structural analysis of autogenous anterior cruciate ligament graft biopsies [Abstract]. *In* Proceedings of the International Society of the Knee, Sydney, Australia, 1987.
17. DeLee J, Allman F, Howe J, et al: Therapeutic Exercise Modalities. *In* Drez D Jr (ed): Therapeutic Modalities for Sports Injuries, pp. 49–79. Chicago: Year Book Medical, 1986.
18. Fardy PS: Exercise testing and exercise prescription. *In* Grana WA, Kalenak A (eds): Clinical Sports Medicine, pp. 37–65. Philadelphia: WB Saunders, 1991.
19. France EP, Paulos LE, Jayaraman G, Rosenberg TD: The biomechanics of lateral knee bracing: Part II. Impact response of the braced knee. Am J Sports Med 15:430–438, 1987.
20. Garrick JG, Requa RK: Prophylactic knee bracing. Am J Sports Med 15:471–476, 1987.
21. Goletz TH, Henry JH: Continuous passive motion after total knee arthroplasty. South Med J 79:1116–1120, 1986.
22. Gose JC: Continuous passive motion in the postoperative treatment of patients with total knee replacement. Phys Ther 67:39–48, 1987.
23. Grana WA, Curl WL, Reider B: Cold modalities. *In* Drez D Jr (ed): Therapeutic Modalities for Sports Injuries, pp. 25–32. Chicago: Year Book Medical, 1986.
24. Grana WA, Karr J, Stafford M: Rehabilitation techniques for athletic injury. *In* American Academy of Orthopaedic Surgeons: Instructional Course Lectures, vol 34, pp. 393–400. St. Louis: CV Mosby, 1985.
25. Hewson GF, Mendini RA, Wang JB: Prophylactic knee bracing in college football. Am J Sports Med 14:262–266, 1986.
26. Huegel M, Indelicato PA: Trends in rehabilitation following anterior cruciate ligament reconstruction. Clin Sports Med 7:801–811, 1988.
27. James SE, Wade PJF: Lateral popliteal nerve palsy as a complication of the use of a continuous passive motion knee machine: A case report. Injury (Guildford) 18:72–73, 1987.
28. Knight KL: Guidelines for rehabilitation of sports injuries. *In* Harvey JS (ed): Clinics in Sports Medicine, pp. 405–416. Philadelphia: WB Saunders, 1984.
29. Knott M, Voss D: Proprioceptive Neuromuscular Facilitation, 2nd ed. New York: Harper and Row, 1968.
30. Laupattarakasem W: Short term continuous passive motion. J Bone Joint Surg 70B:802–806, 1988.

31. Lynch AF, Bourne RB, Rorabeck CH, et al: Deep-vein thrombosis and continuous passive motion after total knee arthroplasty. J Bone Joint Surg 70A:11–14, 1988.
32. Mishra DK, Daniel DM, Stone ML: The use of functional knee braces in the control of pathologic anterior knee laxity. Clin Orthop 241:213–220, 1989.
33. Mooney V, Nickel VL, Harvey JP Jr: Cast-brace treatment for fracture of the distal part of the femur: a prospective controlled study of one hundred and fifty patients. J Bone Joint Surg 52A:1563–1578, 1970.
34. Noyes FR, Butler DL, Paulos LE, Grood ES: Intra-articular cruciate reconstruction I: perspectives on graft strength, vascularization, and immediate motion after replacement. Clin Orthop 172:71–77, 1983.
35. Noyes FR, Keller CS, Grood ES, et al: Advances in the understanding of knee ligament injury, repair and rehabilitation. Med Sci Sports Exerc 16:427–443, 1984.
36. Noyes FR, Mangine RE, Barber S: Early knee motion after open and arthroscopic anterior cruciate ligament reconstruction. Am J Sports Med 15:149–160, 1987.
37. Pipes TV, Wilmore JH: Isokinetic vs. isotonic strength training in adult meniscectomies. Med Sci Sports Exerc 7:262–274, 1975.
38. Radcliffe J, Farentinos R: Plyometrics: Explosive Power Training, 2nd ed. Champaign, IL: Human Kinetics Publishers, 1985.
39. Richardson WJ, Garrett WE: Clinical uses of continuous passive motion. Contemp Orthop 10:75–79, 1985.
40. Richmond JC, Gladstone J, MacGillivray J: Continuous passive motion after arthroxopically assisted anterior cruciate ligament reconstruction: comparison of short- versus long-term use. Arthroscopy 7:39–44, 1991.
41. Rovere GD, Haupt HA, Yates CS: Prophylactic knee bracing in college football. Am J Sports Med 15:111–116, 1987.
42. Ryan EJ III, Stone JA: Specific approaches to rehabilitation of athletic injury. In Grana WA, Kalenak A (eds): Clinical Sports Medicine, pp. 255–263. Philadelphia: WB Saunders, 1991.
43. Shelbourne KD, Whitaker J, McCarroll JR, et al: Anterior cruciate ligament injury: evaluation of intraarticular reconstruction of acute tears without repair. Am J Sports Med 18:484–489, 1990.
44. Singer K, D'Ambrosia R, Graf B, et al: Electrical modalities. In Drez D Jr (ed): Therapeutic Modalities for Sports Injuries, pp. 33–48. Chicago: Year Book Medical, 1986.
45. Sitler M, Ryan J, Hopkinson W, et al: The efficacy of a prophylactic knee brace to reduce knee injuries in football. Am J Sports Med 18:310–315, 1990.
46. Steadman JR: Rehabilitation after knee ligament surgery. Am J Sports Med 8:294–296, 1980.
47. Sutter Biomedical, Inc.: [Advertisement]. Am J Sports Med 17, 1989.
48. Voss DL, Kieuta M, Myers BJ: Proprioceptive Neuromuscular Facilitation, pp. 298–307. Philadelphia: Harper & Row, 1985.
49. Yates CK, McCarthy M, Hirsch HS, Pascale MS: The early effects of continuous passive motion following anterior cruciate ligament reconstruction with autogenous patellar tendon grafts: a prospective randomized study. J Sport Rehab 2:121–131, 1992.

CHAPTER 15

Patellofemoral

Pain Problems

WILLIAM A. GRANA, M.D.

■

PATELLOFEMORAL PAIN DEFINED

The term "internal derangement of the knee" for undiagnosed disorders of the knee has been largely abandoned. However, the term "chondromalacia of the patella" remains the nonspecific diagnosis for a disorder of the patellofemoral joint with the common symptoms of patellar pain, giving way, or crepitation. However, with improvements in diagnosis brought by the use of arthroscopy to correlate clinic findings with gross disease, this term is also becoming passé.[37] Chondromalacia is often asymptomatic and frequently caused by age-related anatomic and mechanical causes. "Patellofemoral pain syndrome" is the best generic term to use until a specific diagnosis is apparent. An accurate assessment of history and the physical examination provide a better understanding of the specific problem of the patellofemoral joint.[5, 37] Patients with patellofemoral pain have peripatellar and subpatellar pain, difficulty in sitting for long periods of time (the so-called movie theater sign), giving way, and crepitation. These problems occasionally produce swelling, particularly when articular surface change or arthrosis is present, and with the swelling there is a certain amount of true quadriceps atrophy with a decreased thigh circumference.[5, 16, 37]

In Chapters 2 and 3, the anatomic and biomechanical reasons for patellofemoral problems are discussed. Extensor mechanism disorders may result from intrinsic, general, or developmental abnormalities of the bone or soft tissue structure of the joint. In addition, extrinsic trauma may play a role in the occurrence of these problems by acute direct injury or by the indirect effects of effusion or chronic repetitive stress.[25, 33] The common result of these factors is their effect on patellofemoral contact force, their effect on tracking of the patella in the trochlear groove, or a combination of these two. Incongruous motion or increased load may result in localized stress and be the first step in producing articular cartilage damage.[14]

Many authors have discussed the effects of increased contact stress on the patella.[7-10, 12, 23, 28] In addition, contact force is markedly increased by a variety of flexed-knee activities. The potential results of this increased contact force include wear and tear changes of the articular cartilage, which produce synovial irritation with resultant inflammation and pain. However, in many patients with patellofemoral pain, the articular surface is intact, with no evidence of significant synovial irritation. Goodfellow and associates described a lesion that they termed "basal degeneration" and that consists of fibrillation of collagen in the middle and deep zones of articular cartilage without first affecting the surface.[12] An increase in subchondral interosseous pressure has been shown to produce pain; therefore, any failure of the articular cartilage and its ability to absorb energy could cause an increase in intraosseous pressure and, consequently, more pain. This basal degeneration might well explain the biomechanical failure of patella articular cartilage and subsequent transfer of load alterations to the subchondral bone, from which it is normally protected, that then result in pain.[14]

A variety of classifications of patellofemoral pain are available, including those developed by Ficat and colleagues, Insall, Merchant, and Radin.[10, 16, 25, 33] For the purposes of this chapter, a modification of Radin's four categories of patellofemoral pain is used: traumatic lesions of the patella, osteoarthritis of the patellofemoral joint, and synovial fringe entrapment (odd facet syndrome), which occur separately or as a result of underlying patellofemoral malalignment.

In a prospective review of the relative frequency of each type of patellofemoral pain, about 65 per cent of cases were caused by tracking and instability problems, 20 per cent by chondromalacia, 10 per cent by extra-articular or synovial problems, and 5 per cent by patellofemoral osteoarthrosis. This study revealed that a majority of patients fail to comply with the physician's recommendation for continued knee rehabilitation, and such failure compromises the success of treatment of patellofemoral disorder.[37]

In this chapter, the extra-articular causes of patellofemoral pain, tracking abnormalities of the patella, and chondromalacia and osteoarthrosis of the patella are described.

EXTRA-ARTICULAR PATELLOFEMORAL PAIN

Medial Shelf Syndrome

Numerous reports support the observation that a plica may be the cause of symptoms.[1, 16, 18, 29] A thickened medial patella plica produces symptoms when it abrades the anteromedial surface of the medial femoral condyle or because a bowstring-like effect over the medial femoral condyle is created. Flexion of the knee causes interposition of the shelf between the patella and femur, which results in patellofemoral pain (Fig. 15–1).[29] Usually, symptoms arise after an acute injury with synovitis and effusion or as the result of repetitive stress as might be seen in a runner. A direct blow may cause such thickening, which is caused by the local edema that results in the impingement or the bowstring effect. Any effusion or

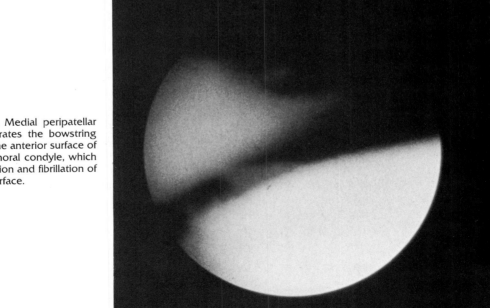

FIGURE 15–1. Medial peripatellar plica demonstrates the bowstring effect across the anterior surface of the medial femoral condyle, which results in abrasion and fibrillation of the articular surface.

synovitis can change an asymptomatic plica to a pathologic shelf and may result in chondromalacia of the medial femoral condyle or the medial facet of the patella. Repeated minor episodes of trauma cause synovitis, which results in a synovial thickening of the plica, which in turn, on flexion, produces the impingement. In addition, a pannus formed on the medial femoral condyle may contact the anterior horn of the medial meniscus, resulting in impingement, or the plica may impinge on the edge of the meniscus, and varying degrees of flexion result in the medial joint line pain as well as femoral condylar and patellar pain.

In a review of 51 knees in 42 patients, Muse and associates examined this problem. More than 90 per cent of patients had pain that was localized to the anteromedial femoral condyle, the medial joint line, or the anterior lateral femoral condyle. Eighty per cent had a snapping or catching sensation localized over the femoral condyle, and about 33 per cent had a momentary sensation of locking. The combination of snapping and medial femoral condyle pain was found more frequently than any other combination of symptoms. Two thirds of the patients had swelling, and two thirds had a palpable fold over the femoral condyle. In a smaller percentage, patellar crepitation and free fluid effusion were noted in the joint.[29]

The nonoperative management of this problem comprises complete rest or limitation of strenuous physical activities, a nonsteroidal anti-inflammatory medication for a period of 2 to 3 weeks, and an exercise program that includes progressive resistive exercise through a painless range of motion. If the symptoms subside, the patient may resume more strenuous activity. However, if after a period of 12 to 16 weeks of this type of management the patient continues to be symptomatic even with restricted activity, operative management is considered.[29]

Operative management has consisted of a variety of methods.[1] Some authors recommend arthroscopic release, and some recommend total excision. In the author's review of 51 knees, it was believed that better results were obtained by the complete excision of the shelf than by a release alone. Therefore, his preferred method of treatment is complete excision. This is accomplished by an arthroscopic technique through an inferolateral portal with a 30° angled arthroscope and with operating instruments either inferomedial or superolateral. A basket is usually used to trim the thickened bank down to the wall of the joint, and then a shaver is used through the inferomedial portal to smooth this cut edge. Small bleeding vessels are cauterized. In patients who have significant chronic synovitis or effusion, a Hemovac drain is left in place for 24 hours. Concomitant chondromalacia of the medial femoral condyle or the patella, if present, is treated by chondroplasty as indicated.[29]

Of patients treated in this way, approximately 90 per cent return to unrestricted activity or strenuous activity with nonlimiting pain. About 25 to 33 per cent of the patients may have some recurrence of mild pain. The presence of chondromalacia tends to compromise the result and to be associated with recurrent discomfort.[29]

Synovial Fringe Entrapment

Synovial fringe entrapment, or the "odd facet" syndrome, was described by Radin,[33] who noted in the evaluation of cadaver knee that in about 30 per cent of people, the extreme medial edge of the patella has an extra or odd articular facet. This facet is in contact with femur only in hyperflexion—more than 120° of flexion—of the knee. This odd facet is crossed by a synovial fringe in about 40 per cent of people who have them, and in cadaver studies, there was evidence of old synovial inflammation as a result of entrapment. According to the author's experience, the fat pad may also be entrapped by the patellofemoral joint and produce impingement and symptoms similar to the impingement and symptoms of the medial shelf syndrome. The author views this entity as similar to the problems caused by a symptomatic medial plica, and nonoperative treatment is therefore the same for both conditions. Operative treatment consists of resection of the hypertrophic synovium and the fat pad as well as chondroplasty of the patella if articular cartilage damage is present. The patient is also instructed to avoid hyperflexion of the knee. As in the symptomatic shelf, a small amount of residual problems can be expected for these patients.

Reflex Sympathetic Dystrophy

Any injury or surgery of the patella may be complicated by an abnormality that is recognized radiographically as an acute regional osteoporosis of the bone. This finding is a result of reflex sympathetic dystrophy (RSD) of the patella and is a poorly understood problem that seems to be associated with several factors. But undertreatment and overtreatment of injuries and postoperative rehabilitation have a role in the precipitation of RSD. In addition, such patients often have a passive-aggressive personality that affects their ability to participate in a rehabilitation program; a significant degree of hostility is present in many of these patients. Although the mechanism of RSD is not understood, abnormal or dysfunctional sympathetic vasomotor control is believed by most investigators to have a role in the onset of this problem.[8]

Clinically, patients have pain that occurs after the inciting injury or surgery and is out of proportion to the stimulus. Normal improvement does not occur. The pain continues or even increases. Active motion of the knee becomes difficult. The pain is localized to the patella or the peripatellar area. The skin is shiny, exhibits hyperesthesia, and may be cyanotic and cool. The joint is stiff, and there is often a feeling of fullness in the retinacular areas that restricts patellar movement.

Evaluation of this problem includes plain radiographs, which show regional osteoporosis with radiolucent changes and demineralization of the patella (Fig. 15–2). Bone scintigraphy with technetium 99m shows increased uptake in the patella (Fig. 15–3).[6] Although these radiographic evaluations may be of help, the main tool is a high index of suspicion for the presence of the characteristic clinical and physical findings. RSD is difficult to characterize and must be constantly kept in mind for the patient whose pain is unresponsive and out of proportion to the usual treatment regimen.

Treatment of RSD is frequent active range-of-motion exercises of the knee within comfortable range and alternating contrast treatments with hot and cold. A nonsteroidal anti-inflammatory agent is also useful, as is nonnarcotic pain medication. Lumbar sympathetic block with a local

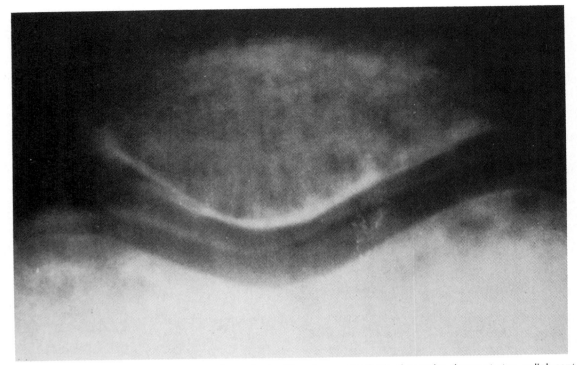

FIGURE 15–2. Patellofemoral joint view of a patient with reflex sympathetic dystrophy demonstrates radiolucent changes and demineralization of the patella, which are characteristic of this disorder.

anesthetic is beneficial because a positive response with relief of pain is diagnostic and may also be therapeutic, providing a long duration of relief of the pain. A skilled anesthesiologist can use multiple lumbar sympathetic blocks with a longer acting local anesthetic to break the cycle of pain and restricted motion. Relief enables the patient to have full participation in an exercise program. As a last resort, lumbar sympathectomy may be used to relieve these symptoms in the patient who responds well to sympathetic block.[8]

Quadriceps Dysfunction

Acute or repetitive trauma of the extensor mechanism may produce muscle imbalance with hamstring tightness and relative weakness of the quadriceps muscle.[11] Any effusion results in reflex inhibition of the quadriceps muscle, which potentiates this problem. Patellofemoral pain results from quadriceps muscle dysplasia and patellar malalignment and compression. In children, muscles and ligaments become stretched during longitudinal skeletal growth. Tightness and loss of flexibility about the joints occur. Restoration of flexibility and muscle balance in the antagonistic quadriceps and hamstring muscles preserves the normal patellar tracking.[30] By far the most common cause of patellofemoral pain syndrome is quadriceps muscle weakness in relation to the hamstring muscles with lateral tracking and increased patellofemoral joint reaction force. Thigh circumference measurement and isokinetic testing are useful in the evaluation of these

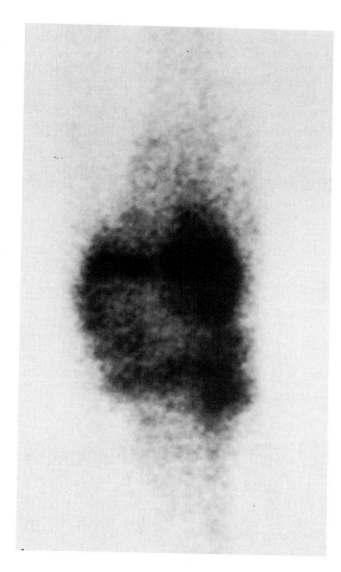

FIGURE 15–3. Technetium 99m scan in the patient referred to in Figure 15–2, showing the increased uptake in the patella.

problems. An aggressive resistive quadriceps exercise program along with hamstring stretching, decreased impact loading, and decreased bent-knee function relieves these symptoms.[11, 14] The patellofemoral rehabilitation program in Chapter 14 is appropriate for this problem.

TRACKING ABNORMALITY OF THE PATELLOFEMORAL JOINT

Patellar Malalignment and Patellar Compression Syndrome

Patellar malalignment is the presence of excessive lateral tracking of the patella in the trochlear groove without evidence of subluxation or excessive capsular tightness. Patellar compression syndrome includes these findings along with excessive tightness of the lateral retinaculum, which increases the patellar contact force on the femur. Insall postulated that this lateral tightness is an adaptation to lateral tracking, which supports the concept that patellar compression is part of the continuum of extensor mechanism disorders. Insall also classified patellar pain and pointed out the difficulty in differentiating its causes.[13, 16] Pain secondary to patellar instability is usually recognized from a careful history and physical examination, but when subluxation or dislocation is not present, the cause of the pain is difficult to determine from clinical and radiographic appraisal alone.[34, 35] The presence of lateral tracking of the patella as the cause of patellofemoral pain has been called patellar malalignment or patellar compression syndrome, depending on the findings.[16, 20]

The symptom in these tracking problems is subpatellar or peripatellar pain that is related to activity, which is often athletic; symptoms of giving way occur during athletic participation, but there is no problem in normal daily activities. Physical examination reveals that the patient has pain with patellar compression in addition to excessive lateral motion in the first 45° of flexion. There may be restricted medial motion as well. There is sufficient synovial irritation to produce joint line tenderness, and this may be confused with meniscus disease. Physical examination reveals the presence of lateral tracking of the patella in the first 45° of flexion or the "grasshopper eye" appearance on observation of the patella at 90° of flexion (Fig. 15–4). With the patient standing, the alignment of the extremity often demonstrates femoral anteversion with the squinting patellar appearance (Fig. 15–5). There may be increased lateral excursion

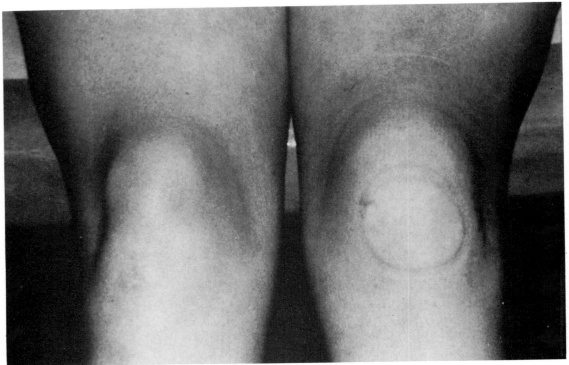

FIGURE 15–4. "Grasshopper eye" appearance of the patella seen at 90° of flexion illustrates the tendency for the patella to subluxate and tilt laterally.

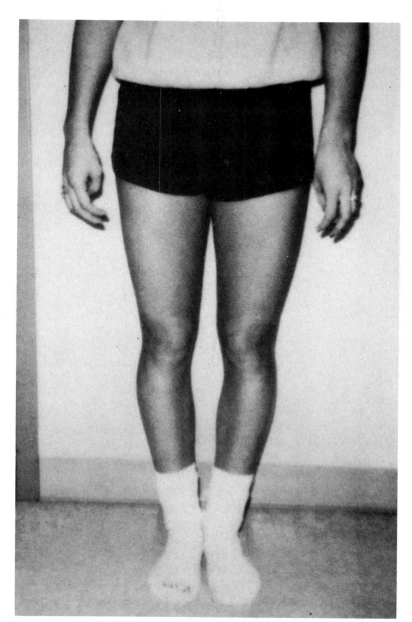

FIGURE 15–5. Femoral anteversion with inward or squinting patellar appearance is often associated with patellofemoral pain and patellar malalignment.

of the patella with decreased medial excursion in response to applied manual pressure.

Radiographic evaluation of the patellofemoral joint may help demonstrate an abnormality in the patellofemoral relationship. The patellofemoral radiographs show lateral incongruity of the patella with lateral tilt and, in rare instances, lateral subluxation. Merchant's congruence angle and Laurin's lines are useful but not diagnostic in this evaluation.[21, 26] Both Casscells and Metcalf emphasized the importance of viewing the patellofemoral joint arthroscopically during flexion and extension of the knee, and this is an important diagnostic method for recognizing the presence of lateral tracking as a cause of patellofemoral pain.[3, 27] It is best done from the suprapatellar pouch area through a superomedial puncture.

Nonoperative management of this problem consists of nonsteroidal anti-inflammatory medication for a period of about 1 month. In two studies, this treatment, if helpful, was continued for 8 to 12 weeks. Patients began an exercise program that consisted initially of straight-leg raising and, as tolerated, gradually progressed to include short-arc and long-arc quadriceps exercise and functional activities as outlined in Chapter 14. A failure was defined as an inability to tolerate straight-leg exercise, accompanied by persistent pain with daily activity, climbing stairs, and sitting for more than 15 or 20 minutes. If a patient showed no improvement after at least 8 to 12 weeks of nonoperative management, arthroscopy was indicated.[13, 37]

The operative management of this problem consists of open or arthroscopic lateral retinacular release with or without medial imbrication of the vastus medialis to the edge of the patella. The author's preferred approach to this problem includes complete arthroscopic evaluation of the knee with careful attention to the patellofemoral relationship viewed from the medial suprapatellar portal. The knee is passively moved through a range of motion from 0° to 90° or until the patellofemoral joint closes sufficiently to prevent further visualization of the two articular surfaces. A tilt or a tracking of the patella laterally in the first 45° of flexion confirms the diagnosis of patellar malalignment. The author defines lateral tracking as a failure of the central ridge of the patella to seat in the trochlear groove of the femur in the first 45° of flexion. In the knee that tracks normally, the patella usually seats by 20° to 30° of flexion. The central ridge tracks along the lateral femoral condyle, and there is a concomitant tilt of the patella with widening of the medial patellofemoral joint space, which forces the lateral facet and central ridge against the lateral femoral condyle. If the central ridge does not seat at 45° of flexion, then the diagnosis of lateral tracking is confirmed. The tilted appearance of the patella at arthroscopy is described as Casscells' sign (Fig. 15–6).

With the arthroscope in the inferomedial portal and with the inflow cannula in the inferolateral portal, an arthroscopic cautery is placed through the superomedial portal. Under direct vision, a lateral release is accomplished. The extent of the lateral release is from the inferior pole of the patella to 1 to 2 cm above the superior pole of the patella. Care is taken to identify the geniculate vessel and any other significant blood vessels in order to cauterize them. A fluid pump is used, and the pump pressure is decreased sufficiently to allow easy visualization of bleeding vessels.

Postoperative management includes a compression dressing with a foam horseshoe-shaped pad over the lateral retinaculum in order to keep pressure on this area. A Hemovac drain is left in place, and the patient is seen by the physical therapist within 24 hours after surgery. The Hemovac drain is removed, and the dressing is changed. A smaller lateral compression pad is put in place. The wounds are dressed with adhesive bandages, and a woven elastic wrap is used to hold the pad in place. As the effusion recedes, the patient begins a patellofemoral rehabilitation program. In approximately 4 to 6 weeks, the patient is allowed to return to full activity if there is no persistent swelling or pain.

After the arthroscopic release, patellar motion is reviewed again. Almost always the patellar tilt is resolved by the lateral release, but if subluxation is still present, a small, straight incision is made over the

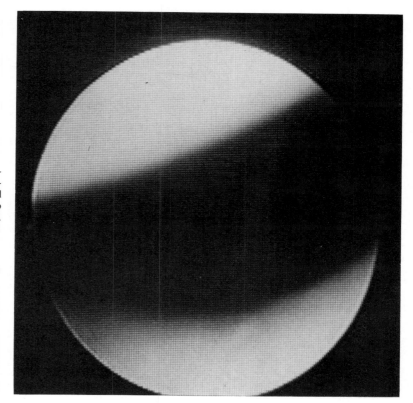

FIGURE 15–6. Widening of the medial patellofemoral joint and narrowing of the lateral patellofemoral joint as the knee flexes from 0° to 90° are described as Casscells' sign.

vastus medialis (Fig. 15–7), and a triangular flap that consists of the vastus medialis obliquus is dissected from the quadriceps tendon, the medial retinaculum, and the capsular lining of the joint (Fig. 15–8). It is advanced just to the edge of the patella and sutured in place with horizontal mattress sutures. Care must be taken not to advance the patella over the edge, because this may produce a medial tilt of the patella or increased medial contact force (Fig. 15–9). In this instance, when a medial imbrication is accomplished, the knee is immobilized for 3 weeks, but passive range-of-motion exercise is begun approximately 7 to 10 days after surgery as the wound heals.

The author's experience is that about 90 per cent of patients treated in this manner have a satisfactory functional result with either unrestricted activity or strenuous activity with nonlimiting pain.[13] The complications that result from lateral release include hemarthrosis that persists more than 3 to 5 days and persistent pain. Hemarthrosis is avoided by the use of a cautery and careful attention to hemostasis before the completion of the arthroscopy. Pain is usually associated with chondromalacia (patellofemoral arthrosis) of the patella, and the severity may compromise the ultimate result, particularly if patients try to continue impact-loading activity. A patient who has lateral tracking of the patella as well as chondromalacia is well advised to avoid impact-loading activity and to participate in activities less stressful to the patellofemoral joint, such as bicycling or swimming. In addition, patients must continue a regular exercise program. Other authors have noted that the results of lateral release show an 85 per cent satisfactory outcome but with some tendency

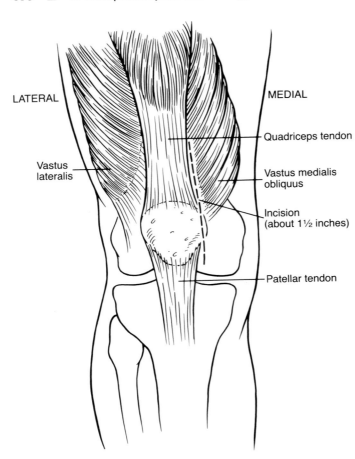

LATERAL

MEDIAL

Quadriceps tendon

Vastus
lateralis

Vastus medialis
obliquus

Incision
(about 1½ inches)

FIGURE 15–7. Incision for a vastus medialis obliquus imbrication.

Patellar tendon

for the result to deteriorate with time if the patient does not adhere to a regular exercise program. For older patients with chondromalacia, the author is selective about the use of lateral retinacular release and frequently addresses only the patellar articular surface problem unless the tracking problem is severe.

Acute Dislocation or Subluxation of the Patella

Acute dislocation occurs as a result of a direct blow to the anteromedial aspect of the patella or as a result of internal rotation of the femur on the fixed, externally rotated tibia during a sudden twisting movement. A common mechanism of the latter is softball batting or forcefully swinging and missing the ball with the back leg planted, resulting in a dislocation of the patella of the back knee. Direct trauma is the usual cause of such problems in men, whereas in women, acute dislocation is more commonly associated with a twisting mechanism with predisposing bony alignment and soft tissue abnormalities, as discussed in Chapter 2.

Marked patellofemoral pain and a large effusion are demonstrated on physical examination. Active motion and passive motion are limited. There is tenderness over the medial retinaculum, and, to a lesser extent, the whole patella is tender to compression glissement. There may be a

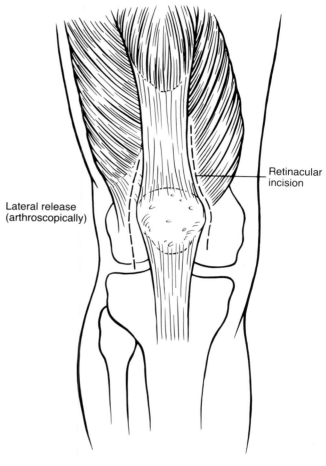

FIGURE 15–8. The triangular flap consists of the vastus medialis obliquus as dissected from the quadriceps tendon medial retinaculum and the capsular lining of the joint for advancement medially and distally.

Lateral release (arthroscopically)

Retinacular incision

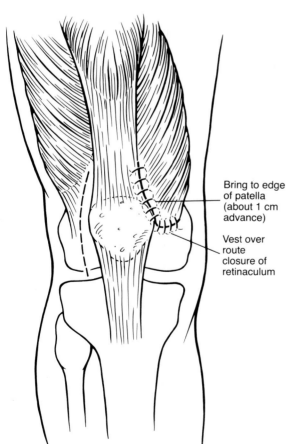

Bring to edge of patella (about 1 cm advance)

Vest over route closure of retinaculum

FIGURE 15–9. The vastus medialis obliquus is advanced to but not over the edge of the patella in order to avoid the production of an increased medial contact force.

palpable defect in the area of the vastus medialis. The patient becomes severely apprehensive with attempts to subluxate the patella laterally.[2]

After dislocation, the patella almost always relocates spontaneously with extension of the knee. Occasionally, a patient comes into the emergency room or the physician's office with a patellar dislocation. Usually, gentle passive extension results in relocation of the patella. Local aspiration and instillation of a local anesthetic are sometimes necessary for reducing the patella. In this instance, reduction is accomplished with gentle extension and manual pressure from lateral to medial on the patella.

Plain radiographs are usually normal, although they may show osteochondral injury to the medial side of the patella or to the lateral femoral condyle (Fig. 15–10). If either of these injuries is present and is documented as a new finding, arthroscopic evaluation of the knee and treatment of the osteochondral injury with removal of any loose fragments are recommended. In addition, if there is any palpable defect, arthroscopy for the evaluation of the joint should be performed, and repair of the vastus medialis and lateral retinacular release are preferred.

On the other hand, in the absence of either radiographic evidence of osteochondral injury or physical evidence of vastus medialis disruption, the patient is managed in a knee immobilizer for a period of 3 weeks; early motion exercise and the patellofemoral rehabilitation program are

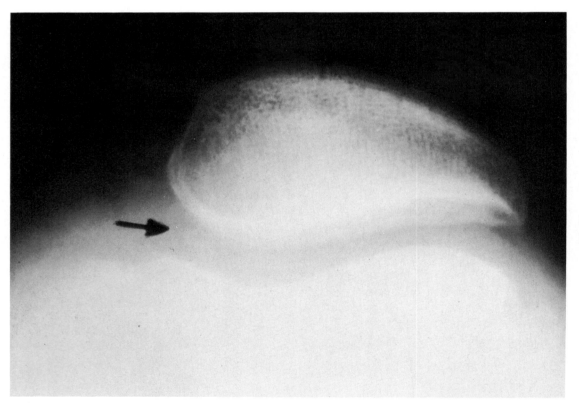

FIGURE 15–10. Radiograph shows an osteochondral fragment (*arrow*) off the medial side of the patella in acute dislocation.

instituted at about 10 days. However, the immobilizer should be worn for a total of 3 weeks, the patient removing it only for exercise during that time. Men do well after such management if there is no underlying alignment abnormality. On the other hand, the vast majority of women continue to experience some degree of recurrent instability.

Recurrent Subluxation

Patients who complain of recurrent giving way with a sensation of patellar hypermobility and apprehension have recurrent patellar subluxation. These patients have, in addition, peripatellar and subpatellar pain, swelling, and crepitation. Radiographs show that such patients have Merchant's congruence angle that is more than 4° to 6°. These patients frequently have abnormalities of extremity alignment with an abnormal Q-angle, femoral anteversion, genu valgum, and external tibial torsion. About 20 per cent of patients with patellofemoral pain have recurrent subluxation.

Like all other patients with patellofemoral pain, these patients are treated nonoperatively with a patellofemoral rehabilitation program and a patellofemoral brace in an attempt to control patellar motion. However, if symptoms persist 3 to 6 months and limit activity so as to produce excessive disability, operative treatment is recommended.

The author's preferred method is arthroscopic lateral retinacular release followed by assessment of patellar motion, and if lateral tracking or lateral tilt persists, proximal realignment is completed by medial imbrication. The patient is then placed in the routine patellofemoral rehabilitation program with a return to activity as tolerated. A small percentage of these patients may have recurrent complaints; for them, distal realignment with transfer of the tibial tubercle medially and elevation of the tubercle are necessary in order to produce a distal realignment to correct the Q-angle and to decrease patellofemoral contact force.

Recurrent Dislocation

About 10 per cent of patients with patellar instability problems note true recurrent dislocations of the patella.[37] Almost all of these patients are female and have significant alignment abnormalities that result in malalignment of the entire extensor mechanism. The complaints and physical findings are similar to those seen in chronic subluxation. Fractures associated with recurrent patellar dislocation occur in the medial facet of the patella or in the lateral femoral condyle. The author's preferred surgical management involves arthroscopic management of any osteochondral injury, lateral release, and medial imbrication of the vastus medialis obliquus. If the Q-angle is more than 15° for a male patient and 20° for a female patient, a distal realignment with medial shift of the patellar tendon and elevation of the tibial tubercle attachment is indicated as well. Surgical intervention is almost always required in order to eliminate the significant disability that true recurrent dislocation of the patella produces.[4, 15, 19, 22] Fortunately, it is relatively rare.

CHONDROMALACIA OF THE PATELLA (PATELLOFEMORAL ARTHROSIS)

The concept that abnormalities of patellar tracking and associated changes in contact force of the patella may eventually result in chondromalacia has been discussed extensively in the literature.[10, 23, 33] Outerbridge and Dunlop listed several possible causes for chondromalacia, noting that malalignment with recurrent subluxation was probably the most common.[31] In a prospective study, Insall and collaborators found patellar malalignment to be the most common cause of chondromalacia of the patella.[17] McNab pointed out that recurrent subluxation of the patella is almost always associated with damage to the patellar articular surface.[22] Values for high tensile stress on the medial facet and particularly the odd facet exceed the values obtained by Weightman for tensile fatigue failure of cartilage collagen.[36] The usual appearance of chondromalacic lesions is of crab meat because the facet is not subjected to the large compression forces seen on the lateral facet. In addition, high sheer stress may result in a closed-type chondromalacic lesion that is similar to the basal degeneration that Goodfellow and associates described.[12] Finally, the lateral facet is often involved with firm sclerotic cartilage as a result of the excessive pressure syndrome seen with the high compressive contact stresses on the lateral facet in this type of patellar tracking abnormality.[23]

Although some authors would argue that patellofemoral arthrosis and chondromalacia are not part of a continuum, the vast majority of authors believe that patellofemoral arthrosis is the final stage in the deterioration of the patellofemoral joint as a result of excessive pressure on the patellar cartilage.[33] The cause of arthrosis is a phenomenon of excessive pressure. Maquet reported that patellofemoral arthrosis results when the patellofemoral pressure is unevenly distributed or too high for the resistance of the tissues.[23] As noted, early changes in proteoglycan content are associated with degeneration of the articular surface, and Ficat and Maroudas observed that the combination of high contact pressure and lower glycosaminoglycan content of the articular cartilage is an important factor in the occurrence of chondromalacia of the patellar cartilage. The chondrolytic enzymes that are released from the open chondromalacic lesions result in the progression to osteoarthritis.[9]

Patients with arthrosis have patellofemoral pain, crepitation, and swelling with disability during impact-loading activity, such as running or jumping, or with any bent-knee activity, such as squatting or bending. Mechanical symptoms, which occur often, involve primarily the knee in full extension, which results in catching and pseudolocking. Physical examination shows abnormalities in alignment that are consistent with those described previously in this chapter. In addition, patients may experience mild to moderate apprehension if the patella is manipulated. The joint is tender on patellar compression (glissement) or with forced flexion of the knee or with squatting. Palpating the knee cap through a range of motion from 90° to full extension often elicits crepitation, which may be increased if the tibia is loaded through this range. There is often a painful click in the last 20° to 30° before full extension. Although there may not be any asymmetry in the thigh circumference unless the patient has had recurrent effusions, there is often dysplasia of the vastus medialis, which is poorly developed or has a high insertion.

Plain radiographs may show some evidence of osteophytic changes of the joint and narrowing of the patellofemoral joint, which are consistent with patellofemoral arthrosis. More often than not, the only abnormalities noted are those associated with the patellar tracking problems. The author has not found computed tomographic scans or magnetic resonance imaging to be useful in the evaluation of these patients, although other authors have.[32, 33] Arthroscopy remains the best method for defining the depth and extent of the problem as well as for determining the best treatment.

Treatment of these problems depends on the understanding of the pathomechanics, which have been described earlier in this chapter and in Chapter 3. This understanding implies a rational approach to treatment, which includes correction of the tracking problem and a reduction in the load on the patellofemoral joint. The methods used include restriction of activity, exercise, rehabilitative exercise, medical management, orthosis, and surgical intervention.[14]

Nonoperative management is successful in 75 to 80 per cent of patients and is based on an alteration in activity, on exercise, and on anti-inflammatory medication. A decrease or a change in activity—for example, from running to swimming or cycling—reduces patellofemoral load and decreases the effect of the tracking problem.[5] Such an alteration may reduce the load two- to threefold and relieve symptoms to the patient's satisfaction.

Rehabilitative exercise, which includes quadriceps strengthening and hamstring stretching, as noted in the patellofemoral exercise program, also reduces patellofemoral contact force and decreases lateral tracking. However, this exercise must be monitored because through a full range of motion it produces loading and may exacerbate symptoms or cause progression of articular cartilage damage. It may be necessary to select a pain-free range of motion for the patient in order to help relieve any symptoms caused by the exercises.

Medical management includes the use of nonsteroidal anti-inflammatory medication for reducing synovial irritation and effusion. In addition, in the farther advanced cases, local steroid injections may also provide symptomatic relief. As often as possible, the author treats these patients with an intermittent course of the nonsteroidal medication in an attempt to reduce their exposure to these medications.

Orthotic devices that decrease lateral tracking, such as braces designed to control patellar motion, may also be of benefit. These devices may be as simple as a felt pad taped in place laterally during activity.

Operative management is aimed at elimination of the tracking abnormality of the damaged articular surface and reducing the increased contact force. These realignment procedures are often performed concomitantly because patellofemoral pain often has multiple causes. As discussed, the use of proximal realignment procedures is often the first step in treatment of tracking disorders. Debridement of the articular lesion is useful if it is confined to one facet and if the severity of chondromalacia is grade II or III. Treatment by removal of loose articular cartilage creates a stable bed, whether this goes down to bone or not, and yields the best chances of a satisfactory result. After debridement, these patients may require a period of non–weight bearing as well as passive motion in order to maximize healing. Progression of the patellofemoral exercise program should be slowed down because active flexion activities, especially with loading, may increase local symptoms immediately after surgery. Indications that the author considers for chondroplasty include a combination of patellofemoral pain and swelling associated with mechanical symptoms and pseudolocking, which usually occurs in full extension and which momentarily interrupts motion. The best results are obtained in patients who have grade II or III chondromalacia and who fail to respond to the general rehabilitation program.[24]

The surgical repair is accomplished arthroscopically with the use of a motorized shaver, free knife blades, and curettes as necessary. The object is to remove loose or unstable cartilage material until a stable bed or bone is reached. No attempt is made to drill holes into the bone, but every effort is made to provide a stable rim to the articular cartilage lesion. In the author's experience, a defect fills in with fibrocartilage if it is less than 2 cm in diameter. Larger defects carry a very poor prognosis for healing; even if the defect heals over a 12- to 18-month period, the patient has recurrent problems unless a realignment procedure and activity modification are undertaken. The only exception to this pattern is a defect in a a patient under 16 years of age. In such a patient, clinical experience indicates that the chance that the defect will heal is good, and therefore the author would consider drilling small holes with a burr or a Kirschner wire as a stimulus to this healing process. The key here is to identify the underlying problem, which is frequently malalignment, and to treat this adequately.

About 85 per cent of patients with grade II or III lesions are subjectively improved at a 2-year follow-up, but only about 66 per cent have a result that is satisfactory according to objective evaluation. Results depend on the severity of the disease, the age of the patient, and the patient's activity. The more severe the disease is, the lower is the probability of satisfactory results. About 70 per cent of patients with grade II lesions experience a satisfactory functional result, whereas 50 per cent or fewer of patients with grade IV disease experience satisfactory results. Moreover, the best results are obtained when a stable bed is provided for the lesion.[23] Both age and activity affect the results. Patients over 50, who place fewer demands on the patellofemoral joint, may have a better chance of reducing symptoms.

In patients who have evidence of patellofemoral arthrosis and for whom nonoperative management or local management of the articular cartilage lesion fails, the preferred method of treatment is to reduce the contact force as well as improve tracking abnormalities. Increased contact forces may be relieved by tibial tubercle elevation or by patellectomy. Both of the procedures have proponents and detractors, and both have clinical and theoretical disadvantages. The purpose of these procedures in the treatment of extensor mechanism disorder is one of salvage. Every effort should be made to keep the patella as bony stock potential for total joint replacement. To this end, the author has curbed the use of patellectomy for patellofemoral arthrosis, reserving it only for the most severe comminuted patellar fractures; therefore, he believes that the management of patellofemoral arthrosis must involve some form of tibial tubercle elevation. Maquet, Radin, and Schutzer and colleagues recommended tibial tubercle elevation and, more recently, tibial osteotomy with medial shift, which provides elevation of the tibial tubercle.[23, 33, 35] The author believes that any distal realignment procedure must involve elevation as well as medial shift of the tibial tubercle, and the guarded early results of distal realignment procedures without such elevation bear this out.

The author's preferred method of tibial tubercle elevation involves modification of the described procedure whereby elevation is achieved by bone block obtained from Gerdy's tubercle. In addition, it has not been necessary in his experience to use the long shingle described by Maquet and others, nor has a 2-cm elevation been necessary.[23] A short shingle with a 1-cm elevation has been used, as advocated by P. Ferguson. The technique is as follows:

The patient is supine, and a tourniquet is used for control of bleeding. An incision that is slightly transverse and oblique proximal to the junction of the patellar tendon and the tibial tubercle is made and is extended laterally over Gerdy's tubercle to a length of approximately 5 cm (Fig. 15–11). The medial edge of the incision should reach the medial border of the patellar tendon. The tubercle is exposed, and the iliotibial band is incised in the line of its fibers. A 1.5 × 1.5 cm bone graft is outlined with a drill. The graft is predrilled for a 6.5-mm cancellous screw or a 4.5-mm malleolar screw (Fig. 15–12). An osteotome is used to harvest the graft. First a cautery and then a drill are used to outline the tibial tubercle so that it can be elevated with an osteotome. The distal extent of the tubercle is not incised but is drilled distally to produce a clysis of the bone in order to leave the soft tissues intact. The tubercle is predrilled centrally for a 6.5-mm cancellous screw or a 4.5-mm malleolar screw (Fig. 15–13). An osteotome is then used to make medial and lateral cuts, elevating the

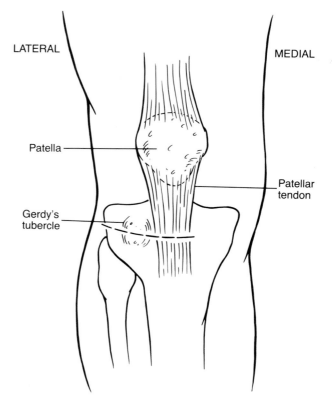

FIGURE 15–11. The incision for the modified tibial tubercle elevation and transfer is made on the lateral and anterior aspects of the proximal leg. It is a slightly transverse oblique incision proximal to the junction of the patellar tendon and the tibial tubercle and extended laterally over Gerdy's tubercle to a length of about 5 cm.

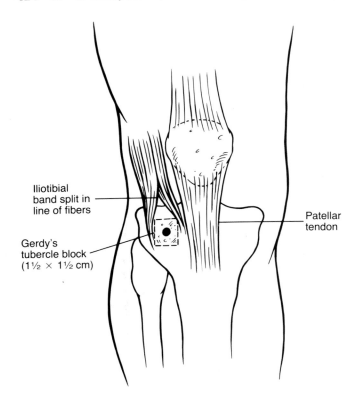

Iliotibial
band split in
line of fibers

Gerdy's
tubercle block
(1½ × 1½ cm)

Patellar
tendon

FIGURE 15–12. A 1.5 × 1.5 cm bone graft is outlined and predrilled for a 6.5-mm cancellous screw or a 4.5-mm malleolar screw. An osteotome is used to harvest the graft.

FIGURE 15–13. The tubercle is predrilled centrally for a 6.5-mm cancellous screw or a 4.5-mm malleolar screw.

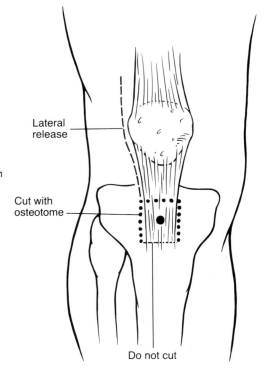

Lateral
release

Cut with
osteotome

Do not cut

tubercle and shifting it on the distal soft tissue hinge (Fig. 15–14). The bone graft is put in place in order to elevate the tendon at least one full centimeter (Fig. 15–15). The transfer medially is approximately half the width of the patellar tendon, but motion of the patella should be checked before the tibial tubercle and the bone graft are fixed with a screw and a flat metal washer. If the incision is planned appropriately, the screw placement should be just below the level of the incision.

Postoperative rehabilitation includes the use of a knee immobilizer with early passive range-of-motion exercise approximately 10 days after surgery. The knee immobilizer is in place for approximately 6 weeks. Weighted resistive exercise is started about 3 to 6 weeks after surgery, depending on the radiographic appearance of healing. The screw and the washer are removed 6 months postoperatively as an outpatient procedure.

In a review by the author of 15 patients who underwent this procedure for patellofemoral arthrosis, there were two failures that resulted in subsequent patellectomy. One of the two patients is now functioning successfully; the other continues to experience pain. Of the remaining 13 patients, seven had excellent functional results, two had good results, one had a fair result, and three had poor results. Of these 13 patients, 12 expressed satisfaction with their surgery and would have undergone the procedure again. There were no problems with wound healing, and there were no fractures or nonunions. One patient fell 2 weeks after surgery, and the screw was bent, but this did not affect the position of the elevation of the graft on radiographs, and the screw was subsequently removed without difficulty. The author believes that this procedure does not have the difficulties of a short shingle in the classic Maquet operation, and it

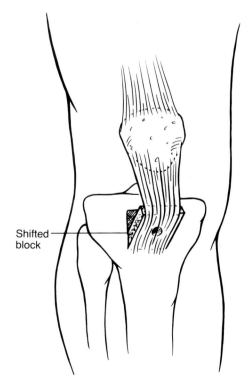

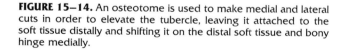

FIGURE 15–14. An osteotome is used to make medial and lateral cuts in order to elevate the tubercle, leaving it attached to the soft tissue distally and shifting it on the distal soft tissue and bony hinge medially.

Shifted block

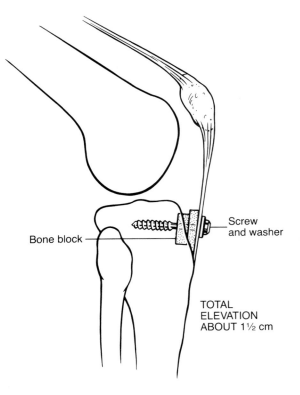

FIGURE 15–15. The bone graft is put into place and held with a 6.5-mm cancellous screw or a 4.5-mm malleolar screw. Each screw is used with a washer.

Bone block

Screw and washer

TOTAL
ELEVATION
ABOUT 1½ cm

also avoids the long incision and bone dissection required for the traditional Maquet procedure.

Patellectomy is the last resort for patellofemoral arthrosis, and in this problem the results are unpredictable, and the physician must apprise the patient of this. Patellectomy is best used after trauma for severely comminuted fractures; the outcome is not as well defined for arthrosis. The technique is performed as follows with the patient supine. A midline incision is made over the patellofemoral joint, extending from about 2 cm above the quadriceps tendon to the inferior pole of the patella and just below. Flaps are undermined, and a medial parapatellar retinacular incision is made. The patella is shelled out of its retinaculum, and the two ends of the tendons are approximated with the use of a suture that inverts the central patella retinaculum. This creates a cosmetic bulge in the area of the patella. Lateral release is accomplished, as is immediate imbrication as well. When the reconstruction is completed, the knee is flexed from 0° to 90°, and this should be done without any tension on the suture lines.

The postoperative management includes the use of a knee immobilizer with ambulation weight bearing as tolerated for 10 days, passive range-of-motion exercise to 45° for the next 10 days to 2 weeks, and straight-leg raising with weights up to 10 to 15 pounds. At 3 weeks the patient may continue passive range-of-motion to 90° as allowed; at 6 weeks, active range-of-motion exercises begin with resistive exercise as tolerated. At 2 to 3 months, the patient is allowed to return to full activity with the exception of impact-loading sports. Bicycling is usually begun at 8 weeks as tolerated.

Function, particularly strength and power in quadriceps function, is diminished after patellectomy. However, patients who have undergone patellectomy for trauma do somewhat better. In a review of function after patellectomy, Peeples and Margo indicated that 85 per cent of patients who underwent patellectomy for fracture achieved satisfactory function; 79 per cent of those with patellofemoral arthrosis achieved satisfactory results. Some quadriceps muscle weakness was usually present, and that the end result depended on a patient's ability to comply with a vigorous rehabilitation program. At least 1 year after surgery was required for securing the maximal benefit for function.[32]

SUMMARY

Patellofemoral disorder is a complex problem that frequently affects both the general population and people involved in sports activities. Whatever treatment is planned depends on an understanding of the pathomechanics of extensor mechanism disorder and which specific components of these mechanics require adjustment in order to effect relief of patellofemoral pain. This understanding is the basis for a rational approach to the management of these problems, regardless of whether the abnormality involves soft tissue, bone, or cartilage pathomechanics.

REFERENCES

1. Broom MJ, Fulkerson JP: The plica syndrome: a new perspective. Orthop Clin North Am 17:279–281, 1986.
2. Carson WG Jr, James SL, Larson RL, et al: Patellofemoral disorders: physical radiographic evaluation. Part I: physical examination. Clin Orthop 185:165–177, 1984.
3. Casscells SW: The arthroscope in the diagnosis of disorders of the patellofemoral joint. Clin Orthop 144:45–000, 1979.
4. Crosby EB, Insall J: Recurrent dislocation of the patella: relation of treatment to osteoarthritis. J Bone Joint Surg 58A:9–13, 1976.
5. DeHaven KE, Dolan WA, Mayer PJ: Chondromalacia patellae in athletes: clinical presentation and conservative management. Am J Sports Med 7:5–11, 1979.
6. Dye SF, Boll DA: Radionuclide imaging of the patellofemoral joint in young adults with anterior knee pain. Orthop Clin North Am 17:249–262, 1986.
7. Ficat RP: Degeneration of the patellofemoral joint. *In* Ingwersen B (ed): The Knee Joint. New York: Excerpta Medica, American Elsevier, 1974.
8. Ficat RP, Hungerford DS: Disorders of the Patello-Femoral Joint. Baltimore: Williams and Wilkins, 1977.
9. Ficat C, Maroudas A: Cartilage of the patella: topographical variation and glycosaminoglycan content in normal and fibrillated tissue. Ann Rheum Dis 34:515–519, 1975.
10. Ficat RP, Phillippe J, Hungerford DS: Chondromalacia patellae: a system of classification. Clin Orthop 144:55–62, 1979.
11. Fox T: Dysplasia of the quadriceps mechanism: hypoplasia of the vastus medialis muscle as related to the hypermobile patella syndrome. Surg Clin North Am 55:199–225, 1975.
12. Goodfellow J, Hungerford DS, Woods C: Patellofemoral joint mechanics and pathology: chondromalacia patellae. J Bone Joint Surg 58B:291–299, 1976.
13. Grana WA, Hinkley B, Hollingsworth S: Arthroscopic evaluation and treatment of patellar malalignment. Clin Orthop 186:122–128, 1984.
14. Grana WA, Kriegshauser LA: Scientific basis of extensor mechanism disorders. Clin Sports Med 4:247–257, 1985.
15. Grana WA, O'Donoghue DH: Patellar-tendon transfer by the slot-block method for recurrent subluxation and dislocation of the patella. J Bone Joint Surg 59A:736–741, 1977.
16. Insall J: Current concepts review: patellar pain. J Bone Joint Surg 64A:147–152, 1982.
17. Insall J, Falvo KA, Wise DW: Chondromalacia patellae: a prospective study. J Bone Joint Surg 58A:1–8, 1976.
18. Kettelkamp DB, DeRosa GP: Surgery of the patellofemoral joint. *In* American Association of Orthopaedic Surgeons (ed): AAOS Instructional Course Lectures, p. 27. St. Louis: CV Mosby, 1976.
19. Larson RL: Subluxation-dislocation of the patella. *In* Kennedy JD (ed): The Injured Adolescent Knee. Baltimore: Williams and Wilkins, 1979.

20. Larson RL, Cabaud HE, Slocum DB, et al: The patellar compression syndrome: surgical treatment by lateral retinacular release. Clin Orthop 134:158–167, 1978.
21. Laurin DA, Dussault R, Levesque HP: The tangential x-ray investigation of the patellofemoral joint: x-ray technique, diagnostic criteria and their interpretation. Clin Orthop 144:16–26, 1979.
22. MacNab I: Recurrent dislocation of the patella. J Bone Joint Surg 34A:957–967, 1952.
23. Maquet P: Mechanics and osteoarthritis of the patellofemoral joint. Clin Orthop 144:70–73, 1979.
24. McCarroll JR, O'Donoghue DH, Grana WA: The surgical treatment of chondromalacia of the patella. Clin Orthop 175:130–134, 1983.
25. Merchant AC: Classification of patellofemoral disorders. Arthroscopy 4:235–240, 1988.
26. Merchant AC, Mercer RL, Jacobsen RH, Cool CR: Roentgenographic analysis of patellofemoral congruence. J Bone Joint Surg 56A:1391–1396, 1974.
27. Metcalf RW: An arthroscopic method for lateral release of the subluxating or dislocating patella. Clin Orthop 167:9–18, 1982.
28. Minns RJ, Birnie A, Abernethy PJ: A stress analysis of the patella and how it relates to patellar articular cartilage lesions. J Biomech 12:699–711, 1979.
29. Muse GL, Grana WA, Hollingsworth S: Arthroscopic treatment of medial shelf syndrome. Arthroscopy 1:63–67, 1985.
30. O'Neill DB, Micheli LJ: Overuse injuries in the young athlete. Clin Sports Med 7:591–610, 1988.
31. Outerbridge RE, Dunlop J: The problem of chondromalacia patellae. Clin Orthop 110:177–196, 1975.
32. Peeples RE, Margo MK: Function after patellectomy. Clin Orthop 132:180–186, 1978.
33. Radin EL: A rational approach to the treatment of patellofemoral pain. Clin Orthop 144:107–109, 1979.
34. Schutzer SF, Ramsby GR, Fulkerson JP: Computed tomographic classification of patellofemoral pain patients. Orthop Clin North Am 17:235–248, 1986.
35. Schutzer SF, Ramsby GR, Fulkerson JP: The evaluation of patellofemoral pain using computerized tomography: a preliminary study. Clin Orthop 204:286–293, 1986.
36. Weightman B, Chappell DJ, Jenkins EA: A second study of tensile fatigue properties of human articular cartilage. Ann Rheum Dis 37:58–63, 1978.
37. Yates CK, Grana WA: Patellofemoral pain in children. Clin Orthop 255:36–43, 1990.

CHAPTER 16

Problems of

the Menisci

and Their

Treatment

W. Dilworth Cannon, Jr., M.D.

■

In 1883, a century ahead of his time, Thomas Annandale performed a suture repair of a torn anterior horn of a medial meniscus in a laborer.[3] The patient was able to return to work 10 weeks later. This achievement was not appreciated during Annandale's lifetime. Certainly Sutton[93] in 1897 did not recognize the importance of the menisci when he said that they were only the "functionless remains of leg muscle origins."

Don King was the first to relate excision of the meniscus to the development of degenerative arthritis. The idea first came to him while he was examining a patient with unicompartmental gonarthrosis who had undergone a medial meniscectomy 20 years earlier. This led to King's research and eventually to his now famous 1936 publications. In "The Function of Semilunar Cartilages,"[57] he showed that regeneration of the canine meniscus occurred if excision was near the synovial margin; nevertheless, degenerative arthritis occurred. He concluded that "the amount of degeneration appears to be roughly proportional to the size of the segment removed, being greatest when a complete meniscectomy has been done." In another publication, "The Healing of Semilunar Cartilages,"[56] King produced a variety of meniscal tears in canine knees and showed that intrasubstance meniscal tears probably never heal. Tears that communicate with the synovial membrane, however, heal by means of connective tissue originating from the periphery. Partial peripheral tears healed without difficulty. Transverse tears healed with connective tissue ingrowth but spread approximately 2 mm. It is doubtful whether the larger diameter of the meniscus would provide protection from arthritis.

In 1948, Fairbank[29] described three early degenerative changes that followed meniscectomy: (1) the formation of an anteroposterior ridge projecting downward from the margin of the femoral condyle, (2) generalized flattening of the marginal half of the femoral articular surface, and (3) narrowing of the joint space. He found no correlation between clinical and radiographic findings.

Since then, many investigators have determined the deleterious effects of meniscectomy on the knee joint.[2, 4, 13, 16, 35, 45, 50, 52, 54, 59, 63, 64, 66–69, 76, 94, 96, 101] Johnson and co-workers[52] obtained better results after medial meniscectomies than after lateral meniscectomies or removal of both menisci. Overall, 74 per cent of the knees had at least one Fairbank change after meniscectomy and these changes were significantly correlated with clinical result.

Children do not do particularly well after meniscectomy. Medlar and colleagues[68] showed that after a mean follow-up of 8.3 years, only 15 per cent had excellent or good results. In contrast, Northmore-Ball and Dandy[75] in 1982 reported no failures after arthroscopic partial meniscectomy in patients under age 20, but the mean follow-up interval was only 3 years. Perhaps a longer follow-up interval with these patients would have yielded an increasing incidence of knee problems. Johnson and co-workers[52] found that patients under age 21 had fewer excellent results after meniscectomy than did those over 21, although the difference was not significant.

In 1975, Cox[13] demonstrated that the degree of degenerative change in the canine knee was correlated with the amount of meniscus removed. Smillie[90] believed that the best results occurred with complete meniscectomy because meniscal regeneration would produce a replica of the original meniscus. Tapper and Hoover[94] showed that patients who under-

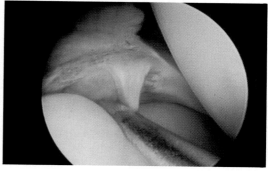

FIGURE 16–1. Radial split tear through the posterior horn origin of the medial meniscus in a right knee. The posterior horn origin is at the lower left. The remaining posterior horn has subluxated posteriorly, providing limited protection against stresses.

went removal of only the bucket-handle fragment instead of a complete meniscectomy had better results. Henning[64] reported that 88 per cent of patients who had either a partial or a total meniscectomy with an anterior cruciate ligament (ACL) reconstruction developed at least one Fairbank radiographic change by 3 years after surgery. O'Brien and associates[76] also reported no major difference between partial and complete meniscectomy in ACL-deficient knees 3 years postoperatively. A different conclusion was reached by McGinty and collaborators.[67] They found that Fairbank's changes were present in 60 per cent of patients who had undergone a complete meniscectomy. In contrast, only 30 per cent who had undergone partial meniscectomy showed such changes at follow-up examination after an average of 5.5 years. Surprisingly, there was no correlation of these radiographic changes with symptomatology. This superiority of partial over complete meniscectomy is further supported by the work of Shrive and co-workers.[88] They showed "that a radial cut through a meniscus, so that no circumferential tension can be developed, is equivalent to meniscectomy in load bearing terms" (Fig. 16–1).

ANATOMY AND BIOMECHANICS

The menisci are semilunar cartilages that act as shims, producing a biconcavity to the tibial plateaus and enabling the femoral condyles to articulate congruently. The medial meniscus has a firm bond to the medial collateral ligament. The thicker lateral meniscus, however, has no ties to the lateral collateral ligament (Fig. 16–2). Because the popliteal tendon

FIGURE 16–2. Drawing of the human tibial plateau, showing the attachments of the medial and lateral menisci and anterior and posterior cruciate ligaments. (Reproduced with permission from Warren RF, Arnocsky SP, Wickiewicz TL: Anatomy of the knee. *In* Nicholas JA, Hershman EB [eds]: The Lower Extremity and Spine in Sports Medicine, pp. 657–694. St Louis: CV Mosby, 1986.)

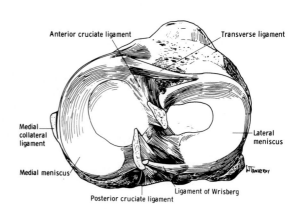

Anterior cruciate ligament

Transverse ligament

Medial collateral ligament

Lateral meniscus

Medial meniscus

Posterior cruciate ligament

Ligament of Wrisberg

courses through the posterolateral corner of the lateral meniscus, there is some additional mobility and decreased vascularity in this location.[5] The popliteal tendon has an attachment to the posterior horn of the lateral meniscus. Both medial and lateral menisci have firm attachment sites at the anterior and posterior horns to resist the hoop tension stresses that occur with axial loading of the joint. The menisci cover substantial areas of the tibial plateaus. The medial meniscus occupies 51 to 74 per cent of the medial plateau, and the lateral meniscus, 75 to 93 per cent of the lateral plateau.[12] The transverse ligament joins the two anterior horns. Despite these attachment sites, the menisci are mobile, especially the lateral meniscus because of the convex shape of the lateral tibial plateau. The rolling and gliding motion of the femoral condyles during flexion results in a femoral rollback of approximately 10 mm on the medial side and 24 mm on the lateral side,[28] with a concomitant similar posterior movement of the menisci. Thompson and colleagues[95] demonstrated the considerable mobility of the menisci during knee motion by using dynamic magnetic resonance imaging (MRI) techniques.

The incidence of certain meniscal tear types varies with age. Vertical longitudinal tears, including displaced bucket-handle tears, tend to occur in the second and third decades of life. Degenerative flap tears and horizontal cleavage tears tend to occur in the fourth decade and beyond. Vertical longitudinal tears are usually amenable to meniscal repair. Degenerative flap tears and horizontal cleavage tears are rarely reparable, and partial meniscectomy is the treatment of choice. In most degenerative menisci, mucoid degeneration is present. Crystalline deposition, such as chondrocalcinosis, may occur in degenerative menisci; the occurrence rate has been reported to be as high as 25 per cent in meniscal tears in patients over age 50.[8]

DIAGNOSIS OF MENISCAL TEARS

The use of MRI and arthrography should not replace a careful history and a thorough physical examination in the diagnosis of a torn meniscus or in the planning of the appropriate treatment. These tools should be used as adjuncts to the clinical workup.

Arthrography

A good-quality double-contrast arthrogram is a highly accurate means of diagnosing medial meniscal disease. Reports in the literature have indicated that the accuracy of an arthrogram in diagnosing meniscal tears ranges from 60 to 97 per cent.[14, 17, 27, 33, 36–38, 48, 55, 58, 87] Accuracy is less for the lateral side than for the medial side because of the presence of dye around the popliteal tendon and hiatus.

Magnetic Resonance Imaging

MRI is the more definitive diagnostic tool for knee joint disease. Although MRI is noninvasive in comparison with arthrography, it is still expensive and is no doubt overused in clinical practice. If a patient exhibits significant clinical findings suggestive of a meniscal tear, a negative MRI scan may not dissuade the arthroscopic surgeon from performing diagnostic arthroscopy. The accuracy of arthroscopy in evaluating meniscal and ACL tears is reported to be 95 per cent.[87]

MRI performed on a 1.5-Tesla imager in 5-mm sections with a dedicated surface coil can provide excellent details of meniscal disease in T1- and T2-weighted images. Reports of the accuracy of MRI in diagnosing meniscal disease, when correlated with subsequent arthroscopic findings, are within a range from 45 to 98 per cent.[32, 49, 62, 65, 78, 82, 89] More recent studies (Mandelbaum et al.,[65] Jackson et al.,[49] Fischer et al.,[32] and Polly et al.[78]) have shown accuracy, sensitivity, and specificity for the medial meniscus to be 92.5 per cent, 95.5 per cent, and 88.7 per cent, respectively. For the lateral meniscus, these values were 91.4 per cent, 73.8 per cent, and 95.7 per cent, respectively. Unlike arthrography, MRI can demonstrate intrameniscal degeneration within intact surfaces (Fig. 16–3). A large amount of degeneration may explain a patient's persisting joint line pain. Fischer and colleagues[32] found that 17 per cent of patients with grade 2 meniscal signals on MRI had a grade 3 tear at arthroscopy.

A primary reason for performing MRI is to assess preoperatively whether a torn meniscus is likely to be reparable. If a tear appears reparable, the pros and cons of meniscal repair versus excision, and the differing postoperative regimens, can be discussed with the patient. In this way, the patient can make an informed choice of treatment before arthroscopy.

In patients with postmeniscectomy symptoms, MRI scans must be interpreted with caution. In most patients who have previously undergone partial meniscectomy MRI shows signals that are suggestive of a persisting or new tear. Only in instances of unstable flaps should the surgeon perform another arthroscopy.[15, 24, 71]

Both MRI and arthrography are useful in confirming the presence of popliteal cysts and cysts of the menisci.

Meniscal Repair Healing Assessment

Unfortunately, MRI has been shown to be misleading in the evaluation of meniscal repair healing. It often produces a grade 3 signal despite lack of clinical and arthroscopic correlation.[15, 25, 53] Arthrography, however, remains an important tool in the assessment of medial meniscal repair healing.

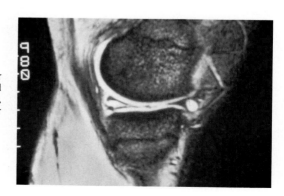

FIGURE 16–3. Magnetic resonance image of the posterior horn of the medial meniscus shows a massive grade 2 signal within the substance of the meniscus. For lesions of this size, there should be a high index of suspicion that a grade 3 tear may be present.

ARTHROSCOPIC MENISCECTOMY: PREFERRED TECHNIQUE

Flap Tear

The flap tear involving the inner meniscal edge is typically a complex oblique tear and not merely a radial cleavage through the meniscus. The inferior surface of the posteromedial corner of the medial meniscus is often involved. The flap is usually anteriorly based at the posterior portion of the middle third of the meniscus (Fig. 16–4). Frequently, it comprises a large portion of the inferior leaf of the posterior horn. The superior leaf is often intact but thinned to the extent that its protective benefit may be marginal.

After identifying a flap tear of the medial meniscus, the surgeon should make certain that there is not a second flap at the posterior horn origin of the medial meniscus. This could occur if there were a broken bucket-handle fragment involving an inferior or superior leaf or the entire posterior horn, which would create a partially hidden flap at the origin of the posterior horn (Fig. 16–5). If missed, a large flap could cause late symptoms of catching.

The surgeon should become facile at inspecting the posteromedial compartment and the origin of the posterior horn from the anterolateral portal. Flap tears at the origin of the posterior horn can easily be identified from this approach. If a tear of the origin of the posterior horn is present, the author treats it first. The probe is placed underneath the posterior horn origin of the medial meniscus. The arthroscope is passed through the intercondylar notch medial to the posterior cruciate ligament into the posteromedial compartment. The probe can be withdrawn easily and moved to the superior surface of the posterior horn of the meniscus. The flap tear is then probed. A 4-mm 30° oblique arthroscope is adequate for accomplishing this visualization. Although a 70° arthroscope is recommended by other authors, this author finds that it is not necessary.

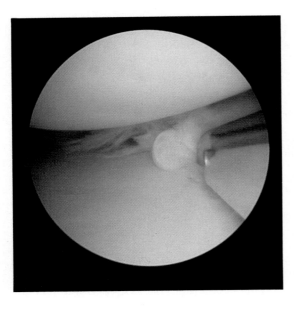

FIGURE 16–4. Typical flap tear of the posterior horn of the medial meniscus in a right knee.

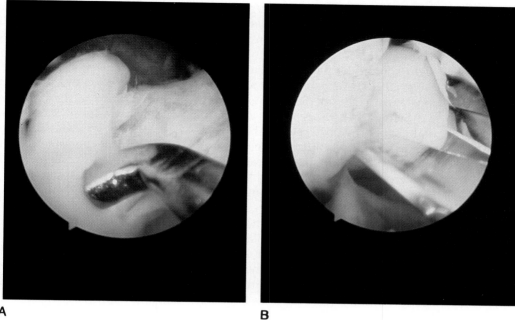

A   B

FIGURE 16–5. (*A*) Vertical flap tear of the origin of the posterior horn. This type of tear may be missed unless the arthroscope is brought through the intercondylar notch to the posteromedial compartment. (*B*) Resection of this fragment is carried out with a small rongeur that is introduced from the anteromedial portal and brought back to the origin of the posterior horn in the medial meniscus.

While the origin of the posterior horn is visualized through the intercondylar notch, the anteromedial portal should be widened with the use of a blunt obturator. A 1-mm straight basket rongeur is introduced and directed to the flap tear of the posterior horn in the same manner as for the previously passed probe. If the flap is lying in a vertical orientation, as many do, the rongeur should be rotated to a horizontal position. The base of the flap is carefully resected until approximately 80 to 90 percent of the base is transected. The mobile flap can then be grasped with a small clamp, avulsed from the posterior horn origin, and withdrawn from the joint. If the flap is not in a vertical orientation, it may be morselized with a basket rongeur. The author occasionally finds a 15° up-biting rongeur to be useful in this location. By rotating the rongeur, access can be gained to a larger portion of the medial meniscus.

If the meniscal fragment is completely transected by mistake and falls into the posteromedial compartment, the surgeon should try pulling it anteriorly in order to avoid the necessity of making a posteromedial incision. An attempt might be made to suck out the fragment anteriorly by inserting a neurosurgical sucker tip through the intercondylar notch from the anteromedial portal into the posteromedial compartment and then applying suction. Sometimes, the meniscal fragment may stick to the sucker tip. If this happens, the fragment should be withdrawn slowly through the intercondylar notch, and the meniscal fragment should be dragged to the anterior part of the joint, where it can be easily removed.

Sometimes digital pressure in the popliteal fossa may accomplish positioning of the fragment near the origin of the posterior horn, where it might be grasped from an anterior portal. If this cannot be accomplished and the meniscal fragment remains in the posteromedial compartment, it is necessary to make a posteromedial portal in order to remove the fragment. With the knee in 90° of flexion, the arthroscope is passed through the intercondylar notch as previously described. It produces a light spot at the posteromedial corner of the knee. This spot is visualized most clearly in a partially darkened room. After palpation of the soft spot posterior to the medial collateral ligament and anterior to the hamstring tendons, an 18-gauge spinal needle then can be introduced through the light spot. The portal should be only skin deep in order to avoid damaging the saphenous vein or nerve. While full distension of the knee is maintained, a blunt or sharp trocar can be used to make an opening into the posteromedial compartment. A pituitary rongeur or a grasping clamp is used to remove the fragment, just as a loose body would be removed from this location.

After the posterior horn has been inspected and the pathologic process attended to, the remaining flap tear at the posteromedial corner of the medial meniscus is brought into view. Placing a straight or an angled rongeur through the anteromedial portal rarely provides a good angle for resection. Therefore, the arthroscope is switched to the anteromedial portal, and the joint is crossed from the anterolateral portal with a 1-mm basket rongeur. This technique consistently enables the surgeon to produce an initial cut into the central portion of the medial meniscus that is smooth and gently tapering from the inner edge of the anterior horn (Fig. 16–6). A right-angled rongeur introduced through the anteromedial portal cannot accomplish this resection as well as this technique.

The resection then continues posteriorly to the base of the flap tear. The cut is brought to the tear site by the rongeur from the anterolateral portal. Before removing the rongeur, the surgeon must make sure that there are no additional small flaps or oblique cleavage tears on the inferior surface of the middle third of the meniscus. Use of the rongeur is the best means of resecting and smoothing off small tears in this area. The arthroscope is moved back to the anterolateral portal, and a small rongeur

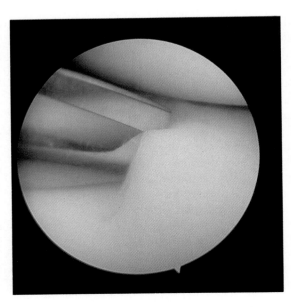

FIGURE 16–6. The author's preferred technique in resecting a flap tear (see Fig. 16–4) is to switch the arthroscope to the anteromedial portal and bring a small rongeur in from the anterolateral portal. This allows excellent contouring of the inner edge of the middle third of the meniscus.

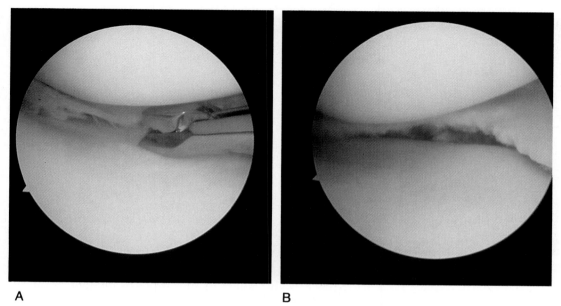

A   B

FIGURE 16–7. (A) After removal of the flap tear (see Fig. 16–4), the posterior horn irregularity is smoothed off and resected back to stable meniscal tissue. (B) The final appearance of the tear after partial medial meniscectomy.

is introduced anteromedially. The cut is continued posteriorly and blended with the remaining posterior horn (Fig. 16–7). If the flap is sizable, it should be cut just enough to allow a small tag of meniscal tissue to remain, just as with flaps of the origin of the posterior horn. A grasper can be used to avulse the fragment and remove it through the anteromedial portal.

Any remaining irregularity of the inner edge of the meniscus can be trimmed with a rongeur or a shaver. If the remaining rim of the meniscus has a vertical inner edge, the surgeon should attempt to make the superior surface of the meniscus slightly beveled. This beveling creates a triangular shape to the inner meniscal edge. Any irregularity remaining on the posterior horn of the meniscus should be trimmed back with a broad-nosed rongeur or shaver. If the tear involves the superior leaf, and if the inner edge of this leaf is difficult to reach because of obstruction by the medial femoral condyle, an up-biting rongeur should be used.

If the surgeon encounters difficulty in a tight medial compartment, the superior leaf can be brought down, by several methods, to a position at which it can be trimmed back. For example, by firm digital palpation posteromedially in the popliteal fossa, the meniscus can occasionally be pushed further anteriorly into the joint. A uniformly successful technique involves introducing an 18-gauge spinal needle through an accessory anteromedial portal, approximately 2 cm medial to the usual anteromedial portal, in order to depress the posterior horn. If visualization of the posterior horn is still not adequate, a nerve hook can be introduced in order to accomplish the same task (Fig. 16–8). Further trimming from the conventional anteromedial portal can then be performed.

The accessory anteromedial portal can be placed further posteriorly if there is difficulty. If necessary, the portal can be placed far enough posteriorly so that a 1-mm straight basket rongeur can be passed over the

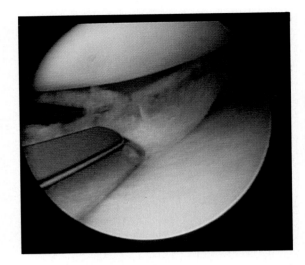

FIGURE 16–8. When posterior horn visualization is difficult as in the case of this torn left medial meniscus, a nerve hook can be introduced through an accessory medial portal in order to pull the posterior horn fragment anteriorly for better visualization. Notice the nerve hook to the left just above the rongeur.

posteromedial surface of the meniscus and brought parallel to the inner edge of the posterior horn to trim off any remaining flaps. If the medial compartment is tight, the surgeon should stand and exert a continuous valgus force with the patient's knee in approximately 15° of flexion. The medial collateral ligament and capsule have some amount of viscoelasticity. Constant valgus force applied for several minutes usually opens the medial compartment enough to enable passage of instruments to the posterior horn. At the end of the meniscal resection, each compartment of the joint should be thoroughly irrigated. This procedure cleanses the joint of meniscal debris, which if not removed may cause chronic synovitis.

The author prefers to use hand instruments rather than power cutters to accomplish meniscal resection. He occasionally uses a power cutter to smooth a frayed meniscal rim, especially a torn anterior horn of the lateral meniscus that is difficult to approach from the conventional anterior portals. He does not use electrocautery for meniscal resection; he believes that it is slower than hand-held mechanical cutting tools and may pose some risk of damage to underlying articular cartilage. In addition, Miller and associates[70] showed retardation of meniscal healing after electrocautery in animal models.

Some authors have advocated laser surgery for meniscal excision. In addition to the high up-front expense of purchasing a laser unit, the author does not believe that it is significantly faster, in view of its required set-up time. The argument by laser surgeons that posterior horn disease that is difficult to reach can easily be handled with the laser probe is controversial. A tight medial compartment in which resection of the posterior horn cannot be accomplished by the conventional techniques just described is extremely rare.

Displaced Bucket-Handle Tears

A displaced bucket-handle tear of the medial meniscus can be clinically diagnosed preoperatively by the presentation of a locked knee, by MRI, or by arthrography. The alternatives of treatment, including the possibility of meniscal repair, should be thoroughly discussed with the patient preoperatively. In patients under the age of 50, serious consideration should be given to meniscal repair of displaced bucket-handle tears unless the anatomic aspects of the tear dictate excision. Considerations for excision include (1) a significant radial split tear in the substance of the displaced bucket-handle fragment, (2) a rim size of 5 mm or more (which would place the tear well within the avascular zone of the meniscus), and (3) a grossly deformed, twisted-on-itself, chronic tear in which the meniscus cannot be pushed back to its normal position against the rim.

One of the author's patients presented with a chronically displaced, deformed bucket-handle tear. The patient wanted meniscal repair and ACL reconstruction, but not at the time of initial arthroscopy. The bucket-handle fragment was displaced in a position that partially locked the knee. With the patient under local anesthesia, the meniscus was pushed back to its normal location and the knee was kept fully extended in an immobilizer for 2 weeks postoperatively. At the time of meniscal repair and ACL reconstruction 4 months later, the patient had experienced no further locking episodes. The meniscus was not displaced and had remodeled itself to look like a normal meniscal segment, which is typical of a nondisplaced vertical-longitudinal tear. Repair was easily accomplished. Even in chronically displaced, deformed meniscal bucket-handle fragments, a certain amount of remodeling of the meniscal fragment occurs once it has been reattached at its orthotopic location.

Excision of the bucket-handle fragment of the medial meniscus (Fig. 16–9) requires pushing the displaced bucket-handle fragment back to its normal position by a nerve hook through the anteromedial portal (Fig. 16–10). If difficulty in accomplishing this is encountered, the surgeon must make sure that the patient's knee is in a position of 15° or less of extension. This usually provides a wider medial compartment opening and allows the displaced bucket-handle fragment to reduce. Difficulty in accomplishing reduction is usually the result of too much knee flexion.

The arthroscope is passed through the intercondylar notch from the anterolateral portal to the posteromedial compartment to the origin of the posterior horn of the medial meniscus. From an anteromedial portal, the posterior horn can be manipulated and the exact location of the origin of the vertical longitudinal tear can be located easily. The origin of the posterior horn of the handle fragment is resected by passing a 1-mm

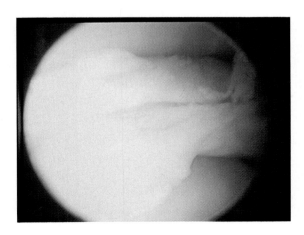

FIGURE 16–9. Anterior visualization of a displaced bucket-handle tear of the medial meniscus in a right knee.

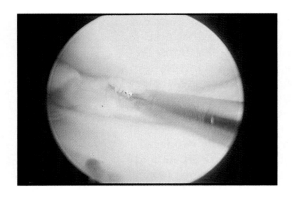

FIGURE 16–10. Reduction of the displaced bucket-handle tear is accomplished with a nerve hook and with the knee in approximately 10° to 15° of flexion.

straight basket rongeur from the anteromedial portal to the origin of the posterior horn. The cut should begin from the origin of the posterior horn and should continue in a peripheral direction to coincide with the exact location of the beginning of the tear cleft (Fig. 16–11).

Once the final cut has been made, the posterior horn attachment of the bucket-handle fragment becomes loose. The arthroscope is moved to the anteromedial portal so that the anterior attachment site of the handle fragment is visualized. A probe is inserted anterolaterally, and the anterior attachment site is palpated. A 1-mm straight basket rongeur or a 15° up-biting rongeur is brought across from the anterolateral portal. A cut is begun in the anterior horn and is aimed toward the origin of the tear (Fig. 16–12). Once this incision is made, the handle fragment is completely mobile. The author usually finishes trimming the nubbin of tissue that remains anteriorly at the tear site before grasping the handle fragment, because the position of the instrument is ideal. A right-angle basket rongeur introduced from the anterolateral portal is occasionally needed for removing the nubbin of tissue on the anterior horn.

Once selection of either the anteromedial or anterolateral portal is made, the surgeon should make sure that it is enlarged enough to enable withdrawal of the fragment. The knife can be used to widen the portal, and the synovial slit can be widened further by opening the jaws of a grasping clamp while it is withdrawn. The bucket-handle fragment is grasped at its end and withdrawn (Fig. 16–13). If there is difficulty in locating the end of the fragment, it should be manipulated until the end is grasped (grasping the midportion of the fragment leads to unnecessary difficulty). The author uses this technique on the less commonly encoun-

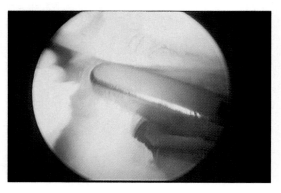

FIGURE 16–11. Resection of the bucket-handle tear should start at the origin of the posterior horn after reduction of the fragment. The arthroscope is adjacent to the posterior cruciate ligament and provides excellent visualization of the posterior horn origin. Transection of the posterior horn attachment is accomplished with a small rongeur introduced through the anteromedial portal.

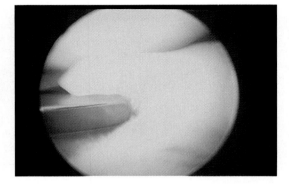

FIGURE 16–12. After the posterior horn attachment of the fragment has been transected, the anterior horn attachment is cut with a rongeur that is introduced through the anterolateral portal.

tered displaced bucket-handle tear of the lateral meniscus. Resecting the anterior horn attachment of the bucket-handle fragment, however, may be more difficult because of the smaller radius of curvature of the lateral meniscus and its posteriorly situated anterior horn. In this situation, the handle fragment should be released from its anterior attachment site with a right-angled up-biting rongeur. An accessory anterolateral portal made 1 or 2 cm lateral to the conventional anterolateral portal may allow a better angle of resection of the anterior horn.

Single Vertical Longitudinal Tears

This tear pattern is most amenable to meniscal repair. It is again emphasized that preoperative discussion with the patient about this option eliminates the dilemma of not knowing the patient's attitude toward meniscal repair and the different postoperative regimens. If excision is elected, the same technique as described for the displaced bucket-handle tear should be used.

Double and Triple Bucket-Handle Tears

For the double bucket-handle tear (Fig. 16–14) and the more rare triple bucket-handle tear, the author recommends using the same approach as

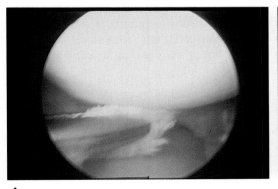
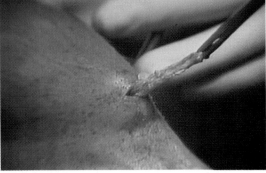

A   **B**

FIGURE 16–13. (A) The bucket-handle fragment is now free in the joint, and a rongeur is shown grasping its cut anterior end. (B) Removal of the bucket-handle fragment through the anterolateral portal.

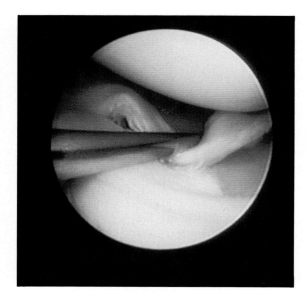

FIGURE 16–14. Displaced double bucket-handle tear of the medial meniscus in a left knee. The probe is on the posterior section of the two fragments. The tear was deemed irreparable, and both fragments were excised.

with the single vertical longitudinal tear. Displaced fragments should be repositioned in their normal location. On occasion, meniscal repair can be carried out. If not, the author recommends release of the posterior horn attachment of the first bucket-handle fragment. The author follows this with an incision of the anterior horn attachment site and removal of the fragment. A second or third bucket-handle fragment can be removed in an identical manner.

Horizontal Cleavage Tears

Horizontal cleavage tears have been thought to be frequently associated with tears of the posterior horn or the middle third of the lateral meniscus (Fig. 16–15). Nevertheless, it is not uncommon to encounter them in the posterior horn of the medial meniscus. Wherever their location, they should be thoroughly probed in order to determine the more substantial and stable leaf. An unstable or torn segment can then be resected back with basket rongeurs to the point at which it will no longer cause mechanical symptoms. The resection should not be carried back to the periphery of the meniscus. If the remaining segment is stable, it should remain asymptomatic. There is a tendency for surgeons to resect too much meniscal tissue for horizontal cleavage tears. Leaving a tear with a depth of up to 3 mm is usually quite acceptable.

Radial Split Tears

Many radial split tears involving either the medial or lateral meniscus may be asymptomatic and discovered only when arthroscopic surgery is performed for a different condition. In 1978 the author performed arthroscopic surgery on a young adult. A radial split tear was found in the middle third of the lateral meniscus, penetrating to a depth of approximately 4 mm from its inner rim (Fig. 16–16). The patient had no lateral

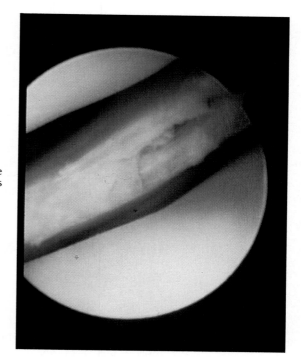

FIGURE 16–15. A partially resected horizontal cleavage tear of the lateral meniscus in a left knee is shown. It is usually safe to leave a cleavage up to 3 mm deep.

symptoms, and the tear was left alone. Four years later, at the time of a second arthroscopy, there was no change in the extent of the tear. The patient remained asymptomatic on the lateral side.

If a symptomatic radial split tear is encountered, simple trimming back of the anterior and posterior leaves immediately adjacent to the tear should be sufficient treatment. Radial split tears of the posterior horn of the lateral meniscus near its origin are frequently associated with ACL tears. An attempt should be made to repair rather than excise them. Because there is a rich blood supply to the posterior horn of the lateral meniscus, repair is usually successful and results in the maintenance of meniscal continuity and function. On occasion, a radial split tear may be part of a complex tear in which the peripheral component of the tear is part of a vertical longitudinal tear or an L-shaped tear.

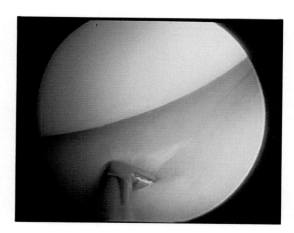

FIGURE 16–16. Four years after a radial split was noted in the middle third of a right lateral meniscus, there was no change in its appearance, and the knee was asymptomatic.

Degenerative Tears

Degenerative tears typically occur in older patients, and associated joint space narrowing is documented on a posteroanterior bent-knee, weight-bearing radiograph.[84] Patients may have loading type pain or mechanical symptoms such as catching. At arthroscopy, a conservative approach with the purpose of preservation of meniscal tissue should be the guideline. Older patients with significant joint space narrowing should be warned before surgery that partial meniscectomy does not offer as high a degree of success as in younger patients with an intact joint space and that progression of the arthritic process can be expected. If indicated, an extensive synovectomy and removal of any impinging osteophytes should be part of the procedure.[8]

THE DISCOID LATERAL MENISCUS

The incidence of discoid lateral menisci has been reported to be between 1.4 and 15.5 per cent.[1] Ikeuchi[47] reported an incidence of 16.6 per cent in the Japanese population. This figure includes patients with different types of discoid lateral menisci, and the true incidence of complete discoid lateral menisci is considerably lower. Watanabe and collaborators[98] divided discoid lateral menisci into three types: the complete, the incomplete, and the Wrisberg types. The complete type (Fig. 16–17) covers almost the entirety of the lateral tibial plateau. The complete discoid lateral meniscus may be thickened, and mucoid degeneration is more extensive within its substance than in normal menisci. In the Wrisberg type, a lateral meniscofemoral ligament, or ligament of Wrisberg, provides attachment to the origin of the posterior horn. There is a deficiency in meniscotibial attachment of the posterior horn, leaving the meniscus hypermobile. The incomplete type is more difficult to define. The diagnosis depends on the arthroscopist's subjective evaluation of the width of the meniscus; thus it is possible that the incidence of the incomplete type is overreported.

Symptoms include pain, swelling, giving way, clicking, and snapping. Kroiss[60] coined the term "snapping knee syndrome" to describe a torn discoid lateral meniscus.

Aichroth and associates[1] showed an association between discoid

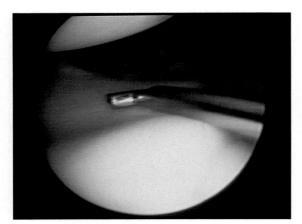

FIGURE 16–17. Complete discoid lateral meniscus in a right knee. The inner edge of the meniscus is adjacent to the intercondylar notch.

lateral meniscus and osteochondritis dissecans that affected the lateral femoral condyle in 7 of 62 knees with discoid lateral menisci. Therefore, osteochondritis dissecans should be ruled out in children with lateral compartment symptoms in the presence of a discoid lateral meniscus.

The diagnosis can be established by a good-quality arthrogram, MRI, or arthroscopy. Treatment may consist of leaving the meniscus alone, partial excision, total excision, or repair. The incidental finding of a discoid lateral meniscus during arthroscopy should not tempt the surgeon to remove it.

Partial discoid lateral meniscectomy may provide reasonable results in the complete and incomplete types.[34, 41] It is not a treatment option for the Wrisberg type unless posterior horn peripheral reattachment is performed at the same time. Hayashi and co-workers[41] recommended leaving a 6-mm rim for complete discoid menisci and an 8-mm rim for the incomplete type; they found no new tears developing in the rim in follow-up.

Ikeuchi[47] reported better results in patients undergoing total meniscectomy than in those with partial meniscectomy after an average follow-up interval of 4.3 years.

Kurosaka and colleagues,[61] in a follow-up of 33 patients with 35 open complete discoid lateral meniscectomies and a minimum follow-up interval of 20 years, found that of the patients under the age of 20 when surgery was performed, more than 85 per cent showed excellent or good results. However, radiographic assessment revealed moderate to severe joint degeneration in 75 per cent of the patients.

Arthroscopic or open repair of a torn discoid lateral meniscus may provide the best protection against later degenerative arthritis and provide the patient with a functional knee. In his series of 24 knees, Ikeuchi[47] performed peripheral meniscal repair under arthroscopic control in three patients but did not report long-term results. Rosenberg and co-workers[83] reported successful arthroscopic repair of a Wrisberg type of discoid lateral meniscus after central partial arthroscopic meniscectomy. A 1-year second-look arthroscopy revealed successful healing. Neuschwander and associates[74] reported seven patients with the Wrisberg type of discoid lateral menisci who underwent open attachment at the meniscocapsular junction. After an average follow-up interval of 2.4 years, none of the patients were having clinical symptoms of catching, swelling, or giving way.

MENISCAL CYSTS

Popliteal cysts were once thought to be associated with tears of the posterior horn of the medial meniscus, although they do not connect with the medial meniscus. The cyst orifice is usually in the posteromedial capsule below the origin of the medial head of the gastrocnemius muscle. The cysts may develop with any condition that causes an increase in intra-articular pressure, such as a meniscal tear, chondromalacia, arthritis, loose bodies, and synovitis. If a popliteal cyst is associated with a torn meniscus, taking care of the meniscal problem should resolve the popliteal cyst. Rarely is surgical excision of the cyst necessary. The technique of Rauschning[80] is preferred.

Lateral meniscal cysts typically include the middle third of the meniscus. They invariably are associated with a horizontal cleavage tear or are combined with a radial split tear.[7, 30] Patients usually have a tender lump along the lateral joint line, with or without intra-articular symptoms laterally. If the condition fails to improve after an appropriate conservative regimen, arthroscopic surgery is indicated. If a typical pathologic process is found, partial lateral meniscectomy usually results in resolution of intra-articular symptoms and the disappearance of the cyst. The latter is more likely to occur if an attempt is made to eviscerate or externally press the cyst contents through its communicating orifice through the meniscal cleavage tear and into the joint (Fig. 16–18). On occasion, a motorized small shaver may be introduced through the orifice of the cyst in order to accomplish its ablation. The objective of surgery is to remove enough of the meniscal unstable flaps that the low-grade synovitis is eliminated, but to conserve as much of the meniscus as possible. Some surgeons[81, 100] have recommended extra-articular excision of the cyst; the author does not find that this is necessary.

Parisien[77] reported 22 lateral and 3 medial meniscal cysts that were treated by arthroscopic partial meniscectomy; there was no recurrence of the cysts after an average follow-up interval of 33.5 months. The average age of the patients was 30 years. Ferriter and Nisonson[31] reported similar excellent results in a group of 18 patients treated by partial lateral meniscectomy for symptomatic lateral meniscal cysts.

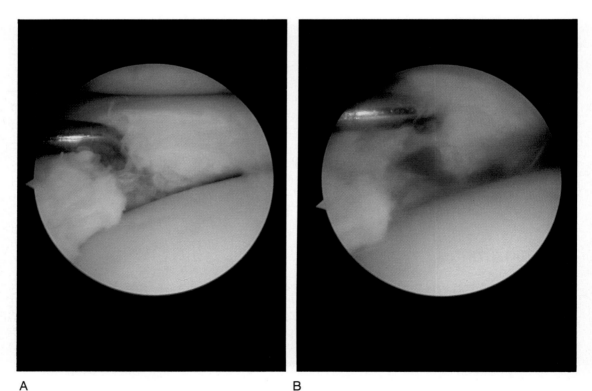

A   B

FIGURE 16–18. (A) A cyst along the lateral joint line of a right knee and a communicating horizontal cleavage tear through the lateral meniscus. (B) After partial resection of the tear, external pressure on the cyst resulted in the exiting of yellowish fluid through the orifice into the joint.

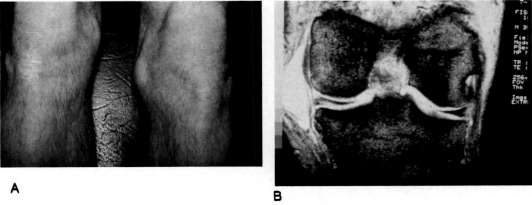

FIGURE 16–19. (*A*) Photograph of a cyst of the medial meniscus of a left knee. (*B*) Magnetic resonance image demonstrating communication between a tear of the posterior horn of the medial meniscus and the cyst.

The pathogenesis of medial meniscal cysts is similar to that of lateral meniscal cysts. They usually occur more posteriorly in the meniscus, typically at the posteromedial corner of the knee (Fig. 16–19). The incidence of medial meniscal cysts is lower than that of lateral cysts, but the symptoms are the same, and treatment should be the same as for the lateral side.

OPEN MENISCAL REPAIR

In the late 1970s, several surgeons began to repair peripheral tears of the meniscus through an open technique.[10, 22, 26, 39, 79] Price and Allen[79] in 1978 reported on repair of peripheral medial meniscal disruptions associated with medial collateral ligament tears. A follow-up of 36 patients revealed that 33 had no limitations caused by knee impairment. Cassidy and Shaffer[10] reported encouraging results in open meniscal repair of 29 menisci torn in the peripheral third. Hamberg and collaborators[39] in 1983 reported clinically apparent healing after open meniscal repair of 84 per

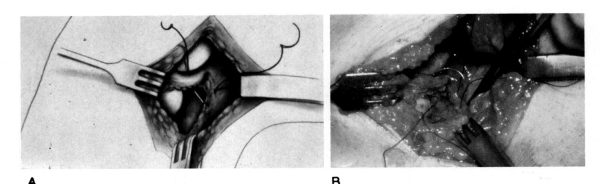

FIGURE 16–20. (*A* and *B*) DeHaven's technique of open medial meniscal repair. The meniscal rim is sutured to its attached synovial bed with the use of vertically placed absorbable 4-0 mattress sutures. With double-armed sutures, a small needle is passed from the inferior to the superior surface of the meniscus, and a larger needle is passed from below up through the capsular bed. (From DeHaven KE, Black JP, Griffiths HJ: Open meniscus repair: technique and two to nine year results. Am J Sports Med 6:788, 1989.)

cent of 50 torn menisci. Arthroscopy was repeated in 64 per cent of the patients, and there was evidence of healing in all of them. In the eight patients who had a second tear, four tears occurred at a new area of the meniscus and were associated with new trauma. DeHaven and co-workers[21-23] started to repair peripheral meniscal tears (up to a 2.5-mm rim size) in 1976. DeHaven's technique for repair of medial meniscal tears in the posterior horn involves a 2-inch vertical posteromedial skin incision and an oblique capsular incision just posterior to the trailing edge of the medial collateral ligament. The edges of the meniscus are debrided and freshened with a curette. Double-armed 4-0 polyglactin 910 (Vicryl) sutures containing a small needle on one end and a larger needle at the other are used. The small needle is passed inferiorly through the meniscal rim. The larger needle is passed from below through the capsular bed, and the suture is tied (Fig. 16–20). DeHaven also used a "king stitch" consisting of a boxlike horizontal mattress suture of 2-0 Vicryl through the most vulnerable portion of the tear site.

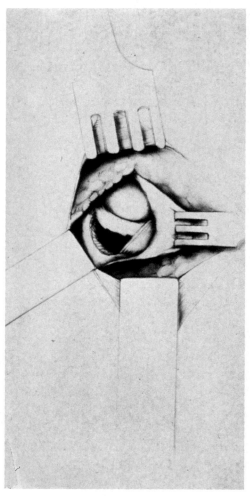
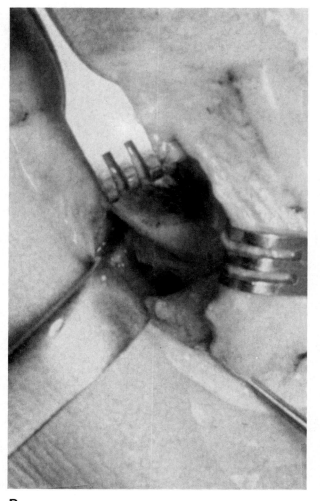

A   **B**

FIGURE 16–21. (*A* and *B*) DeHaven's technique for a repair of a peripheral tear of the posterior horn of the lateral meniscus that extends to the popliteus hiatus.

For repairs of the posterior horn of the lateral meniscus, the iliotibial band is split in line with its fibers. The capsule is opened vertically along the posterior border of the popliteal tendon. The first suture is passed from the superior surface of the meniscus to emerge inferiorly. It then passes through the fibers that run from the popliteal tendon to the lateral meniscus and through the synovial bed (Fig. 16–21).

Rehabilitation consists of touchdown weight bearing for 6 weeks. Two weeks after surgery, limited active motion from 30° to 70° is initiated. Four weeks after surgery, free motion is allowed. From 3 to 6 months, patients begin to jog and swim. Full speed running, agility maneuvering, and full squatting start at 6 months.

DeHaven and Lohrer[23] reported on long-term follow-up results of 33 open meniscal repairs; the average follow-up interval was 11 years. No patients were lost to follow-up. Meniscal survival rate in this study was 79 per cent, in contrast to 89 per cent reported in an earlier series[21] of 80

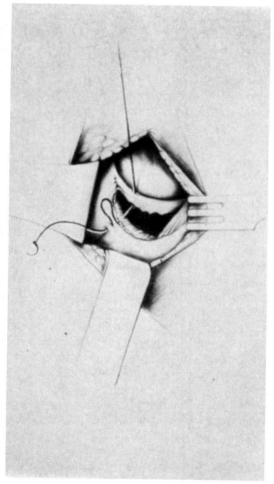
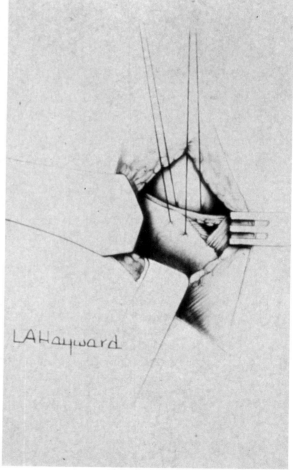

C

D

FIGURE 16–21. *Continued.* (*C* and *D*) The suture is passed from the superior to the inferior surface of the meniscus through the popliteal fibers to the lateral meniscus and then through the synovial bed. (From DeHaven KE, Black JP, Griffiths HJ: Open meniscus repair: technique and two to nine year results. Am J Sports Med 6:788, 1989.)

repairs followed for at least 2 years. DeHaven and Lohrer divided the knees into stable knees (3 mm or less involved-uninvolved difference), nearly stable knees (greater than 3 mm and less than 4.5 mm involved-uninvolved anterior displacement difference), and unstable knees (more than 4.5 mm involved-uninvolved difference). Among nine stable knees repaired, there was one meniscal retear; among nine nearly stable knees, there was one retear; and among the 12 unstable knees, there were five retears (42 per cent). The average time to meniscal retear was 4 years (the range was 1.2 to 9.4 years). All but one were new tears in the meniscus. Retears occurred in three (14 per cent) of 21 acute meniscal tears and in four (33 per cent) of 12 chronic meniscal tears. There was no significant difference in the retear rate between lateral and medial meniscal repairs. Radiographic follow-up in all 33 knees revealed no or mild changes (less than 2-mm joint space narrowing or sclerosis). None had moderate or severe changes.

Sommerlath,[91] in a study of 50 patients with follow-up intervals of 6 to 9 years, noted a 24 per cent failure rate after meniscal repair. She also noted the same incidence of repeated surgery after partial meniscectomy. Knee function was significantly better after meniscus repair than after meniscectomy ($p < .025$). Radiologic evaluation in 96 per cent of the patients revealed that patients with meniscal repair had less osteoarthritis than did patients with partial meniscectomy ($p < .05$).

Open meniscal repair is an established alternative to arthroscopic meniscal repair for vertical longitudinal peripheral tears (rim size less than 2.5 mm) of the posterior horns of the menisci.

ARTHROSCOPIC MENISCAL REPAIR

Except for the most peripheral type of meniscal tear, most surgeons consider arthroscopic meniscal repair easier to perform than open meniscal repair.[9, 40] For rim sizes that are 3 mm or larger, arthroscopic meniscal repair is the only technique to use (Fig. 16–22). Since Ikeuchi[46] reported the first four arthroscopic meniscal repairs, performed from 1969 to 1974, the technique has undergone significant changes and improvements. Henning[42] in 1980 performed the first arthroscopic meniscal repair in North America. At present, there are three techniques for arthroscopic meniscal repair: the inside-outside, outside-inside, and inside-inside techniques. For each of these basic techniques, a variety of meniscal repair sets are commercially available. Ideally, more than one technique and more than one set of instruments should be at the surgeon's disposal. Particular meniscal tear patterns may lend themselves to repair by a technique other than the surgeon's usual one. Suturing should start near or at the origin of the posterior horn for tears in this location. Sutures should be placed in a vertical orientation near the periphery of the meniscus in order to get a good hold on as many circumferentially oriented collagen bundles as possible (Fig. 16–23). Adjacent sutures should be placed close together so that a partially unstable tear is not left at the end of suturing, which could lead to a retear. In addition, sutures should be alternated between the inferior and superior surfaces so as to provide better coaptation of the meniscal fragment against the rim.

Adequate preparation of the rim and the handle or fragment portion

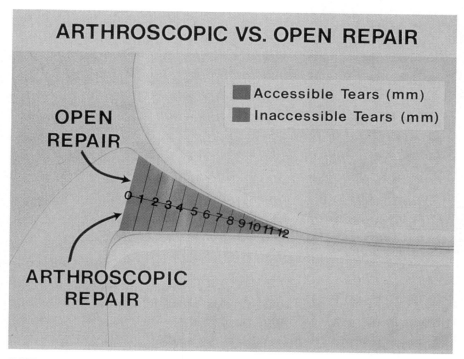

FIGURE 16–22. Arthroscopic versus open repair. The upper half of the meniscus shows the accessibility of the meniscus to open repair; the green area reveals that the surgeon cannot gain access to tears that have rim widths of more than 2.5 to 3.0 mm. In contrast, arthroscopic techniques can repair meniscal tears with rim widths of more than 4.0 mm. (From Cannon WD: Arthroscopic meniscal repair. *In* McGinty JB [ed]: Operative Arthroscopy, p. 237. New York: Raven Press, 1991.)

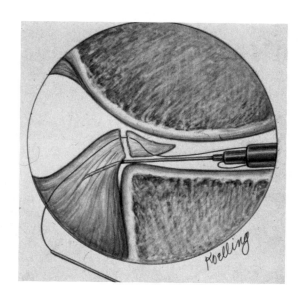

FIGURE 16–23. Diagram of Henning's technique shows the placement of divergent vertically oriented mattress sutures. (From Cannon WD: Arthroscopic meniscal repair. *In* McGinty JB [ed]: Operative Arthroscopy, p. 240. New York: Raven Press, 1991.)

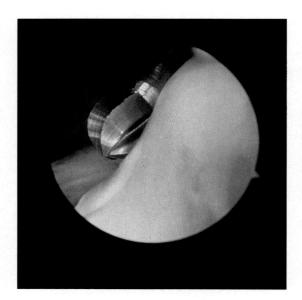

FIGURE 16–24. A 2-mm burr-type rasp has been introduced through the posteromedial incision while viewing is accomplished through the intercondylar notch in a right knee. Parameniscal synovial abrasion is carried out over the superior surface of the meniscus and in the tear site. (From Cannon WD: Arthroscopic meniscal repair. *In* McGinty JB [ed]: Operative Arthroscopy, p. 239. New York: Raven Press, 1991.)

of the tear is necessary. Abrasion of the synovium and the meniscal tear site with rasps 3 mm and smaller is now standard practice (Fig. 16–24). The neovascular response produced provides an adjunct to the healing process.[9] After meniscal repair, second-look arthroscopy may reveal a synovial pannus growing over the meniscus to the previous site of the tear.

The question of whether to use nonabsorbable or absorbable suture material for meniscal repair is still a subject of debate. More surgeons currently are using nonabsorbable than absorbable suture material. Because meniscal healing goes on for many months, these surgeons believe that the presence of nonabsorbable suture material is important during this period. Jokl and colleagues[53] performed an MRI study after meniscal repair with the use of absorbable sutures. They found several cases of widening of the grade 3 signal zone at the repair site 3 to 6 months after surgery. They recommended the use of nonabsorbable sutures.

MODIFIED HENNING TECHNIQUE

Medial Meniscal Repair

The author prefers to keep the patient flat on the table and not to "break" the end of the table. This procedure may lessen the incidence of well-leg nerve palsies and thromboembolic complications. A tourniquet is placed high on the thigh, and a leg holder is distal to the tourniquet. A gel-filled pad is placed posteriorly in order to distribute pressure evenly, and the hip is flexed approximately 30° to 45° (Fig. 16–25). This enables free access to both the posteromedial and posterolateral corners of the knee. ACL reconstruction can be performed without repositioning the leg. Rarely is the tourniquet used during meniscal repair. Because 80 per cent of meniscal repair cases in the author's practice are associated with ACL reconstruction, he tries to save tourniquet time for the ACL reconstruction.

An arthroscopic sweep of the knee is performed in order to substantiate the need for medial meniscal repair. The posterior horn is adequately probed from an anterior portal. The arthroscope is passed from the anterolateral portal medial to the posterior cruciate ligament to the posteromedial compartment in order to directly visualize the posterior horn. A posteromedial incision is made; this is best accomplished by visualizing the light spot at the posteromedial corner of the flexed knee with the arthroscope in the posteromedial compartment. The posteromedial longitudinal incision is approximately 5 to 6 cm in length and centered at the joint line.

Dissection must be performed carefully so as to avoid injury to the saphenous vein and the sartorial branch of the saphenous nerve. The pes anserinus should be retracted posteriorly by making the dissection anterior to the sartorius. Dissection should be between the posteromedial capsule and the direct head of the semimembranosus muscle to approximately halfway across the medial head of the gastrocnemius muscle. Blunt dissection enables the specially designed popliteal retractor to be placed immediately behind the posterior horn of the medial meniscus, in an extra-articular position. Posteromedial dissection is more difficult to accomplish than posterolateral dissection because the direct head of the semimembranosus muscle may push the retractor in a proximal direction. It is occasionally necessary to cut part of the attachment of the direct head of the semimembranosus muscle in order to retrieve sutures exiting below the joint line posteriorly. While visualizing the posteromedial corner of the joint, the surgeon introduces a spinal needle through the synovium for determining accurate placement of a 3- or 4-mm nick in the synovium for rasp introduction.

A rasp 3 mm or smaller is introduced under direct visualization. Abrasion of the meniscosynovial junction is performed over the superior

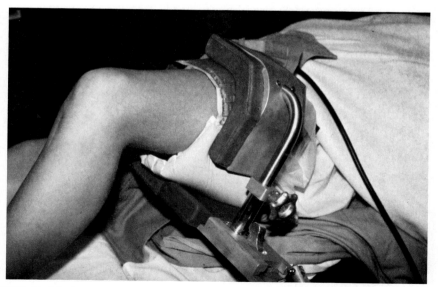

FIGURE 16–25. A thigh holder placed distal to the tourniquet and well padded posteriorly maintains thigh flexion at 45°, providing excellent access to the posteromedial and posterolateral corners of the knee. (From Cannon WD: Arthroscopic meniscal repair. *In* McGinty JB [ed]: Operative Arthroscopy, p. 238. New York: Raven Press, 1991.)

surface of the meniscus and into the tear cleft. Henning[42] showed that it is important to use the rasp on both sides of the tear for removing any amorphous material, which might interfere with meniscal healing from the handle part of the meniscus in chronic tears. The inferior surface of the meniscus at the synovial junction can be abraded by passing a small, angled burr (Bowen & Co.) from the anteromedial portal back underneath the posterior horn of the meniscus, or a small nick can be made in the synovium at the posteromedial corner and the burr introduced underneath the meniscus. Adequate time for freshening up all surfaces of the tear should be allowed.

An external joint distractor (Fig. 16–26) is used for repairs of the medial meniscus when more than two sutures are placed through the posterior horn. The author does not use a joint distractor for repair of the lateral meniscus. Steinmann pins (3/16 inch) are inserted just proximal to the medial femoral epicondyle and into the anteromedial flare of the tibia, and the joint is distracted. If posterior horn visualization is still inadequate, the surgeon should wait a few minutes and distract the joint still further. An additional few millimeters can be gained by transversely "pie-crusting" the medial collateral ligament, as suggested by C. E. Henning (personal communication).

Nonabsorbable sutures of 2-0 Ethibond (Ethicon, Inc., special order D-6702) with double-armed taper-ended Keith needles are used for all suturing. Each needle is bent twice: 4 mm from its tip, approximately 10° to 15°, and 1 cm from the first bend, 10° to 15°. These bends allow the needle to be angled into the meniscus and directed to the posteromedial corner of the joint. The needle is press fitted into a special needle holder (Stryker Corporation). A cannula is inserted through the anteromedial portal close to the patellar tendon and just above the superior surface of the anterior horn of the medial meniscus. The suture needle is passed

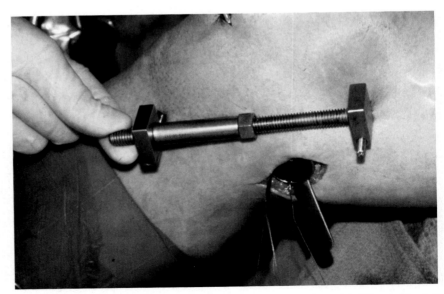

FIGURE 16–26. A knee distractor is used for medial meniscal repairs. This enables better visualization of the posterior horn. The popliteal retractor can be seen in the posteromedial incision. (From Cannon WD: Arthroscopic meniscal repair. *In* McGinty JB [ed]: Operative Arthroscopy, p. 239. New York: Raven Press, 1991.)

through this cannula and aimed into the intercondylar notch in order to avoid inadvertent damage to the articular surfaces in the medial compartment. Once the end of the needle is seen exiting the cannula, it can be redirected to the posterior horn while the knee is maintained in approximately 10° to 15° of extension. For best results, the first suture should be placed near the origin of the posterior horn from the inferior surface and directed superiorly.

Once the needle is introduced up to the second bend, the cannula is levered into the intercondylar notch, creating a third bend in the needle close to the junction of the needle holder (Fig. 16–27). Without this third bend, the needle gets lost in the midline structures behind the joint. As the needle advances from close to the inner border of the intercondylar notch, the point of the needle should exit posteromedially against the popliteal retractor. An extra arthroscopic light cord is useful for illuminating the inside of the popliteal retractor and picking up the needle point. Turning off the inflow into the joint also may be of some help. Once the needle point is grasped posteromedially, the needle holder can be released from the end of the needle anteriorly and withdrawn. The needle is pulled out through the posteromedial corner of the knee and tagged (Fig. 16–28).

The second needle of the first suture is inserted into the needle holder and passed into the joint. The technique has evolved over the years to the point at which the author now places vertical mattress sutures instead of horizontal mattress sutures (Fig. 16–29).[40] In contrast to the first throw that was directed upwards into the meniscus tissue, the second throw is passed underneath the meniscus and out through the meniscosynovial junction, passing by the tear site. The retrieval technique is as described earlier. A third bend in the needle is usually necessary for the first sutures placed close to the posterior horn origin. The author tries to stagger the sutures superiorly and inferiorly at approximately every 3 to 4 mm. (Fig. 16–30). If the vertical longitudinal tear extends anteriorly to the posteromedial corner, suturing should be performed from the anterolateral portal

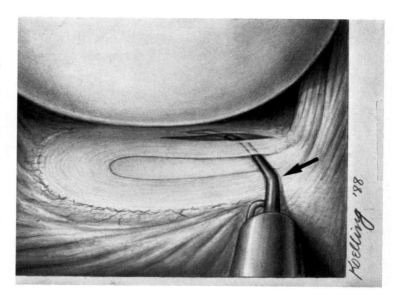

FIGURE 16–27. The first suture, which is placed close to the origin of the posterior horn of either the medial or the lateral meniscus, can be difficult to retrieve posteriorly. Hence a third bend in the needle is made by levering the cannula and the needle holder into the intercondylar notch. The additional bend in the needle enables the surgeon to guide the needle into the popliteal retractor with more ease. (From Cannon WD: Arthroscopic meniscal repair. *In* McGinty JB [ed]: Operative Arthroscopy, p. 240. New York: Raven Press, 1991.)

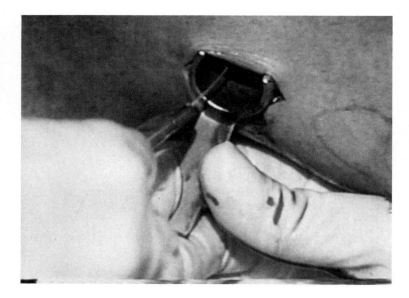

FIGURE 16–28. Once the needle has been passed through the meniscus and out through the posterior capsule, it is deflected off the popliteal retractor and withdrawn with a needle holder.

through a long cannula. The arthroscope is then moved over to the anteromedial portal (Fig. 16–31). Before suture placement, the surgeon should be sure to dissect anteriorly along the superficial portion of the medial collateral ligament from the posteromedial incision so that the needle can be retrieved.

For extensive bucket-handle type tears of the medial meniscus, the author has found that the most anterior sutures are more easily retrieved through a second small incision made midway between the posteromedial incision and the anteromedial portal (Fig. 16–32). The only disadvantage of this accessory incision is that the knots remain prominent postoperatively. In contrast to the more conventional approach just described C. E. Henning used a system of stacked vertical mattress sutures (personal communication). A pair was placed inferiorly and superiorly at each point

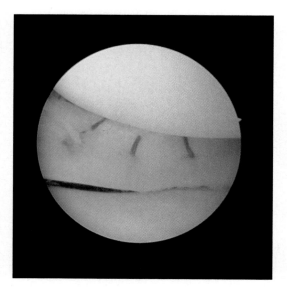

FIGURE 16–29. Appearance of a tear of the posterior horn of the lateral meniscus after placement of vertically oriented mattress sutures. The inferior surface also contains comparably placed sutures.

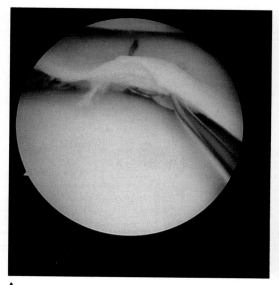
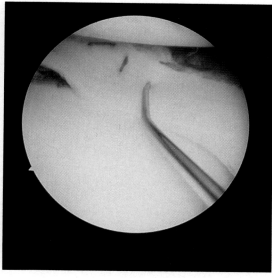

A   B

FIGURE 16–30. (*A* and *B*) Vertically oriented mattress sutures being placed through both inferior and superior aspects of the posterior horn of the medial meniscus in a right knee. (From Cannon WD: Arthroscopic meniscal repair. *In* McGinty JB [ed]: Operative Arthroscopy, p. 241. New York: Raven Press, 1991.)

along the repair zone of the meniscus. This procedure frequently involved the placement of more than 20 sutures per meniscal tear. Henning has placed as many as 42 sutures in one meniscal repair.

Once suturing is completed and all sutures have been tagged and cross-clamped, ACL reconstruction is performed if required.

For meniscal tears that are isolated injuries, the author always inserts fibrin clot into the tear cleft. Arnoczky and associates[6] showed that fibrin clot contains growth factors that can stimulate production of fibrochondrocytes in the repair process. Fibrin clot is prepared by the anesthesiologist by removing approximately 75 mL of venous blood under strict sterile conditions. The blood is placed in a plastic or glass container in the operative field and stirred with a pair of barrels from 10- or 20-mL glass

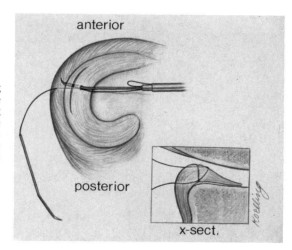

FIGURE 16–31. Diagram shows the technique for repairing the middle third of the medial meniscus. The arthroscope has been moved to the anteromedial portal, and suturing is accomplished through the anterolateral portal. Note again the divergent needle placement, which creates excellent coaptation of the meniscus. (From Cannon WD: Arthroscopic meniscal repair. *In* McGinty JB [ed]: Operative Arthroscopy, p. 241. New York: Raven Press, 1991.)

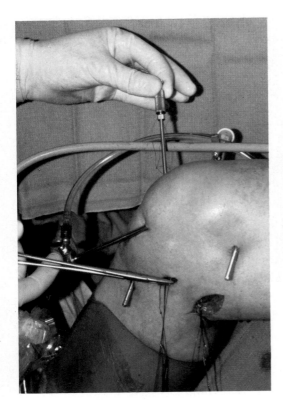

FIGURE 16–32. When the middle third of the medial meniscus is sutured, a second incision occasionally may be made anterior to the posteromedial incision and sutures brought directly through this wound. These sutures have a more radial orientation than if they had been brought through the posteromedial incision. The knee distractor has been temporarily removed. (From Cannon WD: Arthroscopic meniscal repair. *In* McGinty JB [ed]: Operative Arthroscopy, p. 242. New York: Raven Press, 1991.)

syringes (Fig. 16–33). After approximately 5 minutes, fibrin clot should be observed to adhere to the sintered glass barrels. The clot is removed, washed with moistened pads, and shaped into a tubelike structure.

Introduction of the clot into the tear site remains difficult. Henning preferred to inject it through a 13-gauge needle. This author prefers to use two 2-0 Ethibond meniscal repair sutures with one suture tied at either end of the clot (Fig. 16–34). Each remaining needle of the double-armed suture is passed under the meniscus at the most posterior extent of the tear. The second needle passes under the meniscus at the anterior pole of the tear. When both needles have been retrieved, the fibrin clot

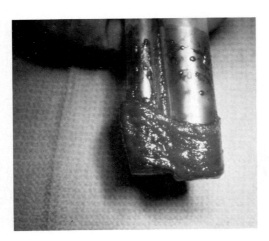

FIGURE 16–33. The appearance of the fibrin clot adhering to two glass syringe barrels after 75 mL of venous blood is stirred for 5 minutes. (From Cannon WD: Arthroscopic meniscal repair. *In* McGinty JB [ed]: Operative Arthroscopy, p. 243. New York: Raven Press, 1991.)

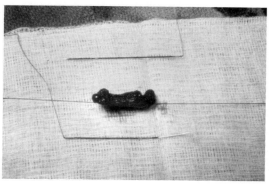

FIGURE 16–34. A 2-0 Ethibond suture is placed through both ends of the fibrin clot, facilitating its stable placement under the inferior surface of the meniscus at the tear site.

can be passed through a 5- or 6-mm cannula and snugged up underneath the inferior surface of the meniscus at the tear site (Fig. 16–35). The previously placed meniscal sutures, having been loosened for the clot insertion, are pulled tight, trapping the clot in the tear site.

In meniscal repairs associated with ACL reconstruction, the author elects not to use fibrin clot unless the rim width is 4 mm or more or unless the tear pattern is complex.

Lateral Meniscal Repair

The technique of lateral meniscal repair is similar to but easier than that of medial meniscal repair. The posterolateral incision is made more easily than the posteromedial incision. With the knee flexed at approximately 90°, the biceps muscle is split from the posterior border of the iliotibial band. Blunt dissection enables the surgeon to easily locate the lateral head of the gastrocnemius muscle. The peroneal nerve lies posterior to the biceps, and once dissection has been performed deep to the lateral head of the gastrocnemius muscle, the nerve should be out of harm's way. The

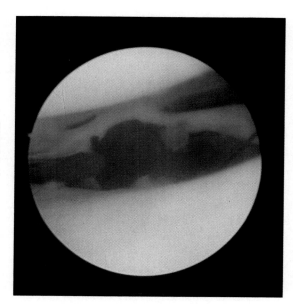

FIGURE 16–35. The fibrin clot is placed under the meniscus throughout the tear length, and the sutures are then pulled tight. Notice the right-hand suture actually holding the clot under the meniscus. (From Cannon WD: Arthroscopic meniscal repair. *In* McGinty JB [ed]: Operative Arthroscopy, p. 243. New York: Raven Press, 1991.)

nerve is not visible. Dissection of the lateral head of the gastrocnemius muscle off the posterior capsule should begin at or below the joint line and worked proximalward. A rasp is used to abrade the periphery of the meniscus and adjacent synovium while being visualized from an antero-medial portal through the intercondylar notch. Although Henning and co-workers[43] used a joint distractor on the lateral side, this author does not.

All meniscal suturing is conducted from the anteromedial portal while the arthroscope is in the anterolateral portal. Suture placement is similar to that used on the medial side. The first suture at the origin of the posterior horn should be placed with care because the popliteal artery lies very close behind the posterior horn origin of the lateral meniscus (Fig. 16–36). At the posterolateral corner, the surgeon should avoid passing sutures through the popliteal tendon, but occasionally this may be necessary.

The origin of the posterior horn of the lateral meniscus is highly vascularized in most patients. Therefore, more complex tears of this area, including radial split tears and complex oblique tears, can be successfully repaired. The technique for repair of radial split tears, including those involving the medial meniscus, consists of placing horizontal mattress sutures through the anterior and posterior leaves of the tear. These sutures should lie closer to the inner edge than in the usual suture placement technique (Fig. 16–37). Tightening the suture approximates the edges of the radial split tear. Radial split tears in the middle third of the lateral meniscus have a poor healing rate. Many can be left alone, but if they are symptomatic, fibrin clot should be used as an adjunct in the repair technique.

For complex tears including flap tears and broken bucket-handle tears, Henning and co-workers[43, 44] sewed a piece of fascial sheath over the meniscus attached superiorly and inferiorly. They then injected the sheath with fibrin clot.

Other Repair Techniques

A double-barreled repair system is commercially available[11] and is generally easier to use and faster than C. E. Henning's technique. The drawback

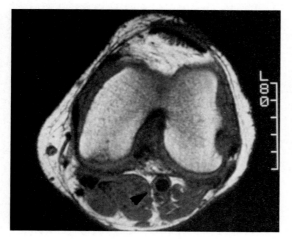

FIGURE 16–36. Magnetic resonance image demonstrates the intimate association of the popliteal artery to the posterior horn of the lateral meniscus. Without the insertion of a popliteal retractor in back of the posterior horn of the lateral meniscus, the artery can be easily injured. The *arrow* indicates the popliteal artery. (From Cannon WD: Arthroscopic meniscal repair. *In* McGinty JB [ed]: Operative Arthroscopy, p. 247. New York: Raven Press, 1991.)

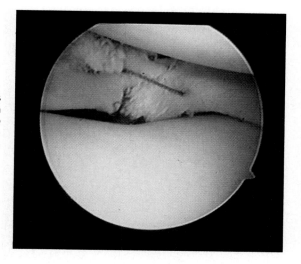

FIGURE 16–37. The technique for repair of radial split tears of the posterior horn involves placement of the suture on both sides of the radial split tear, thus coapting the two edges of the tear. (From Cannon WD: Arthroscopic meniscal repair. *In* McGinty JB [ed]: Operative Arthroscopy, p. 249. New York: Raven Press, 1991.)

with the double-barrel system is that divergent suture placement is difficult. Rosenberg[85] designed a zone-specific curved cannula system with needles introduced one at a time (Fig. 16–38). This creates a divergent suture placement that allows for better meniscal coaptation.

Warren[97] has developed an outside-inside technique in which spinal gauge needles are passed through the skin and the meniscal tear site. A monofilament absorbable PDS suture is passed through the needle and retrieved anteriorly. A double knot tied in the suture anteriorly is pulled back into the joint against the meniscal fragment. A pair of these sutures are tied subcutaneously. Morgan and Casscells[73] reported extensive experience with this system (Fig. 16–39).

In a similar outside-inside technique, developed by Johnson,[51] curved

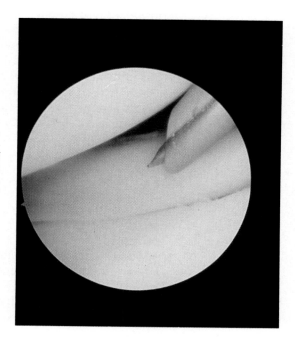

FIGURE 16–38. Arthroscopic view demonstrating an alternative method of meniscal repair. With the use of zone-specific curved cannulas designed by Rosenberg, a pair of long needles are passed through the meniscus in individual throws. (From Cannon WD: Arthroscopic meniscal repair. *In* McGinty JB [ed]: Operative Arthroscopy, p. 244. New York: Raven Press, 1991.)

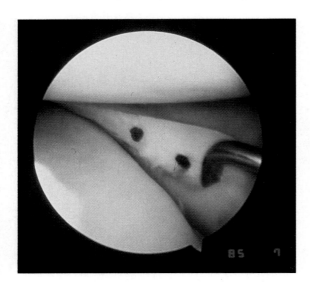

FIGURE 16–39. Another alternative method of meniscal repair, in which knotted sutures are passed from outside in. (From Cannon WD: Arthroscopic meniscal repair. *In* McGinty JB [ed]: Operative Arthroscopy, p. 244. New York: Raven Press, 1991.)

spinal needles and a wire loop are used to retrieve the sutures within the joint.

Morgan[72] reported gaining experience in an all inside-inside technique in which curved suturing needles (Concept, Inc.) are used. Suturing is performed as in an open technique. Knots are passed through a cannula with a special pusher.

POSTOPERATIVE REHABILITATION

The patient with an isolated meniscal repair is allowed to move the knee immediately but is kept on crutches for 6 to 8 weeks. No weight bearing is allowed for the first 4 weeks, and then weight bearing progresses up to full weight bearing from the fourth to the sixth weeks. In most cases, the crutches are used for an additional 2 weeks. Closed kinetic chain quadriceps and unlimited hamstring exercises are commenced at 6 weeks. Running is allowed at 5 months, some sports are allowed at 6 months, but no contact sports are allowed before 9 months.

If ACL reconstruction has been performed in conjunction with meniscal repair, the technique does not differ from that just described. Patients leave the operating room in a brace locked in 0° of extension, but motion is started by the next morning.

RESULTS

Most results reported in the literature have been assessed from a clinical standpoint. Satisfactory results show no joint line pain or tenderness and no locking or catching. Henning[86] devised a precise anatomic definition of success. He recommended second-look arthroscopy 6 months after all lateral meniscal repairs and an arthrogram 6 months after medial meniscal repairs. A residual cleft of 10 per cent or less at the repair site is considered healed. If the cleft is from 10 to 50 per cent of the thickness of the meniscus, it is considered partially healed. If the cleft is more than 50 per cent of the thickness of the meniscus, even if only in one small area of the repair, the outcome is considered to be a failure (Fig. 16–40). Because anatomic failures may not result in clinical failures, surgeons who report results that are based on anatomic assessment report fewer satisfactory results than those who report clinical results. Approximately two thirds of Henning's anatomic failures (personal communication) and approximately half of this author's are clinically asymptomatic.

Since 1982, the author has performed 145 meniscal repairs. Since 1984, only Henning's system has been used. There were 79 medial meniscal repairs and 66 lateral meniscal repairs. Both medial and lateral meniscal repairs were performed in 15 patients. The average age of the patients was 27 years. The average time from injury was 19 months. Most of the patients underwent meniscal repair for chronic tears; 70 per cent of the tears were repaired after more than 1 month from the time of injury, and 80 per cent were associated with ACL surgery.

Arthroscopic or arthrographic results were assessed in 110 patients. The arthroscopic second-look group was composed of 82 patients. The reason for this high number is that some of the repairs were bilateral and were assessed simultaneously. Also, if there was a need for arthroscopic debridement after ACL reconstruction, medial meniscal repairs were assessed at this time.

Henning (personal communication) and the author have found that patients with incompletely healed meniscal tears have done as well as those with healed tears. Therefore, the satisfactory group is composed of healed and the incompletely healed patients. Overall, 78 of the tears were satisfactorily healed, and 22 per cent were failures. In an assessment of the same patients from a purely clinical standpoint, 92 per cent of the tears were healed, and 8 per cent were symptomatic or had come to further meniscal surgery.

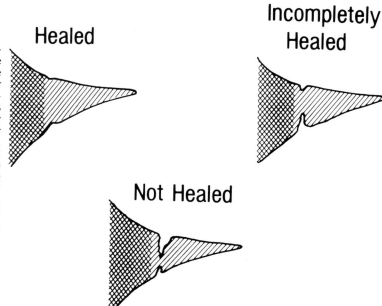

FIGURE 16–40. Six months after repair, the degree of healing can be determined by arthrogram for the medial side and by arthroscopy for the lateral side. A meniscus is classified as "healed" (*top left*) if it is healed over the full length of the tear with a residual cleft less than 10 per cent of the thickness of the meniscus. A tear that is healed over its full length with a residual cleft from 10 to 50 per cent of its vertical height is classified as "incompletely healed" (*top right*). A residual cleft more than 50 per cent of the thickness of the meniscus at any point over the length of the tear is classified as "failed" (*bottom*). (From Cannon WD: Arthroscopic meniscal repair. *In* McGinty JB [ed]: Operative Arthroscopy, p. 245. New York: Raven Press, 1991.)

The results of meniscal repair were statistically significantly better in patients who underwent ACL reconstruction concomitantly than in patients with an intact ACL. Satisfactory healing occurred in 85 per cent of meniscal repairs performed with ACL reconstruction and in only 56 per cent of isolated meniscal repairs. Because fibrin clot has been used only since late 1987 on patients who had isolated meniscal repair, the effects of fibrin clot have not yet been established.

Increasing rim widths and tear lengths also adversely affected the incidence of healing. Meniscal repairs in patient with rim widths of 3 mm or less produced satisfactory healing in 84 per cent, but in rim widths of 4 to 5 mm, the incidence of healing dropped to 46 per cent. The two menisci with 5-mm rim widths that healed are probably aberrations. Of patients who underwent meniscal repair of tears less than 2 cm in length, 88 per cent had satisfactory healing; in contrast, of tears 4 cm or longer, only 41 per cent healed satisfactorily. The rate of satisfactory healing in patients with chronic meniscal tears (i.e., tears that had occurred more than 8 weeks from the time of injury) was 75 per cent; among meniscal repairs conducted within 8 weeks of injury, the rate of satisfactory healing was 88 per cent. These differences were not statistically significant. There was a difference between lateral and medial meniscal repairs, the incidences of satisfactory healing being 86 and 71 per cent, respectively ($p <$ .04).

Interestingly, the author observed better healing rates in older patients. Among patients aged 19 years and older, the incidence of satisfactory healing was 81 per cent, whereas in patients aged 18 years and younger, this rate was only 63 per cent. Among patients over age 35, the rate of satisfactory healing was 91 per cent.

Surgical experience was also related to successful outcomes. During the early years of learning this technique, before 1984, only 60 per cent of patients had satisfactory healing. The results improved to successful healing in 81 per cent of menisci repaired after January 1984.

COMPLICATIONS

No infections or wound healing problems were noted. One case of transient phlebitis was noted 4 weeks after surgery. One patient had a partial peroneal nerve palsy that resulted from the passing of a suture through 25 per cent of the nerve; this suture was released within a week of surgery, and the patient experienced a full recovery. There were no vascular complications. There was no loss of motion in the isolated group. Any loss of motion in the ACL-associated meniscal repair group was more likely attributable to the ACL reconstruction.

DISCUSSION

Most surgeons recommend both meniscal repair and ACL reconstruction in patients with a reparable meniscus tear and an ACL-deficient knee. Rehabilitation after meniscal repair and the time before return to sports are almost as long as after ACL reconstruction; therefore, it makes sense to perform both procedures together. DeHaven and co-workers[20] followed a group of ACL-deficient patients for whom only an open meniscal repair had been performed. Over several years, the failure rate of meniscal repair rose and reached a plateau of approximately 38 per cent. This outcome is in contrast to that of Hanks and collaborators,[40] who reported an 87 per cent satisfactory healing rate in patients who had undergone only meniscal repair and not ACL reconstruction.

An important finding in the author's series was the startlingly large difference in successful results between meniscal repair in knees undergoing simultaneous reconstruction of grade 3 ACL tears and isolated meniscal repair ($p < .00005$). It is the author's opinion that the main reason for this difference is that patients who have a torn meniscus in association with an ACL tear usually have had a major subluxation of the tibia. This has caused the femoral condyle to crunch down on the posterior horn of the medial or lateral meniscus, creating the tear. After successful stabilization of the knee, the meniscal repair site is protected from comparable forces because the tibia no longer subluxates anteriorly. In isolated meniscal tears, it is possible that the biomechanical forces that created the tear could occur again after meniscal repair.

Another explanation is that ACL reconstruction increases the trauma to the knee joint. This creates additional fibrin clot in the joint, which may provide further stimulation to meniscal healing. The author once thought that a reason for the difference in these results was that meniscal tears, resulting from ACL disruption, were more peripheral and in an area of the meniscus that had a better blood supply than were isolated meniscal tears. Analysis of the data did not bear this theory out. The average rim width in meniscal tears associated with an ACL disruption is 2.4 mm; in isolated meniscal tears, it is 2.3 mm.

In 1986, Arnoczky and associates[6] showed that fibrin clot introduced into punched-out holes in the avascular zone of a canine meniscus resulted in fibrocartilaginous healing. Because satisfactory healing of isolated meniscal tears is far from ideal, it made sense to study patients with isolated tears. Therefore, Henning[42] started to introduce fibrin clot into the repair site of these tears as an adjunct to his surgical technique; his successful healing rate rose to 92 per cent. Before the use of fibrin clot, successful healing had occurred in only 59 per cent of his isolated meniscal repairs. Henning thereafter used fibrin clot in all meniscal repairs. The author has used fibrin clot for all isolated meniscal repairs and selectively for more complex meniscal tears associated with ACL reconstruction. He does not use fibrin clot in instances in which the rim size is less than 3 mm when ACL reconstruction is performed concomitantly.

Additional techniques developed by Henning that have increased the incidence of successful healing include the abrasion of both sides of vertical longitudinal tears, spending time to freshen up the handle side of the tear cleft, and use of the stacked suture technique. In another complex technique, Henning[44] showed improved results in repairs of complex flap tears and broken bucket-handle tears with segmental defects by sewing a fascial sheath over the superior surface and under the inferior surface of the meniscus and injecting fibrin clot into the sheath. This technique should not be attempted by the arthroscopic surgeon with only beginning or intermediate surgical skills.

It was predictable that the results of arthroscopic repair would be related to rim width and tear length. As rim width and tear length increased, the failure rate increased. A surprising finding was the successful healing rate in older patients. In patients 36 years of age and older, the incidence of successful healing was 91 per cent. The author believes that serious consideration should be given to meniscal repair and ACL reconstruction in patients up to age 50 who have a significant vertical longitudinal tear of the meniscus associated with an ACL tear.

The placement of vertically oriented sutures appears more biomechanically sound than does that of horizontal mattress sutures. The sutures should be retrieved through an open posterior incision. The author is aware of some instances of injuries to the sartorial branch of the saphenous nerve and the peroneal nerve after arthroscopic meniscal repair. These injuries are avoidable if open retrieval of needles is performed.

MENISCAL TRANSPLANTATION AND FUTURE TRENDS

Beginning in 1984, Milachowski and colleagues[69] began to transplant meniscal allografts into humans. In 1987, they reported on 20 medial meniscal transplantations, of which 14 were lyophilized menisci and six were deep frozen. The initial follow-up after 1.6 years revealed that only one transplant was not healed and was rated a failure. In contrast, Wirth and associates[99] in 1991 reported on the results of 23 allografts, of which 17 were lyophilized and six were deep frozen. Of the 17 lyophilized menisci, 13 were subjected to second-look arthroscopy. One appeared normal, four had undergone a one-third reduction in size, five had undergone a two-thirds reduction in size, and three were absent. Of the six deep frozen menisci, three appeared normal, one had undergone a one-third reduction in size, and two had undergone a two-thirds reduction in size by the time of follow-up.

J. C. Garrett (personal communication) has performed 17 meniscal allograft transplantations. He harvested the menisci under sterile conditions, stored them at 4°C in tissue culture solution, and transplanted them within 5 days. Most of these transplants were performed with ACL reconstruction, osteochondral allografts, or both. Second-look arthroscopy of 13 menisci revealed healing in all cases. In contrast to the experience with frozen or lyophilized menisci, no shrinkage was noted. Long-term follow-up is needed for determining whether these transplants will protect the joint from late degenerative changes.

There is a need to be able to replace the menisci in young patients whose menisci are so badly torn that meniscectomy may be the only choice of treatment. Proper attention to methods of preservation and appropriate sizing of the meniscus to fit the recipient are necessary. An alternative direction of research involves the use of collagen-based prostheses that act as resorbable regeneration templates to induce regrowth of new menisci. Some promising work has been done in animals, but work on humans awaits further research.[92]

REFERENCES

1. Aichroth PM, Patel DV, Marx CL: The congenital discoid lateral meniscus in children: a follow-up study and evolution of management. J Bone Joint Surg, in press.
2. Allen PR, Denham RA, Swan AV: Late degenerative changes after meniscectomy. Factors affecting the knee after operation. J Bone Joint Surg 66B:666–671, 1984.
3. Annandale T: An operation for displaced semilunar cartilage. Br Med J p. 779, 1885.

4. Appel H: Late results after meniscectomy in the knee joint: a clinical and roentgenologic follow-up investigation. Acta Orthop Scand 133:Suppl 133:1+, 1970.
5. Arnoczky SP, Warren RF: Microvasculature of the human meniscus. Am J Sports Med 10:90–95, 1982.
6. Arnoczky SP, Warren RF, Spivak JM: Meniscal repair using exogenous fibrin clot—an experimental study in dogs. J Bone Joint Surg 70A:1209–1220, 1988.
7. Barrie HJ: The pathogenesis and significance of meniscal cysts. J Bone Joint Surg 61B:184–189, 1979.
8. Baumgaertner MR, Cannon WD, Vittori JM, et al: Arthroscopic debridement of the arthritic knee. Clin Orthop 253:197–202, 1990.
9. Cannon WD: Arthroscopic meniscal repair. *In* McGinty JB (ed): Operative Arthroscopy, 1st ed, pp. 237–251. New York: Raven Press, 1991.
10. Cassidy RE, Schaffer AJ: Repair of peripheral meniscus tears: a preliminary report. Am J Sports Med 9:209–214, 1981.
11. Clancy WG, Graf BK: Arthroscopic meniscal repair. Orthopedics 6:1125–1128, 1983.
12. Clark CR, Ogden JA: Development of the menisci of the human knee joint: morphological changes and their potential role in childhood meniscal injury. J Bone Joint Surg 65A:539–547, 1983.
13. Cox JS: The degenerative effects of medial meniscus tears in dog's knees. Clin Orthop 125:236–242, 1977.
14. Crabtree SD, Bedford AF, Edgar MA: The value of arthrography and arthroscopy in association with a sports injuries clinic: a prospective and comparative study of 182 patients. Injury 13:220–226, 1981.
15. Crues JV, Ryu R, Morgan FW: Meniscal pathology: the expanding role of magnetic resonance imaging. Clin Orthop 252:80–87, 1990.
16. Dandy DJ, Jackson RW: The diagnosis of problems after meniscectomy. J Bone Joint Surg 57B:349–352, 1975.
17. Daniel D, Daniels E, Aronson D: The diagnosis of meniscus pathology. Clin Orthop 163:218–224, 1982.
18. DeHaven KE: The knee. *In* Goldstein LA, Dickerson RC (eds): Atlas of Orthopaedic Surgery, 2nd ed, pp. 405–477. St. Louis: CV Mosby, 1981.
19. DeHaven KE: Meniscus repair in the athlete. Clin Orthop 198:31–35, 1985.
20. DeHaven KE, Black KP, Griffiths HS: Meniscus repair. Orthop Transact 2:469, 1987.
21. DeHaven KE, Black KP, Griffiths HJ: Open meniscus repair: technique and two to nine year results. Am J Sports Med 17:788–795, 1989.
22. DeHaven KE, Hales W: Peripheral meniscus repair: an alternative to meniscectomy. Orthop Transact 5:399–400, 1981.
23. DeHaven KE, Lohrer WA: Long Term Results of Meniscus Repair. *Presented at* the meeting of the International Arthroscopy Association, Toronto, May 1991.
24. Deutsch AL, Mink JH: MR imaging of the postoperative meniscus. Radiology 169:20, 1988.
25. Deutsch AL, Mink JH, Fox JM, et al: Peripheral meniscal tears: MR findings after conservative treatment or arthroscopic repair. Radiology 176:485–488, 1990.
26. Dolan WA, Bhaskar G: Peripheral meniscus repair: a clinical pathological study of 75 cases. Orthop Transact 7:503–504, 1983.
27. Dumas JM, Edde DJ: Meniscal abnormalities: prospective correlation of double-contrast arthrography and arthroscopy. Radiology 160:453–456, 1986.
28. Dye SF, Cannon WD: Anatomy and biomechanics of the anterior cruciate ligament. Clin Sports Med 7:715–725, 1988.
29. Fairbank TJ: Knee joint changes after meniscectomy. J Bone Joint Surg 30B:664–670, 1948.
30. Ferrer-Roca O, Vilalta C: Lesions of the meniscus. Part II: horizontal cleavages and lateral cysts. Clin Orthop 146:301–307, 1980.
31. Ferriter PJ, Nisonson B: The role of arthroscopy in the treatment of lateral meniscal cysts. Arthroscopy 1:142–151, 1985.
32. Fischer SP, Fox JM, Del Pizzo W, et al: Accuracy of diagnoses from magnetic resonance imaging of the knee: a multi-center analysis of one thousand and fourteen patients. J Bone Joint Surg 73:2–10, 1991.
33. Freiberger RH, Killoran PJ, Cardona G: Arthrography of the knee by double contrast method. Am J Roentgenol 97:736–747, 1966.
34. Fujikawa K, Iseki F, Mikura Y: Partial resection of the discoid meniscus in the child's knee. J Bone Joint Surg 63B:391–395, 1981.
35. Gear MW: The late results of meniscectomy. Br J Surg 54:270–272, 1967.
36. Gillies H, Seligson D: Precision in the diagnosis of meniscal lesions: a comparison of clinical evaluation, arthrography and arthroscopy. J Bone Joint Surg 61A:343–346, 1979.
37. Hall FM: Methodology in knee arthrography. Radiol Clin North Am 19:269–275, 1981.
38. Hall FM: Pitfalls in the assessment of the menisci by knee arthrography. Radiol Clin North Am 19:305–328, 1981.

39. Hamberg P, Gillquist J, Lysholm J: Suture of new and old peripheral meniscus tears. J Bone Joint Surg 65A:193–197, 1983.
40. Hanks GA, Gause TM, Sebastianelli WJ, et al: Repair of peripheral meniscal tears—open versus arthroscopic technique. Arthroscopy 7:72–77, 1991.
41. Hayashi LK, Yamaga H, Ida K, et al: Arthroscopic meniscectomy for discoid lateral meniscus in children. J Bone Joint Surg 70A:1495–1500, 1988.
42. Henning CE: Arthroscopic repair of meniscus tears. Orthopedics 6:1130–1132, 1983.
43. Henning CE, Lynch MA, Yearout KM, et al: Arthroscopic meniscal repair using an exogenous fibrin clot. Clin Orthop 252:64–72, 1990.
44. Henning CE, Yearout KM, Vequist SW, et al: Use of the fascia sheath coverage and exogenous fibrin clot in the treatment of complex meniscal tears. Am J Sports Med 19:626–631, 1991.
45. Huckell JR: Is meniscectomy a benign procedure? A long-term follow-up study. Canad J Surg 8:254–260, 1965.
46. Ikeuchi H: Surgery under arthroscopic control. Rheumatology (special issue), 1976.
47. Ikeuchi H: Arthroscopic treatment of the discoid lateral meniscus. Clin Orthop 167:19–28, 1982.
48. Ireland J, Trickey EL, Stoker DJ: Arthroscopy and arthrography of the knee: a critical review. J Bone Joint Surg 62B:3–6, 1980.
49. Jackson DW, Jennings LD, Maywood RM, Berger PE: Magnetic resonance imaging of the knee. Am J Sports Med 16:29–38, 1988.
50. Jackson JP: Degenerative changes in the knee after meniscectomy. Br Med J 2:525–527, 1968.
51. Johnson LL: Meniscus mender II [Technical bulletin]. Okemos, MI: Instrument Makar, Inc., 1988.
52. Johnson RJ, Kettlekamp DB, Clark W, et al: Factors affecting late results after meniscectomy. J Bone Joint Surg 56A:719–729, 1974.
53. Jokl P, Lynch KJ, Kent RH, et al: Arthroscopic surgical repair of the meniscus—twelve month follow-up with MRI. *Presented at* AANA ninth annual meeting. Orlando, FL: Arthroscopy Association of North America, April 1990.
54. Jones RE, Smith EC, Reisch JS; Effects of medial meniscectomy in patients older than forty years. J Bone Joint Surg 60A:783–786, 1978.
55. Kaye JJ, Nance EP: Meniscal abnormalities in knee arthrography. Radiol Clin North Am 19:277–286, 1981.
56. King D: The healing of semilunar cartilages. J Bone Joint Surg 18:333–342, 1936.
57. King D: The function of semilunar cartilages. J Bone Joint Surg 18:1069–1076, 1936.
58. Klenerman L, Butcher C: Double contrast arthrography in the diagnosis of lesions of the menisci. J Bone Joint Surg 56B:564, 1974.
59. Krause WR, Pope MH, Johnson RJ, et al: Mechanical changes in the knee after meniscectomy. J Bone Joint Surg 58A:559–604, 1976.
60. Kroiss F: Die verletzungen der kniegelenkoszwischenknorpel und ihrer verbindungen. Beitr Klin Chir 66:598–801, 1910.
61. Kurosaka M, Yoshya S, Ohno O, et al: Lateral discoid meniscectomy—a 20 year follow-up study. *Presented at* the meeting of the American Academy of Orthopaedic Surgeons, San Francisco, January 1987.
62. Lee JK, Yao L, Phelps CT, et al: Anterior cruciate ligament tears: MR imaging compared with arthroscopy and clinical tests. Radiology 166:861–864, 1988.
63. Lufti AM: Morphological changes in the articular cartilage after meniscectomy. J Bone Joint Surg 57B:525–528, 1975.
64. Lynch MA, Henning CE, Glick KR: Knee joint surface changes: long-term follow-up meniscus tear treatment in stable anterior cruciate ligament reconstructions. Clin Orthop 172:148–153, 1983.
65. Mandelbaum BR, Finerman GA, Reicher MA, et al: Magnetic resonance imaging as a tool for evaluation of traumatic knee injuries. Am J Sports Med 14:361–370, 1986.
66. McDaniel WJ, Dameron TB: untreated ruptures of the anterior cruciate ligament: a follow-up study. J Bone Joint Surg 62A:695–705, 1980.
67. McGinty JB, Geuss LF, Marvin RA: Partial or total meniscectomy: a comparative analysis. J Bone Joint Surg 59A:763–766, 1977.
68. Medlar RC, Mandiberg JJ, Lyne ED: Meniscectomies in children: report of long term results (mean, 8.3 years) of 26 children. Am J Sports Med 8:87–92, 1980.
69. Milachowski KA, Weismeier K, Wirth CJ, et al: Meniscus transplantation—experimental study and first clinical report. Am J Sports Med 6:626, 1987.
70. Miller DV, O'Brien SJ, Arnoczky SP, et al: Use of the contact Nd:YAG laser in arthroscopic surgery: effects on articular cartilage and meniscal tissue. Arthroscopy 5:245–253, 1989.
71. Mink JH, Levy T, Crues JV: Tears of the anterior cruciate ligament and menisci of the knee: MR imaging evaluation. Radiology 167:769–774, 1988.
72. Morgan CD: The "all-inside" meniscus repair. Arthroscopy 7:181–186, 1991.

73. Morgan CD, Casscells SW: Arthroscopic meniscal repair: a safe approach to the posterior horns. Arthroscopy 2:3–12, 1986.
74. Neuschwander DC, Finney T, Proffer DS, et al: The Wrisberg type lateral meniscus. *Presented at* the meeting of the International Society of the Knee meeting, Toronto, May 1991.
75. Northmore-Ball MD, Dandy DJ: Long-term results of arthroscopic partial meniscectomy. Clin Orthop 167:34–42, 1982.
76. O'Brien WR, Warren RF, Friederich NF, et al: Degenerative arthritis of the knee following anterior cruciate ligament injury: a multi-center, long-term follow-up study. Am J Sports Med 17:15–16, 1989.
77. Parisien JS: Arthroscopic treatment of cysts of the menisci: a preliminary report. Clin Orthop 257:154–158, 1990.
78. Polly DW, Callaghan JJ, Sikes RA, et al: The accuracy of selective magnetic resonance imaging compared with the findings of arthroscopy of the knee. J Bone Joint Surg 70A:192–198, 1988.
79. Price CT, Allen WC: Ligament repair in the knee with preservation of the meniscus. J Bone Joint Surg 60A:61–65, 1978.
80. Rauschning W: Popliteal cysts (Baker's cysts) in adults: II. Capsuloplasty with and without a pedicel graft. Acta Orthop Scand 51:547–555, 1980.
81. Reagan WD, McConkey JP, Loomer RL, et al: Cysts of the lateral meniscus: arthroscopy versus arthroscopy plus open cystectomy. Arthroscopy 5:274–281, 1989.
82. Reicher MA, Hartzman S, Duckwiler GR, et al: Meniscal injuries: detection using MR imaging. Radiology 159:753–757, 1986.
83. Rosenberg TD, Paulos LE, Parker RD, et al: Discoid lateral meniscus: case report of arthroscopic attachment of a symptomatic Wrisberg-ligament type. Arthroscopy 3:277–282, 1987.
84. Rosenberg TD, Paulos LE, Parker RD, et al: The forty-five degree posteroanterior flexion weight-bearing radiograph of the knee. J Bone Joint Surg 70A:1479–1483, 1988.
85. Rosenberg TD, Scott S, Paulos LE: Arthroscopic surgery: repair of peripheral detachment of the meniscus. Contemp Orthop 10:43–50, 1985.
86. Scott GA, Jolly BL, Henning CE: Combined posterior incision and arthroscopic intra-articular repair of the meniscus. J Bone Joint Surg 68A:847–861, 1986.
87. Selesnick FH, Noble HB, Bachman DC, et al: Internal derangement of the knee: diagnosis by arthrography, arthroscopy, and arthrotomy. Clin Orthop 198:26–30, 1985.
88. Shrive NG, Phil D, O'Connor JJ, Goodfellow JW: Load-bearing in the knee joint. Clin Orthop 131:279–287, 1978.
89. Silva I, Silver DM: Tears of the meniscus as revealed by magnetic resonance imaging. J Bone Joint Surg 70A:199–202, 1988.
90. Smillie IS: Injuries of the Knee Joint, 5th ed. New York: Churchill-Livingstone, 1978.
91. Sommerlath KG: Clinical and radiologic evaluation after meniscus repair and partial meniscectomy in stable knees: a seven year follow-up study. *Presented at* the meeting of the American Academy of Orthopaedic Surgeons, Anaheim, CA, March 1991.
92. Stone KR, Rodkey WG, Webber RJ, et al: Future directions: collagen-based prostheses for meniscal regeneration. Clin Orthop 252:129–135, 1990.
93. Sutton JB: Ligaments, Their Nature and Morphology, 2nd ed. London: HK Lesis, 1897.
94. Tapper EM, Hoover NW: Late results after meniscectomy. J Bone Joint Surg 51A:517–526, 1969.
95. Thompson WO, Thaete FL, Fu FH, et al: Tibial meniscal dynamics using 3D reconstruction of MR images. *Presented at* the Fifteenth Annual Meeting of the American Orthopaedic Society for Sports Medicine, Traverse City, MI, June 1989.
96. Veth RPH: Clinical significance of knee joint changes after meniscectomy. Clin Orthop 198:56–60, 1985.
97. Warren RF: Arthroscopic meniscus repair. Arthroscopy 1:170–172, 1985.
98. Watanabe M, Takeda S, Ikeuchi H: Atlas of Arthroscopy, 3rd ed, p. 88. Tokyo: Igukushion, 1979.
99. Wirth CJ, Kohn D, Milachowski KA: Meniscus transplantation in knee joint instability. *Presented at* the meeting of the International Society of the Knee, Toronto, May 1991.
100. Wroblewski BM: Trauma and the cystic meniscus: review of 500 cases. Injury 4:319–321, 1973.
101. Yocum LA, Kerlan RK, Jobe FW, et al: Isolated lateral meniscectomy: a study of 26 patients with isolated tears. J Bone Joint Surg 61A:338–342, 1979.

CHAPTER 17

Osteochondritis

Dissecans

JOHN C. GARRETT, M.D.

■

Osteochondritis dissecans is an uncommon disorder. Most juvenile cases heal spontaneously, making surgical intervention rarely necessary. Adult forms exhibit a tendency to instability with loosening of the osteochondral fragment and sloughing of loose bodies. In situ lesions may be drilled or bone grafted. Loose bodies are easily extracted but should be replaced and pinned if possible. Articular surface defects may be reconstructed through abrasion arthroplasty with osteochondral allografts when they are large.

The origin of osteochondritis dissecans remains obscure.[2, 20, 32] Growth disorder,[5, 36, 38] epiphyseal abnormality, endocrine imbalance, and familial predisposition[31, 34] are noted in some cases of the juvenile form. Trauma[1, 10, 11] and avascular necrosis[13] continued to be touted as explanations for the adult form.

PATHOLOGY

Of more value than defining the causes has been defining precisely what constitutes osteochondritis dissecans. Bradley and Dandy contend that the adult form of osteochondritis dissecans is a lesion composed of cartilage with an underlying thin shell of bone and classically of the lateral aspect of the medial femoral condyle. Symptoms usually develop during the teenage years, but gross manifestation may occur in the early 20s, although a few cases remain silent until a loose body is extruded in the 30s or 40s (Fig. 17–1).[4] They stated that the process should be distinguished

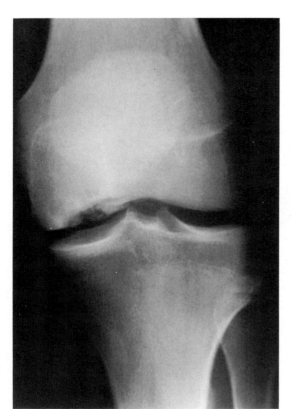

FIGURE 17–1. Osteochondritis dissecans of the medial femoral condyle. Large lesion with multiple foci of calcification, which are correlated with a tendency to fragment and a poor prognosis.

from chondral delamination, in which cartilage separates from underlying bone in the environs of the tide mark, leaving large areas of denuded subchondral bone exposed as a result. Chondral delamination plagues persons in their 20s or 30s but is not evident in routine roentgenographs. It occurs typically in the midportion of the medial femoral condyle, but the margins are indistinct, and progression beyond original bounds often occurs. It defies attempts at repair because of the lack of bony backing that might be used as a vehicle for reattachment. Similarly, osteochondritis should be distinguished from acute chondral fracture, which is often associated with rupture of the anterior cruciate ligament. In an older population, osteochondritis dissecans and chondral delamination are superseded by avascular necrosis, which usually affects the medial femoral condyle but occasionally affects the lateral femoral condyle or the tibial plateau. This disorder occurs most often in women, typically in their 50s and 60s. Large lesions have a relentless course, resulting in steadily increasing pain, collapse, and disintegration (Fig. 17–2). Because avascular necrosis occurs at an advanced age, prosthetic replacement is the usual mode of surgical treatment.

In osteochondritis dissecans, there is an articular cap with an underlying flake of bone. Gross clinical examination may show the bone to vary in thickness, usually being several millimeters thick but sometimes composed of but a few trabeculae; in some areas, there may be none at all. Histologic studies reveal the bone to be largely avascular with segments of revascularization that are suggestive of a reparative process.[7, 28, 42] It is grossly dense and brittle, in comparison with the suppleness of viable trabecular bone. The layer of bone appears to be of a moderately low-intensity signal on T1-weighted MRI (Fig. 17–3).[29] Beneath it is a layer of fibrous tissue several millimeters thick that appears as an encircling ring of extremely low-intensity signal. Beneath this fibrous ring, in turn, is a second layer of sclerotic bone that blends with normal trabeculae; on MRI it appears as a blurred zone of intermediate density. This inert "wasteland" has the appearance and behavior of established nonunion as might occur in a long bone after fracture. The lack of normal solidity or

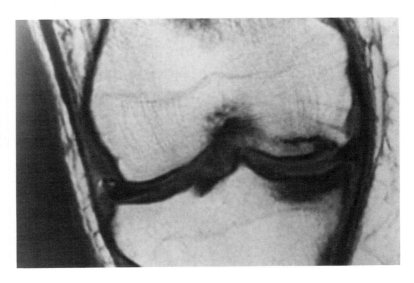

FIGURE 17–2. Osteonecrosis of the medial femoral condyle in a 64-year-old woman. The crescent sign is indicative of subchondral fracture and reactive sclerosis of the opposing tibial plateau.

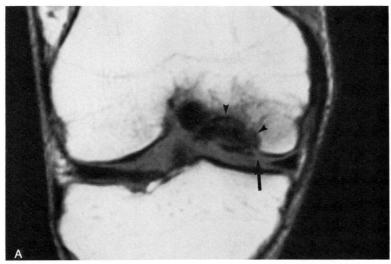

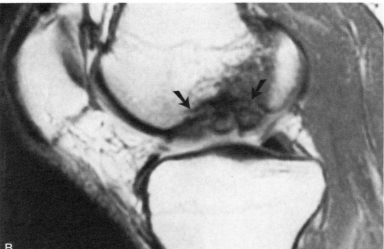

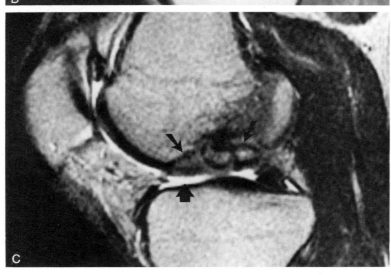

FIGURE 17–3. (*A*) Osteochondritis dissecans in a 25-year-old man. A coronal T1-weighted (TR 800/TE 20) magnetic resonance image reveals an interruption in the normal black cortical signal of the medial femoral condyle (*arrow*). A region 2 cm in diameter (outlined by *arrowheads*) of abnormal signal loss is seen within the spongiosa of the medial femoral condyle. (*B*) An intermediately weighted (TR 2000/TE 20) sagittal image through the lesion reveals abnormal interruption of the black cortical line with irregularity of the articular surface. Abnormal signal loss is seen in the subcortical bone (*arrows*). (*C*) A T2-weighted (TR 2000/TE 80) sagittal image through this lesion reveals irregular signal intensity in the subcortical region of the medial femoral condyle (*arrows*). Of note, however, is that no fluid of high signal intensity is seen extending into the subcortical region of the bone. Thus the joint fluid appears to be contained within the joint space proper (*arrowhead*) without evidence of extension through a defect in the overlying articular cartilage. Despite the large size of this osteochondritis fragment, the overlying articular cartilage was intact at arthroscopy, and the fragments were considered stable. The lack of fluid extending into the osteochondritis dissecans defect correlates well with stability, whereas the presence of fluid of high signal intensity deep to the cortical fragments on a T2-weighted magnetic resonance image correlates well with instability and disruption of the overlying articular cartilage. (Courtesy of John V. Crues III, M.D., Santa Barbara Radiology Medical Group, Inc., Santa Barbara, California.)

adhesiveness explains why adult forms appear to be biologically inert with little tendency toward healing and why these osteochondritis fragments are easy to dislodge.

Serial MRI scans may be a means of studying the healing of juvenile osteochondritis dissecans. Serial bone scans have been used in a similar manner.[6] Adult lesions have not been studied serially, and MRI may have a lesser role in that regard. These lesions have a propensity toward instability, with articular fracture followed by extrusion of loose articular fragments. This event is poorly imaged with computed tomography (CT) or arthrography. Although in some instances MRI may indicate when articular surface fracture has occurred, arthroscopy probably remains the best means of assessing this phenomenon and commonly must be used to determine whether surgical intervention is necessary in the case of the painful knee.[3] However, once fragments have been extruded, the size and the shape of the remaining defect are most vividly demonstrated with three-dimensional CT.

Further insight into osteochondritis dissecans is gained from the behavior of the various anatomic lesions. The majority of the lesions exist on the lateral aspect of the medial femoral condyle; others occur in the midportion of the medial femoral condyle (where they often occur as bilateral lesions before epiphyseal closure), the midportion of the lateral femoral condyle, and the lateral aspect of the trochlear groove.[1, 30] Occasionally, lesions occur in the patella (Fig. 17–4).[9, 41] It has been noted that medial and lateral lesions differ in subtle but significant ways.[16] In fact, lesions of the lateral femoral condyle may be conceptualized as a separate

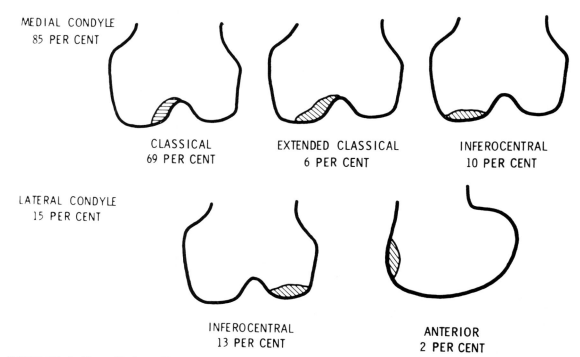

MEDIAL CONDYLE
85 PER CENT

CLASSICAL
69 PER CENT

EXTENDED CLASSICAL
6 PER CENT

INFEROCENTRAL
10 PER CENT

LATERAL CONDYLE
15 PER CENT

INFEROCENTRAL
13 PER CENT

ANTERIOR
2 PER CENT

FIGURE 17–4. Sites of lesions. (From Aichroth P: Osteochondritis dissecans of the knee. J Bone Joint Surg 53B:440, 1971. Courtesy of Paul Aichroth.)

disease entity: not because of etiology but at least because of behavior. Lesions of the medial condyle typically are more anterior and face away from the main tibiofemoral articular surface, cause derangement of the patellofemoral joint as well as of the tibiofemoral articulation, and readily produce popping, clicking, and buckling of the knee joint (Fig. 17–5). These lesions usually are 2.0 to 2.5 cm in diameter, or roughly 4.0 to 6.0 cm² in surface area. They have a reasonably thick bony backing and, when loose, often can be pinned.

Contrariwise, lateral lesions occur further posteriorly, directly on the tibiofemoral weight-bearing surface, and lead to tibiofemoral rather than patellofemoral derangement (Fig. 17–6). Lesions tend to be large; diameters of 3 to 4 cm and surface areas up to 12 to 16 cm² are not uncommon. The massive nature of some lesions has led to a special appellation, "gigantic osteochondritis dissecans," a label not fully deserved and not entirely reserved to lesions of the lateral femoral condyle (Fig. 17–7). Such lesions often have a slim underpinning of bone, if any at all, and are more prone to fragmentation, whereby small segments disengage one at a time, which make replacement impractical (Fig. 17–8). Craters resulting from lateral femoral condylar lesions are large and invariably symptomatic; many patients experience a painful "clunk" each time the knee is flexed or extended. Degenerative changes occur readily (Fig. 17–9).

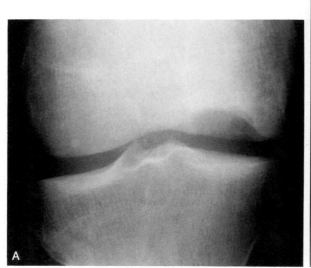
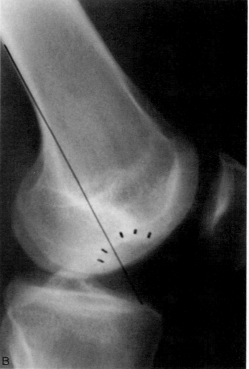

FIGURE 17–5. (*A*) Osteochondritis dissecans of the medial femoral condyle. A large defect is typically situated eccentrically toward the lateral aspect of the medial femoral condyle. (*B*) A lateral view of the same lesion demonstrating the anteroposterior position of the lesion, which typically straddles the line drawn as an extension of the posterior cortex of the femur.

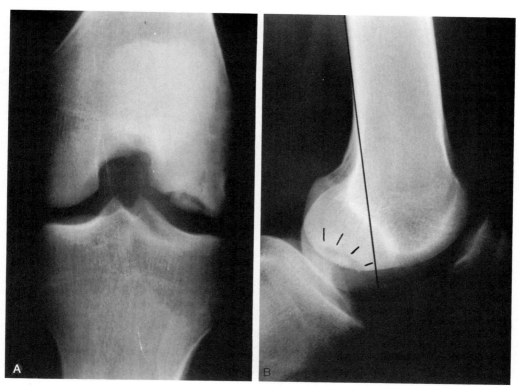

FIGURE 17—6. (A) Osteochondritis dissecans of the lateral femoral condyle. Note the location of the defect, in the midportion of the weight-bearing surface. (B) The lateral view demonstrates the typical position of osteochondritis dissecans of the lateral femoral condyle, posterior to a line drawn as an extension of the posterior cortex of the femur.

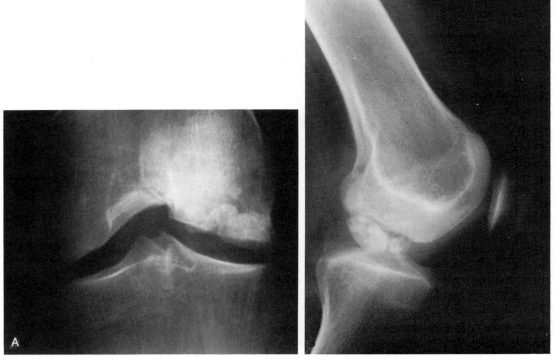

FIGURE 17–7. (*A*) Gigantic lesion of osteochondritis dissecans of the lateral femoral condyle. Note multiple areas of calcification, apparent flattening of the lateral femoral condyle, and widening of the lateral joint space. (*B*) Lateral view in the same patient, demonstrating the lesion.

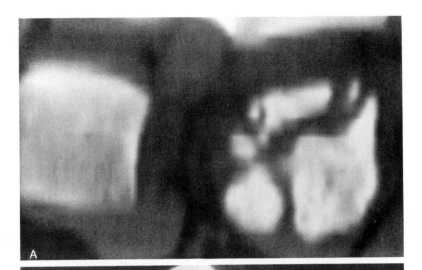

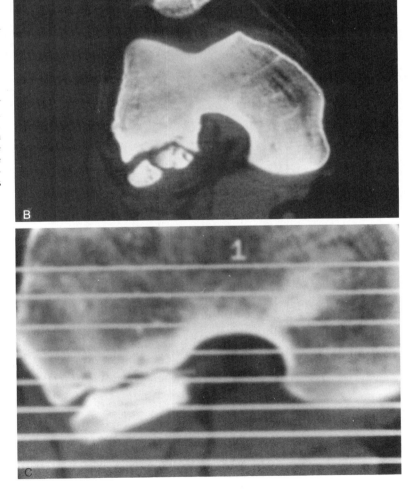

FIGURE 17–8. (*A*) Sagittal view of the image of the distal femur reveals even more extensive fragmentation with multiple minute islands of calcification in large interspersed areas of fibrous tissue. (*B*) Coronal view of the distal femur reveals multiple bony islands with intervening areas of fibrous tissue. (*C*) Computed tomographic scan of osteochondritis dissecans of the lateral femoral condyle. Note single island of bone of reasonable thickness with an underlying fibrous layer that simulates nonunion.

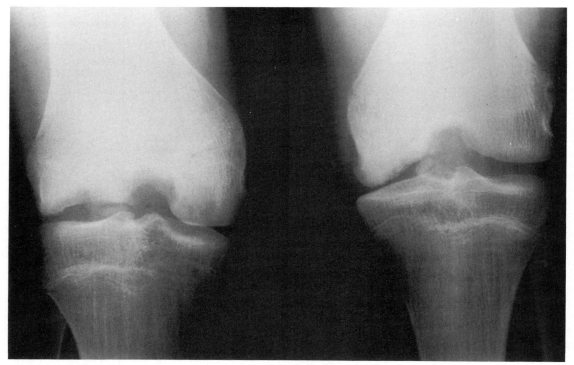

FIGURE 17–9. A rare case of bilateral osteochondritis dissecans that affects the lateral femoral condyle of the right knee and the medial femoral condyle of the left knee in a 15-year-old boy.

CLINICAL COURSE

The majority of the juvenile cases proceed to spontaneous healing (Fig. 17–10). Age 15 or skeletal maturity have been offered as the watershed age for healing.[13, 21, 32, 34] What is not perfectly understood is what happens in adult forms. Patients with intact articular cartilage may suffer intermittent symptoms, especially when vigorously active, presumably because of the presence of the nonunion represented by the sclerotic bone and the fibrous tissue interface beneath the avascular fragment. Once the articular cartilage fractures, symptoms increase and swelling often ensues. It is recognized that adult lesions have a propensity for sloughing loose bodies.[22] Whereas some orthopaedic surgeons regard the subsequent principal problem to be locking of the disengaged fragment, others regard the loss of major portions of the articular surface and resultant arthritis as more worrisome.[22, 24, 26]

Lateral femoral condylar lesions tend to be larger and, therefore, more troublesome. Although a crater may transiently remain clinically silent, degenerative changes eventually develop in the affected compartment (Fig. 17–11). These changes occur earlier in the diseased knee than in the contralateral knee and earlier in affected patients than in age-matched peers.[26] Patients who as teenagers suffer loss of an osteochondral fragment may develop significant degenerative disease in middle age. The degenerative process appears to be multifactorial. Loss of meniscal tissue within the compartment, excess weight or activity, and angular deformity undoubtedly add to the problem. All these findings seem to refute the

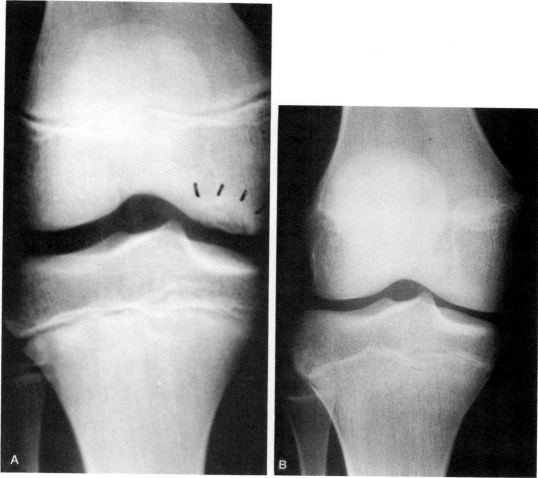

FIGURE 17–10. (*A*) Osteochondritis dissecans of the lateral aspect of the medial femoral condyle in a 13-year-old girl. (*B*) Follow-up films at age 16 reveal healing of the defect.

arguments of authors who have promoted simple extraction of the osteochondral fragment and suggest instead that, when feasible, replacement is preferable.

TREATMENT

Juvenile Osteochondritis Dissecans

Juvenile osteochondritis dissecans differs from the adult form in that the majority of the lesions heal spontaneously. Thus treatment is typically nonoperative. The first task is to determine whether a patient has an epiphyseal growth defect, which often involve multiple joints and should not be confused with osteochondritis dissecans. True clinically silent lesions can be monitored with standard roentgenographs and typically demonstrate healing within 6 to 12 months. Lesions that are painful cause more anxiety, but they too exhibit a propensity for healing spontaneously.

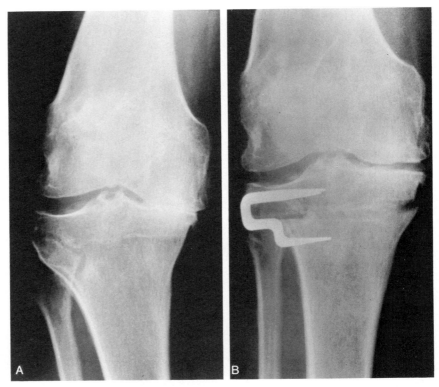

FIGURE 17–11. (*A* and *B*) High tibial osteotomy performed because of medial compartment osteoarthritis in a 37-year-old man, 22 years after removal of osteochondral fragment of the medial femoral condyle for osteochondritis dissecans.

Often these lesions occur during adolescence, when the veracity of the complaint and the intensity of the pain are difficult to ascertain. Nevertheless, for symptomatic patients, treatment with rest for 3 to 6 months usually suffices; immobilization is rarely necessary. Refractory cases can be studied with serial bone scans or MRI. Arthroscopy is rarely necessary; the exception seems to be large lesions that occur directly on the face aspect rather than on the lateral aspect of the medial femoral condyle. Often such lesions are bilateral and occur in late adolescence, thus mimicking adult type rather than the juvenile type of osteochondritis dissecans.

Adult Forms

Adult forms of osteochondritis dissecans vary clinically: those that are recognizable roentgenographically but clinically silent; those that are in the process of fracture and disengagement; and those in which loose bodies have been extruded and articular defects manifest themselves. Whether any lesion is truly solid, innocent, and free of potential harm is a matter of debate. Once recognized, most can be followed clinically, albeit with caution. Pain is a typical hallmark of fracture either of the subchondral plate or of the articular surface and prompts both patient and orthopaedic surgeon to apply more aggressive treatment. Some authors argue that even clinically silent lesions should be treated aggressively in order to prevent fracture and subsequent sloughing of loose bodies.

With the advent of arthroscopy a number of new procedures, some mere revisions of classical forms of treatments and others relatively novel, have appeared.

Drilling of osteochondral lesions with an intact articular surface is quite popular.[8, 26, 38, 39] However, the precise effect of this procedure on the lesion has probably never been fully evaluated. Whether lesions truly heal or simply lie dormant is difficult to ascertain in many instances. Unfortunately, frequently within 1 or 2 years of drilling, the osteochondral fragment is extruded, which suggests that the procedure, although simple to perform and of little morbidity, may be ineffectual.

A more promising and yet technically much more demanding procedure is that of retrograde drilling and bone grafting. Today it is fashionable to perform the procedure arthroscopically (Fig. 17–12).[15, 19] It requires retrograde drilling with a 5- to 10-mm bit over a Kirschner wire that has previously been driven arthroscopically through the center of the defect. The bit is typically advanced until the articular cartilage is seen to vibrate. Remaining fibrous tissue may be removed with a curette. Extra care must be taken in removing the sclerotic bone and the fibrous tissue at the base of the defect without penetrating the articular surface. Bone graft removed from the immediate vicinity is packed into the cylindrical defect. The procedure is innovative but demanding. For lesions that extend far posterior, as is common with those of the lateral femoral condyle, the procedure may be technically impossible. The constant fear is of broaching

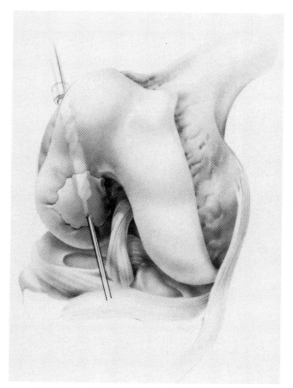

FIGURE 17–12. Retrograde drilling of an osteochondral defect of the medial femoral condyle.

the articular surface with the drill bit, and thus the technique may be more than the inexperienced arthroscopic surgeon may wish to entertain.

Of all the forms of arthroscopic treatment, probably the most facile and useful is extraction of loose bodies. When osteochondral lesions have fragmented, lack adequate bony backing, or have circumambulated for long periods within the joint and lost their original shape, simple extraction is the best treatment; arthroscopic treatment allows extraction with relative ease and little morbidity.

The gold standard of treatment of the intact and congruous loose fragment is replacement and pinning (Fig. 17–13).[26, 43, 44] In addition, the underlying fibrous tissue and sclerotic bone should be excised. Once these

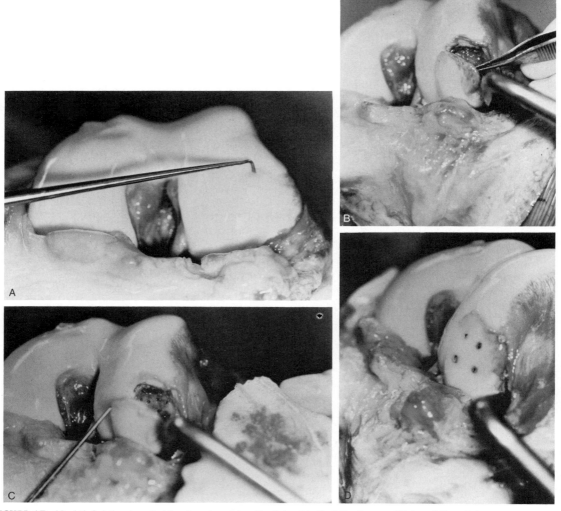

FIGURE 17–13. (A) Subtle chondral fracture involving the lateral half of the image. (B) Instability of the osteochondral fragment, which was obvious at the time of probing. Adequate bony backing was present, and therefore fibrous tissue was removed, and the sclerotic subchondral bone was drilled. (C) Bone graft was obtained from the adjacent femoral condyle, as shown on the gauze pledget held at right. This graft was packed beneath the fragment, which was then fixed with Herbert screws. (D) Osteochondritis dissecans with a 3-cm defect of the lateral femoral condyle in a 20-year-old man.

tissues have been removed, a congruent surface can be achieved with bone grafting, which is used to restore the proper height of the articular surface. Johnson performed this feat arthroscopically.[18] Arthroscopic bone grafting is a most demanding procedure and entails many technical difficulties, including precise incision of the margin of the osteochondral defect without wandering into normal articular cartilage, thorough removal of the underlying fibrous tissue and sclerotic bone, and pinning; bone grafting is almost impossible. In order to complete treatment with facility and thoroughness, it is probably better for inexperienced surgeons to perform the procedure with arthrotomy and depend on physical therapy for enabling the patient to recoup strength and motion.

Fixation of extruded fragments has been achieved by numerous means. Smillie and other authors have reported the use of smooth Kirchner wires,[26, 38] which have no inherent compressive quality; bone pegs,[12, 17, 38] which are relatively fragile; and nails, which must be removed, always with some difficulty and often with damage to the articular surface. More recently, biodegradable pins have been used, but they lack compressive qualities and have proved flimsy. Smillie reported the use of screws. Johnson inserted cannulated screws with arthroscopic technique, but the heads remain prominent and may scratch the opposing tibial articular surface.[18] They should be removed before motion is initiated.

Thomson popularized the use of Herbert screws (Fig. 17–14).[43] Designed for treatment of nonunion of fractures of the navicular bone, these screws have excellent compressive characteristics and heads that may be countersunk below the articular surface, enabling early range of motion, which favors nutrition of the articular cartilage. Although Thomson typically used only one screw per osteochondral fragment, it is probably better to use three or four per fragment in order to ensure proper grip of the entire graft and congruous margins. If the rim of the graft is slightly proud, the graft can be inset 1 or 2 mm simply with the compression

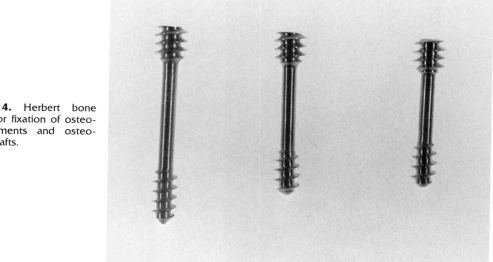

FIGURE 17–14. Herbert bone screws used for fixation of osteochondral fragments and osteochondral allografts.

afforded by the screw. If the rim is slightly recessed, cancellous bone graft may be added beneath the graft.

Because of the stiffness of screws in comparison with the articular cartilage, all screws except those deeply embedded in bone should be removed. Extraction is performed early before bone develops along the shank of the screw and prevents retrograde removal of the screw because of entrapment of the distal threads.

Arthroscopic surgeons have been optimistic about managing craters with abrasion arthroplasty, the arthroscopic version of Pridie spongialization.[10, 12, 43] Small lesions, typically those less than 2 cm in diameter (4 cm^2 in area), especially those with a firm margin or those which occur in younger patients, often respond well.[10] Histologic section reveals fibrous tissue or fibrocartilage with type I rather than type II collagen of hyaline cartilage.[36] A true lamina splendans and collagen arcades are not present. Once covered with fibrous tissue or fibrocartilage, these lesions are relatively silent clinically. Even some larger lesions occasionally fill rather uniformly and at least initially are clinically silent. Even though the fibrous layer may not prove durable and may fail to forestall arthritis, it is difficult not to accept treatment with abrasion arthroplasty as having at least qualified success. However, with lesions larger than 2 cm (4 cm^2), especially those in older patients or in patients who have failed to produce fibrous tissue after abrasion arthroplasty, pain, buckling, and swelling are

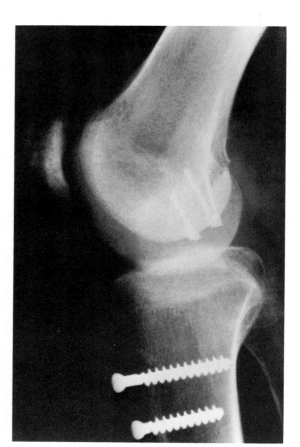

FIGURE 17–15. Treatment with a crescent-shaped osteochondral allograft.

common, and arthritis with joint space narrowing occurs in an accelerated fashion.

An alternative treatment before significant abrasion of the meniscus and tibial articular surface occurs is to patch these defects with an osteochondral graft (Fig. 17–15). Some surgeons[19] have advocated use of heterotopic autogenous grafts from distant sites within the knee; unfortunately, this typically results in symptomatic areas at the donor site, especially when large grafts are used. Allografts are a more plausible form of treatment.

The aims are to restore reasonable joint mechanics with segmental replacement of normal articular cartilage, which is superior to fibrocartilage, and to recreate the normal microarchitecture, including the excellent gliding surface of the lamina splendans, normal compliance of the collagen arcades, and solid anchorage to subchondral bone.

REFERENCES

1. Aichroth P: Osteochondritis dissecans of the knee: a clinical survey. J Bone Joint Surg 53B:440–447, 1971.
2. Barrie HJ: Osteochondritis dissecans 1887–1987: a centennial look at König's memorable phrase. J Bone Joint Surg 69B:693–695, 1987.
3. Bots RA, Slooff TJ: Arthroscopy in the evaluation of operative treatment of osteochondrosis dissecans. Orthop Clin North Am 10:685–696, 1979.
4. Bradley J, Dandy DJ: Osteochondritis dissecans and other lesions of the femoral condyles. J Bone Joint Surg 71B:518–522, 1989.
5. Caffey J, Madell SH, Royer C, Morales P: Ossification of the distal femoral epiphysis. J Bone Joint Surg 40A:647–654, 1958.
6. Cahill BR, Berg BC: 99m-Technetium phosphate compound joint scintigraphy in the management of juvenile osteochondritis dissecans of the femoral condyles. Am J Sports Med 11:329–335, 1983.
7. Chiroff RT, Cooke CP 3d: Osteochondritis dissecans: a histologic and microradiographic analysis of surgically excised lesions. J Trauma 15:689–696, 1975.
8. Clanton TO, DeLee JC: Osteochondritis dissecans: history, pathophysiology and current treatment concepts. Clin Orthop 167:50–64, 1982.
9. Desai SS, Patel MR, Michelli LJ, et al: Osteochondritis dissecans of the patella. J Bone Joint Surg 69B:320–325, 1987.
10. Ewing JW, Voto SJ: Arthroscopic surgical management of osteochondritis dissecans of the knee. Arthroscopy 4:37–40, 1988.
11. Fairbank HAT: Osteochondritis dissecans. Br J Surg 21:67–82, 1933.
12. Gillespie HW, Day B: Bone peg fixation in the treatment of osteochondritis dissecans of the knee joint. Clin Orthop 143:125–130, 1979.
13. Green WT, Banks HH: Osteochondritis dissecans in children. J Bone Joint Surg 35A:26–47, 1953.
14. Gross A, Langer F: Allotransplantation of partial joints in the treatment of osteoarthritis of the knee. J Bone Joint Surg 56A:1540, 1974.
15. Guhl JF: Arthroscopic treatment of osteochondritis dissecans. Clin Orthop 167: 65–74, 1982.
16. Hughston JC, Hergenroeder PT, Courternay BG: Osteochondritis dissecans of the femoral condyles. J Bone Joint Surg 66A:1340–1348, 1984.
17. Johnson EW Jr, McLeod TL: Osteochondral fragments of the distal end of the femur fixed with bone pegs: report of two cases. J Bone Joint Surg 59A:677–679, 1977.
18. Johnson L: Arthroscopic repair of osteochondritis dissecans [Arthroscopy vido digest]. Okemos, MI: Instrument Makar, August 1984.
19. Johnson RP, Aaberg TM Jr: Use of retrograde bone grafting in the treatment of osseous defects of the lateral condyle of the knee: a preliminary report of three knees in two patients. Am J Knee Surg 1:89, 1988.
20. König F: Ueber freie Korper in den Gelenken. Disch Z Fuer Chir 27:90, 1887–1888.
21. Langer F, Percy EC: Osteochondritis dissecans and anomalous centres of ossification: a review of 80 lesions in 61 patients. Can J Surg 14:208–215, 1971.
22. Linden B: Osteochondritis dissecans of the knee. J Bone Joint Surg 53B:448–454, 1971.
23. Linden B: Osteochondritis dissecans of the femoral condyles: a long-term follow-up study. J Bone Joint Surg 59A:769–776, 1977.

24. Linden B, Telhag H: Osteochondritis dissecans, a histologic and autoradiographic study in man. Acta Orthop Scand 48:682–686, 1977.
25. Lindholm S, Pylkkänen P: Internal fixation of the fragment of osteochondritis dissecans in the knee by means of bone pins: a preliminary report on several cases. Acta Chir Scand 140:626–629, 1974.
26. Lindholm TS, Osterman K: Long-term results after transfixation of an osteochondritis dissecans fragment to the femoral condyle using autologous bone transplants in adolescent and adult patients. Arch Orthop Trauma Surg 97:225–230, 1980.
27. Lipscomb PR Jr, Lipscomb PR Sr, Bryan RS: Osteochondritis dissecans of the knee with loose fragments: treatment by replacement and fixation with readily removed pins. J Bone Joint Surg 60A:235–240, 1978.
28. Mesgarzadeh M, Sapega AA, Bonakdarpour A, et al: Osteochondritis dissecans: analysis of mechanical stability with radiography, scintigraphy, and MR imaging. Radiology 161:24, 1986.
29. Milgram JW: Radiological and pathological manifestations of osteochondritis dissecans of the distal femur: a study of 50 cases. Radiology 126:305–311, 1978.
30. Mink JH, Reicher, MA, Crues JV III: Magnetic Resonance Imaging of the Knee. New York: Raven Press, 1987.
31. Mollan RA: Osteochondritis dissecans of the knee. Acta Orthop Scand 48:517–519, 1977.
32. Mubarak S, Carroll NC: Familial osteochondritis dissecans of the knee. Clin Orthop 140:131–136, 1979.
33. Outerbridge RE: Osteochondritis dissecans of the posterior femoral condyle. Clin Orthop 175:121–129, 1983.
34. Paget J: On the production of some of the loose bodies in joints. St Bartholomew's Hosp Rep 6:1–4, 1870.
35. Pappas AM: Osteochondritis dissecans. Clin Orthop 158:59–69, 1981.
36. Phillips HO 4th, Grubb SA: Familial multiple osteochondritis dissecans: report of a kindred. J Bone Joint Surg 67A:155–156, 1985.
37. Reicher MA, Bassett LW, Gold RH: High-resolution magnetic resonance imaging of the knee joint: pathologic correlations. AJR 145:903–909, 1985.
38. Ribbing S: The hereditary multiple epiphyseal disturbance and its consequences for the aetiogenesis of local malacias—particularly the osteochondrosis dissecans. Acta Orthop Scand 24:286–299, 1955.
39. Smillie IS: Treatment of osteochondritis dissecans. J Bone Joint Surg 39B:248–260, 1957.
40. Smillie IS: Osteochondritis Dissecans. London: E. & S. Livingstone, 1960.
41. Sontag LW, Pyle SI: Variations in the calcification pattern in epiphyses; their nature and significance. Am J Roentgenol 45:50–54, 1941.
42. Stougaard J: Osteochondritis dissecans of the patella. Acta Orthop Scand 45:111–118, 1974.
43. Thomson NL: Osteochondritis dissecans and osteochondral fragments managed by Herbert compression screw fixation. Clin Orthop 224:71–78, 1987.
44. Yamashita F, Sakakida K, Suzu F, Takai S: The transplantation of an autogenic osteochondral fragment for osteochondritis dissecans of the knee. Clin Orthop 201:43–50, 1985.

PART IV

Orthopaedic

Sports

Traumatology:

Laxity of the

Knee

CHAPTER 18

Evaluation and

Decision

Making for

Ligamentous

Injury

ROBERT L. LARSON, M.D.

■

Ligamentous injury to the knee is generally categorized into two broad classifications: acute and chronic. Although there are some differences in the time references for acute and chronic injuries, acute injuries are defined as injuries that have occurred within 3 weeks before diagnosis or treatment is sought, and chronic injuries are those that occurred more than 3 weeks earlier. Some authors prefer to classify injuries up to 6 weeks in duration as acute, and others use a third category of "subacute" to differentiate injuries approximately 3 to 12 weeks old. The rationale for limiting the acute category to the 3-week time period is that it is during this period that the effects of the joint trauma are most predominant. Intra-articular attachment sites of the cruciate ligament may still be viable and contribute to the repair or the reconstruction of the ligament. Degenerative changes will not have had a chance to play a part in the outcome of joint function. In the chronic ligamentous injury, the patient will have had a chance to test the functional use of the knee and the limits that the ligamentous laxity places on knee use. Further damage to knee structures may have occurred, such as meniscal damage, degenerative changes, or further ligamentous stretching of secondary stabilizing structures.

ACUTE LIGAMENTOUS INJURY

Many factors influence the decision concerning the treatment of the knee with an acute injury. These factors include the severity and the type of ligament damage that has occurred, the age of the patient, the condition of the joint, associated collateral ligament injuries, meniscal injuries or osteochondral injury, and the activity level of the patient. Medial collateral ligament injuries (MCL) that do not involve either the meniscus or the anterior cruciate ligament (ACL) can usually be treated by nonsurgical methods.

Isolated Medial Collateral and Capsular Injuries

Many studies have shown that rupture of the MCL without an associated injury to the ACL heals satisfactorily with little residual laxity.[5, 9, 11, 22] Inoue and associates[12] studied dogs in which the MCL had been cut. The functional deficit of valgus laxity was compensated for by remaining structures, especially the ACL. A study on cadaver knees showed that when the MCL was cut, a valgus, external torque, and an anterior tibial force (when the tibia is externally rotated) caused increased stress forces to the ACL.[18] The authors of that study suggested that a patient with residual valgus laxity from a previous injury is at risk of producing injurious forces to the ACL by these loading modes.

Treatment by protective mobilization and maintenance of muscle strength is necessary for proper healing of the MCL. These measures diminish the chance of residual valgus laxity and the resultant generation of excessive forces to the ACL.

When the ACL has been torn in addition to the medial supporting structures, surgical repair of the acutely torn tissue is usually appropriate. If a peripheral tear of the meniscus is determined by arthrography, magnetic resonance imaging, or arthroscopy, surgical repair of the meniscus is necessary. This may be accomplished through arthroscopic methods.

A decision of whether to surgically repair the MCL rupture is influenced by the site of the tear. Tears of the proximal portion of the ligament heal without surgical intervention. Ruptures of the distal attachment often require surgical reattachment in order to ensure maximal stability.

The decision of operative versus nonoperative treatment is also influenced by the degree of rupture and the level of athletic activity or the presence of an osteochondral injury. Evidence of a complete midsubstance tear of the MCL with 3+ joint opening on valgus stress testing in a high-level competitive athlete may sway the decision toward an operative repair with autogenous augmentation of the disrupted tissue. An osteochondral injury producing a loose body or a symptomatic articular lesion may also require a surgical approach, which may or may not include surgical repair of the ligament, depending on the severity of the injury. Selectivity of the treatment of ligamentous injuries is necessary. No one approach is correct for every individual.

Lateral Collateral Ligament Injuries

Injuries to the lateral collateral ligament and the structures of the posterolateral corner provide a different perspective for the treating physician. The residual laxity and the resultant instabilities that are produced are often very difficult to correct by reconstructive methods. Isolated lateral collateral injuries are significantly less common than are isolated medial collateral injuries. Particularly troublesome are the posterolateral instabilities that result from injury to the arcuate complex. Many reconstructive procedures have been described for the correction of the functional disability produced by such laxity. The surgical reconstruction is extensive, and the results are not as satisfactory as on the medial side. Approximation of the acutely torn tissue is much easier and more successful than is later reconstruction. Augmentation of disrupted tissue may be required at the time of the acute repair.

Isolated ACL Injury

The existence of an isolated ACL injury has been debated for some time. Joint displacement must be considerable in order to cause tearing of ligamentous structures. The collateral and capsular ligaments and the cruciate ligaments contribute in some part to the major stabilizing function of one another. Meniscal injury is present in more than 60 per cent of those patients in whom the ACL is torn.[3, 14, 15] Often at arthroscopy, additional evidence of joint injury, such as capsular rents or evidence of bleeding in the capsular tissue suggestive of tearing, is found.[2] Thus the assumption that an isolated ACL injury has occurred is probably unfounded; nevertheless, in many patients, the only significant injury detected within the knee joint is the ACL lesion.[14]

There are differing opinions about the treatment of these "isolated" ACL injuries. Jackson[14] evaluated 21 knees that were thought to have isolated lesions of the ACL. In half, there were complete ruptures, and in the other half, there were partial ruptures. At a 10-year follow-up, only 5 per cent of the patients had undergone further surgery, and another 80 per cent were actively involved in sports. This group was compared with another group involving 42 knees that sustained damage to other supporting structures in addition to the ACL tear. Of these patients, 25 per cent underwent further surgery, and only 10 per cent were involved in competitive sports.

In an animal study, the ACL was transected either completely or partially in order to determine the amount of healing that had occurred over a 2- to 52-week period. No regeneration was present after complete transection. Partially sectioned ligaments exhibited slow and incomplete regeneration. Although normal stiffness had returned, the defect was filled with tissue that was histologically different from the normal ligamentous tissue. The strength of the healed ligament was only two-thirds that of the contralateral ACL in the immature rabbit and three-fourths that of the contralateral ACL in the mature animal.[10]

Such studies influence the judgment of repair of ACL ruptures in the acute stage. The patient who wishes to remain athletically active or whose work demands vigorous knee use is a candidate for surgical repair and augmentation or reconstruction. Further meniscal damage may be prevented, and the functional usefulness of the knee will be improved. The older patient whose lifestyle does not entail excessive twisting or impact loading stresses to the knee might instead undergo nonsurgical treatment consisting of muscle strengthening, bracing, and activity modifications that do not stress the knee. The activity level is the factor determining the necessity for surgery, not age. Patients with good joint surfaces who demand an active lifestyle should be able to regain as much function as possible no matter what their age.

If from history and clinical examination there is good reason to suspect that an ACL injury has occurred, an examination with the patient under anesthesia and an arthroscopic evaluation to assess the amount of damage are appropriate. Maruyama and Jackson[14] found that of patients with a torn ACL, 81 per cent have combined injuries to the menisci, capsule, or collateral ligaments, and 19 per cent have an apparently isolated lesion. One third of the ACL tears are partial with some functional bands remaining. Of patients in whom more than half the fibers are ruptured, 75 per cent develop symptomatic instability. A report on arthroscopically confirmed partial tears of the ACL divided the patients into two groups: those with KT-1000 side-to-side differences of less than 3 mm and those with differences of 3 mm and more. Those with more laxity had less functional ability and less subjective satisfaction than did patients with more stable ACLs.[6]

In a prearthroscopy discussion with the patient, a decision should be made as to whether a surgical procedure to correct the ACL deficiency should be conducted at the time of arthroscopy.

Association with Meniscal Tear

Preservation of as much meniscal tissue as possible is now recognized as a protective factor in the prevention of joint wear. In a peripheral rim tear in which the body of the meniscus is still intact, the meniscus should be reattached. Studies by DeHaven and colleagues[4] have shown that in such repairs, the incidence of retear is much higher among patients who have an unstable knee. In a patient with high-demand activities, ACL stabilization is recommended if meniscal repair is performed.

Arthroscopic partial meniscectomy in an ACL-deficient knee was reported by Aglietti and collaborators.[1] A follow-up study of 100 patients after 3.5 years showed a 52 per cent satisfactory result; 41 per cent were able to participate in strenuous sports activities. Complete ACL lesions had a poorer prognosis than did partial tears.

The timing of surgery after an ACL rupture has been determined to be related to postoperative restricted motion. Strum and associates[21] compared a group of acute repairs with a group of chronic reconstructions. Arthrofibrosis was present in 35 per cent of patients in the acute surgical group and in only 12 per cent of patients in the chronic group. Among ACL reconstructive procedures performed as a primary treatment within 1 week of ACL ruptures, there was an increase in the incidence of restricted motion.[7, 16, 19]

Flow charts that help in evaluation and treatment are given in Chapter 20. The steps in the charts are not absolute indications, inasmuch as considerations for the individual patient are part of the decision-making process. These charts are provided only to initiate and aid in determining a proper evaluation and treatment program.

CHRONIC LIGAMENTOUS INSTABILITY

Chronic ligamentous instability usually involves a cruciate injury, a meniscal injury, or unrecognized muscle weakness. A mild instability may become a functional problem after a knee injury with subsequent development of muscle weakness from disuse. MCL injuries without an associated ACL or meniscal tear generally do not result in any residual functional disability.

A chronic instability that produces a functional instability is nearly always associated with an insufficient cruciate ligament. The unrecognized ACL rupture with a resultant pivot shift is the most common type of chronic instability that causes a patient to seek medical help.

More than 60 per cent of acute ACL injuries are associated with a meniscal tear; however, among such patients with a chronic instability that was not diagnosed until 10 years after the original injury, there was a 90 per cent incidence of meniscal tear.[14] Many of these patients seek medical help because of the catching and locking associated with the meniscal tear. Removal of the torn meniscus, although improving the symptoms of catching, locking, and joint irritation, may produce an increase in the instability.

A group of ACL-deficient knees in which chronic meniscal tears were treated by meniscectomy were reviewed by Patterson and Trickey.[17] Removal of the bucket-handle tear provided good results, whereas complete meniscectomy for posterior horn tears yielded poor results. Of the 40 patients studied, 22 experienced relief from instability symptoms by meniscectomy. An additional eight needed no further surgical treatment. The remaining 10 required surgical procedures for stabilizing the knee because of persistent symptoms.

The surgeon faced with the problem of meniscal tears must make a decision with the patient as to whether arthroscopic partial meniscectomy with a relatively quick rehabilitation time or meniscectomy and ligament reconstruction with a much longer period of recovery is appropriate for that patient. For a peripheral tear in a young, active patient, reattachment of the meniscus and an ACL reconstruction provide the best chance of successful result. When a partial meniscectomy is required, the addition of a ligament reconstruction would also be indicated in a patient who wants to continue with a very active lifestyle. In patients who are willing to modify their activity level, the arthroscopic partial meniscectomy may be the procedure of choice. Shields and colleagues[20] reported a series of 45 patients with a 2- to 9-year follow-up who had undergone partial meniscectomy and had an ACL deficiency. They found that 65 per cent with a positive Lachman sign and a 1+ pivot shift returned to their previous activity level with no limitation. Only 20 per cent of those with an instability of more than 1+ were able to perform without limitation.

DEGENERATIVE JOINT DISEASE. This condition may also be associated with chronic ligamentous instability. Often when enough osteophytic proliferation has occurred, the joint becomes more stable. The examiner must differentiate the pain associated with use of a degenerated joint from that associated with any instability that remains. Stabilizing a joint that has undergone degenerative changes may not eliminate the pain.

There are situations in which a marked pivot shift occurs in a joint with degenerative changes or gonarthrosis confined to one side of the joint. The pain is localized to that side and obviously results from the wear changes present. In such a case, a high tibial osteotomy to treat the unicompartmental problem and an ACL reconstruction to resolve the ACL deficiency can be performed in one surgical session.

MUSCLE WEAKNESS. This condition may be a cause of functional disability in a patient with instability. It is sometimes seen in a patient who has a chronic ACL deficiency and who has tolerated the loss well either because of self-imposed restriction of activity level or because of lack of symptoms. An injury to the knee occurs, and because of the lack of use, muscle weakness develops. This results in the emergence of a functional instability that was not manifest when the muscles were at their normal strength. Recognition of the problem as being the development of muscle weakness secondary to the injury and treatment designed to restore muscle strength may enable the patient to return to the preinjury status of function without disability.

If joint changes, such as degenerative joint disease, or marked instability prevents the patient from developing muscle strength through an exercise program, the instability may become a functional problem that requires a surgical correction.

NONSURGICAL TREATMENT

In the acute injury, the nonsurgical treatment is indicated in patients with an MCL injury without associated meniscal or ACL injury. A physical therapy program designed to maintain muscle strength and yet protect the ligament from undue stress is provided. Specifics of this program are described in Chapter 20.

For patients with a chronic problem of ligamentous instability for whom surgical reconstruction is not appropriate or who do not want surgery, a specific exercise program is required for developing and maintaining muscle strength. Activity modification in order to prevent repetitive impact loading to the joint or exposure to situations that may cause the knee to give way is also advised. Bracing may provide enough stability or confidence in the joint that the patient can participate in some recreational athletic endeavors without manifesting the clinical problems of instability.

SURGICAL TREATMENT

Functional instability is the sine qua non of surgical correction for providing active use of the knee. Modifying factors must be considered in order to determine the type of surgery. Degenerative changes in the joint, extremity alignment, age, and activity level influence the decision of which type of surgery would be best for a given patient. Osteotomy, extra-articular procedures, and intra-articular procedures and their indications are discussed in other chapters.

A final judgment concerns the status of the menisci and the activity level of the patient. If the menisci are still intact and the patient with an unstable knee continues to participate in activities that will endanger the integrity of the menisci, thoughtful consideration and advice to the patient of the consequences of meniscal loss should be given. Surgical stabilization in such a situation may protect the knee in the long term.

STANDARD EVALUATION OF KNEE LIGAMENT SURGERY

A uniform method of evaluating results and rating the success of ligamentous surgery of the knee has been lacking. Subjective evaluation has the disadvantage of the variables of interpretation by patients. Objective testing relies on the examiner's definition of laxity and the level of severity as determined by the examiner at the time of testing. This definition and the grading are variable not only from examiner to examiner but also for the same examiner on different days. P. J. Fowler (personal communication) suggested defining the evaluation as "subjective-subjective," "subjective-objective," and "objective-objective." Clinical tests such as the Lachman test, the pivot shift test, and drawer testing are subjective-objective in that performance is rated according to the examiner's interpretation of the degree of laxity and cannot be measured precisely. Only tests that can actually be measured are considered to be objective-objective. Range of motion, instrumented measurement of laxity, and the functional hop test are examples.

The International Knee Documentation Committee,[13] which is made up of members of the American Orthopaedic Society of Sports Medicine and the European Society of the Knee and Arthroscopy, worked for several years to develop a universal system of knee evaluation so that results of different surgeons or studies could be compared. The Committee provided a standardized form for recording the data that was believed to best enable such a comparison. The data are graded according to the guidelines as normal, nearly normal, abnormal, and severely abnormal (Fig. 18–1).

Seven variables—the patient's subjective assessment, symptoms, range of motion, results of ligament examination, compartmental findings

KNEE LIGAMENT STANDARD EVALUATION FORM

Patient Name _____ Date _____/ _____/ _____ Medical Record# _____

Occupation _____ Sport: 1st Choice _____ 2nd Choice _____

Age _____ Sex _____ Ht _____ Wt _____ Involved Knee: ☐ Right ☐ Left   Contralateral Normal: ☐ Yes ☐ No

Cause of injury: ☐ ADL   Date of Injury: ___/ ___/ _____   Procedure _____
        ☐ Traffic
        ☐ Contact Sport   Date of Index Operation: ___/ ___/ ____   Postop Dx _____
        ☐ Noncontact Sport

ACTIVITY

	Pre-injury	Pre-Rx	Post-Rx
I. Strenuous Activity jumping, pivoting, hard cutting (football, soccer)			
II. Moderate Activity heavy manual work (skiing, tennis)			
III. Light Activity (jogging, running)			
IV. Sedentary Activity (housework, ADL)			

PREVIOUS SURGERY

Arthroscopy: Date (1) _____ (2) _____ (3) _____

Meniscectomy: Dx   _____   _____   _____

Stabilization: Procedure   _____   _____   _____

MENISCAL STATUS

	N1	1/3	2/3	Total
Med				
Lat				

SEVEN GROUPS / FOUR GRADES / *GROUP GRADE

SEVEN GROUPS	A. Normal	B. Nearly Normal	C. Abnormal	D. Sev. Abnorm.	A	B	C	D
1. Patient Subjective Assessment How does your knee function?	☐0	☐1	☐2	☐3				
On a scale of 0 to 3, how does your knee affect your activity level?	☐0	☐1	☐2	☐3	☐	☐	☐	☐
2. SYMPTOMS (Grade at highest activity level with no significant symptoms. Exclude 0 to slight symptoms.)	**I.** Strenuous Activity	**II.** Moderate Activity	**III.** Light Activity	**IV.** Sedentary Activity				
Pain	☐	☐	☐	☐				
Swelling	☐	☐	☐	☐				
Partial Giving Way	☐	☐	☐	☐				
Full Giving Way	☐	☐	☐	☐	☐	☐	☐	☐
3. RANGE OF MOTION Ext/Flex: Index side: ___/ ___/ ___ Opposite side: ___/ ___/ ___								
Lack of extension (from 0°)	☐<3°	☐3 to 5°	☐6 to 10°	☐>10°				
Lack of flexion	☐0 to 5°	☐6 to 15°	☐16 to 25°	☐>25°	☐	☐	☐	☐
4. LIGAMENT EXAMINATION (manual, instrument, x-ray) LACHMAN (25° flex)	☐–1 to 2mm	☐3 to 5mm –1 to –3 stiff	☐6 to 10mm < –3 stiff	☐>10mm				
Endpoint: firm/soft	☐firm		☐soft					
Total A.P. Transl. (70° flex)	☐0 to 2mm	☐3 to 5mm	☐6 to 10mm	☐>10mm				
Post. sag (70° flex)	☐0 to 2mm	☐3 to 5mm	☐6 to 10mm	☐>10mm				
Med jt opening (20° flex)(valgus rot)	☐0 to 2mm	☐3 to 5mm	☐6 to 10mm	☐>10mm				
Lat jt opening (20° flex)(varus rot)	☐0 to 2mm	☐3 to 5mm	☐6 to 10mm	☐>10mm				
Pivot shift	☐neg.	☐+ (glide)	☐++ (clunk)	☐+++ (gross)				
Reversed pivot shift	☐equal	☐glide	☐marked	☐gross	☐	☐	☐	☐
5. COMPARTMENTAL FINDINGS Crepitus patellofemoral	☐none		☐moderate	☐severe				
Crepitus medial compartment	☐none		☐moderate	☐severe				
Crepitus lateral compartment	☐none		☐moderate	☐severe palpable & audible	☐		☐	☐
6. X-RAY FINDINGS Med Joint space narrowing	☐none		☐<50%	☐>50%				
Lat Joint space narrowing	☐none		☐<50%	☐>50%				
Patellofemoral joint narrowing	☐none		☐<50%	☐>50%	☐		☐	☐
7. FUNCTIONAL TEST One leg hop (% of opposite side)	☐100 to 90%	☐90 to 76%	☐75 to 50%	☐<50%	☐	☐	☐	☐
****FINAL EVALUATION**					☐	☐	☐	☐

*Group Grade: The lowest grade within a group determines the group grade. **Final Evaluation: The worst group determines the final evaluation. In a final evaluation, all 7 groups are to be evaluated. For a quick knee profile, the evaluation of groups, 1 to 4 are sufficient.

IKDC — INTERNATIONAL KNEE DOCUMENTATION COMMITTEE, Members of the Committee:
AOSSM: Anderson, AF, Clancy, WG, Daniel, D, Dehaven, KE, Fowler, PJ, Feagin, J, Grood, ES, Noyes, FR, Terry, GC, Torzilli, P, Warren, RF.
ESKA: Chambat, P, Eriksson, E, Gillquist, J, Hefti, F, Huiskes, R, Jakob, RP, Moyen, B, Mueller, W, Staeubli, H, Vankampen, A.

FIGURE 18–1. Knee Ligament Standard Evaluation Form developed by the International Knee Documentation Committee. (From International Knee Documentation Committee: Meeting, Abstracts, and Outlines, 117–120. *Presented at* the 17th annual meeting of the American Orthopaedic Society for Sports Medicine, Orlando, FL, July 1991.)

(crepitation), radiographic findings, and results of functional tests—are recorded and assigned one of the four grades just described. The patient's function is graded on the highest activity level attained: level I is jumping, pivoting, and hard cutting; level II is heavy manual work or sports activity such as skiing or tennis; level III is light manual work or activities such as jogging or running; and level IV is sedentary work or activities of daily living (ADL). Symptoms of pain, swelling, partial giving way, or full giving way are also related to the activity level engaged in.

Range of motion is measured and assigned a grade (Fig. 18–1). Ligament examination includes the Lachman test and its end point, total anterior-posterior translation at 70° flexion, medial joint opening (valgus rotation), lateral joint opening (varus rotation), pivot shift, and reverse pivot shift (Chapter 4).

A "Quick Knee Profile" consisting of only the patient's subjective assessment, symptoms, range of motion, and results of ligament examination can be used. For a more thorough evaluation, compartmental findings, radiographic findings, and a functional test (one-leg hop test) can be included.

The evaluation of knee ligament surgery by the use of a standardized form and with an agreed method of grading enables a more valid comparison of various surgical techniques.

Confidence in the accuracy of the assessment of the individual patient and in surgical abilities to reconstruct the ACL remains somewhat shaky because of current clinical testing methods. Harter and associates[8] tested 51 patients with previously reconstructed ACLs for whom the postsurgery follow-up interval averaged 48 months. The patients' perceptions of postoperative knee status were independent of results of static and dynamic clinical tests. Deficits in the reconstructed knee of up to 30 per cent of function and stability in comparison with the normal contralateral knee did not influence the patients' perception of knee function.

REFERENCES

1. Aglietti P, Buzzi R, Bassi PB: Arthroscopic partial meniscectomy in the anterior cruciate deficient knee. Am J Sports Med 16:597–602, 1988.
2. Cerabona F, Sherman MF, Bonamo JR, et al: Patterns of meniscal injury with acute anterior cruciate tears. Am J Sports Med 16:603–609, 1988.
3. DeHaven K: Diagnosis of acute knee injuries with hemarthrosis. Am J Sports Med 8:9–14, 1980.
4. DeHaven K, Black K, Griffiths H: Open meniscal repair technique and two to nine year results. Am J Sports Med 17:788–795, 1989.
5. Ellsasser J, Reynolds F, Omohundro J: The non-operative treatment of collateral ligament injuries of the knee in professional football players: an analysis of 74 injuries treated non-operatively and 24 injuries treated surgically. J Bone Joint Surg 56A:1185–1190, 1974.
6. Foreman K, Daniel D: Determining the partial tears of the anterior cruciate ligament by displacement measurements. *Presented at* the annual meeting of the American Orthopaedic Society for Sports Medicine, Palm Springs, CA, June 1988.
7. Harner C, Paul J, Fu F, et al: Loss of motion following arthroscopic anterior cruciate ligament reconstruction. *Presented at* the annual meeting of the American Academy of Orthopaedic Surgeons, Anaheim, CA, March 1991.
8. Harter RA, Osternig LR, Singer KM, et al: Long-term evaluation of knee stability and function following surgical reconstruction for anterior cruciate ligament insufficiency. Am J Sports Med 16:434–443, 1988.
9. Hastings D: The non-operative management of collateral ligament injuries of the knee joint. Clin Orthop 147:22–28, 1980.
10. Hefti F, Kress K, Fasel J, et al: Healing of the transected anterior cruciate ligament in the rabbit. J Bone Joint Surg 73A:373–383, 1991.

11. Indelicato P: Non-operative treatment of complete tears of the medial collateral ligament of the knee. J Bone Joint Surg 65A:323–329, 1983.
12. Inoue M, McGurk-Burleson E, Hollis M, et al: Treatment of the medial collateral ligament injury: I. The importance of anterior cruciate ligament on the varus-valgus knee laxity. Am J Sports Med 15:15–21, 1987.
13. International Knee Documentation Committee: Meeting, Abstracts, and Outlines, 117–120. *Presented at* the 17th annual meeting of the American Orthopaedic Society of Sports Medicine, Orlando, FL, July 1991.
14. Jackson R: The torn ACL: Natural history of untreated lesions and rationale for selective treatment. *In* Feagin J (ed): The Crucial Ligaments, pp. 341–000. New York: Churchill Livingstone, 1988.
15. Noyes FR, Bassett RW, Grood ES, et al: Arthroscopy in acute traumatic hemarthrosis of the knee: incidence of anterior cruciate tears and other injuries. J Bone Joint Surg 62A:687–695, 1980.
16. Ott J, Graf B, Keene J, et al: Risk factors for restricted motion after anterior cruciate ligament reconstruction: a reconstructive study of 373 patients. *Presented at* the annual meeting of the American Academy of Orthopaedic Surgeons, Anaheim, CA, March 1991.
17. Patterson F, Trickey E: Meniscectomy for tears of the meniscus combined with rupture of the anterior cruciate ligament. J Bone Joint Surg 65B:388–390, 1983.
18. Shapiro M, Markolf K, Finerman G, et al: The effect of section of the medial collateral ligament on forces generated in the anterior cruciate ligament. J Bone Joint Surg 73A:248–256, 1991.
19. Shelbourne K, Whitaker J, McCarroll J, et al: Anterior cruciate ligament injury: evaluation of intra-articular reconstruction of acute tears without repair. Am J Sports Med 18:484–489, 1990.
20. Shields CL, Silva I, Yee L, et al: Evaluation of residual instability after arthroscopic meniscectomy in anterior cruciate deficient knees. Am J Sports Med 15:129–131, 1987.
21. Strum G, Friedman M, Fox J, et al: Acute anterior cruciate reconstruction: analysis of complications. Clin Orthop 253:184–189, 1990.
22. Woo S, Inoue M, McGurk-Burelson E, et al: Treatment of medial collateral ligament injury: II. Structure and function of canine knees in response to differing treatment regimens. Am J Sports Med 15:22–29, 1990.

CHAPTER 19

Acute

Dislocations

ROBERT S. BURGER, M.D.

ROBERT L. LARSON, M.D.

■

Acute traumatic knee dislocations are rare. Many cases that occur go unrecognized because of spontaneous relocations before admission to the hospital.[9] Hoover[8] identified only 14 knee dislocations of 2 million admissions to the Mayo Clinic over a 50-year period. The highest incidence was reported by Quinlan and Sharrard,[19] who reviewed injuries at a regional medical center in England and reported six knee dislocations of 48,000 bone and joint injuries. Shields and associates[22] reported 26 cases admitted to the Massachusetts General Hospital during a 28-year period. Meyers and Harvey[13] reported 53 cases during a 10-year period at the Los Angeles County Hospital. An acute traumatic dislocation of the knee is a true orthopaedic emergency, and rapid diagnosis and treatment are therefore essential.

CLASSIFICATION

Classification is based on the relationship of the position of the tibia to the femur (Fig. 19–1).

TYPE

1. Anterior dislocations.
2. Posterior dislocations.
3. Lateral dislocations.
4. Medial dislocations.
5. Rotational dislocations. Posterolateral is the most common rotational dislocation. Although it rarely occurs, it is usually irreducible.[7, 9, 19] It is associated with a high incidence of peroneal nerve injuries.

OPEN VERSUS CLOSED INJURY

Injuries are also subcategorized as open or closed. Traumatic dislocations of the knee must be differentiated from so-called floating knee, in which fractures occur in both the femur and the tibia. These injuries are complex and must be treated with bone-fixation procedures and are beyond the scope of this chapter (see Chapter 7).

MECHANISM OF INJURY

The majority of traumatic dislocations of the knee occur in motor vehicle accidents. Other causes are high-velocity injuries (such as falling from a height), sporting activities, and severe twisting injuries.

Anterior dislocations are often caused by hyperextension. Kennedy[9] found that the posterior capsule was torn at 30° of hyperextension; at further extension, the posterior cruciate ligament (PCL) was torn, and then the knee dislocated anteriorly. He noted that the popliteal artery ruptured at approximately 50° of hyperextension. Such extremes are not necessary to produce similar injuries in vivo.[10] Girgis and colleagues[5] found that the PCL tears only after the anterior cruciate ligament (ACL) has torn.

Posterior dislocations are caused by a blow to the anterior proximal portion of the tibia, and the extensor mechanism is often disrupted concurrently. Medial and lateral dislocations are caused by varus and valgus stresses, respectively.

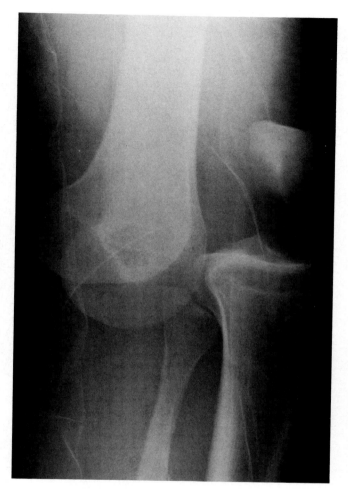

FIGURE 19–1. Anterior dislocation of right knee sustained by a 19-year-old male in a vehicle accident. Initial examination showed absence of posterior tibial and dorsalis pedis pulsation, foot dusky with poor capillary refill. Reduction with the patient under anesthesia followed by arteriogram was performed (see Fig. 19–3). (Courtesy of K. M. Singer, M.D., Eugene, Oregon.)

Posterolateral dislocation is caused by a valgus medial rotational force on the proximal tibia. These types of injuries are often irreducible because of the buttonhole effect of the medial femoral condyle as it passes through the medial capsule.[2, 19, 25] The clinical manifestation is a skin dimple that is produced on the medial side of the knee. Posterolateral dislocations rarely produce arterial injury, but the peroneal nerve is frequently injured.

ANATOMY

The popliteal artery is the main extension of the superficial femoral artery as it passes through the adductor hiatus on the distal medial side of the thigh (Fig. 19–2). The popliteal artery is anchored at two points: proximally at the adductor hiatus and distally at the soleal arch. The artery is tethered at both these sites, causing a limited excursion during any kind of injury. The genicular branches that arise between these two points are insufficient for maintaining viability of the leg.[3, 14] Any injury to the major artery severely compromises the viability of the leg.

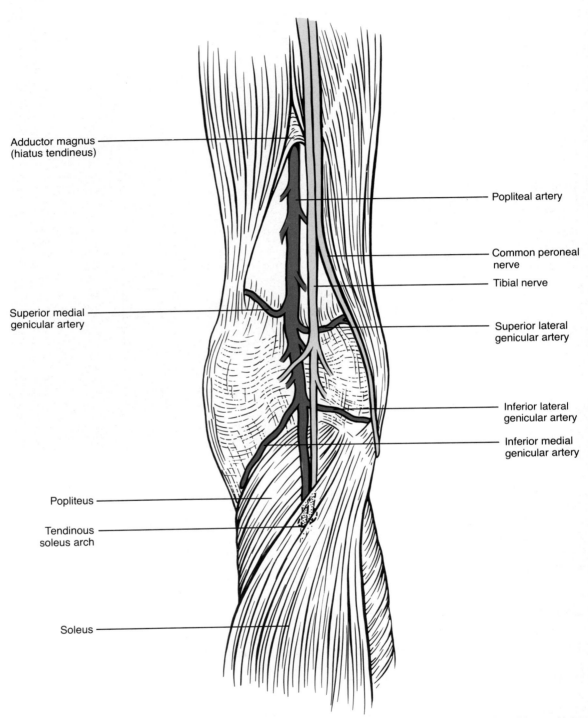

Adductor magnus
(hiatus tendineus)

Superior medial
genicular artery

Popliteus

Tendinous
soleus arch

Soleus

Popliteal artery

Common peroneal
nerve

Tibial nerve

Superior lateral
genicular artery

Inferior lateral
genicular artery

Inferior medial
genicular artery

FIGURE 19–2. Popliteal artery and its branches in posterior aspect of knee. Note artery fixed at adductor hiatus proximally and at soleal arch distally. Fixation points subject the artery to possible injury with knee dislocation.

ASSOCIATED INJURIES

LIGAMENTS. Ligaments are involved in all knee dislocations. Both the ACL and the PCL are involved in most knee dislocations.[10, 15, 20, 23] Meyers and Harvey[13] reported five cases in which the ACL was torn but the PCL was intact. Usually the medial collateral ligament (MCL) or the lateral collateral ligament (LCL) or both are torn. Capsular disruption is often extensive. Tendons are often involved with ligament injury. Injury to the medial gastrocnemius tendon is often associated with MCL injury; injury to the popliteal tendon, with LCL injury.[15] Thorough understanding of the complexities of the anatomy of the posteromedial and postero-lateral complexes is essential before any surgical repair is performed (see Chapter 2).

Associated fractures occur in 20 to 60 per cent of dislocations, usually with fractures of the ipsilateral tibia and femur and exclusive of avulsion fractures.[12, 13, 14, 23, 26] The tibial plateau is often fractured.[12]

ARTERIAL INJURIES. These injuries occur in approximately 40 per cent of anterior and posterior dislocations.[6, 8, 13, 22, 23, 25] Anterior dislocations have the highest rate of vascular compromise and are associated with intimal damage to the vessel, which leads to thrombosis or rupture.[11] Posterior dislocations frequently cause disruption of the artery.[6, 9, 22]

NERVE INJURY. This injury is present in approximately 22 per cent of dislocations.[9, 10, 13, 14, 20, 22, 23] Posterolateral dislocations have the highest incidence of nerve injury. The nerve most commonly injured is the peroneal nerve, followed in frequency by the tibial nerve; both are branches of the sciatic nerve (see Fig. 2–23). The nerves are not as firmly fixed to the surrounding structures as are the arteries; this lack of firm fixation accounts for the lower incidence of injury.

EVALUATION AND TREATMENT

A thorough history and physical examination as well as a high level of suspicion help diagnose a knee dislocation. The patient may have no swelling around the knee, and the position of the leg may appear normal. This occurs when a spontaneous reduction has occurred either at the time of injury or during transport to the hospital. A history from the first person who saw the patient or the people who brought the patient into the hospital (paramedics, trainers, coaches) is necessary in order to ascertain the prehospitalization condition. Pertinent questions include the time of injury, whether there was any immediate swelling, whether a reduction was performed or occurred spontaneously, and whether there had been a change in the hospitalization status from the prehospitalization status. When ischemia lasts more than 6 hours, the prognosis for limb salvage declines from good to poor. The amputation rate is exceptionally high among dislocations in which ischemia extends past 8 hours.[6, 12]

Inspection should include the position of the leg, the condition of the skin, determination of whether the injury is open or closed, and the extent of swelling. Dimpling of the skin, especially on the anteromedial side of the knee, should arouse suspicion of a posterolateral dislocation.

A vascular examination for evaluating the anterior tibial pulse, the posterior tibial pulse, capillary refill, and temperature of the skin is essential. The findings must be documented in order to provide a clear comparison as sequential examinations are performed. No or minimal swelling about the knee may signify severe capsular disruption with extravasation of blood and fluid into the surrounding soft tissues. Palpation of the calf and thigh musculature is necessary for detecting compartmental syndromes. A pressure catheter may be needed for determining increased pressures within any of the compartments.[16]

The vascular examination determines the viability of the leg and the need for immediate surgery. Normal pulses in the uninjured limb must be palpated and compared with those in the injured limb in order to ensure adequate vascular flow is present. A warm foot does not by itself indicate vascular sufficiency.[1, 4, 6, 9, 26]

A Doppler study may be performed, but the arteriogram (Fig. 19–3) is the most specific test and should be performed if there is any question as to the vascular status. Sequential physical examinations are important for documenting the vascular status or any change that may occur for up to 1 week after injury as a result of thrombus formation.[4, 23]

A thorough neurologic examination, both motor and sensory, should

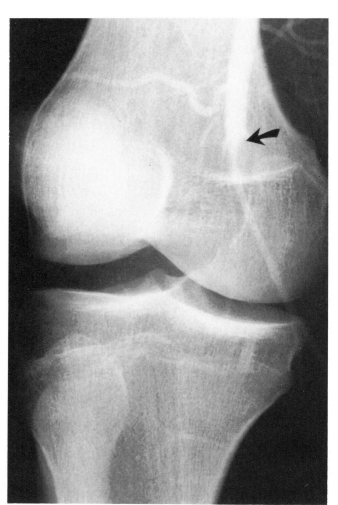

FIGURE 19–3. Postreduction arteriogram of right leg on patient described in Figure 19–1. Complete thrombosis of proximal popliteal artery required surgical exploration for revascularizing the right lower extremity. At surgery, partial avulsion of popliteal artery with thrombosis was treated by popliteal artery repair with reverse saphenous vein bypass graft *(arrow)*. No ligamentous repair was performed.

be performed. This neurologic assessment may be difficult to assess the presence of ischemia. An electromyogram or a nerve conduction velocity study in the nonacute situation may assist in rendering the diagnosis and the future prognosis of the limb.

A general examination for trauma must be performed in order to rule out any additional injuries that the person may have sustained.

Routine radiographs should consist of an anteroposterior, a lateral, and two oblique views of the knee as well as full-length anteroposterior views of the entire femur and tibia in order to rule out an ipsilateral fracture or the possibility of a floating knee. If there was any type of high velocity trauma, a standard anteroposterior radiograph of the pelvis and the chest is indicated. The position of the tibia in relation to the femur should be noted, as should the presence of avulsion fractures, which may indicate capsuloligamentous damage. Stress films are rarely necessary. Additional views such as computed tomograms or magnetic resonance images are probably not indicated in the initial evaluation.

Sequential examinations for up to 1 week after injury are essential in order to detect any change in the neurovascular status. In multitrauma or unconscious patients taken immediately to the operating room for life-saving surgical procedures, a thorough examination of the extremities should be performed. If an instability of the knee (dislocation or subluxation) is discovered, a femoral arteriogram with 45 mL of contrast material should be performed before the patient leaves the operating room.[26] Use of a large cassette and multiple exposures may be needed in order to visualize the artery from above the knee past the trifurcation.

MANAGEMENT

Knee dislocation is an emergency situation that requires immediate reduction in order to provide the best chance of limb survival. This is usually performed, if possible, with the patient under anesthesia so that the stability of the knee can be assessed after reduction. If there is any delay in getting the patient to the operating room, a reduction should be performed in the emergency room, but the patient should nevertheless be taken to the operating room in order to assess stability under anesthesia. Immediate reduction may decrease the extent of vascular or nerve injury and protect skin viability.[7]

During the manipulation to reduce the dislocation of the knee, pressure should not be placed in the popliteal area and the knee must not be hyperextended because both of these maneuvers may injure the vessels. An anterior dislocation is reduced by longitudinal traction on the leg while the femur is pulled forward. A posterior dislocation is reduced by longitudinal traction while anterior translation is applied to the midportion of the tibia. Medial and lateral dislocations require appropriate pressure over the distal femur and the proximal tibia in order to produce reduction.

The leg should be immobilized in 10° to 15° of flexion with a removable splint or a hinged brace in order to allow the reevaluation of the neurovascular status. A circumferential cast should not be used. In very unstable knees, either crossed pinning with Steinmann pins or external fixation may be needed initially in order to maintain reduction.[12, 23] At times, a re-reduction may be necessary. Radiographs, an immediate neurovascular check, and an assessment for compartmental syndrome should be routine after reduction. Some authors believe that for all dislocated knees, a postreduction arteriogram should be obtained in order to rule out intimal damage (Fig. 19–3).

SURGICAL INDICATIONS

The decision of whether to operate depends on multiple factors. Absolute indications for immediate surgery are the following:

1. Open dislocation.
2. Arterial injury.
3. Irreducible dislocation.
4. Compartmental syndrome.

Surgery for a vascular injury or for an open dislocation may require that a vascular surgeon be present at the time of reduction in order to assist in the evaluation of the vascular status and in the treatment of the vascular injury. If vascular surgery is indicated, the orthopaedic surgeon should assist the vascular surgeon in planning incisions, providing stabilization of fractures when necessary,[12, 23] reattaching avulsion fractures, and repairing ligaments in an acute situation as long as the extra surgery does not compromise the repair of the vessel.

VASCULAR INJURIES

Vascular repair, if necessary, should be performed within 6 hours of injury in order to afford the best prognosis. Ischemia that lasts beyond 8 hours increases the likelihood of amputation.[6, 12, 14] DeBakey and Simeone[3] reported the results from World War II surgeries on dislocated knees. They showed that the amputation rate was higher than 49 per cent among patients who did not undergo immediate vascular repair. Green and Allen[6] reported an amputation rate of 11 per cent when immediate surgery was performed. Strong pulses, a warm foot, and a normal finding on Doppler examination are indicative of good vascular flow.[26] If the pulses are weak or absent, an arteriogram (Fig. 19–3) should be performed if it will not jeopardize the outcome of a vascular repair within the crucial period of time. Some authors[11, 18, 27] have recommended arteriography for all knee dislocations, whereas others[6] have recommended exploration without further studies, particularly if there has been a delay in transportation to the hospital, because the area of injury is believed to be between the adductor hiatus and the soleal arch. Consultation with a vascular specialist may assist in the decision-making process. Vascular injuries may occur in patients who sustain major ligamentous injuries without dislocations.

Varnell and collaborators[26] and Frassica and associates[4] recommended femoral arteriogram (with an 18-gauge catheter and 45 mL of contrast) in the operating room just before exploration and reconstruction of the artery because it is accurate and quick and helps localize the site of injury. If the catheter is left in place, it can be used again intraoperatively and postoperatively to assess the patency of the repair or reconstruction. Frassica and associates[4] reported that in two of nine patients who had a reversed saphenous vein graft, the intraoperative arteriogram showed a narrowed anastomosis that required revision.

The current treatment of vascular injuries is exploration and repair or reconstruction with a reverse saphenous vein graft, usually from the other leg in order to avoid additional swelling and morbidity to the already injured leg.[20, 21, 27] Some vascular surgeons prefer an in situ venous bypass, but this may further jeopardize the recovery of an already injured venous system. Repair of the popliteal vein, if injured, has been recommended.[4, 27] If primary arterial repair is performed, postoperative thrombosis may occur. A four-compartment fasciotomy should be performed at the time of arterial repair in order to avoid the possibility of a compartmental syndrome.[16] An arteriogram and a radiograph are needed intraoperatively for ascertaining the patency of the artery and the position of the reduced joint.

NERVE INJURIES

Nerve injuries associated with dislocations of the knee occur less frequently than vascular injuries.[6, 20, 23, 25] A review of the literature[10] revealed 32 nerve injuries in 143 knee dislocations. Twenty-seven of the nerve injuries were treated closed, and the other five were treated with a surgical procedure to decompress the nerve. In seven injuries, there was a complete recovery; in one, there was a partial recovery; in the remaining 24 there was no recovery after long-term follow-up. Improvement occurred in seven of those injuries treated closed and in one treated by exploration and decompression. On the basis of this evaluation, there appeared to be no difference between the patients treated by an open method and those treated by a closed method. If the nerve injury is incomplete (neuropraxia, axonotmesis), recovery is more common; if nerve injury is initially complete (neurotmesis), it is often a permanent condition, and exploration with decompression does not seem to be effective.[10, 13, 14, 23] The nerve is seldom avulsed. Sisto and Warren[23] suggested that neurolysis or nerve repair be performed if surgery is necessary for a vascular injury and only if the vascular status is not jeopardized. Nerve injury that produces a foot drop requires immediate bracing with the expectation that the injury is permanent. This bracing prevents later contractures.

LIGAMENT INJURIES: REPAIR AND RECONSTRUCTION

There are conflicting opinions in the literature as to how to treat ligament injuries associated with knee dislocations.[4, 9, 10, 14, 17, 20, 23, 24, 25] Both nonoperative and operative treatments have been advocated. The decision depends on the extent of injury, the patient's age, the patient's activity level, and the presence of associated injuries. It must be kept in mind that repair of ligaments in the acute stage may jeopardize vascular repair.

Taylor and colleagues[24] showed that 18 of 26 patients treated nonsurgically had good results but regained only 90° of flexion. These patients were able to perform activities of daily living but were not able to participate in sports.[13, 14] Meyers and co-workers, comparing nonoperative with operative treatment, found that of 13 patients treated nonsurgically, one had good results, two had fair results, and 10 had poor results. Twenty patients were treated with some type of surgery; in four, some but not all ligaments were repaired, whereas 16 underwent repair of all injured ligaments. Of those treated by partial repairs, one had good results, one had fair results, and two had poor results. Of those who underwent repair of all torn ligaments, three had excellent results, 10 had good results, two had fair results, and one had poor results. Sisto and Warren[23] found that stiffness was more of a problem than instability in the operative group in comparison with the nonoperative group; of the operative group, a surprisingly large percentage (75) were able to resume some type of sports participation.

Roman and collaborators[20] also found that stiffness was a problem in the operative group, whereas instability was a problem in patients treated nonoperatively. They believed that early surgical repair of the ligaments offered the best results in younger, active patients and in patients of all age groups in whom all four of the major ligaments were torn. Older and sedentary patients with fewer than four ligaments torn were more apt to experience satisfactory results with nonoperative treatment.[20, 23, 25] PCL insufficiency has been shown to be the most common cause of long-lasting instability and disability.

Montgomery[15] summed up ligament surgery by saying that closed treatment can provide good results, but the only way to obtain excellent results is through open ligamentous surgery. Few patients with these severe injuries are able to resume vigorous activity.

TIMING OF SURGERY

The timing of surgery depends on whether the injury is open or closed. Immediate surgical indications previously mentioned are open dislocations, arterial injury, irreducible dislocations, and compartmental syndrome.

An open injury with ligaments exposed in the surgical field should be repaired if it does not delay treatment or jeopardize the vascular status. If possible, ligaments or capsule should be repaired without extension of the incision.

Stabilization or immobilization is required in order to protect the repaired tissue. The foot should be splinted and put through range-of-motion exercises early in order to avoid contractures if associated nerve injury is noted.

If there is no vascular injury or nerve injury, and if a closed reduction is performed successfully, the patient should be observed for 5 to 10 days in the hospital. The leg should not be placed in a circumferential cast. As the swelling resolves and motion returns, repair or reconstruction of the ligaments should be performed. Most authors believe that in active, healthy patients and in patients with injuries to all four major ligaments, repair or reconstruction should be accomplished after the vascular status has been returned to normal and usually within 2 weeks after injury. The decision regarding which ligaments to repair or reconstruct depends on the instability. Restoration of anterior and posterior stability by ligament repair or reconstruction is a major goal in achieving functional use of the knee.

SURGERY*

Arthroscopy is contraindicated in the immediate surgical setting because the extravasation of fluid resulting from soft tissue damage may predispose the patient to a compartmental syndrome.

Early decisions must be made about repair or reconstruction of ligaments in order to provide for the best possible environment for rehabilitation of the injured extremity. If ligament repair is elected, a systematic approach should include evaluation of the capsule, the menisci, the patellar tendon, and the retinaculum; inspection of the ACL and the PCL; and evaluation of the MCL and the LCL. All peripheral structures should be repaired. The ACL and the PCL should be repaired or reconstructed. A surgical finding sometimes seen is avulsion of the LCL and the popliteal tendon from their femoral attachments. Surgery that is delayed requires one or more incisions (medial and lateral utility) that allow repair of all injured ligaments. Peroneal or tibial nerve injuries can be explored, and a neurolysis or nerve repair performed if indicated.

Postoperatively, early protected motion is recommended in order to avoid loss of motion as long as the reduction is stable. Some recommend continuous passive motion in the immediate postoperative setting within the range of brace and ligament stability. A functional brace is used in conjunction with active exercises in order to maximize motion and minimize disability. If vascular repair has been performed, motion and weight bearing are dictated by the protection that this surgery requires. In any course of treatment elected, the priority is to obtain and maintain a competent vascular supply, inasmuch as this supply determines limb viability.

The salient features in handling patients with a possible knee dislocation are summarized as follows:

1. High level of suspicion.
2. Early diagnosis.
3. Neurovascular assessment.
4. Early immediate knee reduction.
5. Arteriogram if vascular status is in question.
6. Vascular consultation if needed.
7. Reconstitution of neurovascular flow within 6 hours.
8. Capsuloligamentous repair or reconstruction as indicated (immediate or delayed).
9. Early controlled knee motion, which does not compromise vascular flow, capsuloligamentous repair, or both.
10. Counseling the patient and a family relative with regard to future activity level.

---

*Surgical techniques are described in Chapter 20.

REFERENCES

1. Bell WW, Jacocks MA, Carmichael DH: Popliteal artery injury associated with knee dislocation. J Okla State Med Assoc 77:418–421, 1984.
2. Brennan JJ, Krause ME, MacDonald WF: Irreducible posterolateral dislocation of the knee joint with grossly intact cruciate ligaments. Am J Surg 104:117–119, 1962.
3. DeBakey ME, Simeone FA: Battle injuries of arteries in World War II; analysis of 2,471 cases. Am J Surg 123:534–579, 1946.
4. Frassica F, Sim F, Staeheli J, Pairolero P: Dislocation of the knee. Clin Orthop 263:200–205, 1991.
5. Girgis FG, Marshall JL, Monajem ARJ: The cruciate ligaments of the knee joint: anatomical, functional, and experimental analysis. Clin Orthop 106:216–231, 1975.
6. Green N, Allen B: Vascular injuries associated with dislocation of the knee. J Bone Joint Surg 59A:236–239, 1977.
7. Hill J, Rana N: Complications of posterolateral dislocation of the knee: case report and literature review. Clin Orthop 154:212–215, 1981.
8. Hoover NW: Injuries to the popliteal artery associated with fractures and dislocations. Surg Clin North Am 41:1099–1112, 1961.
9. Kennedy JC: Complete dislocation of the knee joint. J Bone Joint Surg 45A:889–904, 1963.
10. Kremchek T, Welling R, Kremchek E: Traumatic dislocation of the knee: review paper. Orthop Rev 18:1051–1057, 1989.
11. McCoy G, Hannon D, Barr R, Templeton J: Vascular injuries associated with low velocity dislocations of the knee. J Bone Joint Surg 69B:285–287, 1987.
12. Mendonca J, Matos A: Arterial injuries associated with trauma to the knee. Am J Surg 147:210–211, 1984.
13. Meyers MH, Harvey JP Jr: Traumatic dislocation of the knee joint: a study of eighteen cases. J Bone Joint Surg 53A:16–29, 1971.
14. Meyers M, Moore T, Harvey J: Follow-up notes on articles previously published in the journal: traumatic dislocation of the knee joint. J Bone Joint Surg 57A:430–433, 1975.
15. Montgomery J: Dislocation of the knee. Orthop Clin North Am 18:149–156, 1989.
16. Mubarak SJ, Owen CA: Double incision fasciotomy of the leg for decompression in compartment syndromes. J Bone Joint Surg 59A:184–187, 1977.
17. O'Donoghue DH: Surgical treatment of fresh injuries to the major ligaments of the knee. J Bone Joint Surg 32A:721–738, 1950.
18. Pearsall AW, Schueller D: Anterior knee dislocation: case report and discussion. J Orthop 186:231–233, 1990.
19. Quinlan AG, Sharrard WJW: Posterolateral dislocations of the knee with capsular interposition. J Bone Joint Surg 40B:660–663, 1958.
20. Roman P, Hopson C, Zenni E: Traumatic dislocations of the knee: a report of 30 cases and literature review. Orthop Rev 16:917–924, 1987.
21. Settembrini P, Spraefico G, Zannini P: Popliteal artery injuries associated with knee dislocations. J Cardiovasc Surg 22:135–140, 1981.
22. Shields L, Mital M, Cave EF: Complete dislocations of the knee: experience at the Massachusetts General Hospital. J Trauma 9:192–215, 1969.
23. Sisto D, Warren R: Complete knee dislocation: a follow-up study of operative treatment. Clin Orthop 198:94–101, 1985.
24. Taylor AR, Arden GP, Rainey HA: Traumatic dislocation of the knee: a report of forty-three cases with special reference to conservative treatment. J Bone Joint Surg 54B:96–102, 1972.
25. Thomas P, Rud B, Jensen U: Stability and motion after traumatic dislocation of the knee. Acta Orthop Scand 55:278–283, 1984.
26. Varnell R, Coldwell D, Sangeorzan B, Johansen K: Arterial injury complicating knee disruption. Am J Surg 55:699–704, 1988.
27. Welling R, Kakkasseril J, Cranley J: Complete dislocations of the knee with popliteal vascular injury. J Trauma 21:450–453, 1981.

CHAPTER 20

Acute

Ligamentous

Injury

Robert S. Burger, M.D.

Robert L. Larson, M.D.

■

The evaluation of an acutely injured knee that is not obviously fractured involves determining whether the injury is to ligament, menisci, articular cartilage, or a combination of these structures. The urgency of the evaluation depends on the vascular status (see Chapter 19). If no vascular injury is present, the evaluation of ligamentous continuity, meniscal damage, or osteochondral fracture can be more deliberate.

An immediate evaluation at the time of injury is most helpful in assessing stability before swelling, muscle spasm, and guarding have occurred. Such an examination is often possible during athletic activities at which a trainer or a physician is present and can examine the knee immediately. In the more common scenario, the patient presents a day or two after the injury, holding the swollen knee in flexion with guarding and becoming apprehensive if any movement is attempted.

The evaluation begins with the history of the injury, a description of the mechanism of the injury, and the history of any previous knee injury or conditions. Ligamentous injuries vary from a mild sprain of the medial collateral ligament to significant injuries, including complete tearing of the cruciate or collateral ligaments, or both, along with meniscal injury.

"Natural history" studies of knee ligament injuries have improved physicians' ability to counsel patients about future prognosis. Delineation of injuries into isolated versus combined injuries, whether complete or partial ligamentous disruption, and recognition of avulsion-type injuries help to determine the overall prognosis with both nonoperative and operative treatment.

The actual incidence of knee ligament injuries is not well delineated. The medial collateral ligament (MCL) is the most commonly injured ligament about the knee, but anterior cruciate ligament (ACL) injury is the most common injury to cause pathologic laxity.[11, 77, 230] Hirschman and associates[113] reviewed the incidence of knee ligament injuries in an unselected general population. In 500 acute knee ligament injuries of grade II or III in which pathologic laxity was noted, they reported a 64 per cent incidence of ACL injuries, a 45 per cent incidence of MCL injuries, an 8 per cent incidence of posterior cruciate ligament (PCL) injuries, and only a 3 per cent incidence of lateral collateral ligament (LCL) injuries. Three hundred six grade I MCL injuries and 13 grade I LCL injuries did not display pathologic laxity. Hirschman and associates determined an overall ligament injury rate of 98 knee ligament injuries per 100,000 in an unselected general population per year. Sporting activities accounted for 61 per cent of acute ligamentous injuries associated with pathologic laxity (70 per cent of the isolated ACL injuries, 54 per cent of the isolated MCL injuries, and 61 per cent of combined ACL and MCL injuries). Non–sport-related events (vehicular and other) accounted for the majority of PCL and LCL injuries.

ACUTE KNEE HEMARTHROSIS

In the presence of an acute knee ligament injury, pain, reflex guarding, and hemarthrosis limit the information obtainable by physical examination. Various authors have reported the arthroscopic findings in knees with acute hemarthrosis in which no demonstrable laxity was evident on clinical examination.[31, 58, 213] The ACL was torn in approximately 70 per cent of the cases in which hemarthrosis was present; 65 per cent of these were complete tears. The majority of tears (60 to 80 per cent) were associated with other injuries (meniscal injury, osteochondral fractures, or other ligamentous injury). Of the patients in whom the ACL was torn, 65 per cent had associated meniscal injuries, of which 5 to 17 per cent had bilateral involvement. Osteochondral fractures were found in 15 per cent. In 5 to 10 per cent of the cases of acute hemarthrosis, there was no evidence of ligamentous, cartilaginous, or bony abnormalities.

MENISCAL INJURY ASSOCIATED WITH LIGAMENT INJURIES

Numerous studies have been reported on the association of meniscal lesions and ACL tears. Some investigators have found the lateral meniscus to be more commonly torn,[31, 58, 213, 268] and others have reported the medial meniscus to be more frequently injured.[14, 22, 35, 47, 126, 236]

Meniscal tear patterns associated with ACL injuries have also been described with differing findings.[35, 47, 126] On the medial side, posterior horn longitudinal tears were most frequently seen. On the lateral side, radial tears occurring equally in all thirds were reported in one study,[35] whereas longitudinal tears of the posterior horn were reported as the most frequent lateral tear in another study.[47]

It is important to preserve the shock-absorbing, weight-bearing, and stabilizing function of the meniscus, particularly in the unstable knee.[13, 49, 70, 75, 76, 140, 162, 173, 181, 207, 237, 258, 276, 286, 301, 302] A total meniscectomy in an ACL-deficient knee produces an increase in anterior-posterior translation in comparison with an ACL-deficient knee in which the menisci are intact.[13, 173, 289, 301, 302] Studies have shown less favorable results in patients who have undergone either partial or total meniscectomies in association with ACL tears.[2, 75, 76]

Isolated PCL injuries are associated with a much lower incidence of meniscal injuries.[39, 43, 81, 235] However, meniscal injury occurs in 30 to 50 per cent of cases involving combined PCL and other ligamentous injury.[19, 50, 119, 178, 247, 293, 294]

The status of the menisci must be ascertained in cases of acute ligamentous injury with detectable laxity or in cases of acute hemarthrosis, with or without laxity. In addition to the clinical examination, additional studies such as magnetic resonance imaging (MRI) or arthroscopy may be required.

DIAGNOSIS

History

A history of the mechanism of injury may provide a clue to the structures injured. In sporting activities, non–contact injury usually causes less ligamentous injury than does contact injury. Twisting injuries often associated with a pop may indicate an ACL tear. Hyperextension of the knee may injure the ACL or the PCL or both. A dashboard injury or a fall on the flexed knee may injure the PCL. A blow to the lateral side of the knee or a sudden twist to the opposite direction of the weight-bearing leg causes stress to the MCL or the ACL or both. A sudden giving way or buckling of the knee may indicate loss of ligamentous support.

A feeling of the knee's "going out of place" with a spontaneous reduction is a clue to dislocation or subluxation of the patella. Popping, catching, or clicking after injury may indicate a meniscal tear or an osteochondral injury. Numbness or tingling of the lower leg is suggestive of neurovascular injury. Pain above or below the patella should alert the examiner to the possibility of rupture of the quadriceps or patellar tendon or avulsion of the tibial tubercle. Swelling that occurs immediately or within the first few hours after injury is suggestive of hemarthrosis. Inability to continue activity or bear weight suggests ligamentous involvement.

The history of previous injury to or surgery on the knee is necessary for evaluating the present status. A previous injury that produced a pop in the knee with immediate swelling and a period of disability suggests the possibility of a previous ACL tear, the present injury situation being a manifestation of the residual instability. Feagin (cited by Sherman and co-authors[270]) suggested that in at least 15 per cent of acute ACL disruptions, there existed a partial old tear.

Physical Examination

Various tests used for the evaluation of knee stability are described and illustrated in Chapter 4. The examination should be conducted systematically by inspection, palpation, and ligament testing. The leg should be inspected for deformity (valgus or varus angulation, recurvatum, or flexed position), and status of the skin, swelling in or around the knee, position of the patella, and position of the tibia (sagging posterior to the femur or any gross deformity) should be noted.

Palpation is necessary for checking sensation, pulse, degree of effusion, and areas of generalized or localized tenderness. Specific areas that should be palpated are the patella, the quadriceps muscle, and the patellar tendon for any defects; the tibial tubercle; and the medial and lateral retinacula around the patella. The presence of any apprehension with medial or lateral pressure to the patella should be noted in order to assess any extensor mechanism injury. Tenderness or palpable defects at the insertional sites of the MCL and LCL as well as of the ligaments are clues to whether injury has occurred. Joint line tenderness and the exact location suggest capsular or meniscal injury. The medial and lateral hamstring tendons should be palpated for continuity and tenderness.

Ballottement of the patella is important for determining the amount of effusion that has occurred. The patient is asked to actively contract the quadriceps muscle in order to determine whether there is any dynamic patellar abnormality and to assess the status of the quadriceps mechanism. Active motion of the ankle by the patient and the evaluation of sensation around the foot and ankle help determine whether peroneal nerve injury has occurred. The range of active motion of the knee that the patient can achieve and the range of passive motion are checked by the examiner. These ranges may be limited by pain, swelling, or muscle spasm.

Immediate examination before effusion and guarding reveals the most valid findings concerning ligament laxity.[130] Tense effusion may require aspiration; it also provides both information as to the type of fluid (blood, fat, or joint fluid) and the opportunity to inject lidocaine (Xylocaine) into the joint in order to relieve much of the patient's discomfort and guarding. The noninjured knee is always examined first. This helps assure the patient that the injured leg will be handled gently and also provides the examiner a comparison of the laxity present in the ligaments tested. Physiologic laxity varies in different patients. The difference in side-to-side comparison helps in the assessment of the amount of laxity produced by the present injury.

Manual examination of ligament stability, the mainstay of the physical examination, is a necessary assessment by the examiner of the amount of displacement that occurs with stress testing. Several instrumented testing devices have been produced in order to make this assessment a more objective and reliable evaluation. Daniel and colleagues[55, 57] reported the results of using a KT-1000 arthrometer in evaluating the acutely injured knee. There was a high correlation of side-to-side difference of 3 mm or more on KT-1000 testing and pathologic laxity by examination under anesthesia with arthroscopic findings of an ACL tear. Although the use of instrumented testing for knee laxity in acute ACL injury can provide reliable results, the examiner conducting the testing must be trained and experienced in the use of the instrument, and the patient must relax properly. Manual testing by experienced examiners, especially when performed immediately after injury, can provide an accurate assessment of ligament injury.

The amount of translation and the presence and quality of the endpoint are the criteria used in the evaluation of ligament stability. The various tests are designed to isolate the primary restraint to the particular stress.[101, 218, 219] Translatory motion of the tibia on the femur is tested first because this test is usually less painful and produces less guarding than do the rotatory tests. If there is any question of acute fracture, knee dislocation, or "floating knee," initial roentgenograms should be taken before the manual testing of ligaments. The following is the usual order of testing for ligament stability:

1. The knee is flexed to 20°, and Lachman's test[83, 292] is performed to determine ACL stability.

2. With the knee flexed 0° to 5°, a valgus stress test is performed while the medial joint line is palpated for evidence of joint space opening (MCL, posterior oblique ligament [POL], PCL/ACL).

3. The same stress test is performed with the knee flexed to 30° (MCL).

4. With the knee flexed 0° to 5°, a varus stress test is performed while the lateral joint line is palpated for evidence of joint space opening (LCL, PCL).

5. The same test is performed with the knee flexed 30° (LCL).

6. Active Lachman's test[51]: A small bolster is placed under the thigh to flex the knee 20°. The patient straightens the knee against gravity while the knee is viewed from the side. The examiner looks for anterior subluxation of the tibia as the knee comes into extension and for reduction as the knee flexes (ACL).

7. The knee is passively flexed to 90° (if tolerated by the patient), and the contour of the knee is viewed from the side in order to determine

whether any posterior sag of the tibia is present (see Fig. 4–12*B*). The injured side is compared with the opposite side. The anterior joint line is palpated in order to determine whether the tibia sits approximately 1 cm anterior to the femoral condyles. If there is posterior sag or if the anterior edge of the tibial plateau is even or posterior to the anterior plane of the femoral condyles, rupture of the PCL is likely.

8. An anterior drawer test[165, 189, 279] is performed with the foot in neutral rotation (ACL), with the foot in 30° of external rotation (ACL, POL, and the posterior horn of the medial meniscus), and with the foot in 15° of internal rotation (ACL/PCL, anterolateral complex).

9. A posterior drawer test is performed with the foot in neutral rotation (PCL), external rotation (PCL, LCL, posterolateral complex), and internal rotation (PCL, MCL, POL).

10. With the knee in 90° of flexion, the patient actively contracts the quadriceps muscle,[56] and any forward motion of the tibia is noted by the examiner (PCL).

11. A bolster is placed under the patient's thighs to flex both knees to 30 degrees, and the patient externally rotates the feet. Any tibial sag or excessive external rotation on the injured side should be noted (PCL, posterolateral complex).

12. The rotational tests—pivot-shift test,[90, 116, 118, 179, 180] flexion-rotation-drawer test,[213, 214] anterolateral rotatory instability test,[278] reverse pivot-shift test,[132] and external rotation pivot-shift test[238] (see Chapter 4)—are performed.

13. With the patient's hip and knee flexed 90°, the examiner looks for a posterior tibial sag (PCL) (Fig. 20–1).

14. A dynamic posterior shift test[266] is performed.

15. The external rotation recurvatum test[122] is performed (posterolateral complex).

16. To check for meniscal pathology, the examiner conducts McMurray's and Apley's tests.

Lachman's test is the most consistently reliable evaluation for ACL laxity in the acutely injured knee.[31, 35, 144, 292] It should be performed with

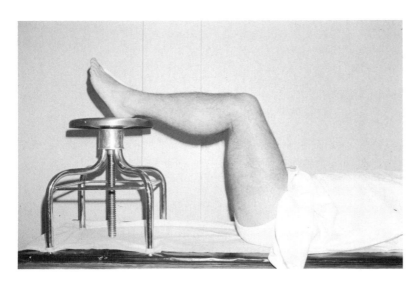

FIGURE 20–1. Position of extremity to take a posterior sag view (Godfrey's view). A 10-pound weight may be hung over the anterior tibial tubercle to increase the stress to posterior displacement of the proximal tibia. A lateral radiograph of the knee is taken.

the examiner standing on the lateral side of the knee to be examined in order to avoid internal rotation of the tibia on the femur, which would tighten the PCL and give a false-negative result.[83]

Hip[9] and knee[90, 116, 118, 179, 214, 219, 277] positions, as well as tibial rotation,[9, 41, 83, 101] affect the results of the pivot-shift test. The hip should be in neutral position with the leg in abduction while the pivot-shift test is performed. The test should be performed successively with the tibia in internal rotation, neutral position, and external rotation. This will improve the rate of true-positive results and reduce the number of false-negative results.[9]

Examination with the patient under anesthesia is consistently more accurate (95 per cent) than manual examination of the unanesthetized patient.[21, 31, 35, 65, 144, 219, 292] When the diagnosis is in question, examination, often in association with arthroscopic evaluation, may be performed with the patient under anesthesia. In some situations, an MRI study would be appropriate and would provide a more accurate diagnosis.

Radiographic Evaluation

Standard radiographs should include anteroposterior, lateral, bilateral Merchant's views, and either bilateral notch views or bilateral flexion weight-bearing views, depending on whether the patient is able to bear weight.

The examiner should look for osteochondral defects; a lateral capsular sign[312] (Segond's fracture), as seen with ACL injuries; avulsion injuries to the tibial spine, as seen in ACL injuries; medial calcifications, which are consistent with injury to the MCL (either acute avulsion or chronic sign of injury); and posterior tibial avulsion fractures, which are consistent with PCL injuries. The examiner should also check alignment for tibiofemoral subluxation, check patellar alignment in the sulcus on the Merchant view, and look for calcifications within the notch, as seen in ACL and PCL injuries.

Valgus stress radiographs have been used to determine the degree of MCL injury.[107, 296] Usually the extent of the injury is determined on the physical examination. Posterior stress radiographs have been used for PCL injuries; the patient lies in the supine position with the hip and knee flexed to 90°, and a 10-pound weight is hung from the anterior tibia with the heel supported on a stool (see Fig. 20–1). Comparative views of both knees reveal an increase in posterior tibial translation on the femur if the PCL is injured. This finding is more frequent in chronic PCL injury.

Arthrography and Magnetic Resonance Imaging

In evaluations of ACL tears, double-contrast arthrography has been reported to be 95 per cent sensitive and 98 per cent specific.[239] Reider and co-authors[243] reported an accuracy rate of 85 per cent and a sensitivity rate of 85 per cent in 212 knees when single-contrast arthrography was used. In evaluations of the menisci, arthrography[129, 161, 172, 210, 259, 288] has been shown to have a diagnostic accuracy rate ranging from 73 to 97 per cent, with greater accuracy on the medial side.

MRI has been used as a diagnostic tool for determining the status of the bony and soft tissue components in knee injuries. Variance in technical factors such as relaxation times, the different knee coils used, and varying capabilities of the different hardware systems affects the diagnostic efficacy of the MRI in evaluating ligament and meniscal injuries. Continued improvement in equipment and techniques and the increased expertise in MRI interpretation have enhanced the diagnostic reliability.

In evaluations of injuries to the ACL, the accuracy has ranged from 72 to 100 per cent; eight of nine studies have shown an accuracy rate higher than 93 per cent.[95, 131, 155, 171, 184, 202, 203, 241, 299] In 1988, Mink and colleagues[203] reported the largest series of 94 ACL tears; using T1-weighted images, they showed that the accuracy of MRI was 85 per cent and the sensitivity was 95 per cent. When they used T2-weighted images the accuracy rose to 100 per cent and the sensitivity to 96 per cent. A T2 mode is recommended for imaging the ACL. The ACL can best be visualized in a single sagittal slice taken with the knee in 10° to 15° of external rotation, but both coronal and sagittal images are necessary for complete visualization of the ACL.

Mandelbaum and co-workers,[184] comparing physical examination with MRI evaluation of suspected ACL tears in 35 patients, showed that the accuracy of the physical examination was 94 per cent, the sensitivity was 92 per cent, and the specificity was 96 per cent. With MRI, the accuracy was 100 per cent, and both sensitivity and specificity were 100 per cent. MRI provides a clear visualization of PCL continuity.

MRI has been found to have an accuracy rate of 90 per cent in evaluations of all meniscal lesions (89 per cent sensitivity and 90 per cent specificity).[28, 29, 52, 95, 131, 155, 184, 203, 241, 242, 275] The accuracy rate is higher (94 per cent) in evaluations of acute, as opposed to chronic, meniscal injuries[28, 29] and also when there is a simultaneous ACL injury.[28, 29] This phenomenon may be the result of the effusion[17, 28, 29, 242] present in acute injuries, which may act as a natural contrast-enhancing agent. Evaluation of the integrity of the ACL or the PCL by physical examination is less accurate in acutely injured knees than in chronically injured knees.[144] MRI thus has a role in the diagnosis of acute knee injuries. With further experience and technical improvements, MRI will play a greater role in the evaluation of the injured knee.

Arthrography has the disadvantage of being an invasive procedure with a low risk of infection and often is uncomfortable for the patient. It is less expensive than MRI, and the accuracy of results is more operator dependent. The advantages of MRI are that it is noninvasive, no ionizing radiation is used, and both the bony and the soft tissue structures are visualized. Patients who are obese, are claustrophobic, or have metallic implants such as pacemakers cannot undergo MRI evaluation.

MEDIAL INJURIES

The chief components providing stability to the medial side of the knee are the MCL and the semimembranosus complex. The latter consists of the semimembranosus muscle and its divisions, the POL, and the posterior horn of the medial meniscus. The importance of this functioning unit has been emphasized by Müller[208] (Fig. 20–2). As the foot bears weight, an anterior thrust of the tibia occurs. This translation is prevented by the ACL. This action causes the femoral condyle to slide back on the tibial plateau, and the sliding in turn is checked by the wedge-shaped posterior horn of the medial meniscus. The meniscus is prevented from being pushed back by its attachment to the posterior oblique ligament. Tears or stretching of the POL or loss of the posterior horn of the medial meniscus allows increased anterior translation of the medial tibial plateau in relation to the medial femoral condyle. Increased anterior translation of the tibia occurs if there is associated ACL deficiency. This synergistic action among various stabilizing structures is a characteristic of the biomechanics of knee function.

The primary static stabilizer of the medial side of the knee is the MCL.[101, 102, 121, 157, 219, 304, 305] When the knee is flexed 20° to 30°, the MCL provides 80 per cent of the resistance to medial joint opening. The ACL provides 10 to 15 per cent, and the capsule 10 per cent, of the stabilization.[102, 116, 127, 157, 186, 310] At 0° to 5° of knee flexion, the MCL provides only 60 per cent of the medial stability; the contribution of the POL increases to 20 per cent, and the cruciate ligaments contribute 15 per cent. The structures injured by stresses to the knee vary with the force of the injury and the angle of the knee at the time of injury.

The most common mechanisms of injury are a direct blow to the lateral aspect of the knee and a twisting while turning away from the weight-bearing leg. The patient feels a tearing or an inward buckling of the knee associated with the feeling of lack of support when attempting to push off the leg to the opposite direction. Examination may reveal some swelling but more often tenderness at the site of the torn tissue. A careful evaluation for the most tender spot, particularly during the immediate examination, is helpful for differentiating injury to the MCL, the medial meniscus, the medial retinaculum, or other structures.

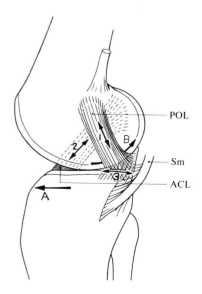

FIGURE 20–2. Synergistic action of the anterior cruciate ligament (ACL) and posterior oblique ligament (POL). As the tibia is thrust forward on foot strike (A), its anterior displacement on the femur is restrained by the ACL (2). The femoral condyle must push posteriorly on the posterior horn of the medial meniscus or ride upward on it (B). The POL with its meniscotibial attachment to the meniscus (3) prevents backward displacement of the meniscus. This functions with the femoromeniscal portion of the POL (1), which comes under tension as a wedge brake against anterior displacement of the tibia. (From Müller W: The Knee: Form, Function, and Ligament Reconstruction, p. 69. New York: Springer-Verlag, 1983.)

Examination and Classification

MCL injuries have been classified into grades I, II, and III, depending on the extent of joint opening of the medial side with valgus stress.[48] A valgus stress is applied with the patient's knee flexed to 30° and at 0° while the examiner's fingers palpate the joint line to determine the amount of joint opening and the firmness of the endpoint. In grade I injury, there is tenderness over the MCL with 0 to 5 mm of medial opening and a good endpoint. In grade II injury, the tenderness is over the ligament with 5 to 10 mm of joint opening and a softer endpoint. In grade III injury with more disruption, there may be less tenderness but some swelling and 10 to 15 mm of joint opening with no discernible endpoint. When the joint opening is wider than 10 mm, there is most likely injury to other structures such as the cruciate ligaments, the posteromedial complex, and the meniscus. When joint opening can be demonstrated with the knee at 0°, cruciate injury should be suspected. Tests for the integrity of the ACL, PCL, and menisci and for patellar stability should be performed in all cases.[165, 218, 279]

Imaging should consist of standard radiographs in order to rule out fracture or avulsion injuries. Stress views are usually not necessary.[105, 107, 109, 296] MRI should be considered only when meniscal symptoms such as locking and clicking have occurred or in grade III injuries so as to rule out associated ACL or meniscal tears. Arthroscopy may be appropriate in grade III tears for evaluating the menisci and cruciate ligaments.[12, 124]

Incidence

The MCL is the most commonly injured ligament about the knee. Hirschman and associates[113] reported on 819 acute ligamentous injuries of the knee. Of these, 306 were grade I MCL injuries and 144 were grades II and III MCL isolated injuries. In addition, 64 patients had combined MCL and ACL injuries. MCL injuries accounted for 63 per cent of the total number of ligament injuries; 55 per cent of the injuries in this series were isolated MCL injuries, and 8 per cent were combined MCL and ACL injuries. Grades II and III MCL injuries in which pathologic motion was present accounted for 42 per cent of 500 cases. Derscheid and Garrick,[64] in a prospective series of college football players, found that of 70 knee injuries that caused loss of playing time, 84 per cent involved the MCL. Eighty-six per cent were isolated grades I and II injuries, 8 per cent were isolated grade III injuries, and 6 per cent were combined with ACL injuries.

The incidence of meniscal tears associated with MCL injuries varies between 0 and 5 per cent in grades I and II MCL injuries and between 2 and 22 per cent in grade III MCL injuries.[64, 116, 147, 244, 250] Meniscocapsular separation was reported in 70 to 88 per cent of patients treated for grade III injuries in two large series.[12, 116]

Grade III injuries often are associated with other major ligamentous injuries to the knee. The MCL-ACL injury pattern is the most common combination and has been reported in 44 to 100 per cent of cases in which there is a grade III MCL tear.[205, 250, 296] Fetto and Marshall[77] reported associated ACL injury in 53 per cent of grade II MCL injuries and in 20 per cent of grade I injuries.

Treatment and Its Rationale

ISOLATED MCL INJURY

An acute isolated injury to the MCL is usually a nonsurgical problem, whereas combined injuries of the MCL and the ACL, PCL, and postero-lateral complex (PLC) are more controversial (Fig. 20–3).

Laboratory animal studies have revealed that in isolated MCL injuries, the intact ACL provides the secondary restraint to medial stability necessary for allowing appropriate healing of the MCL.[26, 103, 127, 232, 310] Additional studies have proved the beneficial effects of early motion[84, 212, 248, 308, 309] and exercise[20, 45, 85, 86, 170, 290] on ligament healing. On the basis of these two concepts, the current approach to isolated MCL injuries is nonoperative treatment and early protected motion for all grades of MCL injuries.

Ellsasser and collaborators[67] reported a 98 per cent success rate with nonoperative treatment and early motion of isolated grades I and II injuries in professional football players. In 1978, Fetto and Marshall[77] reported no difference in outcome between surgical and nonsurgical treatment of grades I and II MCL injuries, but a slightly better functional level was produced in grade III injuries treated with surgery. Hastings[105] reported that of 29 patients treated nonoperatively for isolated grades II and III MCL injuries, 28 returned to sports without disability; these 28 included 14 professional hockey players. In 1983, Indelicato[124] reported the first prospective study, stating that there was no difference between the results of operative and nonoperative treatment of grade III isolated MCL injuries; both afforded a 90 per cent success rate. Patients treated

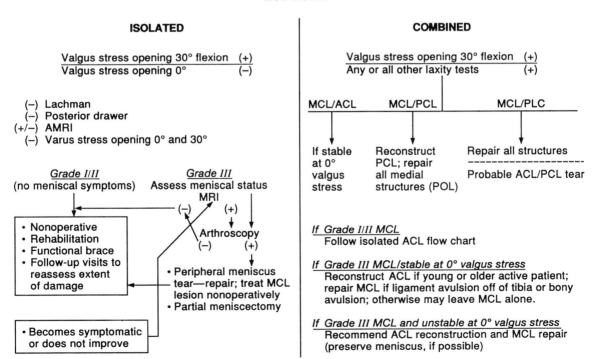

FIGURE 20–3. Flow chart to aid in determining evaluation and treatment of patients with a medial collateral ligament injury.

both operatively and nonoperatively had a residual 1- to 5-mm laxity that did not seem to alter overall function. Sandberg and associates,[250] in another prospective study, confirmed Indelicato's findings. They compared operative with nonoperative treatment for grades II and III MCL injuries and concluded that there was no difference in the final outcome between the two groups; however, patients in the nonoperative group experienced more rapid recovery of function, strength, and range of motion without undergoing the risks of surgery.

Other authors have verified the success rate of nonoperative treatment of both grades I and II injuries[12, 48, 64, 114, 147, 244] as well as isolated grade III MCL injuries.[125, 143] In general, the time before resumption of sports was between 2 and 8 weeks in grades I and II injuries and between 4 and 12 weeks in grade III injuries. Those authors stress that if the patients are not improving over a normal period of time, an arthroscopic evaluation may be necessary in order to rule out additional meniscal, osteochondral, or ligamentous damage.

If there is any question in the diagnosis or if the patient is not permitted the luxury of observation in cases thought to be isolated MCL injuries, MRI or arthroscopy should be used to rule out associated injuries. These techniques are required most frequently in grade III MCL injury (see Fig. 20–3).

MCL INJURIES ASSOCIATED WITH OTHER MAJOR LIGAMENTOUS INJURIES

In grade II and grade III MCL injuries, there is a high incidence of associated ligamentous damage, the ACL being the most frequently injured.[77, 78, 113, 250, 296] In 1950, O'Donoghue[229] provided convincing evidence that acute repair of the so-called unhappy triad (ACL, MCL, medial meniscal tear) provided better long-term results than did nonoperative treatment in terms of stability and function. Although in additional reports[11, 118, 147, 151, 209, 230, 231, 238, 265, 278, 280, 281, 305] the advantages of operative treatment have been discussed, other authors have reported favorable results with the nonoperative treatment of this combined instability.[141, 205, 250]

Laboratory studies have shown that the intact ACL provides a major secondary restraint to medial stability of the knee. Simultaneous injury to the MCL and the ACL adversely affects the healing of the MCL and, therefore, leads to increased abnormal valgus laxity.[26, 32, 101–103, 127, 175, 218, 219, 310] These findings are consistent with those of clinical studies in which increased valgus laxity and external rotation have been noted after nonoperative management of combined ligament injuries.[77, 78] Woo and coauthors[310] noted that the structural properties of the bone-ligament-bone complex in the MCL returned to normal values more rapidly than usual and formed an excessively large mass of reparative tissue in the MCL- and ACL-injured knees, in comparison with the knees in which only the MCL was severed. This may explain the favorable functional clinical outcome reported by other authors who elected nonoperative treatment of MCL-ACL combined injuries.

A comparison of a group of patients with partially transected ACLs to a group with completely transected ACLs revealed a marked difference in results, suggesting that partial tear of the ACL did not alter the kinematics of the joint to an appreciable extent. This has been found to be the case in numerous reports of clinical studies on isolated partial and complete ACL injuries.[15, 27, 79] The POL, the posteromedial capsule, and the medial meniscus may be injured along with the ACL and MCL.[116, 118, 121, 229–231] At physical examination and arthroscopy, it is essential to determine which of the structures or which combination of structures is injured in order to establish appropriate treatment.

There are conflicting reports concerning the success rates of both nonoperative and operative treatment of combined MCL-ACL injuries. Mok and Good[205] reported on 25 patients with combined MCL-ACL grade III injuries that were treated by a nonoperative protocol, which consisted of cast-bracing, early motion, and weight bearing. Of these injuries, 11 were complete ACL tears and 14 were partial tears. Average follow-up was 24 months. Four patients had mild and four had moderate medial instability, and 17 had no instability. At 1-year follow-up, only patients with complete ACL tears had residual anterior laxity and a positive pivot-shift test result, although these findings were not deemed functionally relevant. All 12 patients involved in sports before the injury returned to sports after treatment; two reinjured their knees as a result of instability (both had a diagnosis of complete ACL tear at the time of initial injury).

Jokl and co-workers,[141] in a series of 28 patients with combined MCL and ACL injury, reported a 60 per cent return to full activity with nonoperative treatment. The failures usually occurred within 6 months. Operative reconstruction of the ACL and repair of the MCL in these patients were recommended in the failed group. Sandberg and associates[250] compared nonoperative to operative treatment. The operative treatment consisted of primary repair of the ACL and MCL. They found that patients treated nonoperatively had more anterior translation and larger pivot shifts, as well as higher rates of clinical symptoms and episodes of giving way (17 per cent), than did the operative group (3 per cent). There was no functional difference between the operative and nonoperative groups.

Sandberg and associates[250] reported that 76 per cent of players in both the operative and nonoperative groups discontinued playing after 1 year because of instability. Overall satisfaction with the results of treatment went down from 67 per cent at 1 year to 41 per cent in 2 years with no differences between the groups. None of the patients in this series had ACL reconstructions—only primary repairs.

Fetto and Marshall[77, 78] compared nonoperative with operative treatment in grade III MCL-ACL injuries. The results in terms of stability showed that operative treatment was superior to nonoperative treatment, and Fetto and Marshall stated that "spontaneous recovery of the integrity of the MCL will be hampered by the presence of instability, resulting from other associated ligamentous injuries—specifically the ACL. In mixed ligament injuries, factors other than MCL stability more dramatically determine the overall result of the knee function post-injury." Good-to-excellent results were more closely correlated with the recovery of the ACL than of the MCL.

Other authors have reported on the advantage of the operative treatment of both the ACL and MCL.[11, 230, 238, 303] In 1983, Hughston and Barrett[118] reported on 154 patients with acute anteromedial rotatory instability, of whom 59 per cent had combined ACL tears and grade III injuries of the medial structures. In this series, with regard to repairs of only the medial structures (the POL, the posteromedial capsule, the MCL, the medial meniscus, and the semimembranosus tendon), Hughston and Barrett reported 73 per cent objective, 88 per cent subjective, and 90 per cent functionally satisfactory results. Other authors[77, 230, 281, 303] were unable to corroborate these results and recommended treating both lesions operatively.

Shelbourne and Baele[265] reported the only series in which the operative treatment of both the ACL and the MCL was compared with reconstruction of the ACL alone in patients with the combined injury. They concluded that there was no difference in overall outcome regardless of whether the MCL was repaired. Knees in which the MCL was repaired had slightly decreased range of motion and more symptoms than those in which the MCL was not repaired. Shelbourne and Baele's conclusions substantiate the findings of other authors[77, 78, 310]: that the ACL appears to be the key structure in stabilizing the knee when there is a combined MCL-ACL injury.

In the decision on appropriate treatment of a patient with combined MCL-ACL injury, the future demands on knee function must be considered. Active patients usually require a functioning ACL in order to provide satisfactory stability and to lessen the chance of further injury to other joint structures.

Injuries involving the MCL and PCL are less frequent than those involving the ACL. These injuries are discussed in the section on combined PCL injuries.

Authors' Preferred Treatment

In acute situations, isolated grades I, II, and III MCL injuries can usually be treated nonoperatively. In grade III injuries, either arthroscopy or MRI should be used to rule out associated meniscal or cruciate ligament injury. Patients in whom nonoperative treatment fails require surgery.

If the MCL is injured along with posteromedial structures, as evidenced by a positive valgus stress test result at 0° or anteromedial instability, primary repair of all medial structures is indicated.

If the MCL is injured along with a complete ACL tear, the treatment depends on the need for a functioning ACL (see ACL section for indications and technique). In low-demand patients, nonoperative treatment may be appropriate. In moderate- or high-demand patients, an ACL reconstruction is indicated. The indications to repair the medial structures along with the ACL are as follows:

1. The POL, the posterior capsule, and the MCL all are torn (anteromedial instability).
2. Grade III MCL tears at the tibial insertion.
3. Occasionally in association with medial meniscus repair.

If there is a partial ACL tear with a negative pivot shift, the injury should be treated as an MCL tear only.

Although the MCL heals if the combined MCL-ACL injury is treated nonsurgically, there is a higher risk of residual medial and anterior instability, which will be poorly tolerated by the moderate- and high-demand patient.

FIRST-DEGREE MCL INJURIES

Patients with these injuries are treated with restriction of activities until the soreness has subsided. Throughout the rehabilitation, they should work on range of motion and strengthening the muscles. Immobilization is not necessary and may delay recovery. A functional brace is used throughout the entire season if a player is involved in contact sports.

SECOND-DEGREE MCL INJURIES

Patients with these injuries require protected mobilization with an exercise program in order to maintain muscle strength. They should advance from partial to full weight bearing as tolerated. A rehabilitation program should begin immediately with work on passive and active range of motion, strengthening muscles against resistance, and stationary bicycling as tolerated, and it should advance to running and cutting as pain subsides and strength improves. Only when tenderness has resolved, no abnormal laxity is present, and muscle strength in the injured leg is near equal to that in the opposite leg is return to full activity allowed. Bracing is used for vigorous sports. In most cases, abstention from vigorous activity lasts from 2 to 6 weeks.

THIRD-DEGREE MCL INJURIES: ISOLATED

Before the patient undergoes any treatment, additional injuries to other ligaments and the menisci must be ruled out.

If nonoperative treatment is elected, reexaminations are necessary because injuries to the menisci and the cruciate ligaments are often masked in the acute situation. A hinged brace locked at 30° is used with early partial weight bearing. Advance to full weight bearing as tolerated. Passive and active motion is encouraged as tolerated, and isometric exercises are performed regularly. Protected mobilization in the brace is allowed as soreness and muscle spasm subside.

Advancement in the rehabilitation process depends on the amount of pain, the range of motion, and improvement in stability. Full weight bearing is allowed in the brace when there is no pain and there is full range of passive and active motion. Stationary bicycling should begin as soon as pain subsides. The knee should be gently tested for stability in order to ascertain whether pain, tenderness, and laxity are decreasing. Usually this occurs over 2 to 4 weeks. A functional brace is applied as the knee becomes clinically stable. Isotonic, isokinetic, and slide-board exercises are begun. Non–contact sports may be resumed when agility is obtained. The patient may progress to contact sports when the knee is completely stable without pain and has full range of motion and when muscle strength is at least 90 per cent of normal, in comparison with the contralateral side. A brace for the entire season is required if the patient returns to sports activity.

Authors' Preferred Surgical Technique

In the acute situation, medial repairs are more common than reconstructions. The type of repair is determined by the structures injured.

The goals of surgical treatment are to preserve the medial meniscus, establish tension in the POL, semimembranosus attachments, and appropriate tension in the MCL.[133, 157, 278, 280, 281] It should be kept in mind that one half to two thirds of the fibers of the POL pass directly from the femur to the tibia, forming a true femorotibial ligament. Repair or restoration of these fibers often requires imbrication or reefing in order to establish the normal tension of this structure.

If meniscal repair is indicated, repairing a peripheral meniscal tear is easier when performed during rather than after the course of the open procedure. Meniscal tears with rim widths of more than 3 mm are more easily treated by arthroscopic suture placement and tying the sutures down during the open repair than by pulling sutures through the open incision. If only the ACL is reconstructed, arthroscopic repair of the menisci should be performed.

POSITIONING

The patient is positioned supine with the leg draped free. A tourniquet is placed on the upper thigh. The knee may be flexed and the hip externally rotated in order to allow access to the medial side of the knee. The authors' preference is to drop the foot of the operating table so as to allow knee flexion past 90° (Fig. 20–4). A bolster or a leg holder is used to maintain this position and allows free access to the posteromedial structures. Arthroscopy may be carried out from this position to assess intra-articular pathology.

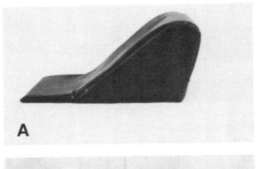

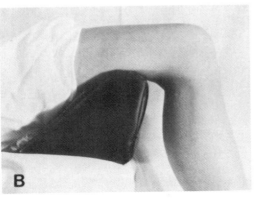

FIGURE 20–4. (*A*) A bolster used under the proximal thigh to allow knee flexion past 90°. (*B*) Note space between top edge of bolster and the popliteal crease, which allows room to approach the posterior aspect of the knee through either medial or lateral incisions. (From Larson RL: Dislocations and ligamentous injuries to the knee. *In* Rockwood CA, Green DP [eds]: Fractures in Adults, 2nd ed, vol 2, p. 1528. Philadelphia: JB Lippincott, 1984.)

INCISION

The stability of the knee, as determined with the patient under anesthesia, and arthroscopic evaluation of the knee joint help in determining the type of incision necessary. A reattachment of a peripheral meniscal rim tear and reefing or repair of the POL require a vertical incision over the posteromedial aspect of the knee. If an ACL is to be reconstructed with arthroscopic assistance, a short incision over the area of tear of the MCL might be used. More extensive surgery on the medial side requires the use of a gently curved anteromedial incision (Fig. 20–5).

The incision is started just above the medial femoral epicondyle and extended distally in a curved line toward the medial patella and medial edge of the patellar tendon, ending just below and medial to the tibial tubercle. A full-thickness posterior skin flap can then be developed to allow exposure of the medial side of the knee from the patellar tendon to the posteromedial corner of the knee. The area of the tear is often identifiable from bleeding at the site. If fascial planes are difficult to identify, it is helpful to find the lower edge of the pes anserinus insertion (identified by the semitendinosus tendon) and to elevate this insertion from below upward. This elevation exposes the tibial insertion of the MCL—which may be torn—and allows the exposure of the more proximal portions of the MCL in the proper plane. Repair of the MCL can be accomplished; reefing of the POL or any peripheral repair of the medial meniscus can be performed through this incision.

If the POL is lax, a reefing procedure is needed. A vertical incision is made posterior to the trailing edge of the MCL. The posterior capsule is

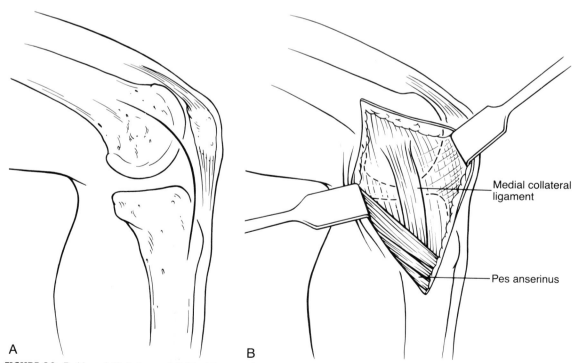

Medial collateral
ligament

Pes anserinus

A   B

FIGURE 20–5. (*A* and *B*) Anteromedial incision used to expose medial structures and allow access to the joint through an anteromedial capsular incision (see text).

pulled forward through the use of mattress sutures and pulled beneath the anterior edge (Fig. 20–6). The anterior portion is brought over the top of the posterior section in a double-breasted manner so as to duplicate the physiologic action of the POL with knee flexion.

The meniscotibial ligament or the meniscofemoral ligament needs to be repaired with sutures when torn (Fig. 20–7). Two small drill holes may be required for suture placement and reattachment.

Reconstruction procedures[133, 166, 208, 209, 278, 280, 281] on the medial side in the acute situation are rare. If the superficial MCL is shredded, it may be possible to use a sartorial slide procedure, which consists of freeing up the sartorius tendon proximally and suturing it along the line of the deficient MCL (Fig. 20–8). Care should be taken to protect the sartorial branch of the saphenous nerve proximally. Additional procedures may be required, such as a pes anserinus[107, 166, 278, 280, 281] transplant or advancement of the anteromedial limb of the semimembranosus muscle anteriorly (Fig. 20–9).

After surgery, patients are placed in a hinged brace locked at 45°. This brace can be removed for range-of-motion exercises when operative discomfort has subsided. The brace is worn when the patient is up on crutches. Weight bearing is allowed as determined by the patient's comfort. Range-of-motion exercises are gradually increased, with caution to avoid motion past 20° to 90°. The brace is removed after 6 weeks. Rehabilitation progresses as described in Chapter 14.

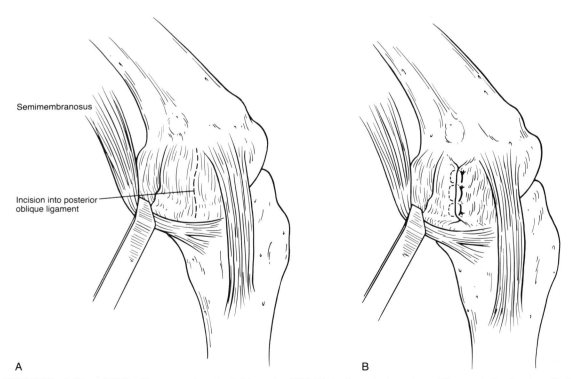

Semimembranosus

Incision into posterior oblique ligament

A

B

FIGURE 20–6. (*A* and *B*) Reefing procedure to tighten a lax POL. Note the anterior edge of the posterior flap is pulled beneath the anterior flap (*B*). The amount of imbrication must be determined so that it does not limit knee flexion.

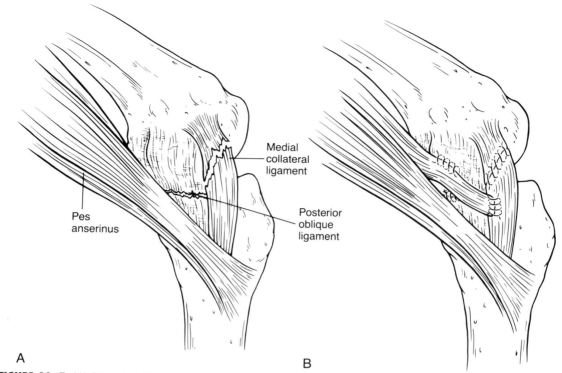

FIGURE 20–7. (*A*) Disrupted fibers of the medial collateral ligament (MCL) and POL. (*B*) Direct repair of torn tissue with advancement of anterior limb of semimembranosus used to reinforce repair.

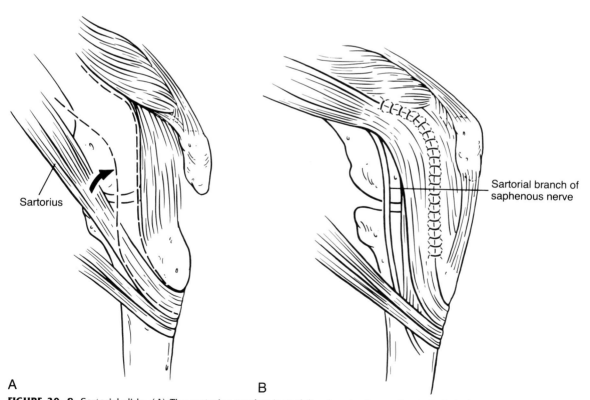

FIGURE 20–8. Sartorial slide. (*A*) The sartorius tendon is mobilized and advanced anteriorly in line with the MCL. (*B*) The tendinosus anterior edge of the sartorius is sutured to the distal fascia of the vastus medialis obliquus. The tendons of the semitendinosus and gracilis muscles may be advanced proximally in the manner of a pes anserinus transplant for additional medial support.

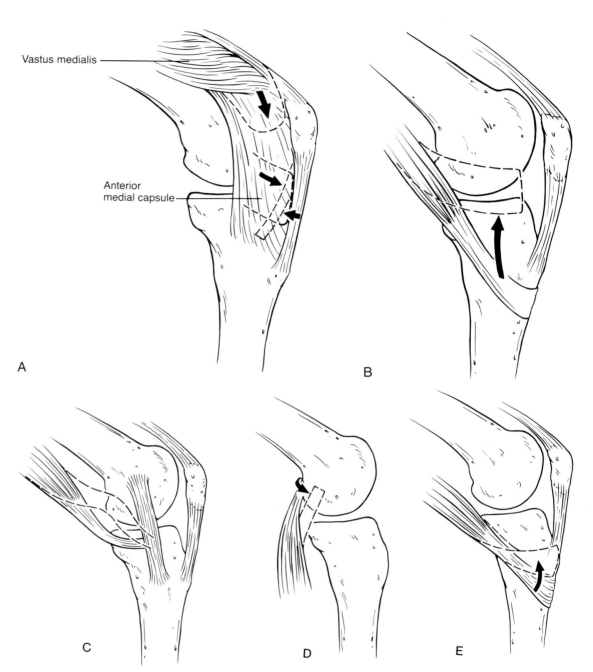

FIGURE 20–9. Additional procedures that may be used to augment deficient tissue. (*A*) Distal advancement of the vastus medialis obliquus (*top arrow*); medial transplant of medial half of patellar tendon and anterior advancement of anterior medial capsule. (*B*) Pes anserinus used as a patch over deficient tissue. (*C*) Anterior proximal advancement of anterior tendon of semimembranosus muscle. (*D*) Medial anterior advancement of medial half of tendinosus to medial head of the gastrocnemius muscle. (*E*) Pes anserinus transplant.

ANTERIOR CRUCIATE LIGAMENT INSTABILITY

Advances in diagnostic and therapeutic capabilities, as well as better controlled follow-up studies in both the nonoperative and operative treatments of ACL injuries, have revealed the advantages of operative reconstructive procedures in the high- and moderate-demand patient populations in comparison with the nonoperative methods of treatment. Age and sex should no longer be major determinants in decisions about the indications for surgery. Activity level as desired or required by the patient is probably the most important aspect in determining mode of treatment. High-demand patients (strenuous labor workers, competitive athletes, intensive recreational athletes) have been shown to function or perform better with fewer symptoms after ACL surgical reconstruction than did patients treated nonoperatively[3, 14, 22, 27, 42, 82, 106, 150, 221, 222, 236, 261, 306] (decreased giving-way episodes, decreased pain, and decreased hesitation). Low-demand patients—those with sedentary lifestyles and athletes in low-demand sports (e.g., bicycling, golfing) that do not involve jumping, cutting, or twisting—have a higher level of success with nonoperative treatment than do high-demand patients.[3, 14, 22, 106, 113]

Defining the extent of the injury (partial versus complete tear of the ACL; associated meniscal injury; associated major ligamentous injury) is equally important for determining the overall method of treatment. Patients with partial ACL tears have been found to have fewer meniscal injuries and less objective laxity, both initially and at follow-up examination, than do patients with complete ACL tears. Those with partial tears have a higher rate of returning to preinjury level of sports, a lower reinjury rate, a higher performance level, a lower reconstruction rate, and lower rates of pain and giving way than those treated nonoperatively with complete ACL tears.[15, 79, 194, 223, 228]

Improvement of diagnostic capability (physical examination, MRI, arthroscopy), technical advances (graft strength,[215–217, 296] graft positioning,[97, 108, 240, 256, 313] isometry, graft tensioning, fixation methods[54, 164, 165]), and advances in rehabilitation[30, 54, 220, 267, 283] (early complete motion, early weight bearing) have all contributed to the markedly improved results obtained with ACL surgery.

Functional Anatomy

The adult ACL has been measured to be approximately 3.5 cm in length.[5, 7, 94, 160, 211] It has a semicircular attachment at the posterior portion of the medial aspect of the lateral femoral condyle and courses in an anteromedial and distal direction, making an outward spiral and inserting in the region of the anterior spine of the tibial plateau. The tibial attachment is usually 1.5 cm posterior to the anterior articular surface of the tibial plateau. The ACL, like the PCL, is an extrasynovial structure and yet intra-articular.

The ACL provides a primary restraint to anterior tibial translation on the femur[26, 32, 88, 94, 101, 102, 186, 246] and acts as the major secondary restraint to medial tibial displacement.[26, 101, 127, 310] It provides stabilization to valgus and varus opening as well as to internal and external rotation.[26, 89, 94]

The ligament itself is a collective bunch of fascicles that fan out over broadened insertion areas. Depending on the author, the fascicles have been divided into either two[1, 89] or three[211] functional bands that vary in tension in accordance with the angle of knee flexion.[94, 160] The anteromedial bundle provides restraint during flexion, whereas the posterolateral bundle functions in extension.[89, 94, 211]

The ACL receives its blood supply from the middle, medial, and lateral inferior genicular arteries.[5, 6, 254] In addition, neurofibers providing vasomotor, mechanoreceptor, and possibly proprioceptive functions have been identified in the periligamentous as well the ligamentous tissue of the ACL.[156, 160, 255]

Understanding of this functional anatomy forms a diagnostic basis for the physical examination (Lachman's maneuver, the pivot-shift phenomenon, and anterior drawer).

Mechanism of Injury

Various mechanisms can produce rupture of the ACL. The most common contact injury is a valgus force applied to the flexed externally rotated knee, producing the triad of ACL, MCL, and associated medial meniscal injury[229] or lateral meniscal[268] injury. Non–contact injuries (skiing, jumping) occur when the knee is in extension and the tibia is internally rotated on the femur.[89, 138, 159] Other authors have described a varus force that, when applied to the knee with the tibia internally rotated, causes the ACL to tear.[213]

Incidence

Although the MCL is the most commonly injured ligament about the knee, the ACL is the most common ligament injury causing abnormal knee laxity.[11, 58, 77, 113, 301] Isolated injuries to the ACL without other associated major ligamentous injuries occur in approximately 60 per cent of cases,[21, 31, 57, 213] although meniscal injuries are associated with acute ACL injury in an average of 66 per cent of the cases.[21, 31, 35, 47, 57, 113, 213]

History

The classic history of an ACL rupture, whether a non–contact or contact injury, is a sudden twisting of the knee accompanied by the sensation of feeling or hearing an audible pop or snap[78, 106] and an associated feeling of hesitation, instability, and giving way of the knee. Many patients continue to participate in the activity that caused the injury (skiing), although usually by the end of the day swelling produced by hemarthrosis and the sensation of instability have occurred.[213] Patients may describe this instability by using what is called the double-fisted sign,[78] which consists of placing one clenched fist on top of the other and showing a back-and-forth motion similar to Lachman's or the pivot-shift phenomenon. A differential diagnosis would include a meniscal tear, a retinacular tear caused by a dislocated patella, an intra-articular fracture, or injury to one of the other major ligaments about the knee.

Physical Examination

All examinations, regardless of maneuvers performed, should be conducted on both the injured leg and the uninjured leg and recorded as side-to-side differences. Variations in laxity exist among individuals, and loose-jointed or hyperelastic patients may display what appears to be a positive test result when, in fact, it is the same phenomenon displayed in the uninjured leg. Markolf and collaborators[186] showed that normal uninjured persons may routinely exhibit a 3- to 5-mm side-to-side difference. Daniel and colleagues[55, 57] reported that a 3-mm side-to-side difference may be present in normal knees when tested with a KT-1000 arthrometer. The amount of increased anterior translation with the anterior drawer test and Lachman's test should be graded in terms of side-to-side difference in millimeters because there are variations in what each examiner describes as grade 1, 2, or 3 or grade 1+, 2+, or 3+. The authors' grading is as follows: 0 to 1+, less than 5 mm; 2+, 6 to 10 mm; 3+, more than 10 mm.

The degree of rupture of the ligament, ability of the patient to relax, joint configuration, positions of the hip[9] and knee,[90, 116, 118, 179, 214, 219, 277] and rotation of the tibia[9, 41, 83, 101] all are important parameters that, when varied, may change the results of each test. An understanding of the mechanics of the various tests as the maneuvers are accomplished enables the examiner to diagnose ACL injuries more accurately.

The accuracy of the physical examination in detecting an ACL injury is higher in the chronically deficient ACL than in the acutely injured knee.[144] In the acute situation, the patient displays apprehension and guards against the maneuvers involved in the physical examination because of swelling, pain, limitation of motion, or hamstring spasm.[130] In the chronically injured knee, secondary restraints may have stretched, producing more laxity. Studies have shown a higher diagnostic accuracy rate with complete ACL tears than with partial ACL tears.[21, 79, 213, 223] Finsterbush and colleagues[79] and others[71, 194, 223, 225] have stated that most patients with partially torn ACLs have a history and physical examination findings that are more consistent with a meniscal tear (catching and pseudolocking along with a positive McMurray's test). A higher diagnostic accuracy rate occurs when the ACL is injured along with another major knee ligamentous structure.[293] The diagnostic accuracy of all tests is higher in anesthetized patients than in unanesthetized patients.[21, 31, 35, 65, 144, 219, 292] In patients who are considered candidates for surgery, an examination with anesthesia and arthroscopy should be performed.

Specific Tests*

ANTERIOR DRAWER TEST.[189] The patient is supine with the knee flexed from 70° to 90°. The tibia should be in neutral rotation and be stabilized by keeping the patient's foot close to the examiner's buttock while the examiner sits just off to the side of the patient's foot. The proximal tibia is encircled by the examiner's two hands, the thenar

---

*See Chapter 4.

eminences are kept near the tibial tubercle, and the examiner's thumbs are placed at the joint line. The thumbs should palpate the distal femur and the tibial plateau. A firm, anteriorly directed force is applied in order to determine the amount of anterior translation of the tibia on the femur as palpated by the tips of the examiner's thumbs. If the PCL is damaged, the tibia may be sitting slightly subluxed posteriorly, and this maneuver will yield a false-positive result. The bent knee should always be viewed from the side to determine whether any posterior sag of the tibia is present at the time of examination (see Fig. 4–12*B*). The anterior drawer test is more reliable in the acute case when performed with the patient under anesthesia.

LACHMAN'S MANEUVER.[83, 292] To perform Lachman's maneuver, the examiner stands on the side of the patient's injured knee, keeping the knee flexed approximately 20°. The examiner uses the hand farthest away from the patient to stabilize the femur and uses the hand closest to the patient to apply an anterior transitory force to the posterior aspect of the proximal tibia. A positive result is one in which there is proprioception or visualization of anterior tibial translation in relation to the femur, with a characteristic mushy or soft endpoint. When the anterior horizon of the knee is viewed from the lateral aspect, the normal slope of the infrapatellar tendon becomes obliterated. Slight flexion of the injured knee helps negate the effect of the hamstring spasm and removes the obstructive wedge posed by the posterior horn of the medial meniscus, which is present when the knee is kept at 90° of flexion. The anterior drawer test is positive in 24 to 52 per cent of cases when performed in an unanesthetized patient with an acute ACL injury.[31, 82, 144, 213, 292] Lachman's test is positive in 68 to 100 per cent of unanesthetized patients with an ACL injury.[21, 31, 35, 144, 292] In the anesthetized patients, these examinations have consistently shown 90 to 100 per cent accuracy.[9, 31, 35, 144, 292]

Internal rotation of the tibia decreases the amount of anterior tibial translation during Lachman's test.[83] The examiner should always stand on the lateral side of the patient's knee in order to avoid reaching across the table and grabbing the tibia, which would cause internal rotation to occur. The tibia should be in slight external rotation somewhere between neutral and maximal external rotation, and the anterior transitory force should be placed posteromedially on the proximal tibia.

ACTIVE LACHMAN'S TEST.[51] The active Lachman's test is conducted with the patient lying supine with a firm bolster under the thigh of the injured leg in order to let the knee flex from 30° to 40°. While the examiner observes from the lateral aspect, the patient raises the heel off the table by extending the knee and then rests it back down on the table, relaxing the quadriceps muscle. When there is an isolated rupture of the ACL, the lateral tibial plateau gently subluxes or slides forward on the femoral condyle as extension occurs. In a report[51] of 212 patients with a history of an ACL tear, 182 had a positive active Lachman's test result. Of these 182 patients, 144 underwent surgery, and all 144 were found to have torn ACLs; of the remaining 38 patients, who did not undergo surgery, all developed a positive pivot-shift test result over time. Of the other 30 patients with negative active Lachman's test results initially, only two went on to develop a positive pivot-shift test result with time. These tests may be helpful in patients who are apprehensive and in patients with extremely obese or muscular legs.

PIVOT-SHIFT PHENOMENON.[90, 116, 118, 179, 180, 277] The pivot shift is both a clinical phenomenon that gives rise to the complaint of giving way and a physical sign that can be elicited during examination of the injured knee. It is characterized by an anterior subluxation of the lateral tibial plateau on the femoral condyle as the knee approaches extension and the spontaneous reduction during flexion. The pivot-shift phenomenon has been shown to be pathognomonic for an injury to the ACL. The speed of the subluxation-reduction phenomenon is instantaneous, as confirmed by radiographic analysis. Four clinical tests are used to demonstrate the pivot-shift phenomenon (the pivot-shift test,[90, 180] Losee's test,[179] the anterolateral rotatory instability test,[277] and the jerk test[116, 118]). All these tests demonstrate the subluxation-reduction of the lateral tibial plateau in relation to the lateral femoral condyle. In Losee's test and the jerk test, the knee starts in flexion (a reduced position) and subluxes as it is placed into extension. In the pivot-shift test and the anterolateral rotatory instability test, the knee starts in the extended (subluxed) position and reduces as flexion reaches 30° or 40°. In order for reduction to occur, the iliotibial band must be intact. Relaxation is essential for obtaining an accurate test. These tests are described in detail in Chapter 4.

In conscious, unanesthetized patients with an acute knee injury, the pivot-shift test has not been found to be as accurate as Lachman's test.[31] In anesthetized patients, however, the pivot-shift test has been consistently found to be more than 95 per cent accurate.[9, 35, 180]

Accurate testing for the pivot-shift phenomenon may be difficult because of hamstring spasm and apprehension by the patient in the acute situation. This prompted Noyes and associates[213, 214] to describe the flexion-rotation drawer test, which is a modification of the pivot-shift test for anterior subluxation of the lateral tibial plateau. It differs from the pivot-shift test in that the subluxation is produced by the weight of the thigh as the leg is held with the knee in 20° to 30° of flexion and with neutral tibial rotation. The femur is allowed to rotate freely between the subluxed and reduced positions as the knee is extended and flexed with a slight anterior force on the proximal tibia. Noyes and associates believed that this test brings out the rotational component of the ACL laxity. This test, although more subtle than the pivot-shift test, is gentler and more reproducible in patients with acute knee injury. Of unanesthetized patients with complete disruption, 38 per cent had positive flexion-rotation drawer test results, whereas of patients who underwent the test under anesthesia, 89 per cent had positive results. For partial ruptures of the ACL, the test result was positive in only 8 per cent of unanesthetized patients, as opposed to 62 per cent of the patients examined under anesthesia.

Clancy and Ray[41] and Bach and co-workers[9] showed that tibial rotation affects the gradation of the pivot-shift phenomenon and that external rotation consistently yielded higher or equal degrees of the pivot-shift phenomenon in comparison with internal rotation. Furthermore, Bach and co-workers[9] stated that hip positioning may also affect the degree of the pivot-shift phenomenon because of the effect on the length and tension of the iliotibial tract. Hip abduction consistently provided a higher degree of the pivot-shift phenomenon. In the authors' experience, the pivot-shift phenomenon can be reproduced in many positions, and it behooves the examiner to master each of the techniques.

In summary, for the conscious patient in the acute setting, Lachman's test has been found to be the maneuver that most consistently determines the integrity of the ACL. The pivot-shift phenomenon, when present, is pathognomonic for tears of the ACL. For patients under anesthesia, Lachman's test and the pivot-shift maneuvers have consistently been shown to be 98 per cent accurate, sensitive, and specific in diagnosing ACL injuries.

In cases in which the leg is extremely obese or muscular and there is difficulty in adequately stabilizing or cradling the leg, the active Lachman's test, the anterior drawer test, the anterolateral rotatory instability test, and the flexion-rotation drawer test all may be useful. Patients whose history is consistent with that of a torn ACL but with negative or suspicious findings on physical examination should be considered candidates for examination under anesthesia and for arthroscopy if surgical intervention is indicated. In patients likely to be treated by nonoperative methods and for whom the examination result is still in question, MRI should be considered in order to assess the status of the menisci.

Treatment

The treatment of an ACL-injured knee depends on numerous variables. The prognosis for isolated ACL lesions is different from that for combined lesions of the ACL and other major ligaments. Partial ACL injury and the extent of associated abnormal laxity must be differentiated from the complete ACL lesion because the overall prognoses when treatment is nonoperative are different.[15, 223, 310] Because the rate of meniscal injury associated with ACL tears is very high, it is necessary to approach the ACL not as an isolated structure but as a combined functional unit with the meniscus in terms of diagnostic workup and treatment (Fig. 20–10).

PARTIAL ACL TEARS. Partial ACL tears represent 10 to 43 per cent of all ACL injuries.[11, 27, 58, 78, 79, 174, 194, 213, 223, 228, 249] The literature emphasizes the difference objectively, subjectively, and functionally between partial and complete ACL tears.[15, 79, 194, 213, 223, 310] A partial ACL tear may be clinically difficult to differentiate from a meniscal tear in that minimal or no hemarthrosis is often present.[71, 194, 223] There may be a history of pseudolocking[71, 79, 194, 223, 225] or locked knee; rarely has there been a description of a popping or snapping sensation as seen with complete ACL tears. Most authors have shown a decreased incidence of objective laxity during the physical examination in both conscious and anesthetized patients.[15, 21, 71, 223] This may hamper the actual diagnosis. The use of the arthroscope enables determination of a partial or complete tear with or without associated meniscal pathology.[15, 21, 27, 223] Although disruption is detectable through arthroscopy, the amount of microscopic ligamentous disruption and plastic deformation is difficult to assess.[37, 159, 213, 216, 223]

In one study, Noyes and associates[216] found the ultimate failure strength of an intact ACL to be 1700 newtons when loading was along the tibial axis and 2400 newtons when loading was along the ACL axis. It has been estimated that the working load on the ACL during normal activities is approximately 500 newtons and that it is significantly higher in the more demanding activities. When stressed, the ACL can be elongated to more than 150 per cent of its resting length before ultimate

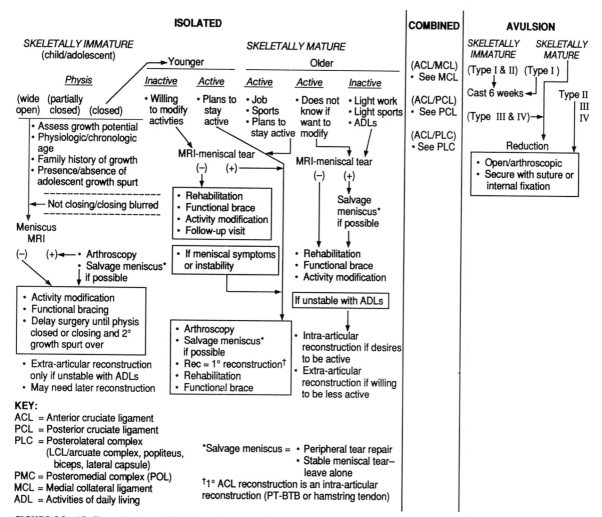

FIGURE 20–10. Flow chart to aid in determining evaluation and treatment of patients with an anterior cruciate ligament injury.

failure. This is defined as the point at which the ligament is unable to support load. Noyes and associates found that at this point, the ligament was macroscopically intact, although physiologically and functionally worthless. Kennedy and colleagues[160] demonstrated microscopic wide-spread disruption of the collagen fibrils in macroscopically intact ligaments when stressed just to the point of ultimate failure.

There is a difference of opinion in the literature regarding correlation of the percentage of tear and the overall clinical outcome.[27, 223] Buckley and collaborators[27] evaluated partial ACL tears involving 10 to 75 per cent of the ligament as visualized through the arthroscope. The patients had a maximum of 5 mm of laxity on Lachman's test and the anterior drawer test as well as the absence of pivot shift when examined under anesthesia. At follow-up, no correlation was found between the percentage of tear and the overall subjective or functional outcome.

Noyes and associates[223] classified patients with partial ACL tears into two categories: those with partial tears that are objectively stable and those with abnormal objective laxity. For tears of one quarter of the ligament or less, there was a lower incidence of progression from objective stability to objective laxity of the knee. Of the patients with tears of half the ligament, 75 per cent went on to experience objective instability of the knee, and of the patients in whom three fourths of the ligament was torn, 100 per cent went on to experience objective laxity of the knee. The finding of abnormal objective laxity did not alter the percentage of patients who returned to a preinjury level of sports. Of those considered to have objective stability of the knee, 40 per cent continued to play at the same level of sports; only half of them were symptomatic. Of the patients with objective laxity of the knee, 58 per cent continued participating at the same level of sports, but all were symptomatic. Those with objective stability had a better chance of having few or no symptoms.[15, 27, 223]

A higher number of associated meniscal injuries occur with complete ACL tears than with partial tears.[14, 15, 27, 79, 213, 223] Partial tears have been associated with meniscal injuries in 12 to 50 per cent of patients,[15, 27, 79, 223, 228] whereas complete tears have been associated with meniscal injuries in 50 to 72 per cent in the same studies.[14, 15, 31, 35, 58, 213] In terms of the need for additional surgery, there is clearly a higher rate of secondary meniscal injury and the need for an ACL reconstruction in patients with complete tears.[14, 15, 27, 79]

Of the patients whose symptoms do not warrant a reconstructive procedure, approximately 45 per cent will be able to participate at the same level of athletics, 20 per cent of whom will be asymptomatic.[11, 27, 223, 228, 249] This is especially true of patients who are willing to modify their activities if symptoms do occur.[27, 223] Some patients reinjure the knee or progress to subjective and functional instability and require a secondary surgical procedure.[11, 15, 79, 223, 228]

Nonoperative treatment should consist of obtaining full range of motion and muscle strengthening as well as functional retraining and maintaining endurance capabilities. Appropriate follow-up in all patients, whether treated operatively or nonoperatively, is essential because approximately 15 to 20 per cent of these patients reinjure the meniscus and have further problems with the knee.

COMPLETE ACL TEARS. The treatment of isolated complete ACL tears is different from that of other ACL tears associated with other major ligamentous injuries.

Of patients with acute hemarthrosis of the knee,[21, 31, 126, 213] approximately 66 per cent have an ACL tear. Of patients who have an acute ACL injury, 60 per cent have an associated meniscal injury.[14, 22, 31, 35, 58, 59, 113, 126, 213, 236, 311] There is an associated chondral lesion in 20 per cent of the cases.[21, 113, 126, 213] In comparison, symptomatic, chronic ACL-deficient knees, when subjected to arthroscopy, have been found to have an 80 per cent rate of meniscal tear (more on the medial than on the lateral meniscus) and a 50 per cent rate of chondral lesions (more on the medial side than on the lateral).[2, 59, 82, 113, 126, 311] This review implies that the natural progression of a nonreconstructed ACL-deficient knee would be one of increasing meniscal damage, chondral degeneration, and a potential increase in symptoms and subsequent disability.

Articular and periarticular changes noted with ACL insufficiency have been reported in both animal[187, 197] and human[72, 73, 195, 196, 221, 222, 236, 271] studies. Feagin and associates[72, 73] reported that radiographic signs consistent with

ACL insufficiency are (1) peaking of the intercondylar tubercles, (2) spurring and hypertrophy of the intercondylar eminence, (3) osteophytosis of the inferior facet of the patella, (4) stenosis of the intercondylar notch, (5) narrowing of the joint space, and (6) buttressing osteophytosis. In 1988, Sherman and co-authors[271] reiterated that chronic ACL insufficiency causes radiographic signs of degeneration along with decreased functional knee scores. Initially (within the first 5 years), knees with ACL injuries combined with MCL and meniscal injuries show earlier signs of degeneration and lower knee scores, but after approximately 10 years, even the knees with isolated ACL injuries develop degenerative changes and lower clinical knee scores that are no different from those of the combined injuries.

These and other studies[78, 82, 87, 221, 222, 300] that address the natural history frequently report on the symptomatic patients with a chronically ACL-deficient knee and do not include asymptomatic patients. This procedure may inflate the incidence of pathologic objective radiographic and subjective findings, and therefore these findings may not reflect a true natural progression. These studies, along with long-term meniscal studies, have shown that radiographic changes usually occur 7 to 10 years after injury or after total meniscectomy.[70, 140, 150, 162, 271, 286] Symptoms are not necessarily correlated with radiographic findings. The patient's functional status may not be correlated with either radiographic changes or symptoms, because aggressive, determined patients may participate in sports even with pain and instability. Noyes and associates categorized such patients as "knee abusers."[221, 222]

Other investigators[14, 22, 106, 113, 236] have evaluated function and symptoms in terms of activities of daily living, ability to perform work obligations, and recreational and competitive sporting activities in order to determine the success or failure of the treatment method. Patients who had isolated acute ACL injuries with or without associated meniscal injury (which necessitates partial meniscectomy or repair) and who were treated nonoperatively were evaluated. All were provided with a formal rehabilitation program, functional bracing, and counseling of activity modification. A total of 265 patients with an average time to follow-up of 52.4 months (range of 38 to 67 months) were included in these reports. The findings were as follows:

1. In more than 90 per cent of cases, patients were usually able to resume activities of daily living and nonstrenuous work obligations without problems. Jobs requiring excessive climbing or agility sometimes caused more problems, requiring a reconstructive procedure.[14]

2. An average of 75 per cent of all patients were able to resume sporting activity. Of the 25 per cent who were unable to resume sporting activities, most could not because of the knee; others abstained from sports because of either time constraints or lack of desire to continue with the sport. Only 15 per cent of all patients were able to resume their preinjury sporting level without symptoms. Approximately 60 per cent modified their sporting activities. It is not clear whether modification was the result of counseling (self-imposed) or of knee symptoms (inflicted).

3. Meniscal reinjury occurred in 12 per cent of all patients, necessitating a secondary arthroscopy. In addition, 20 per cent of patients either elected or required a late reconstructive surgery for inability to perform

activities of daily living or work obligations, inability to participate in sports at all, or desire to perform at a more competitive level than they were able.

4. The majority of patients were symptomatic at follow-up; instability with giving way was present in 62 per cent, pain in 57 per cent, and swelling in 36 per cent. Although symptoms appeared to be directly related to activity and type of sports, approximately 10 to 15 per cent of patients experienced these symptoms even during activities of daily living.

Activities involving quickness, speed, and agility (cutting, lateral movement, twisting, jumping, fast running) caused the most problems (instability, pain, swelling). More than 50 per cent of the patients gave up high-demand sports (such as racquetball, handball, basketball, snow skiing, water skiing, football, wrestling, ice hockey, and soccer). The extent of objective abnormal laxity in the presence of the pivot-shift phenomenon has been correlated directly with a poor overall functional result.

5. Although all of these authors agreed that the presence or absence of a unilateral meniscal tear did not affect results, Barrack and co-workers[14] showed that bilateral meniscal tears associated with complete ACL tears clearly produced poor functional results and a higher rate of reconstruction. Two groups of authors[106, 236] noted early degenerative changes on radiographs and yet could not find a correlation of these changes either to the presence of a meniscal injury or a partial meniscectomy or to the overall objective or functional result. These findings have been substantiated by other authors.[272, 300]

6. Thigh girth, quadriceps strength, and hamstring strength were directly correlated with overall functional rating in reduced symptoms. These findings have been well documented in both acute and chronic situations.[3, 82, 87, 93, 195, 196, 221, 222, 226, 260, 300]

7. Functional bracing improved symptoms in one study.[22] Those authors postulated that more patients may have participated in some athletic endeavor because they felt more secure using the brace, and yet in the same study more than 60 per cent of the patients believed that the brace limited their overall performance level. Other authors[106, 113, 236] have contended that most patients choose not to use a brace even when it is prescribed.

8. Patients in their early 20s seem to have more symptoms and a higher reconstruction rate than do patients in their late 20s, probably as the result of an unwillingness to modify their activities and an increased desire to compete at higher levels and in more demanding sports. Nevertheless, age was not considered a determining factor in terms of overall results.

9. Bonamo and colleagues[22] reported that overall functional results worsened with time from initial injury.

These and other studies[2, 8, 36, 87, 93, 150, 195, 196, 221, 222, 226, 253] suggest that the conservative treatment of the acute, isolated, complete ACL injury with or without a unilateral meniscal injury offers acceptable results at medium-range follow-up (5 years). Such treatment should be offered to the nonathlete, the noncompetitive recreational athlete who is willing to modify sporting activities, and patients who are unwilling to risk the potential morbidity of ligament reconstruction. Professional or highly competitive athletes and recreational athletes who are unwilling to modify participation in high-demand sports should be considered for early ACL reconstruction. Failure of conservative treatment may also be an indication for reconstruction.

Conservative treatment consists of determining the status of the menisci, either by MRI or by arthroscopy, and repairing or partially excising the torn meniscus. A supervised therapy program that combines strengthening of hip, thigh, and calf muscles with endurance and agility training should be provided. A home maintenance program should be taught, and its value in avoiding reinjuries should be stressed. Counseling on activity modification and on the use of a functional brace, as well as educating the patient about early signs of worsening symptoms, is appropriate. Repeated arthroscopies are necessary because the studies previously mentioned show a 12 per cent meniscal reinjury rate, and approximately 20 per cent of the patients ultimately undergo an ACL reconstructive procedure. High-level athletes such as those in high-demand (professional, college, and highly competitive recreational) sports place greater demands on their knees. The nonoperative approach would not provide the same results as have been described with operative procedures.[42, 269, 306]

Surgical Treatment of Acute ACL Disruption

Advocates of early surgical intervention for acute ACL disruptions have stated that the ACL serves as an important guide in determining knee motion (screw-home mechanism), stability (pivot-shift phenomenon), and overall function.[42, 112, 115, 269, 306] Results of animal studies and human clinical studies suggest that chronic ACL insufficiency leads to stretching of secondary restraints, rotational instabilities, functional disabilities, increasing meniscal injury rates, and subsequent cartilaginous injuries and premature degeneration of the joint.[42, 59, 72, 82, 87, 126, 187, 198, 221, 222, 271, 311] These studies do not reflect the true natural history, inasmuch as they represent only the symptomatic population of chronically ACL-insufficient patients and not the asymptomatic population. Some of the data from these studies clearly show that patients undergoing reconstructive procedures for chronically symptomatic ACL insufficiency do improve, and perhaps earlier surgical intervention may therefore work prophylactically to reduce the percentage of patients who go on to have chronically symptomatic knees.

Studies have focused on return to preinjury activity levels as a means of determining the success or failure of a treatment modality. The lack of correlation between objective laxity and overall function and symptoms has made it difficult to evaluate the efficacy of different surgical techniques employed in the ACL-injured knee.[104, 261] The presence of a pivot shift greater than grade 1+ is correlated with a decrease in functional activity level.[42, 221, 222, 262, 303]

Palmer[234] in 1938 and O'Donoghue[229] in 1950 were advocates of early primary repair of all major ligamentous injuries around the knee and stressed the efficacy of repair for acute injury in comparison with reconstruction for chronic injury. Follow-up reports on primary surgical repair of a torn ACL have shown promising early objective and functional results with deterioration over time.[3, 74, 112, 154, 190, 191, 227, 230, 270] Feagin and Curl[74] reported that 25 of 30 patients had good results 2 years after primary repair for the ACL, but after 5 years nearly all patients were dissatisfied with the results and unable to participate in sports.

The ACL has poor healing potential. The primary repair of a torn ACL has been unpredictable unless augmented with other tissue.[33, 74] Comparison of various studies is difficult because of differences in rating techniques, subjective evaluation, and different-activity population groups.[104, 261] Several studies reviewed showed elimination of the pivot shift in 54 to 82 per cent of patients. There was a deterioration in stability from the 2- to the 5-year follow-ups.[3, 74, 154, 190, 191, 227, 230, 270]

Andersson and associates[3] conducted a prospective, randomized study of nonoperative treatment, primary repair, and primary repair with augmentation of the ACL carried out to a 4-year follow-up. Return to previous athletic activity was the same in the patients who underwent nonoperative treatment and primary repair but significantly better in the patients who underwent primary repair with augmentation.

The ACL suspended in the joint without surrounding soft tissue and bathed by synovial fluid has a healing environment that is inappropriate for successful primary repair by itself. The case for augmentation of the repaired ACL has been demonstrated by several authors.[3, 33, 38, 40] Theoretically, augmentation accomplishes three goals: (1) transplanted tissue used for augmentation acts as a scaffolding for the disrupted ACL fibers and provides proper alignment; (2) the disrupted ACL fibers and surrounding soft tissue enhance the revascularization of the transplanted tissue; and (3) the stability provided by the transplanted graft acts as a stent to protect against excess stress to the sutured ACL.

In a prospective, nonrandomized study,[40] the results of nonoperative treatment in patients with no or a mild pivot shift were compared with those of the operative treatment of patients with a moderate or severe pivot shift. Operative treatment consisted of a primary repair of the torn ACL ligament and augmentation with a central-third patellar tendon graft. At the 48-month follow-up, the results for 13 of 22 nonoperative patients and for 68 of 70 surgical patients were rated good or excellent. Similar results have been reported by other authors.

Two studies have shown no difference in results regardless of whether an extra-articular procedure was performed in addition to the primary repair and augmentation.[68, 285] One study[285] reported 10 per cent of patients to have a significant loss of motion; 6.9 per cent required manipulation under anesthesia. Results of the longest follow-up study, of 78 months, were compared with the results of an 18-month follow-up. Of the patients with the shorter follow-up, 93 per cent had good or excellent results, whereas of the patients with the longer follow-up, 82 per cent had results in this category. There was no difference in objective stability findings between the two groups.

Various autogenous tissues were used for augmentation, including the semitendinosus-gracilis tendons,[37, 111, 133, 134, 167, 176] the patellar tendon,[40, 42, 74, 134, 139, 142, 191] and the iliotibial band.[3, 145, 154]

Some authors prefer to perform a primary ACL reconstruction after an acute ACL disruption.[42, 224, 269, 306] Delay of surgery for 1 to 3 weeks in order to allow the effects of the acute injury to subside and to restore range of motion of the knee has been found helpful in decreasing the number of patients who have residual loss of motion after acute ACL surgery.[204, 264] A report[269] of 140 athletes with a 4-year follow-up after primary ACL reconstruction with a bone–patellar tendon–bone graft showed that 87 per cent returned to their preinjury level of sports. Ninety-four per cent showed no instability. Minimal loss of motion was reported in 8 per cent of this group.

In another study,[306] a double-looped semitendinosus graft was used for acute primary reconstruction with an extra-articular procedure. Ninety-three per cent of the competitive athletes studied had returned to their preinjury level of sport at a 48-month follow-up.

A primary repair of the ACL ligament with augmentation involving autogenous tissue and a primary reconstruction of the ACL have similar results if strong augmentation is used. A delay in surgery of more than 1 or 2 weeks may favor a primary reconstruction.

SURGICAL TECHNIQUE FOR ANTERIOR CRUCIATE RECONSTRUCTION

The two most commonly used autograft tissues in ACL reconstruction are the patellar tendon (bone-tendon-bone complex) and one or both hamstring tendons. There appears to be no difference in the overall outcome between the use of either of these grafts in reconstruction of the ACL in the acute situation.[42, 104, 115, 135, 185, 285] Either arthroscopically assisted or open techniques can be used. There is no difference in results with the use of either the arthroscopically assisted or the open technique.[104, 115, 135] The open technique[134] may be performed through the defect created in the patellar tendon if this graft is used. No difference in overall results was apparent between the modified over-the-top position for placement of the graft on the femur and the dual tunnel technique (tibial and femoral bone tunnels).

Patellar tendon bone-to-bone fixation appears to provide the best early fixation and is the usual preference for a vigorous athlete. The double-loop semitendinosus tendon with the gracilis tendon in some cases is preferred if an arthroscopically assisted procedure with minimal incisions is desired.

POSITIONING

The patient is placed in a supine position, with the knee flexed 90° over the end of the table, with a bolster placed under the proximal thigh (see Fig. 20–4). A removable lateral post is placed for diagnostic arthroscopy. A tourniquet is placed high up on the thigh over sheet wadding (Webril wrap) to allow access to the lateral side of the distal third of the femur.

Diagnostic arthroscopy is performed with the use of standard antero-medial and anterolateral portals; the inflow-outflow cannula is placed in the superomedial parapatellar portal so as not to interfere with subsequent lateral procedures.

Systematic visualization of the joint is performed in the usual manner. If an adequate ACL stump can contribute blood supply or tensile strength to the augmentation, it should be retained. If reconstruction of the ACL is indicated, the ACL is debrided, and a small amount of the tibial stump, if available, is left to ensure correct location of the tibial guide pin. The PCL must not be injured during the debridement. The integrity of the meniscus must be ascertained, and either partial meniscectomy or meniscal repair should be performed as indicated. If meniscal repair is chosen, placement of the sutures arthroscopically should be performed, but the sutures should not be tied until after the ACL reconstruction or repair is completed.

A notchplasty should be performed if there is any question of adequate space for the graft. Either straight or curved curettes, short-ended rasps, an osteotome or power abraders, and burs may be used for the notchplasty. The complete extent of the notchplasty should be determined interoperatively after graft placement by noting whether the graft is being impinged upon by the notch as the knee goes through a full range of motion. Removal of bone off of the anterior lateral portion and the superior portion of the notch should be performed initially so as to allow adequate visualization of the posterior aspect of the lateral femoral condyle heading toward the over-the-top position. The posterior aspect usually can be identified by placing a probe in the anteromedial portal and the arthroscope in the anterolateral portal. Switching of portals may be necessary for further delineating the need for posterior and superior debridement. Protection of the PCL throughout the procedure is important. Usually the meniscal repair or the partial meniscectomy, as well as the notchplasty, may be performed without the use of a tourniquet.

PATELLAR TENDON (BONE-TENDON-BONE) TECHNIQUE

An anterior incision should be made either directly over the midportion of the patellar tendon or slightly off toward the medial side, extending approximately 3 cm above the inferior pole of the patella to approximately 3 cm below the superior portion of the tibial tubercle (Fig. 20–11). Smaller incisions that require more traction on the soft tissue may be used. Transverse incisions have also been employed.

Full-thickness skin flaps should be made medially and laterally to the extent of the size of the patellar tendon. The medial skin flap is elevated approximately 2 cm further medial to the distal third of the patellar tendon to allow for drilling of the tibial tunnel. The sheath of the patellar tendon in the midportion of the tendon should be carefully incised. The tendon itself must not be injured. The sheath is lifted, and the tendon is separated from the peritenon sheath, both medially and laterally, to expose both sides of the patellar tendon from the insertion on the patella to the tibial tubercle. With the knee flexed to 90°, the width of the patellar tendon is measured, and the middle third is marked with methylene blue. A graft of 10 to 12 mm in width is desirable (Fig. 20–12A). A 1-cm–width oscillating saw is used to cut out a rectangular portion of bone from the distal pole of the patella; this portion follows the outlines previously drawn and has a length of 25 mm, a width of 10 mm, and a depth of approximately 5 to 8 mm (Fig. 20–12B). Care must be taken not to injure the tendon insertion into the patellar bone or to violate the articular surface of the distal patella. The parallel cuts into the patella should be slanted inward to lessen the bone loss from the patella and to retain more structural strength.

The incisions previously marked are carried on the central third of the patellar tendon down to the tibial tubercle. The tibial bone block may be taken either as a rectangular portion of bone if interference fit is to be used in the tibial bone hole (Fig. 20–12C) or as a wedge-shaped piece of

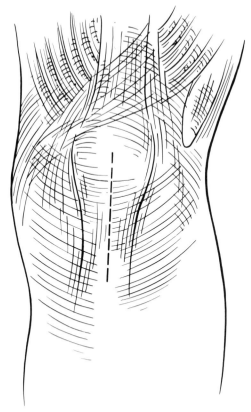
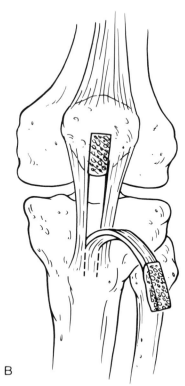

FIGURE 20–11. (*A*) Anterior incision used to expose the patellar tendon. Length of incision can be shortened and skin retracted proximally and then distally in order to allow harvest of bone plugs. (*B*) Proximal patellar bone plug has been harvested and middle third of tendon mobilized before tibial bone plug is taken.

bone if it is to be used with the modified over-the-top reconstruction (Fig. 20–12*D*). The proximal portion of the tibial bone is 10 mm in width, and the distal extent is approximately 20 mm in width, the bone plug being 30 mm in length. The depth of the bone plug to be taken is between 5 and 8 mm. Injury to the insertion of the patellar tendon into the tibial tubercle must be avoided. A 3.5-mm drill hole is drilled proximally and a 2.0-mm drill hole is drilled distally in the midportion of the patellar bone block. These drill holes are used for suture placement in passing of the graft as well as in fixation if a 4.0-mm screw is used (Fig. 20–12*E*). The tibial bone plug is also provided with a 2.0-mm drill hole for suture placement used to manipulate the graft.

The patellar bone plug is lifted carefully out of the patella trough with a small osteotome. The patellar tendon is slowly peeled off of the fat pad as it is elevated from its bed to the tibial tubercle. The tibial tubercle bone plug is lifted carefully from its bed with an osteotome. Number 5 Ethibond sutures are then placed through the drill holes placed in the bone plugs. The patellar bone plug is contoured and sized by commercially available sizing devices. In the modified over-the-top method, the wedge of bone taken off of the tibial tubercle is to be used to wedge into the tibial drill hole. Only the patellar bone plug needs to be measured so as

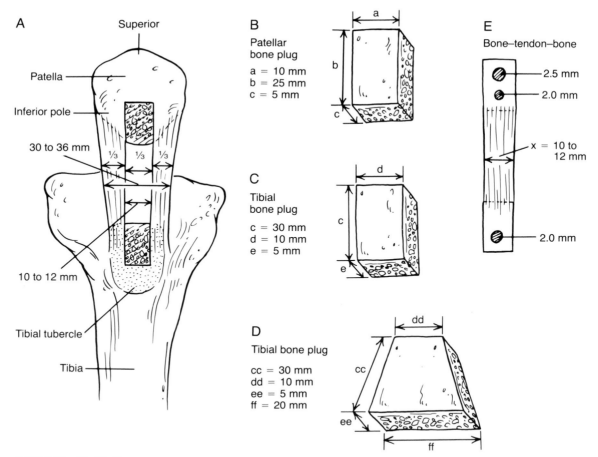

FIGURE 20–12. (*A*) Measurements of patellar tendon graft. (*B*) Size of patellar bone plug. (*C*) Size of tibial bone plug. (*D*) Alternative method of taking tibial bone plug, which enables trapezoid shape of plug to be wedged into tibial tunnel for fixation. (*E*) Drill holes in patellar and tibial bone plugs. Proximal hole in patellar plug is used for screw fixation if the over-the-top method is used. This hole is not necessary if plug is to be taken into a femoral drill hole with interference screw fixation.

to get through the tibial tunnel as the graft is passed into the joint and into the over-the-top position.

The tibial drill hole should be made through the use of a guide wire with cannulated reamers placed over the guide wire. The guide pin should be started approximately 3 cm distal to the joint surface and approximately 1.5 to 2 cm medial to the tibial tubercle. This places the tibial hole above the pes anserinus confluence of tendons and far enough down from the joint line to allow adequate placement of the bone plug without impinging upon the joint itself. With the arthroscope in the anterolateral portal, the tibial guide pin is directed to the anatomic site of the ACL at its insertion on the tibia. Tibial guide systems may be used (Fig. 20–13*B*), or the pin may be directed by focusing on its placement. There have been numerous reports regarding the correct site of this placement. The anatomic site is the best position, and if the surgeon is to err, the placement should be just anterior within 5 mm of the medial intercondylar eminence and just slightly medial to this eminence. The position should stay at least 1 cm posterior to the front of the anterior surface of the medial tibial plateau.

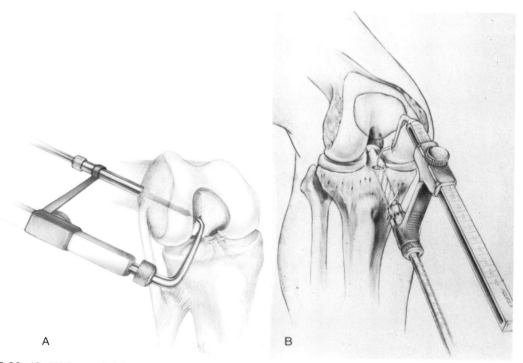

A   B

FIGURE 20–13. (*A*) Femoral drill guide used to drill hole from the outside in. Note very posterosuperior position of drill hole in notch. (From Lambert KL, Cunninghamm RR: Anatomic substitution of the ruptured ACL using a vascularized patellar tendon graft with interference fit fixation. *In* Feagin J [ed]: The Crucial Ligaments, p. 405. New York: Churchill Livingstone, 1988.) (*B*) Tibial drill guide used to place drill hole at anatomic attachment of the ACL. (From Rosenberg TD, Paulos LE, Abbott PJ Jr: Arthroscopic cruciate repair and reconstruction: an overview and descriptions of technique. *In* Feagin J [ed]: The Crucial Ligaments, p. 412. New York: Churchill Livingstone, 1988.)

Arthroscopic visualization is essential for confirming the pin site intra-articularly.

Attention should then be directed toward the lateral incision. Two incisions are described: one for the modified over-the-top position and one for the femoral tunnel placement (Fig. 20–14). For incision placement on the lateral side, with the knee bent at 90°, the superior pole of the patella and the most posterior superior aspect of the lateral femoral condyle at its junction into the distal femur are palpated. The biceps tendon as it goes into the fibula head is also palpated. The incision for the modified over-the-top position placement of the graft should be made 0.5 cm posterior to the condylar-shaft junction and should extend approximately 2 cm distal and 3 cm proximal. When a femoral tunnel is used, the incision should be made approximately 0.5 to 1.0 cm above that junction so as to stay anterior to the lateral intramuscular septum. The incision is carried down through skin, subcutaneous tissue, and to the fascia. Full-thickness skin flaps are developed both anteriorly and posteriorly.

In the modified over-the-top position, the incision through the iliotibial band is along the posterior third of the iliotibial band. The inferior portion of the band is retracted posteriorly, and the superior portion is retracted anteriorly. Adipose tissue in this area is excised through the use of cutting electrocauterization. The anterior genicular artery and veins are identified and cauterized. The lateral intramuscular septum is followed

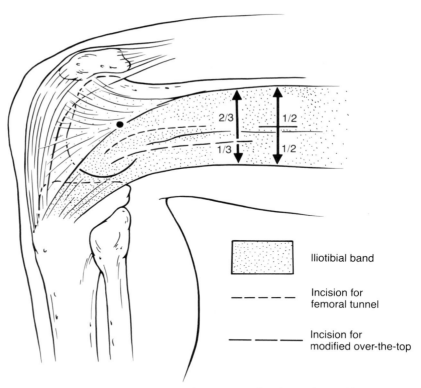

FIGURE 20–14. Lateral incisions necessary for fixing patellar plug to femur. The more anterior incision is used if a femoral drill hole is used. The more posterior incision is used for over-the-top placement.

distally to the insertion of the lateral head of the gastrocnemius muscle on the femur. The superior portion of the insertion of the gastrocnemius muscle is released by cutting electrocauterization, and the distal end of the intramuscular septum is detached. The electrocutting knife is used to incise the periosteum, and a small periosteal elevator is used to lift the periosteum off the posterior aspect of the femur. The surgeon can use a finger to palpate over the posterior aspect of the lateral femoral condyle down to the posterior capsule. A groove is made in the over-the-top position with the use of curved curettes and rasps and is deepened 4 to 5 mm anteriorly. This is the near-isometric position.

Keeping an index finger on the posterior capsule, the surgeon can then penetrate the capsule either by a curved tendon passer or by a commercially available gaf along the medial portion of the lateral femoral condyle intra-articularly and out the over-the-top position. Dilators can then be used to widen the hole in the posterior capsule for graft passage.

The edges of the patellar bone portion of approximately 1 cm in width are beveled in order to aid in passage through the tibial drill hole and the posterior capsule. The tibial guide pin is overdrilled with the proper-sized drill hole, usually a 10- to 12-mm hole (see Fig. 20–13B). The edges of the tibial hole should be chamfered with the use of a curved curette, a rasp, or a power Chamfer bur, particularly at the posterior and lateral aspects of the intra-articular hole. A Gore-Tex smoother can be passed through the tibial hole and out the over-the-top position for smoothing the passageway of the graft.

The isometry of graft placement can be checked by means of the Gore-Tex smoother or a catheter. The catheter or smoother is manually fixed at the attachment point on the lateral femur, and the knee is put through a range of motion in order to see whether there is any excessive excursion (over 2 mm). Commercially available isometers can be used. Before the graft is placed, the catheter is checked for any impingement at the notch as the knee is flexed and extended. If there is, further notch-plasty is necessary.

The patellar bony portion is then pulled through the tibial hole into the joint and out the posterolateral side of the femur to the over-the-top position. The tibial wedge bone plug is engaged into the tibial hole and impacted into position; the bone should not jut into the intra-articular portion of the joint. Tension is placed on the patellar bone block sutures, and the knee is flexed and extended to take out slack and pre-tension the graft. The graft should be held with approximately 5 to 8 pounds of tension while the bone block is fixed. The bone block is secured to the posterior aspect of the femur by using a K-wire into the most proximal bone hole in the patellar bone plug and into the femur.

The knee is again put through the full range of motion to make sure that there is adequate tension on the graft and to check for any impingement. If there is full range of motion with appropriate tension, a cannulated drill is used over the K-wire to provide a hole for a cannulated 4.0-mm screw with ligament washer. The screw is then used to secure the bone plug to the posterior aspect of the femur (Fig. 20–15). Stability of the knee is checked with Lachman's test and a pivot-shift test, and the surgeon should make sure that there is no impingement upon the graft. This technique may be used as the primary ACL reconstruction or in cases in which there has been a breakthrough when drilling a femoral drill hole.

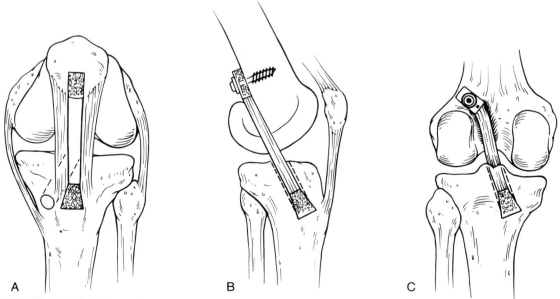

A　　　　　　　　　　B　　　　　　　　　　C

FIGURE 20–15. (*A*) Graft is harvested, and tibial drill hole is made. (*B*) Lateral view showing position of graft through tibial drill hole, notch, and over-the-top with fixation of distal plug by wedging and fixation of proximal bone plug by screw and washer. (*C*) Position of screw and washer in proximal plug as seen from posterior view.

The bone reamings from the tibial drill holes are placed into the patellar defect. The patellar tendon defect is closed with interrupted absorbable suture, and the peritenon sheath is closed over the suture line. The tourniquet is released before closure, and hemostasis is obtained. Drains are used as necessary before closure of fascial and skin incisions.

The wedge graft in the tibia provides firm fixation. The patellar bone plug is usually incorporated into the back of the femur in 6 to 10 weeks.

DUAL TUNNEL TECHNIQUE

This technique is performed by arthroscopically assisted means. Fixation of the bone plug can be accomplished by an interference screw placed through an incision over the lateral femoral condyle or by an endoscopically placed interference screw. The lateral incision is made approximately 0.5 cm to 1.0 cm above the junction of the posterolateral femoral condyle and the posterior portion of the femoral shaft. The incision extends 2 cm distal and 2 cm proximal. The incision is carried down through skin and subcutaneous tissue (see Fig. 20–13). The iliotibial band is incised along its midline. Above the lateral intramuscular septum, the vastus lateralis muscle and tendon are retracted anteriorly. The proximal portion of the lateral condyle and epicondyle is exposed by incising the periosteum.

A drill guide can be used through the anterolateral portal, with the guide tip placed 4 to 5 mm anterior to the posterior wall of the lateral notch (see Fig. 20–13A). A posterior guide system that requires passing the guide tip through the posterolateral capsule for its placement is also available. Usually a bullet type of guide is then placed over the lateral femoral condyle. This is usually a finger's breadth anterior to the lateral intramuscular septum and 4 cm proximal to the lateral epicondyle (see Fig. 20–13). While the joint is visualized arthroscopically, the guide pin is placed, and a cannulated drill, the size of which is based on the previous measurements of the graft harvested, is used to make the femoral drill hole. When there is dense cortical bone, it is helpful to start with a smaller drill and advance to a larger drill.

A red rubber catheter or a Gore-Tex smoother is placed along the course of the graft to check for near-isometric placement, as previously described. Both the tibial and femoral holes are chamfered to smooth their edges. A Gore-Tex smoother is used both to smooth out the edges of the tunnel and as an isometer. Isometers are also commercially available. After it is established that the graft is near isometric and that there is no impingement, the graft may be placed. The patellar bone plug is passed through the tibial hole into the joint and out through the femoral hole. The patellar bone plug is fixed in the femoral hole.

There are a number of techniques for securing the graft once positioning and tension are correct. Sutures tied over unicortical bone screws as posts, sutures through ligament buttons, and interference screw fixation techniques have been described.[164] Kurosaka and collaborators[163] described the self-tapping screw for interference fit, and many commercial self-tapping cannulated interference screws are now available (Figs. 20–16A, 20–16B).

It is important that interference screws be available in multiple widths and lengths so that the ones used do not extend past the end of the bone plug and potentially injure the ligament. The screws should routinely be

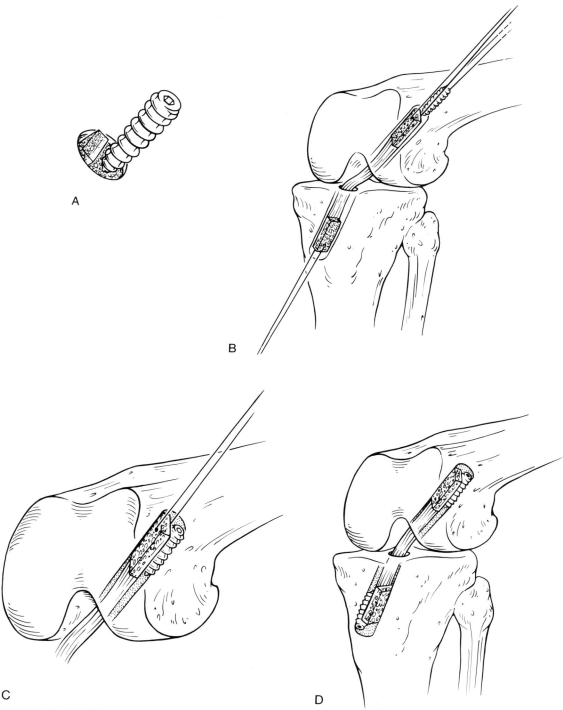

FIGURE 20–16. (*A*) Interference screw is placed on the cortical surface of the bone plugs (see text). (*B*) Femoral interference screw is usually placed on the lateral side of the tunnel, forcing the cancellous bone of the plug into a superior position. The screw must be placed parallel with the bone block. (*C*) With knee in 20° flexion, tension is placed on the graft and knee is put through a range of motion. Check for any impingement of graft. (*D*) Fixation of the tibial bone plug with interference screw while tension is maintained on the graft.

Illustration continued on following page

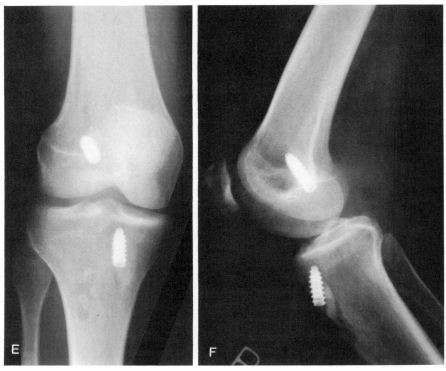

FIGURE 20–16 (*continued*). (*E*) Anteroposterior radiograph showing interference screws in place. (*F*) Lateral radiograph. The tibial screw has been screwed in slightly too far.

placed in the anterior aspect of the tibial tunnel against the cortical surface in the tibial portion and on the lateral side of the bone plug in the femoral hole.

The patellar bone plug is usually secured in the femoral hole first. Tension is placed on the graft, and the knee is put through a range of motion. The graft should be arthroscopically visualized to ensure proper tension. The knee must go through a full range of motion—through flexion and extension—without impingement. Further notchplasty may be necessary. At this time, the tibial bone plug is secured with interference screw fixation. Tension must be kept on the graft while placement of the screw is performed with the knee held in 20° of flexion. Lachman's test and a pivot-shift test are performed to ensure that adequate stabilization has been obtained. The screws should be placed parallel to the bone plugs; any divergence may cause inadequate fixation or migration of the plug or the screw.

The sutures placed through the bone plug may also be used to tie over a screw with ligament washer as a post. This procedure may be used as a means of fixation or as an additional fixation with the interference screw.

HAMSTRING HARVESTING

Hamstring graft placement is performed by an arthroscopically assisted technique. The knee is arthroscopically evaluated, and the ACL tear is confirmed. Arthroscopic procedures are conducted as necessary: repair of meniscal lesions, chondroplasty of articular defects, and notchplasty.

A vertical incision of 5 to 7 cm is made 2 to 3 cm medial to the tibial tubercle. The pes anserinus tendons are identified by finger palpation, and the semitendinosus tendon is isolated (Fig. 20–17).

If the semitendinosus tendon is to be used as an augmentation to the repair of the ACL stump, it is left attached distally and freed proximally through the use of an open-slot tendon stripper. It is important to section fascial bands between the inferior surface of the tendon and the gastrocnemius fascia. This is most efficiently performed by passing scissors parallel to the inferior side of the tendon because the fascial bands may cause the tendon stripper to cut the tendon prematurely, which would result in inadequate length. The tendon stripper is passed proximally past the musculotendinous junction, and the detached tendon is pulled distally into the incision site. The gracilis tendon may be isolated and stripped if additional tissue is needed.

If a double-looped semitendinosus graft is used, the tibial attachment is detached, and a closed tendon stripper is used to harvest the tendon. Cutting of the fascial gastrocnemius bands is necessary before the tendon is stripped.

The tibial tunnel is prepared with a drill guide; a guide wire is

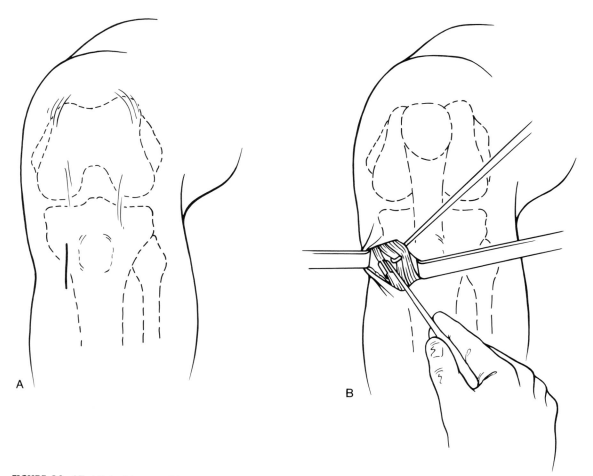

A

B

FIGURE 20–17. (A) Incision used to expose pes anserinus insertion and to make tibial drill hole. (B) Tendon stripper used to harvest the semitendinosus tendon.

introduced just above the pes anserinus insertion medial to the tibial tubercle (Figs. 20–18*A*, 20–18*B*). The size of the graft should be measured, whether it is a single-strand, double-looped, or composite gracilis-semitendinosus tendon, and an appropriate tibial hole is drilled with the use of a cannulated drill. A 6- to 8-mm hole is usually adequate. The size of the drill hole should be identical to or no more than 1 mm larger than the size of the graft.

In an acute tear in which the ACL stump is preserved, the exit site of the tibial tunnel should be just posterior and medial to the tibial attachment. If stump preservation is not required, the exit site of the tunnel should be anterior and slightly medial to the medial tibial spine.

A rasp is used to radialize the edges of the tibial tunnel on the posterior aspect of the exit hole on the tibial surface and the distal edge of the entrance hole on the tibial cortex (Fig. 20–18*C*).

The lateral incision is made as previously described (see Fig. 20–14). The iliotibial tract is incised in the direction of the fibers to expose the posterolateral aspect of the femoral condyle and distal femoral shaft (Fig. 20–19). The distal attachment of the intermuscular septum is identified and elevated proximal to the lateral femoral epicondyle for the area of fixation of the semitendinosus tendon. The posterolateral aspect of the notch is palpated through the posterior capsule.

A groove is made "over-the-top" area of the lateral femoral condyle (Fig. 20–20). A rasp may be used if bare bone contact is possible, or a guide wire may be directed into the posterior aspect of the lateral notch with a cannulated drill to create a 5-mm trough or groove. Retraction of the posterior structures protects against soft tissue injury.

A curved guide is passed through the notch into the anteromedial portal to exit over the top of the lateral femoral condyle and through the posterior capsule (Figs. 20–21*A*, 20–21*B*). The tip of the guide is visualized in the posterolateral area, and a wire loop is passed through the guide tip into the notch. The loop is grasped by a tendon passer introduced into the notch through the tibial tunnel. In some cases, it is easier to pass the guide from the posterolateral corner into the notch, using the fingers posteriorly to guide the curved ligament passer to the appropriate position. The wire loop is recovered with a hook or a grasper through the tibial tunnel and delivered to the anterior aspect of the tibia.

Four-millimeter Mersilene tape is passed through the wire loop, and the Mersilene loop is pulled through the tibial tunnel, through the notch, through the posterior capsule, and over the top of the posterolateral femoral condyle (Figs. 20–21*C*, 20–21*D*). The loop is placed over a K-wire fixed to the femoral shaft at the point of intended fixation (Figs. 20–21*E*, 20–21*F*). The knee is flexed and extended and checked for any pistoning of the Mersilene tape as motion occurs. If there is more than 2- to 3-mm excursion, the posterior aspect of the tibial tunnel should be enlarged.

The Mersilene tape loop is used to pull another loop of 4-mm Mersilene tape or a flexible tube leader from the posterolateral aspect into the notch and out the tibial tunnel. A strong suture is used to attach the looped end of the semitendinosus tendon to the flexible tube leader, or a looped 4-mm tape is passed through the loop of the semitendinosus tendon. The tube leader or the two ends of the Mersilene tape are pulled out posterolaterally, and the graft is pulled through the tibial tunnel, the

Text continued on page 561

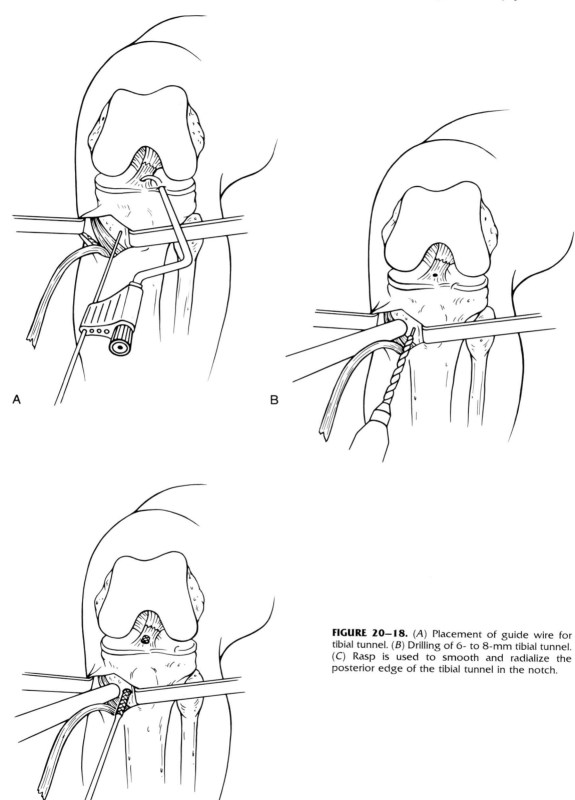

FIGURE 20–18. (*A*) Placement of guide wire for tibial tunnel. (*B*) Drilling of 6- to 8-mm tibial tunnel. (*C*) Rasp is used to smooth and radialize the posterior edge of the tibial tunnel in the notch.

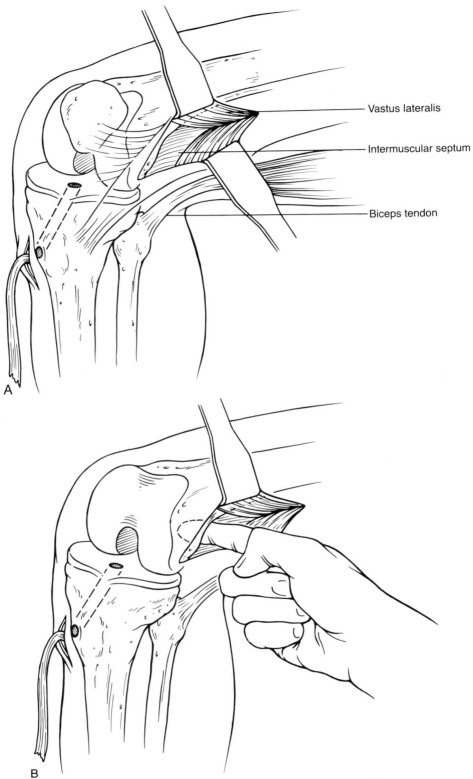

Vastus lateralis

Intermuscular septum

Biceps tendon

A

B

FIGURE 20–19. (*A*) Exposure of intermuscular septum. (*B*) The posterolateral aspect of the posterior capsule should be palpated through incision made in the intermuscular septum.

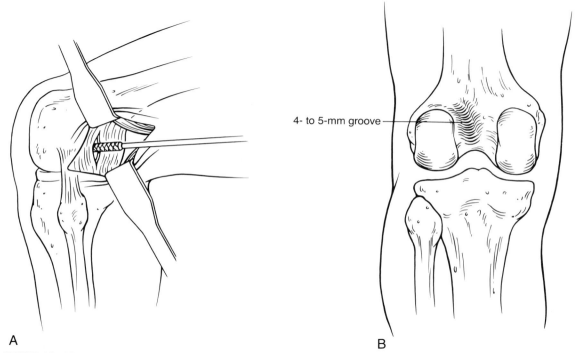

A

B

FIGURE 20–20. (*A*) A trough or a groove is made at the junction of the lateral femoral condyle and the femoral shaft. (*B*) This is carried down to the posterior capsule and into the notch. The groove should be deepened to 4 to 5 mm.

4- to 5-mm groove

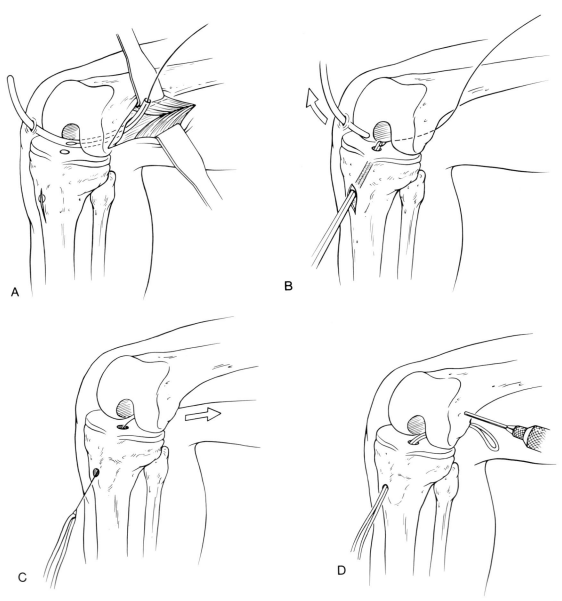

FIGURE 20–21. Preparation for passage of graft through drill hole and notch. (*A*) A curved guide or curved tendon passer is passed through the arthroscopic portal and posterior capsule and out the over-the-top area to the lateral incision site. A wire or a suture can then be delivered into the notch. (*B*) The guide is removed, leaving the suture loop in the joint. (*C*) The loop is recovered with the tendon passer or hook and pulled through the tibial drill hole. Four-millimeter Mersilene tape is placed through the loop. (*D*) The loop of tape is delivered along the course of the graft placement. A K-wire is attached to the area where the graft will be attached.

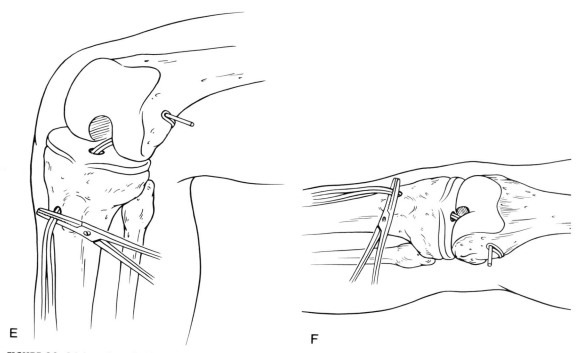

E   F

FIGURE 20–21 (*continued*). (*E* and *F*) The loop of tape is placed over the end of the K-wire, and a clamp is placed at the exit of the tape from the tibial tunnel. The knee is moved from flexion to extension in order to check for any pistoning or impingement.

notch, and the posterior capsule until the loop of semitendinosus tendon is delivered into the posterolateral aspect (Figs. 20–22*A* to 20–22*C*). The knee may need to be flexed or extended to provide a straight pull. If the semitendinosus and gracilis tendons are left attached distally, the free end is passed through the joint in a similar manner.

The semitendinosus loop is fixed to the posterolateral aspect of the femur with a bicortical screw and ligament-spiked washer (Fig. 20–23*A*). Tension is then applied to the free ends of the tendon, and the knee is repeatedly flexed and extended to take out any slack and to pre-tension the ligament. The knee is flexed to 20°, tension is maintained with an approximate 8-pound pull, and a staple is placed over the distal half of the ligament. The remainder of the distal half is folded proximally, and its end is stapled over the proximal half of the ligament in a belt-buckle technique (Fig. 20–23*B*).

When the semitendinosus tendon is left attached distally, the free end that has been delivered posterolaterally is fixed to the posterolateral femoral shaft by means of two staples and the belt-buckle technique (Figs. 20–24*A*, 20–24*B*).

Immobilization in a brace at full extension immediately after surgery is recognized as helpful in preventing flexion contracture.[164a] The brace is removed for a full range of passive motion as tolerated by the patient on the first or second day after surgery. Continuous passive motion machines have been used immediately postoperatively, but their use has not shown any significant difference in range of motion, laxity, and girth in comparison with standard physical therapy, including range-of-motion exercises

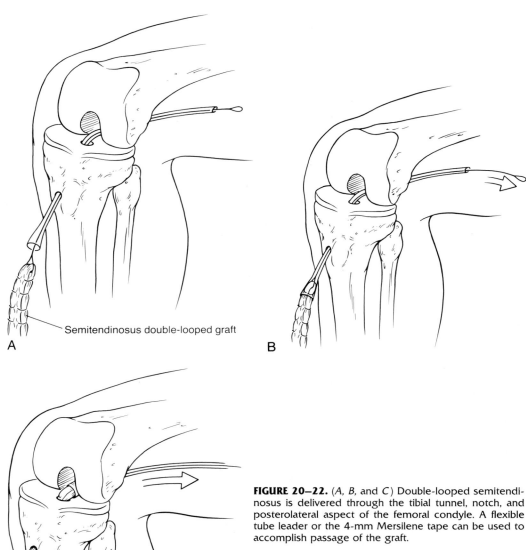

Semitendinosus double-looped graft

A

B

C

FIGURE 20–22. (*A, B,* and *C*) Double-looped semitendinosus is delivered through the tibial tunnel, notch, and posterolateral aspect of the femoral condyle. A flexible tube leader or the 4-mm Mersilene tape can be used to accomplish passage of the graft.

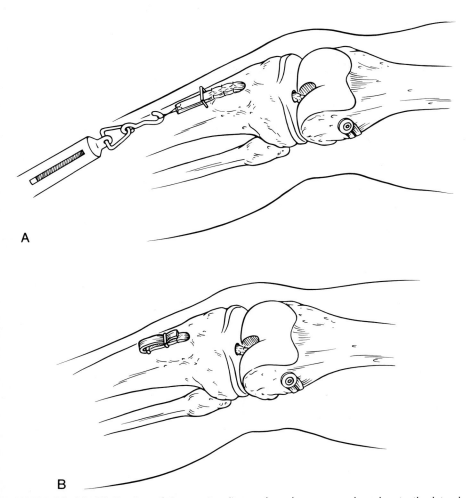

A

B

FIGURE 20–23. (*A*) Fixation of the semitendinosus loop by screw and washer to the lateral aspect of the femur. Five to 8 pounds of tension is applied to the distal end of the graft as the knee is flexed and extended in order to take out any slack and to pre-tension the graft. (*B*) With the knee flexed to 20° and tension maintained, the distal end of the graft is fixed with belt-buckle staple technique.

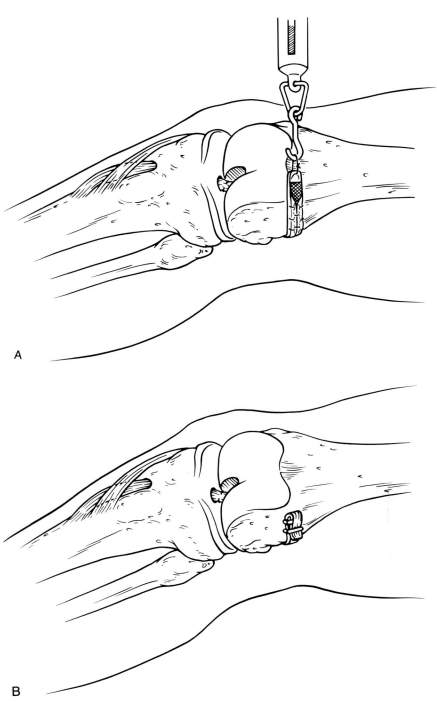

FIGURE 20–24. (*A*) Tension is applied to the proximal portion of the graft when the semitendinosus is left attached distally (used for augmenting a repaired ACL). (*B*) Fixation proximally by belt-buckle staples.

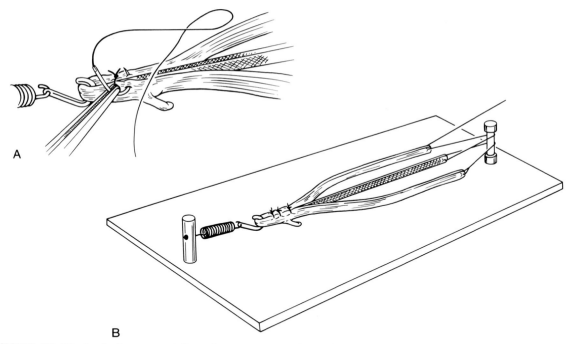

FIGURE 20–25. Synthetic augmentation of autogenous graft. (*A*) LAD is sandwiched between two limbs of the semitendinosus tendon. A loop of tendon is left free for fixation of the tendon only proximally. (*B*) Commercial suture board, which maintains equal tension on limbs of the semitendinosus muscle and the LAD while the composite graft is sutured.

at 30 repetitions three times per day.[129a] Ambulation is allowed with crutches as soon as the patient is comfortable. Protected weight bearing is allowed as tolerated by the patient and is continued for 3 weeks. When the gait is normal with the use of crutches and full weight bearing is achieved, the crutches can be discontinued. Progressive rehabilitation to regain motion, muscle strength, and agility is conducted as discussed in Chapter 14.

Other autogenous ACL reconstructions and augmentations have been described. Synthetic augmentation of the autogenous tissue with a ligament augmentation device (LAD) has been advocated if tissue with poor tensile strength is used or if additional length for fixation is required. Sandwiching an LAD between the two limbs of the semitendinosus loop (Fig. 20–25) has been used to provide increased tensile strength during the early healing phase.

POSTERIOR CRUCIATE AND POSTEROLATERAL INJURIES

PCL and posterolateral injuries occur with much less frequency than ACL or medial side injuries.[46, 58, 63, 113, 116, 117, 119, 120, 136, 137, 182, 229]

Incidence

The incidence of PCL injuries ranges from 2 to 23 per cent in studies of large series of knee ligament injuries.[16, 19, 43, 46, 58, 63, 80, 113, 116, 117, 136, 138, 178, 182, 206, 229, 235, 247] Of these, isolated PCL injuries account for 30 per cent, and

PCL injury in combination with other ligament injury accounts for the remainder. The lower incidence of PCL injury is probably a result of its greater tensile strength.[159, 217] The diagnosis may be missed because of the extrasynovial location and the lack of hemarthrosis,[6, 58, 59] the support provided by an intact ligament of Humphry or Wrisberg (which causes a false-negative posterior drawer test),[24, 39, 110, 117, 146, 235] and the lack of functional instability-disability seen with grade I or II PCL instability.[62, 81, 116, 235]

Isolated posterolateral injury that produces a posterolateral instability is more unusual.[61, 63, 98, 149, 229] DeLee and co-authors[62, 63] reported that in 735 patients with knee ligament injuries, 7 per cent involved the lateral ligament complex; 1.6 per cent were isolated posterolateral structure injuries. Grana and Janssen[98] reported that 16 per cent of 120 knee ligament injuries involved the lateral side, and only one was an isolated injury. Other authors[117, 159, 229] have confirmed the rarity of lateral side injury. Most injuries to the posterolateral complex occur in association with PCL injuries.[10, 39, 62, 63, 80, 117] The structures that may be involved in lateral and posterolateral injury are the LCL, the posterior horn of the lateral meniscus, the arcuate ligament complex, the popliteal tendon, and the lateral head of the gastrocnemius muscle[4, 10, 62, 63, 117, 152, 153, 169, 188, 257, 287] (see Chapter 2).

PCL Injury

The anatomic structure of the PCL is described in Chapter 2. The PCL functions as an axis about which knee rotation occurs.[119] The PCL restrains the femoral condyle from forward movement on the tibia with knee flexion. It is the primary restraint of posterior translation of the tibia on the femur.[32, 88, 96, 101, 186, 257]

MECHANISM OF INJURY

The two most common causes of injury to the PCL are motor vehicle accidents and sporting activities. Three common mechanisms of injury produce a tear of the PCL:

1. The most common is a blow to the proximal anterior surface of the tibia on the flexed knee. The anterolateral portion of the PCL is in a horizontal position, and the posterior capsule is in a relaxed position. The anterior impact drives the tibia posteriorly, tearing the PCL and possibly the capsule. This is the classic dashboard injury, which commonly produces a midsubstance tear of the PCL.

2. A contact hyperflexion injury occurs when the patient falls on the flexed knee with the foot in a plantar-flexed position. A blow to the tibial tubercle drives the tibia posteriorly, injuring the PCL but usually not the capsule. The calf contacts the posterior thigh muscles and, therefore, limits the posterior translation of the tibia.

3. Hyperextension[94] injury produces stress to the posteromedial bundle of the PCL and may cause avulsion of the tibial attachment off the periosteum or with a bone fragment. This particular type of injury is often associated with valgus and varus forces and produces combined collateral ligament disruptions. Severe abduction or adduction stress may injure first the collateral ligaments and then the secondary restraints (cruciate ligaments).

DIAGNOSIS

History

In the acute situation, the history often provides a clue to the correct diagnosis, especially in cases of isolated PCL injuries. A dashboard injury or a hyperflexion injury caused by a fall is an indication of a possible PCL injury. A description of the direction of the force at the moment of impact may help the examiner assess the possibility of a combined ligament injury. Patients sustaining isolated PCL injuries may have minimal pain or pain only after flexing the knee more than 90°. Minimal effusion is caused by the extrasynovial position of the PCL. In dashboard injuries, the possibility of an associated ipsilateral hip injury as well must be ruled out.

Physical Examination

An abrasion over the front of the knee is another clue to a possible injury to the PCL. Mild effusion, as opposed to the tense effusion seen in ACL tears, is usually noted. A posterior sag of the tibia with prominence of the patella may be observed when the knee is viewed from the side with the knee flexed to 90°.[128] The medial tibial plateau should be palpated approximately 1 cm anterior to the plane of the medial femoral condyle with the knee flexed to 90°.[39] Loss of this step-off point should arouse suspicion of a PCL injury. Palpation of the popliteal space may reveal fullness and tenderness.

The alignment of the involved extremity may suggest tibia vara, external tibial rotation, or genu recurvatum, which is consistent with a posterior subluxation of the lateral tibial plateau or posterolateral complex injury. The patient, however, tends to walk with a flexed knee gait in order to avoid terminal extension.[289]

Ligament Testing*

The posterior drawer test performed with the knee at 90° of flexion in neutral rotation is the most sensitive test for straight posterior instability. Before this test, both knees should be flexed to 90° in order to ensure that the tibial tubercles are at equal heights and that there is no posterior sag of the tibia on the femur, which would cause a false-negative posterior drawer sign and a false-positive anterior drawer sign. The posterior drawer test should be performed with the tibia in neutral position, in external rotation (to rule out posterolateral complex injury), and in internal rotation. A positive result in the neutral position may be followed by a negative result in the internally rotated position because of intact accessory meniscofemoral ligaments (ligaments of Wrisberg and Humphry).[146, 235] With the knee at 30° of flexion, a posterior drawer test should also be performed in external rotation (posterolateral complex injury) and in neutral position (PCL injury). Valgus and varus stress tests at 0° and 30° should be performed in order to rule out additional injuries to the medial, lateral, and posterolateral structures as well as to the cruciate ligaments. Additional tests include the reverse pivot-shift test,[132] the quadriceps active drawer test,[56] and the dynamic posterior shift test.[266] Many of these

---

*See Chapter 4 for details of each test.

tests yield positive results in the chronic situation but may yield false-negative results in the acute situation, especially if there is an isolated injury to the PCL.

Imaging Evaluation

Standard radiographs include anteroposterior, lateral, notch, and Merchant's views. A posterior sag, or Godfrey's, view (see Fig. 20–1) is taken with the hip and the knee flexed at 90° and the patient in a supine position. The heel is supported. A weight is hung from the anterior portion of the tibia, and a lateral view of both knees is obtained for comparison. Before any stress views are obtained, a knee dislocation must be ruled out. Avulsion injuries within the notch or posteriorly should especially be looked for.

MRI appears to be the most accurate noninvasive procedure for diagnosing a PCL tear (see section on MRI in this chapter). The PCL is easily identified in the sagittal plane.

Arthroscopy

Lysholm and Gilquist[182] have shown the value of arthroscopy in diagnosing PCL injuries. Of 484 arthroscopies, they were able to inspect the PCL satisfactorily in 96 per cent. Of 28 cases in which the PCL was torn as evidenced at the time of arthrotomy, 27 were diagnosed at the time of arthroscopy, which was performed just before arthrotomy. Both a 30° and a 70° arthroscope should be available for evaluating the integrity of the entire PCL. Delaying arthroscopy 5 to 7 days may avoid fluid extravasation if the capsule is torn.

Meniscal injuries are rarely associated with isolated PCL injuries.[43, 81, 136] In combined injuries of the PCL and other capsuloligamentous structures, the meniscal injury rate is between 30 and 50 per cent.[19, 43, 50, 119, 178, 247, 293, 294] PCL injuries have also been associated with peroneal nerve palsies, chondral and osteocondylar fractures, and vascular injuries.

TREATMENT

Controversy exists with regard to the appropriate treatment of acute PCL injuries.

ISOLATED PCL INJURIES: IN-SUBSTANCE TEARS. There is general agreement that the nonoperative treatment of isolated PCL injuries provides patients with good subjective and functional results, although probably not static stability.[50, 53, 81, 120, 146, 198, 235, 293, 294] This is particularly true of patients with minimal to grade 1+ posterior drawer. Cross and Powell[50] showed 100 per cent good to excellent results in patients with grades 0 to 1+ posterior drawer, whereas among those with grade 2+ to 3+ posterior drawer, 73 per cent had results of this quality. Other studies[80, 81, 146] have shown that more than 80 per cent of patients return to their original sport, even though clinical posterior laxity is present. In one study,[39, 43] radiologic assessment of patients with posterior laxity revealed that 36 per cent had evidence of arthritic changes at an average of 8.4-year follow-up. Another study[146] revealed no radiologic evidence of degenerative changes at a 7.5-year follow-up, but 3 of 17 patients had positive bone scans. The KT-1000 test revealed posterior excursion of 7 to 8 mm, but the excursion decreased when the test was performed with the foot in internal rotation. This suggests that intact meniscofemoral ligaments (Wrisberg and Humphry) contribute some stabilizing function.

Clancy and Ray[39, 43] reported on the degenerative changes found in the medial joint compartment in patients requiring surgery for a chronic PCL-deficient knee. Clancy and Ray advocated a more aggressive approach to the acute PCL injury: a PCL reconstruction involving the central third of the patellar tendon with a bone-tendon-bone unit in patients with significant laxity. They reported good to excellent results in all 10 patients surgically treated with an acute injury.

It is the authors' opinion that the highly active patient with grade 2+ or 3+ posterior instability be considered for acute repair and augmentation or primary reconstruction. If a postponement or delay of surgery is required or desired by the patient a close follow-up to assess both the functional and radiologic status of the knee is appropriate.

AVULSION INJURIES. Bone avulsion occurs in 9 to 34 per cent of PCL injuries[199, 293, 294] (Fig. 20–26). It occurs more frequently in motor vehicle

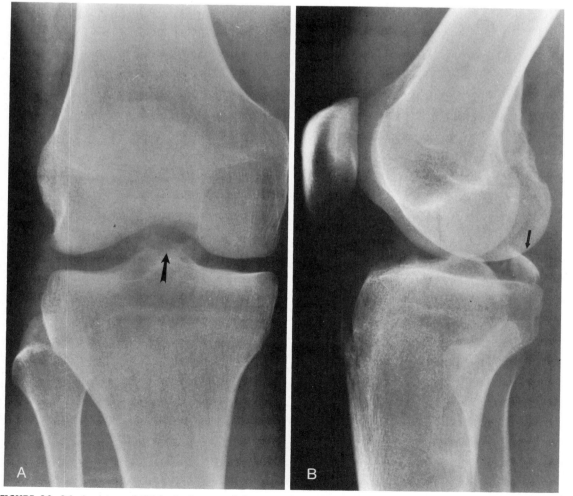

FIGURE 20–26. Avulsion of tibial attachment of the posterior cruciate ligament (PCL) with the bone fragment. (A) Anteroposterior view. (B) Lateral view.

accidents than in athletic injury.[50, 199, 293, 294] The presence of a bone avulsion of the tibial attachment of the PCL is suggestive of more damage within the knee joint than that produced with the in-substance tear associated with athletic injury. Cross and Powell[50] reviewed 116 PCL injuries and reported that 85 per cent of those sustained during athletics progressed to good or excellent results, whereas of those sustained in motor vehicle accidents, only 17 per cent progressed to good or excellent results.

The size of the bone fragment and the amount of displacement are the determinants of the necessity for surgical reattachment.[199, 293, 294] Torisu[293, 294] reported on 21 cases of PCL injuries associated with bone avulsion. Bone fragments that were less than 1.3 cm in size, had less than 3 mm of separation and less than 5 mm of upward displacement, and were not comminuted tended to unite with nonoperative treatment of immobilization. Fragments not meeting these criteria tended to go on to nonunion or delayed union. A larger segment of bone with a greater amount of displacement is usually associated with a capsular tear or meniscal injury and should not be considered an isolated injury to the PCL.[199, 293, 294] Patients with delayed union or nonunion had less satisfactory results than those in whom the fragments united.[199, 284, 293, 294] Cast immobilization for smaller and minimally displaced fragments and surgical reattachment for the larger fragments minimize the chance for delayed union or nonunion and poor results. Delayed union and nonunion are best treated within the first 2 months of injury.

PCL INJURIES IN ASSOCIATION WITH OTHER LIGAMENT INJURIES. PCL injuries combined with other ligament injuries produce both a greater amount of functional disability and a greater propensity for arthritic degeneration.[16, 19, 39, 43, 120, 178, 235, 297, 298] Early surgical repair of all structures or primary reconstruction of the PCL is appropriate.[10, 19, 39, 43, 46, 62, 63, 80, 120, 206]

SUMMARY

Isolated injury to the PCL that produces less than 1 cm of posterior tibial translation on stress testing should be treated nonoperatively; early motion and rehabilitation should be directed toward quadriceps and hamstring strengthening and function.[34, 50, 81, 119, 120, 146, 158, 235, 247, 252] Arthroscopic or MRI evaluation is appropriate for ruling out associated intra-articular pathology. Active patients with 1 cm or more of posterior laxity should be considered for early surgical repair or reconstruction or followed closely for evidence of functional disability or articular wear.[39, 43, 50, 81, 146, 235]

Avulsion injuries of the tibial attachment should be radiologically evaluated for size and amount of displacement. Larger bony fragments meeting the criteria mentioned earlier should be surgically reattached. Immobilization for injuries involving smaller fragments and minimal displacement is appropriate.[199, 293, 294]

PCL injuries combined with other ligament injuries should undergo early surgical treatment with repair or reconstruction of all injured structures.

Surgical treatment rarely restores complete static stability or proprioception. Subjective and functional results are not correlated with objective stability.

Posterolateral Complex (PLC) Injuries

The structures of the lateral and posterolateral corner of the knee work as a unit to stabilize the lateral and posterolateral aspect of the knee. Injury seldom involves only one of the anatomic structures of this posterolateral complex.[10, 39, 62, 63, 80, 98, 117, 120, 149, 158, 229]

CLASSIFICATION

Injuries to the lateral side of the knee have been classified by Hughston and colleagues[117] to be (1) straight lateral instability, (2) anterolateral rotatory instability, (3) posterolateral rotatory instability, and (4) antero-lateral combined with posterolateral instability. Straight lateral instability involves injuries that include the cruciate ligaments as well as posterolateral structures.

MECHANISM OF INJURY

Sports participation and motor vehicle accidents are the leading causes of injury to the posterolateral complex. Injuries to the lateral collateral ligament and capsule are caused by a blow to the medial side of the knee with the leg extended.[62, 63] Injuries to the posterolateral complex are usually caused by a blow to the anteromedial aspect of the tibia with the knee slightly flexed.

Injury to the peroneal nerve and popliteal artery, depending on the severity of force, may also occur. It is important to ascertain whether there is numbness or tingling in the leg. In such severe injuries, a careful history is important for determining whether knee dislocation with spontaneous reduction may have occurred.

PHYSICAL EXAMINATION

Evidence of contusion or tenderness over the medial and anteromedial portions of the tibia suggests possible injury to the lateral structures of the knee. A varus stress test with the knee at 0° and 30° of flexion should be performed. At 0°, the PCL and the PLC are simultaneously contributing to the stability being tested. When the knee is flexed to 30° the LCL is the primary constraint to lateral opening of the joint. Excessive external rotation of the tibia at 90° (posterolateral drawer)[122, 273] in comparison with the other leg, an external rotation recurvatum holding the legs extended by the toes, and reverse pivot shift all attest to incompetency of the posterolateral structures. Grade 3+ varus stress at either 0° or 30° warrants MRI evaluation to check the status of the PCL.

IMAGING STUDIES

Anteroposterior, lateral, notch, and Merchant's roentgenograms should be obtained in order to rule out fractures of the fibular head, lateral capsular fractures (Segond's fracture), and fractures of the tibial plateau. If the latter is suspected, computed tomographic scan or MRI imaging is appropriate for full evaluation of the status of the bone.

TREATMENT

Nonoperative treatment of injuries to the lateral and posterolateral structures should be confined to patients who show less than 10 mm of joint opening with varus stress test results at 30°.[62, 63, 149] Patients with more than 10 mm of joint opening and those with known combined injuries involving other stabilizing structures should undergo an acute repair of all the involved structures.[10, 39, 62, 63, 98, 117, 120, 149] Grana and Janssen[98] found that patients with LCL and posterolateral ligament complex injuries had more functional disability than those with ACL or medial side injuries, an opinion shared by Hughston and colleagues.[117, 120] The biomechanical explanation is that with weight bearing, the medial side bears most of the load on the bony structures, whereas lateral stability depends more on the soft tissues.

Studies[62, 149] have shown that less functional disability and fewer osteoarthritic changes occur in patients with grade III instability (more than 10 mm of joint opening) treated by surgical repair. At surgery, the cruciate ligaments should be carefully evaluated for evidence of partial or complete tears. Findings at surgery may also include bony avulsion injuries of the LCL from the fibular head or, less frequently, from the femur and injuries to the popliteus muscle or tendon.

The nonoperative treatment for grade I or II injuries to the posterolateral aspect of the knee is protection in a brace at 45° of flexion with touch-down weight bearing allowed. Early passive and active range of motion is permitted as pain allows. Avoidance of the last 15° of extension prevents stretching of the injured soft tissues. After 3 weeks, full range of motion can be allowed. Isometric exercises should be started when a full range of painless motion is achieved. Progression to isotonic and agility exercises is allowed as muscle strength and motion return and when not associated with any pain. A protective brace is appropriate as activity is allowed. Full return of quadriceps and hamstring strength and a good endpoint to varus testing, albeit slight varus laxity, is the desired result. The rehabilitation period for nonoperative treatment extends over a 4- to 8-week period, depending on the severity of the injury.

Surgical Techniques for PCL and Posterolateral Ligament Complex Injury

PCL REPAIR AND AUGMENTATION

Repair of a torn PCL is appropriate when a substantial remnant of the PCL remains. The repair should be augmented with additional autogenous tissue. Because of the posterior position of the PCL in the joint, there is a better potential for healing than with the ACL. A report by Moore and Larson[206] of acute repairs in 18 patients revealed a high incidence of associated injuries. With repair of the PCL and other disrupted ligamentous tissue, a functionally good or excellent result was obtained in 78 per cent of patients, although mild residual instability was present in all.

Patellar tendon bone-to-bone tissue,[39, 43] the hamstring tendons,[282, 307] the popliteal tendon,[193] and the medial half of the medial head of the gastrocnemius muscle[46, 120, 128, 158, 206, 247] have been used as augmentation tissue. The patellar tendon bone-to-bone graft is a primary reconstruction and can be used when ligamentous remnants are repaired or removed.[39, 43]

PRIMARY REPAIR WITH AUGMENTATION WITH MEDIAL HEAD OF THE GASTROCNEMIUS MUSCLE. When a reparable stump of PCL is present, a medial utility incision is used to expose the medial ligamentous structures (Fig. 20–5). An anteromedial capsular arthrotomy allows direct visualization of both cruciate ligaments and their palpation with stress. The femoral attachment of the PCL is easily visualized and approached through the anteromedial incision. The tibial attachment and the body of the PCL are exposed through a posteromedial capsular incision with dissection of the tibial attachment of the posterior oblique ligament and the posterior capsule from their bony insertion. Many times these structures are already disrupted by trauma, but if not, they may later be reattached by drill holes in the tibia. The popliteus muscle insertion may be subperiosteally dissected off the posterior aspect of the tibia if it obscures visualization of the tibial attachment of the PCL.

The neurovascular structures lie behind the posterior capsule and popliteus muscle and should be protected by retraction of these structures.

Nonabsorbable sutures are used through the stump of the PCL to reattach it to the anatomic site on the femur or tibia through drill holes (Figs. 20–27A, 20–27B). Drill guides should be used to provide exact placement. The tendinous portion of the insertion of the medial third to half of the medial head of the gastrocnemius muscle provides both tissue bulk to augment the repair and a dynamic anterior thrust to the posterior tibia when the gastrocnemius muscle contracts or the foot is actively or passively dorsiflexed.[158, 206]

The medial portion of the femoral attachment of the gastrocnemius muscle is detached with a block of bone and developed distally approximately 15 cm (Fig. 20–27C). A ⅜-inch drill hole is placed from the medial femoral epicondyle to exit just posterior to the normal attachment site of the PCL by means of a drill guide and a cannulated drill to ensure precise positioning (Fig. 20–27E). A nonabsorbable suture is placed through a small drill hole in the bone block to facilitate passage of the graft. The graft is then passed deep to the still-attached portion of the gastrocnemius muscle and through the posterior capsule at the tibial attachment site of the PCL (Fig. 20–27D). The tendon end and the bone are then brought into the femoral drill hole, where they are fixed with a screw or tied over a button. Care must be taken during passage of the graft not to disrupt the previously placed PCL sutures and to make certain that the bone block is delivered into the femoral tunnel. The sutures in the bone block and the repaired PCL are not tied until associated ligament or meniscal pathology has been repaired and the tibia can be maintained in the neutral position.

PRIMARY PATELLAR TENDON RECONSTRUCTION

Improved drill guide systems and arthroscopic techniques have enabled arthroscopically assisted PCL reconstruction with the use of the middle third of the patellar tendon. The procedure can also be conducted by working through the defect created in the patellar tendon (Fig. 20–28). If the only incision used is the one to harvest the patellar tendon, additional incisions may be necessary for repairing associated ligament injuries. If

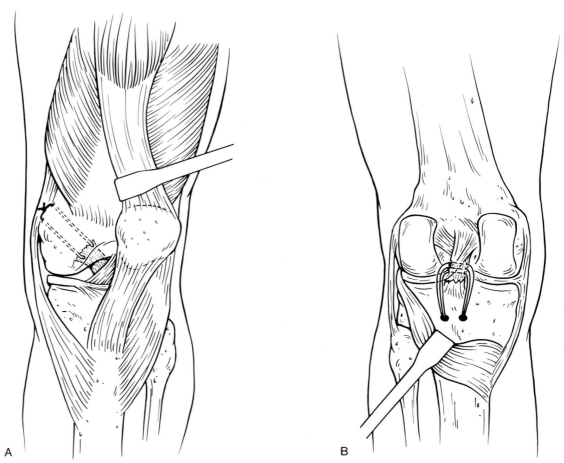

FIGURE 20–27. (*A*) Primary repair of PCL torn from its femoral attachment site. Sutures are passed through drill holes in the medial femoral condyle. (*B*) Repair of PCL torn off tibial attachment without bone avulsion. Sutures are placed in the stump and delivered through drill holes and tied over the front of the tibia.

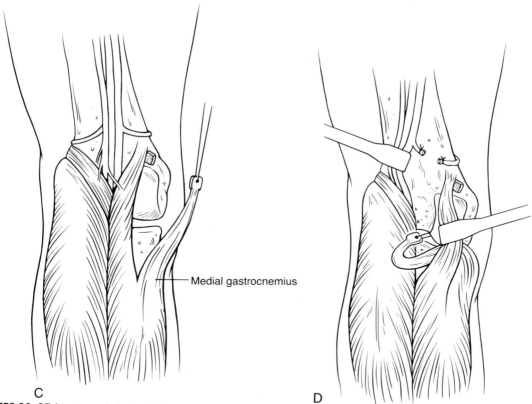

C   D

— Medial gastrocnemius

FIGURE 20–27 (*continued*). (*C*) Medial third of tendinous portion of medial gastrocnemius muscle insertion with bone block. (*D*) Passage of graft through rent created in central portion of posterior capsule. Note ligation of the superior medial genicular artery, which may be necessary.

FIGURE 20–27 (*continued*). (*E*) The bone block is passed through a drill hole created in the medial femoral condyle and fixed in the tunnel with a screw or tied over a button.

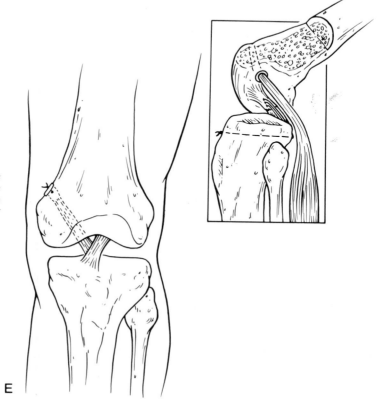

E

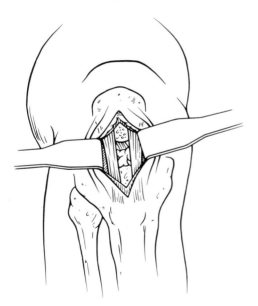

FIGURE 20–28. Exposure of the joint provided through a defect created in the patellar tendon enables tibial drill guide to be positioned over top of the tibial surface.

repair of the medial structures is required, the use of a medial utility skin incision enables harvesting of the patellar tendon, repair of medial structures, and access to the posterior medial capsule, which can be incised to allow visualization and palpation of the PCL at its tibial attachment. When the medial structures are intact, three separate smaller incisions can also be used if arthroscopically assisted techniques are not employed: the anterior incision for harvesting the graft and for visualizing the inside of the joint through the defect created; a posteromedial incision to allow access to the posteromedial capsule and the PCL; and a small incision over the medial femoral epicondyle for placement and drilling of the femoral drill hole. With any of the techniques, an image intensifier used at surgery helps ensure accurate placement of the tibial and femoral drill holes and additional security in avoiding injury to the posterior neurovascular structures.

The patient is placed supine, and the tourniquet is placed high on the thigh. The foot of the table is dropped, and the knee is flexed to 90° and extended over a bolster 5 to 6 inches past the break in the table. This position enables better access to the posteromedial aspect of the knee and allows the neurovascular structures to fall away from the posterior capsule.

Arthroscopic evaluation is conducted, and appropriate arthroscopic surgery is performed. If meniscal repair is needed, the sutures may be placed at this time but not tied until completion of the procedure.

A tibial drill hole is started distal and slightly medial to the tibial tubercle (Fig. 20–29*A*). This allows a more vertical orientation of the tunnel for adequate bone stock anteriorly and prevents marked angulation of the graft as it is passed over the posterior tibia. A drill guide is used for pin placement. Guides that enable the arthroscopic placement of the tip, which can be checked by the image intensifier are available (Fig. 20–29*B*).

The authors prefer to make a posteromedial incision. The medial head of the gastrocnemius muscle is identified by finger palpation and is freed off the posterior capsule and retracted posteriorly. The posterior capsule is dissected off the posterior aspect of the tibia to allow visualization and

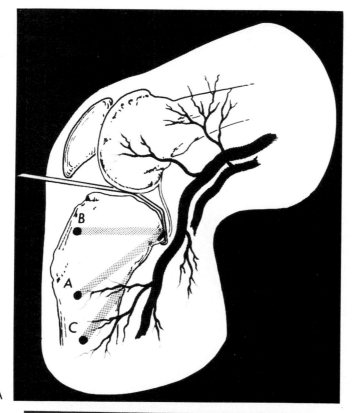

A

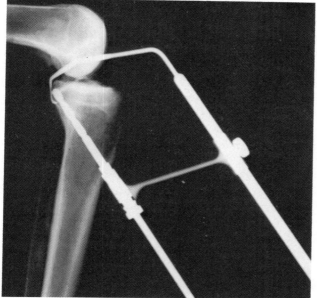

B

FIGURE 20–29. Placement of tibial tunnel for PCL reconstruction. (*A*) Position A is the proper orientation of the tibial tunnel. (Position B is too horizontal, causing marked angulation and a stress riser to graft; position C is too vertical and may cause a double penetration of the tibial cortex distally and proximally.) Note the tip of the drill guide in proper position on the posterior tibia. (*B*) Image intensifier view for checking proper positioning of the drill tip guide and drill to avoid overpenetration. (From Rosenberg TD, Paulos LE, Abbott PJ: Arthroscopic cruciate repair and reconstruction. *In* Feagin JA Jr [ed]: The Crucial Ligaments, p. 417. New York: Churchill-Livingstone, 1988.)

palpation of the posterior tibial sulcus. Partial release of the medial head of the gastrocnemius muscle may be necessary for adequate retraction and visualization in order to protect the neurovascular structures. The tip of the drill guide can be introduced through this incision and placed at the anatomic tibial attachment of the PCL. The guide wire is then directed from the anterior tibial site through the guide to the guide tip on the posterior tibia. Direct visualization, finger palpation, and protective retractors protect the posterior structures against injury from the guide pin and drill.

The femoral drill hole is made through a small incision over the medial epicondyle. The tip of the drill guide is positioned through the defect in the patellar tendon on the medial wall of the notch at the center of the femoral insertion site[100] (Figs. 20–30A, 20–30B). If no cruciate stump is present, the surgeon should use a point 8 mm proximal to the margin of the articular surface of the femoral condyle at the 2 o'clock position for a left knee (or 11 o'clock position for a right knee) on the medial wall of the notch with the knee flexed 90° (Fig. 20–30C). The guide wire is inserted, and a 4-mm trial hole is made. A Gore-Tex smoother can then be placed through the tibial hole from anterior to posterior, brought into the joint and out through the femoral drill hole.

With the knee in 30° of flexion, an anterior drawer is used to bring the tibia to its neutral position. The smoother is then fixed at both ends, and the knee is passed through a full range of motion to determine whether near-isometric position has been obtained and whether any graft impingement occurs. If the position is correct, a larger drill hole appropriate for accommodating the size of the bone plug is made. The drill hole edges are chamfered, and the tunnels are smoothed. The Gore-Tex smoother can then be used to pass the graft from the anterior tibial side to the posterior side, through the notch, and into the femoral tunnel. The patellar tendon bone plug used to go into the femoral tunnel is made 2 cm in length in order to facilitate passage of the graft posteriorly over the tibia and into the notch. A finger placed posteriorly on the tibia and a hook passed through the defect in the patellar tendon to guide the bone plug aid in the passage of the graft around this difficult bend.

The knee is flexed and extended several times to pre-tension and to take slack out of the graft. The knee is placed at 30° of flexion, and an interference screw is placed in the femoral tunnel for fixation (Figs. 20–31A, 20–31B). With the tibia in the reduced position, slight tension (approximately 5 pounds) is placed on the graft, and the tibial side is secured with an interference screw. Alternative methods of fixation with the use of a screw and washer as a post over which to tie the sutures in the bone plugs or tying the sutures over a button can be used.

The patellar defect is loosely approximated and covered with peritenon. The knee is immobilized in complete extension.

In rehabilitation after PCL repair or reconstruction, the knee is kept in a protective brace at full extension. At 3 days, passive range of motion between 0° and 60° is started. Isometric quadriceps exercises, manual patellar mobilization, and hip and ankle exercises are also started at this time. Partial weight bearing with crutches and the knee in extension is allowed as tolerated. Flexion past 60° and hamstring exercises are delayed until 6 weeks after surgery.

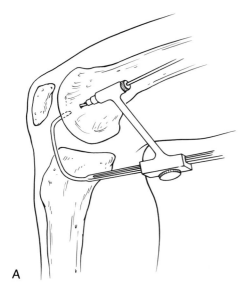

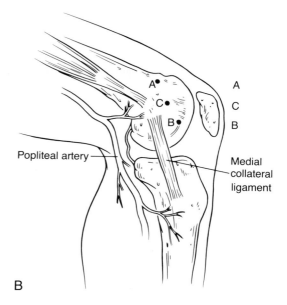

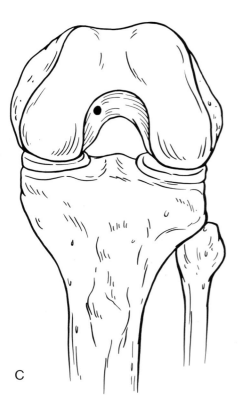

FIGURE 20–30. Placement of femoral drill hole for PCL reconstruction. (*A*) Drill guide tip positioned through a defect in the patellar tendon on the medial wall of the notch at the center of the femoral insertion of the PCL (see text). (*B*) Point C is ideal spot for extra-articular opening of the femoral tunnel in order to minimize tunnel divergence through the full range of motion. Point A provides excessive divergence in flexion, and point B too much divergence in extension (Rosenberg). (*C*) Point of femoral tunnel exit on the medial wall of the notch for a right knee (2 o'clock position for a left knee).

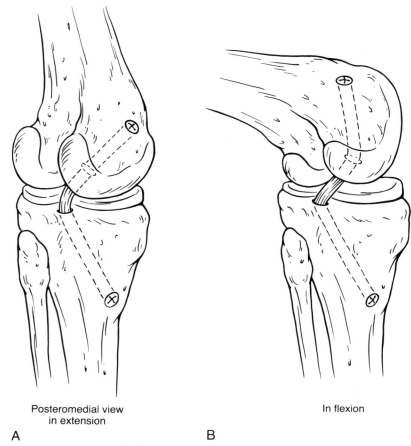

Posteromedial view
in extension

In flexion

A   B

FIGURE 20–31. Direction of the graft as it passes through the tibial tunnel, notch, and femoral tunnel. Fixation of bone blocks in the femoral and tibial tunnels may be by interference screw fixation, tying sutures over a button, or tying them to a screw and a washer as a post. (*A*) Posteromedial view in extension. (*B*) Posteromedial view in flexion.

As with any rehabilitation program, progression has to be tailored to the individual patient's response to the activity (i.e., swelling, pain, and return of motion and strength). Progression to quadriceps-strengthening exercises, hamstring exercises against gravity, closed-chain isometric exercises, and hamstring-strengthening exercises are added as the patient tolerates. Light activity should begin at approximately 3 months. A functional PCL brace can be used with the initiation of activity and continued for 6 to 12 months.

Surgical Treatment of Posterolateral Ligament Complex Injuries

Structures to identify before the incision is made are the lateral and superior borders of the patella, the fibular head, the lateral joint line, the lateral collateral ligament, Gerdy's tubercle, and the biceps tendon. These landmarks help position the incision in the appropriate location so as to allow repair of the involved tissue.

A lateral utility incision 3 cm lateral to the midpatella, extending proximally 7 cm and distally over Gerdy's tubercle, provides adequate access (Fig. 20–32A). Hemorrhage or swelling may be present over the area of maximal injury. Continuity of the biceps tendon and the lateral collateral ligament should be checked. If the biceps tendon has been injured, care should be taken to identify and protect the peroneal nerve, which lies posterior to the fibular head.

The interval between the biceps tendon and the iliotibial band is incised, and the iliotibial band is retracted anteriorly to expose the posterolateral corner, the lateral collateral ligament, and the popliteal tendon (Fig. 20–32B). The lateral inferior genicular vessels run between the lateral collateral ligament and the capsule and may require ligation. In the posterolateral corner, the lateral head of the gastrocnemius muscle is identified by its tendinous insertion into the posterior aspect of the lateral femoral condyle. Retraction of this muscle allows inspection of the posterior capsule, the popliteus muscle and tendon, the arcuate ligament, and the lateral capsule (Fig. 20–32B). The intermuscular septum at the juncture of the shaft of the femur and the lateral femoral condyle is the usual location of the superior genicular artery, which may require ligation.

Before repair or reattachment of any involved structures, the lateral capsule should be inspected and, if not torn, opened for inspection of the capsular attachment of the lateral meniscus. It is sometimes best to make a capsular incision anterior to the lateral collateral ligament above the joint line. The popliteal tendon insertion on the femur and its course through the capsule can be evaluated. This capsular defect created by the popliteal tendon is no more than 1.5 cm in length; elongation of this recess is suggestive of tearing of the capsule and requires repair.

SITES MOST FREQUENTLY TORN. The iliotibial band is frequently torn

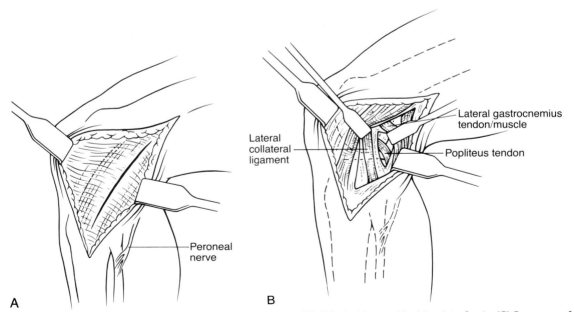

FIGURE 20–32. Lateral incision used to repair torn structures. (A) Skin incision and incision into fascia. (B) Exposure of the lateral collateral ligament and the popliteal tendon through the interval between the biceps tendon and the iliotibial band.

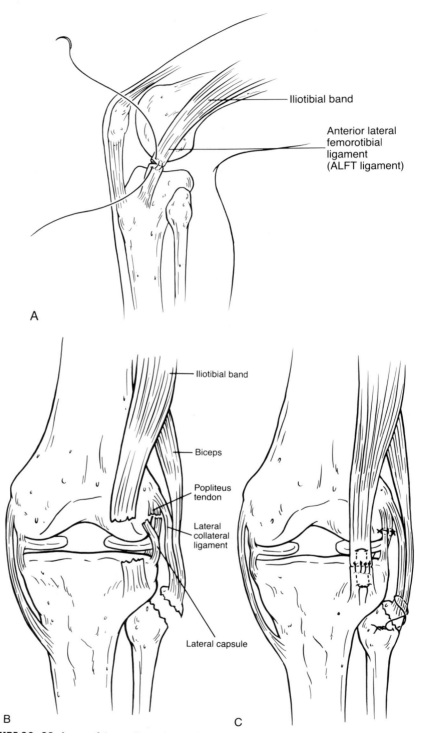

FIGURE 20–33. Areas of tissue disruption on lateral side. (*A*) Repair of anterolateral femorotibial ligament.[208] (*B*) Avulsion of bony attachment of the biceps tendon and lateral collateral ligament, tear of the popliteal tendon, lateral capsule, and iliotibial band. (*C*) Primary repair of torn tissue.

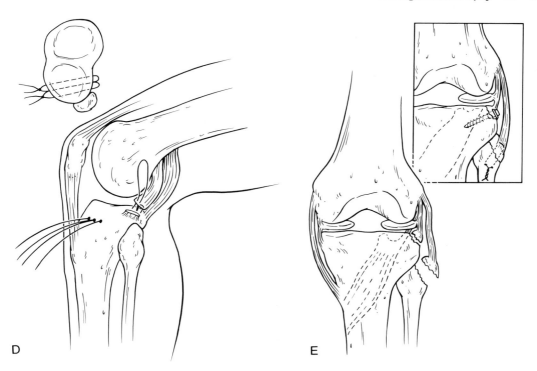

FIGURE 20–33 *(continued)*. *(D)* Repair of torn arcuate ligament, posterior capsule. *(continued)*. *(E)* Screw fixation of lateral capsular fracture (Segond's fracture) and repair of avulsion of lateral collateral ligament. This injury is associated with an ACL tear.

from its attachment to the tibia in its middle third (Fig. 20–33*A*). This band, which extends from the supracondylar tubercle of the femoral condyle to Gerdy's tubercle, was termed the anterolateral femorotibial (ALFT) ligament by Müller.[208] Less frequently, it avulses Gerdy's tubercle. The biceps femoris tendon is most frequently injured at its insertion into the fibular head or avulsed with the LCL along with an avulsed portion of bone from the fibular head (Fig. 20–33*B*). The lateral capsule is usually torn off the tibia, and this tearing off may be identified on radiographs with a fragment of bone (Segond's fracture). The LCL is usually torn at its insertion into the fibular head, but it may be injured anywhere along its course to its attachment on the lateral femoral epicondyle. The popliteal tendon is usually injured within 2 cm of its femoral attachment. Other structures, less well defined, such as the arcuate ligament, the short collateral ligament, and the posterior capsular plate may be disrupted in the severe injuries. Kaplan[152, 153] stated that the "quadruple complex" consisting of the iliotibial tract, the LCL, the popliteal tendon, and the biceps muscle provides the chief stabilizing function to the lateral side of the knee.

In acute injury in which repair is indicated by the amount of instability present, all structures should be repaired anatomically if possible. The repairs should begin from deep to superficial and from the back portion of the joint to the front. Meniscal repair should be performed when possible.

The posterior capsule and the arcuate ligament may be reattached to the posterior portion of the tibia through drill holes made anterolateral to posterolateral (Fig. 20–33*D*). Meniscal sutures can be passed at this time into the posterior capsule. The popliteal tendon should be reattached to the femur by a staple or a screw with a ligament washer. In-substance tears should be approximated and reefed when possible.

The lateral capsule is reattached to the remaining capsule on the tibia or by drill holes in the bone. In-substance tears are approximated by direct suture. If an avulsed piece of bone is present, stapling may be appropriate. The LCL is repaired by direct suture if an in-substance tear is present. If the LCL is avulsed from the tibia or femur, screw fixation can be used (Fig. 20–33*E*). The biceps tendon, the LCL, and the arcuate ligament are often detached as a unit and can be reattached with a cancellous screw and a ligament washer. An in-substance tear of the biceps tendon should be repaired with sutures. Separation of the anterior and posterior portions of the capsule should be repaired and imbricated with nonabsorbable suture. The iliotibial band is approximated or attached back to bone with a staple or a screw and washer. Associated ligamentous injury such as to the ACL, the PCL, or the medial stabilizing ligaments requires repair as discussed in the relevant sections of this chapter.

Rehabilitation

Immobilization in a brace locked at 45° of flexion is used initially to relieve tension of the repaired posterior structures. Passive range of motion directed more on flexion than extension is initiated at 1 week. Passive motion toward full extension is started at 2 to 3 weeks. Isometric exercises are delayed until 4 to 6 weeks to allow healing of the soft tissue. Adjustment of this schedule depends on the severity of injury and the strength of the repaired tissue. Progression of the range of motion and in the exercise program depends on the response of the individual patient. Active range of motion and strengthening exercises of the quadriceps muscles, calf muscles, and hamstrings should be started at about 6 weeks and progressed as tolerated. Touch-down weight bearing with the leg in the brace should be continued for 6 weeks, and full weight bearing should be gradually resumed afterwards. Isotonic exercises and return to activity begin between 8 and 12 weeks and depend on the progress made toward restoration of full joint motion and return of muscle strength.

ACUTE LIGAMENTOUS INJURY IN CHILDREN

Knee ligamentous injury in children younger than 14 years is uncommon.[23, 137, 168, 251] In a skeletally immature patient, the epiphyseal plate is more prone to traumatic injury than is the ligament.[25, 233, 245] The bone-ligament interface has also been shown to be weaker than the ligament itself in animal studies.[183, 229, 309, 310] However, Bertin and Goble[18] found that of 29 epiphyseal injuries about the knee, 38 per cent were accompanied by ACL injury and 10 per cent by associated MCL injury.

The ligamentous injury to the knee in a skeletally immature patient that would present a surgical dilemma is an acute ACL injury. In many children, there is hyperlaxity of the supporting structures or congenital laxity, which makes interpretation of the physical findings after injury confusing and perplexing. Children whose history is consistent with ACL insufficiency must be checked for generalized joint laxity, and a comparison with the opposite knee must be made to establish a base line. Roentgenograms for assessing the presence, absence, or abnormalities of configuration of the tibial spines help determine whether there is a congenital absence of the ACL.[92, 291]

ACL tears have been more frequently diagnosed in adolescents because of an increased involvement in sports and improved diagnostic capabilities.[24, 148, 177, 192, 263] Traumatic injury to the knee in adolescents that results in increased laxity should be radiographed in order to rule out epiphyseal injury. Stress radiographs may be necessary for adequately evaluating the epiphyseal status[60, 61] (Fig. 20–34).

Adolescent patients may manifest findings similar to those in adults with hemarthrosis, lack of flexion and extension, instability and a feeling of giving way, locking caused by meniscal injury, and pain.

Three types of ACL injury occur: avulsion of the intercondylar eminence of the tibia, midsubstance tears, and avulsions of the femoral attachment. Although avulsion of the tibial spine was thought to be more common in this age group,[23, 44, 123, 200, 201] midsubstance tears are being diagnosed with more frequency.[69, 150, 177, 192, 263] Each type presents a different problem.

Avulsions of the Intercondylar Eminence of the Tibia

The ACL is attached to the tibia at a depressed area in front of and lateral to the anterior tibial spine. Because the intracondylar eminence offers less

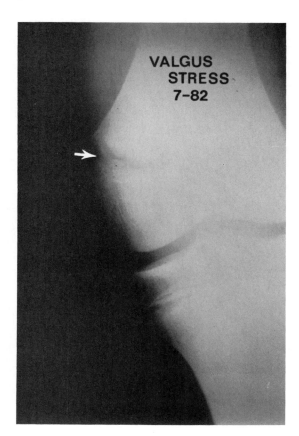

FIGURE 20–34. Anteroposterior radiograph with valgus stress. Adolescent patient had medial laxity after an injury. Laxity was caused by epiphyseal separation of the distal femoral epiphysis (*arrow*).

resistance to traction forces than does the ACL itself, it has been postulated that the most frequent type of injury is an avulsion injury (Fig. 20–35). Meyers and McKeever[200, 201] classified tibial eminence fractures into four groups. In type I, the fragment is minimally displaced from its bed in the tibia, and there is only slight elevation of the anterior margin. In type II, the anterior third to half of the avulsed fragment is elevated from its bony bed, which produced a beaklike appearance in a lateral roentgenogram. In type III, the avulsed fragment is completely lifted from its osseous bed in the intracondylar eminence, and there is no bone apposition. In type III +, the avulsed fragment is completely lifted from its bony bed and rotated so that the cartilaginous surface of the fragment faces the raw bone of the bed, making union impossible. In Meyers and McKeever's series,[200, 201] only one patient exhibited this type. Lack of damage to the other supporting structures was noted with avulsion injury to the ACL.

The 47 avulsion injuries reported consisted of 12 type I, 25 type II, and 10 type III injuries. Types I and II injuries were successfully treated by aspiration of the hemarthrosis and a well-fitting plaster cast from groin to toes with the knee flexed 20°. Union of the fragment required 6 to 12 weeks. Type III injuries required open reduction and fixation with absorbable sutures. Plaster immobilization was used for 6 weeks.

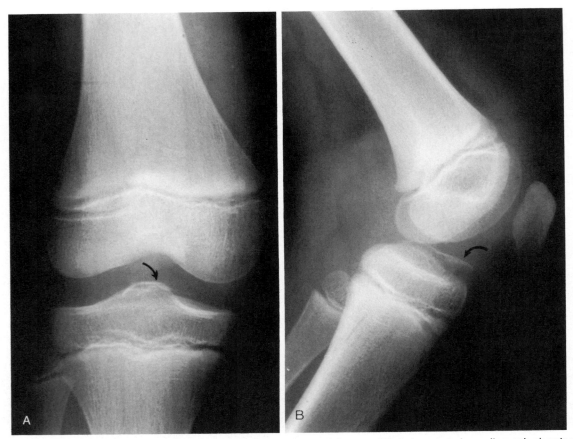

FIGURE 20–35. Avulsion of tibial attachment of the ACL in an adolescent. (*A*) Anteroposterior radiograph showing bone fragment. (*B*) Lateral view showing elevation of anterior half of insertion (type III).

Other authors have recommended closed reduction by extension of the knee, which causes replacement of the fragment by the femoral condyles' pushing down the wings of the articular cartilage that are lifted off with the bony avulsion. There is agreement that anatomic replacement is required regardless of whether it be by closed or open means.[91, 200, 201, 314] Failure of closed reduction is thought to be a result of interposed meniscal tissue or rotation of the fragment.

In all series, authors have reported excellent results with minimal residual laxity as long as good reduction is obtained.

Collateral ligament injuries have been reported with tibial spine avulsions.[44, 61, 123] Also reported is the association of in-substance tears of the ACL with a collateral ligament injury. Patients with medial or lateral laxity in association with a tibial avulsion injury should be evaluated with MRI or arthroscopy in order to fully define the extent of the injury and to plan the appropriate treatment.

Midsubstance Tear of the ACL

Shelbourne[263] reported on 113 skeletally immature athletes who had sustained midsubstance tears of the ACL. Fifty-three were treated non-operatively, and 60 were treated operatively with the use of an autogenic graft of the central third of the patellar tendon. The graft was placed through tibial and femoral drill holes that penetrated the growth plates. At an average 4.2-year follow-up, all patients treated nonoperatively had either experienced episodes of giving way (94 per cent) or developed meniscal pathology that required surgical treatment (63 per cent). Only 42 per cent were able to return to sports, and all reported episodes of giving way while playing. In the operative group, only 5 per cent experienced giving way, and 2 per cent developed meniscal tears. Ninety-two per cent were able to return to their original sporting activity. No patient in the operative group sustained abnormalities of growth. To qualify for surgery, patients required an assessment for potential growth and an evaluation of the epiphyseal plate that indicated that it was blurred or closing.

Other authors have reported on the results of primary repair and extra-articular procedures.[44, 60, 61, 193] Recurrent episodes of giving way and return of laxity was the usual outcome.

Surgical treatment of acute injuries in adolescent patients should be restricted to those who are unwilling to modify their activities, show positive results of Lachman's test and the pivot-shift test, or have a reparable meniscal tear. In a child with wide open epiphyseal plates, the definitive procedure should be delayed until the epiphyseal plates are closing and the child is past the adolescent growth spurt.[99, 263] Modification of the patient's activity level and the use of a functional brace for activity in low-demand sports can be considered until the criteria for surgical repair have been achieved.[263]

Although reports are given of surgery with careful drilling through the open epiphyseal plates with relatively successful results, cases of growth disturbance have occurred.[177, 192, 263] This possible complication should be mentioned if a surgical procedure is required in patients with open epiphyseal plates.

Avulsion of the Femoral Attachment of the ACL

This type of injury has rarely been reported in children or adolescents. It has been recommended that such ligament avulsions be reattached to their anatomic position in young children.[66, 276]

REFERENCES

1. Abbott LC, Saunders JB, Bost FC, Anderson CE: Injuries to the ligaments of the knee joint. J Bone Joint Surg 26A:503–521, 1944.
2. Aglietti P, Buzzi R, Basi P: Arthroscopic partial meniscectomy in the anterior cruciate deficient knee. Am J Sports Med 16:597–602, 1983.
3. Andersson C, Odensten M, Gillquist J: Knee function after surgical or nonsurgical treatment of acute rupture of the anterior cruciate ligament: a randomized study with long-term followup. Clin Orthop 264:255–263, 1991.
4. Andrews J, Baker C, Curl W, Giedumal R: Surgical repair of acute and chronic lesions of the lateral capsular ligamentous complex of the knee. *In* Feagin JA (ed): The Crucial Ligaments, pp. 425–438. New York: Churchill-Livingstone, 1988.
5. Arnoczky S: Anatomy of the anterior cruciate ligament. Clin Orthop 172:19–25, 1983.
6. Arnoczky SP: Blood supply to the ACL and supporting structures. Orthop Clin North Am 16:15–28, 1985.
7. Arnoczky SP, Warren RF: Anatomy of the cruciate ligaments. *In* Feagin JA (ed): The Crucial Ligaments, pp. 174–179. New York: Churchill-Livingstone, 1988.
8. Arnold J, Coker T, Heaton L, et al: Natural history of anterior cruciate ligament tears. Am J Sports Med 7:305, 1979.
9. Bach B, Warren R, Wickwiecz T: The pivot shift phenomenon: results and description of a modified clinical test for anterior cruciate ligament insufficiency. Am J Sports Med 16:571–576, 1988.
10. Baker C, Norwood L, Hughston J: Acute combined posterior cruciate and posterolateral instability of the knee. Am J Sports Med 12:204–208, 1984.
11. Balkfors B: The course of knee ligament injuries. Acta Orthop Scand 198:1–91, 1982.
12. Ballmer PM, Jakob RP: The nonoperative treatment of isolated complete tears of the medial collateral ligament of the knee. Arch Orthop Trauma Surg 107:273–276, 1988.
13. Bargar W, Moreland J, Markolf K, et al: In vivo stability testing of post meniscectomy knees. Clin Orthop 150:247–252, 1987.
14. Barrack RL, Bruckner J, Kneisel J, et al: The outcome of non-operatively treated complete tears of the ACL in the active young adults. Clin Orthop 259:192–199, 1990.
15. Barrack RL, Buckley SL, Bruckner JD, et al: Partial versus complete acute anterior cruciate ligament tears: the results of nonoperative treatment. J Bone Joint Surg 72B:622–624, 1990.
16. Barton T, Torg J: Natural history of the posterior cruciate ligament deficient knee. Am J Sports Med 13:439, 1985.
17. Beltran J, Noto AM, Mosure JC, et al: Joint effusions: MR imaging. Radiology 158:133–137, 1986.
18. Bertin KC, Goble EM: Ligament injuries associated with physeal fractures about the knee. Clin Orthop 177:188–195, 1983.
19. Bianchi M: Acute tears of the posterior cruciate ligament: a clinical study and results of operative treatment in 27 cases. Am J Sports Med 11:308–314, 1988.
20. Binkley JM, Peat M: The effects of immobilization on the ultrastructure and mechanical properties of the medial collateral ligament of rats. Clin Orthop 203:301–308, 1986.
21. Bomberg BC, McGinty JB: Acute hemarthrosis of the knee: indications for diagnostic arthroscopy. Arthroscopy 6:221–225, 1990.
22. Bonamo JJ, Fay C, Firestone T: The conservative treatment of the anterior cruciate deficient knee. Am J Sports Med 18:618–623, 1989.
23. Bradley G, Shives T, Samuelson K: Ligament injuries in the knees of children. J Bone Joint Surg 61A:588–591, 1979.
24. Brantigan OC, Voshell AF: Ligaments of the knee joint: the relationship of the ligament of Humphry to the ligament of Wrisberg. J Bone Joint Surg 28A:66–67, 1946.
25. Bright RW: Physeal injuries. *In* Rockwood CA Jr, Wilkins KE, King RE (eds): Fractures in Children, vol 3, p. 87. Philadelphia: JB Lippincott, 1984.
26. Bryant JT, Cooke TD: A biomechanical function of the ACL: prevention of medial translation of the tibia. *In* Feagin JA (ed): The Crucial Ligaments, pp. 235–242. New York: Churchill-Livingstone, 1988.
27. Buckley SL, Barrack RL, Alexander AH: The natural history of conservatively treated partial ACL tears. Am J Sports Med 17:221–225, 1989.

28. Burger R: Magnetic resonance imaging of the meniscus: how accurate? *Presented at* the 52nd annual meeting of the Western Orthopaedic Association, Honolulu, October 1988.
29. Burger RS, Baciocco E, Conrad S, et al: Magnetic resonance imaging of the meniscus: how accurate? Orthop Trans 13:65, 1989.
30. Buseck M, Noyes FR: Arthroscopic evaluation of meniscal repairs after ACL reconstruction and immediate motion. Am J Sports Med 19:489–494, 1991.
31. Butler DL, Andrews JR: The role of arthroscopic surgery in the evaluation of acute traumatic hemarthrosis of the knee. Clin Orthop 228:150–152, 1988.
32. Butler DL, Noyes FR, Grood ES: Ligamentous restraints to AP drawer in the human knee: a biomechanical study. J Bone Joint Surg 62A:259–270, 1980.
33. Cabaud A, Feagin J, Rodkey W: Acute anterior cruciate ligament injury in augmented repair: experimental studies. Am J Sports Med 8:395–401, 1980.
34. Cain T, Schwab G: Performance of an athlete with straight posterior knee instability. Am J Sports Med 9:203–208, 1981.
35. Cerabona F, Sherman MF, Bonamo JR, Sklar J: Patterns of meniscal injury with acute ACL tears. Am J Sports Med 16:603–609, 1988.
36. Chick R, Jackson D: Tears of the anterior cruciate ligament in young athletes. J Bone Joint Surg 60A:970–973, 1978.
37. Cho K: Reconstruction of the anterior cruciate ligament by semitendinosus tenodesis. J Bone Joint Surg 57A:608–612, 1975.
38. Clancy WG Jr: Anterior cruciate ligament functional instability: a static intra-articular and dynamic extra-articular procedure. Clin Orthop 172:102–106, 1983.
39. Clancy WG: Repair and reconstruction of the posterior cruciate ligament. *In* Chapman MW (ed): Operative Orthopaedics, p. 1651. Philadelphia: JB Lippincott, 1988.
40. Clancy WG Jr, Nelson DA, Reider B, Narechania RG: Anterior cruciate ligament reconstruction using one-third of the patellar ligament, augmented by extra-articular tendon transfers. J Bone Joint Surg 64A:352–359, 1982.
41. Clancy WG, Ray JM: ACL autografts. *In* Jackson DW, Drez D (eds): The ACL Deficient Knee: New Concepts in Ligament Repair, pp. 193–210. St Louis: CV Mosby, 1987.
42. Clancy W, Ray J, Zoltan D: Acute tears of the anterior cruciate ligament: surgical versus conservative treatment. J Bone Joint Surg 70A:1483–1488, 1988.
43. Clancy WG, Shelbourne KD, Zoellner G, et al: Treatment of knee joint instability secondary to rupture of the posterior cruciate ligament: report of a new procedure. J Bone Joint Surg 65A:310–322, 1983.
44. Clanton T, DeLee J, Sanders B, et al: Knee ligament injuries in children. J Bone Joint Surg 61A:1195–1201, 1979.
45. Clayton ML, Miles JS, Abdulla M: Experimental investigations of ligamentous healing. Clin Orthop 61:146–153, 1968.
46. Clendenin M, DeLee J, Heckman J: Interstitial tears of the posterior cruciate ligament of the knee. Orthopaedics 3:764–772, 1980.
47. Coward DB, Endicott MD: Incidence and pattern of meniscal tears seen in acute isolated ACL tears. Orthop Trans 13:67, 1989.
48. Cox JS: Symposium: Functional rehabilitation of isolated medial collateral ligament sprains. Injury nomenclature. Am J Sports Med 7:211–213, 1979.
49. Cox JS, Nye CE, Schaefer WW, Woodstein I: The degenerative effect of partial and total resection of the medial meniscus in dogs' knees. Clin Orthop 109:178–183, 1975.
50. Cross M, Powell J: The long-term follow-up of posterior cruciate ligament ruptures: a study of 116 cases. Am J Sports Med 12:292–297, 1984.
51. Cross MJ, Schmidt DR, Mackie IG: A no-touch test for the anterior cruciate ligament. J Bone Joint Surg 69B:300, 1987.
52. Crues JV III, Mink J, Levy TL, et al: Meniscal tears of the knee: accuracy of MR imaging. Radiology 164:445–448, 1987.
53. Dandy D, Pusey R: The long-term results of unrepaired tears of the posterior cruciate ligament. J Bone Joint Surg 64B:92–94, 1982.
54. Daniel D: Principles of knee ligament surgery. *In* Daniel D (ed): Knee Ligaments: Structure, Function, Injury, and Repair, Chapter 2, p. 11. New York: Raven Press, 1990.
55. Daniel DM, Malcom LL, Lossee G, et al: Instrumented measurement of anterior laxity of the knee. J Bone Joint Surg 67A:720–726, 1985.
56. Daniel DM, Stone ML, Barnett P, Sachs R: Use of the quadriceps active drawer test to diagnose PCL disruption and measure posterior laxity of the knee. J Bone Joint Surg 70A:386–397, 1988.
57. Daniel D, Stone M, Sachs R, Malcom L: Instrumented measurement of anterior knee laxity in patients with acute ACL disruption. Am J Sports Med 13:401–407, 1985.
58. DeHaven KE: Diagnosis of acute knee injuries with hemarthrosis. Am J Sports Med 8:9–14, 1980.
59. DeHaven KE: Arthroscopy in the diagnosis and management of the ACL deficient knee. Clin Orthop Rel Res 172:52–56, 1983.

60. DeLee J: ACL insufficiency in children. *In* Feagin JA (ed): The Crucial Ligaments, pp. 439–447. New York: Churchill-Livingstone, 1988.

61. DeLee J, Curtis R: Anterior cruciate insufficiency in children. Clin Orthop 172:112–118, 1983.

62. DeLee J, Riley M, Rockwood C: Acute posterolateral rotatory instability of the knee. Am J Sports Med 11:199–207, 1983.

63. DeLee J, Riley M, Rockwood C: Acute straight lateral instability of the knee. Am J Sports Med 11:404–411, 1983.

64. Derscheid GL, Garrick JG: Medial collateral ligament injuries in football: Nonoperative management of grade I and grade II sprains. Am J Sports Med 9:365–368, 1981.

65. Donaldson W, Warren R, Wickiewicz T: A comparison of acute ACL examination intact: initial versus exam under anesthesia. Am J Sports Med 13:5–10, 1985.

66. Edeady JL, Cardenas C, Sopa D: Avulsion of the femoral attachment of the anterior cruciate ligament in a 7-year-old child: a case report. J Bone Joint Surg 64A:1376–1378, 1982.

67. Ellsasser JC, Reynolds FC, Omohundro JR: The nonoperative treatment of collateral ligament injuries of the knee in professional football players. J Bone Joint Surg 56A:1185–1190, 1974.

68. Engebretsen L, Benum P, Fasting O, et al: A prospective randomized study of three surgical techniques for treatment of acute ruptures of the anterior cruciate ligament. Am J Sports Med 18:585–590, 1990.

69. Engebretsen L, Svenningsen S, Benum P: Poor results of anterior cruciate ligament repair in adolescents. Acta Orthop Scand 59:684–686, 1988.

70. Fairbanks T: Knee joint changes after meniscectomy. J Bone Joint Surg 30B:664–670, 1948.

71. Farquharson-Roberts M, Osborne A: Partial rupture of the ACL of the knee. J Bone Joint Surg 65B:32–34, 1983.

72. Feagin JA: The syndrome of torn anterior cruciate ligament. Orthop Clin North Am 10:81–90, 1979.

73. Feagin J, Cabaud E, Curl W: The anterior cruciate ligament: radiographic and clinical signs of successful and unsuccessful repairs. Clin Orthop 164:54–58, 1982.

74. Feagin JA, Curl W: Isolated tear of the anterior cruciate ligament: A five-year followup study. Am J Sports Med 4:95–100, 1976.

75. Ferkel RD, Davis JR, Friedman M, et al: Arthroscopic partial medial meniscectomy: an analysis of unsatisfactory results. J Arthroscopy Rel Res 1:44–52, 1985.

76. Ferkel RD, Markolf K, Goodfellow D, et al: Treatment of the ACL absent knee with associated meniscal tears. Clin Orthop 222:239–248, 1987.

77. Fetto JF, Marshall JL: Medial collateral ligament injuries of the knee: a rationale for treatment. Clin Orthop 132:206–218, 1978.

78. Fetto JF, Marshall JL: The natural history and diagnosis of anterior cruciate ligament insufficiency. Clin Orthop 147:29–38, 1980.

79. Finsterbush A, Frankl U, Malen Y, Mann G: Secondary damage to the knee after isolated injury to the ACL. Am J Sports Med 18:478–479, 1990.

80. Fleming R, Blatz D, McCarroll J: Posterior problems in the knee: posterior cruciate insufficiency and posterolateral insufficiency. Am J Sports Med 9:107–113, 1981.

81. Fowler P, Messieh S: Isolated posterior cruciate ligament injuries in athletes. Am J Sports Med 15:553–557, 1983.

82. Fowler P, Reagan W: The patient with symptomatic chronic anterior cruciate ligament insufficiency: results of minimal arthroscopic surgery and rehabilitation. Am J Sports Med 15:321–325, 1987.

83. Frank C: Accurate interpretation of the Lachman test. Clin Orthop 213:163–166, 1986.

84. Frank C, Akeson W, Woo S, et al: Physiology and therapeutic value of passive joint motion. Clin Orthop 185:113–125, 1984.

85. Frank C, Amiel D, Woo S, Akeson W: Normal ligament properties and ligament healing. Clin Orthop 196:15–25, 1985.

86. Frank C, Woo S, Amiel D, et al: Medial collateral ligament healing: a multidisciplinary assessment in rabbits. Am J Sports Med 11:379–389, 1983.

87. Frieden T, Zatterstrom T, Lindstrand A, Moritz U: Anterior cruciate insufficient knees treated with physiotherapy: a three-year follow-up with late diagnosis. Clin Orthop 263:190–199, 1991.

88. Fukubayashi Y, Torzilli PA, Sherman MF, Warren RF: An in vitro biomechanical evaluation of A-P motion of the knee. J Bone Joint Surg 64A:258–264, 1982.

89. Furman W, Marshall J, Girgis F: The anterior cruciate ligament: a functional analysis based on post-mortem studies. J Bone Joint Surg 58A:179–185, 1976.

90. Galway HR, MacIntosh DL: The lateral pivot shift as symptom and sign of anterior cruciate ligament insufficiency. Clin Orthop 147:45–50, 1980.

91. Garcia A, Neer C: Isolated fractures of the intracondylar eminence of the tibia. Am J Surg 95:593–598, 1958.

92. Giorgi B: Morphological variations to the intracondylar eminence of the knee. Clin Orthop 8:209–217, 1956.
93. Giove T, Miller S, Kent V, et al: Nonoperative treatment of the torn anterior cruciate ligament. J Bone Joint Surg 65A:184–192, 1983.
94. Girgis F, Marshall J, Monaghem A: The cruciate ligaments of the knee joint: anatomical, functional, and experimental analysis. Clin Orthop 106:216–223, 1975.
95. Glashow JL, Katz R, Schneider M, Scott WN: Double blind assessment of the value of magnetic resonance imaging and the diagnosis of anterior cruciate and meniscal lesions. J Bone Joint Surg 71A:113–118, 1989.
96. Goelleham DL, Warren RF, Turzilli PA: The role of the posterolateral and cruciate ligaments in stability of the human knee: a biomechanical study. J Bone Joint Surg 69A:233–242, 1987.
97. Good L, Odensten M, Gillquist J: Intracondylar notch measurements with special reference to ACL surgery. Clin Orthop 263:185, 1991.
98. Grana WA, Janssen T: Lateral ligament injury of the knee. J Orthopaedics 10:1039–1044, 1987.
99. Greulich W, Pyle S: Radiographic Atlas of the Skeletal Development of the Hand and Wrist. Stanford, CA: Stanford University Press, 1959.
100. Grood ES, Hefzy MS, Lindenfield TN: Factors affecting the region of most isometric femoral attachments. Part I: the posterior cruciate ligament. Am J Sports Med 17:197–207, 1989.
101. Grood ES, Noyes FR: Physical examination—diagnosis of knee ligament injuries: biomechanical precept. *In* Feagin JA (ed): The Crucial Ligaments, pp. 245–260. New York: Churchill-Livingstone, 1988.
102. Grood ES, Noyes FR, Butler DL, Suntay WJ: Ligamentous and capsular restraints preventing straight medial and lateral laxity in intact human cadaver knees. J Bone Joint Surg 63A:1257–1269, 1981.
103. Hart DP, Dahners LE: Healing of the medial collateral ligament in rats: the effects of repair, motion, and secondary stabilizing ligaments. J Bone Joint Surg 69A:1194–1199, 1987.
104. Harter R, Osternig L, Singer K, et al: Long-term evaluation of knee stability and function following surgical reconstruction for anterior cruciate ligament insufficiency. Am J Sports Med 16:434–443, 1988.
105. Hastings DE: The nonoperative management of collateral ligament injuries of the knee. Clin Orthop 147:22, 1980.
106. Hawkins RJ, Misamore G, Merritt T: Followup of the acute nonoperative isolated anterior cruciate ligament tear. Am J Sports Med 14:205–210, 1986.
107. Hede A, Hejgaard N, Sandberg H, Jacobsen H: Sports injuries of the knee ligaments—a prospective stress radiographic study. Br J Sports Med 19:8–10, 1985.
108. Hefzy MS, Grood ES, Noyes FR: Factors affecting the region of most isometric femoral attachments. Part II: the anterior cruciate ligament. Am J Sports Med 17:208–216, 1989.
109. Hejgaard N, Sandberg H, Hede A, et al: Prospective stress radiographic study of knee ligament injuries in 62 patients treated by acute repair. Acta Orthop Scand 53:285–290, 1982.
110. Heller L, Langman J: The meniscofemoral ligaments of the human knee. J Bone Joint Surg 46B:307–313, 1964.
111. Hey-Groves E: The crucial ligaments of the knee joint: their function, rupture, and the operative treatment of the same. Br J Surg 7:505–515, 1920.
112. Higgins RW, Steadman JR: Anterior cruciate ligament repair in world class skiers. Am J Sports Med 15:439–447, 1987.
113. Hirschman HP, Daniel DM, Miyasaka K: The fate of unoperated knee ligament injuries. *In* Daniel DM (ed): Knee Ligaments: Structure, Function, Injury and Repair, pp. 481–503. New York: Raven Press, 1990.
114. Holden DL, Eggert AW, Butler JE: The nonoperative treatment of grade I and II medial collateral ligament injuries to the knee. Am J Sports Med 11:340–344, 1983.
115. Holmes P, James S, Larson R, et al: Retrospective direct comparison of three intra-articular ACL reconstructions. Am J Sports Med 19:596–600, 1991.
116. Hughston JC, Andrews JR, Cross MJ, Moschi A: Classification of knee ligament instabilities. Part I: the medial compartment and cruciate ligaments. J Bone Joint Surg 58A:159–172, 1976.
117. Hughston JC, Andrews JR, Cross MJ, Moschi A: Classification of knee ligament instabilities. Part II: the lateral compartment. J Bone Joint Surg 58A:173–179, 1976.
118. Hughston JC, Barrett GR: Acute anteromedial rotatory instability: long-term results of surgical repair. J Bone Joint Surg 65A:145–153, 1983.
119. Hughston J, Bowden J, Andrews J, Norwood L: Acute tears of the posterior cruciate ligament: results of operative treatment. J Bone Joint Surg 62A:438–450, 1980.
120. Hughston J, Degenhard T: Reconstruction of the posterior cruciate ligament. Clin Orthop 164:59–77, 1982.

121. Hughston JC, Eilers AF: The role of the posterior oblique ligament in repairs of acute medial (collateral) ligament tears of the knee. J Bone Joint Surg 55A:923–940, 1973.

122. Hughston JC, Norwood LA: The posterolateral drawer test and external rotational recurvatum test for posterolateral rotatory instability of the knee. Clin Orthop 147:82–87, 1980.

123. Hyndman J, Brown D: Major ligamentous injuries of the knee in children. J Bone Joint Surg 61B:245, 1979.

124. Indelicato P: Non-operative treatment of complete tears of the medial collateral ligament of the knee. J Bone Joint Surg 65A:323–329, 1983.

125. Indelicato P: Nonoperative management of complete tears of the medial collateral ligament. Orthop Rev 18:947–952, 1989.

126. Indelicato P, Bittar E: A perspective of lesions associated with ACL insufficiency of the knee: a review of 100 cases. Clin Orthop 198:77–80, 1985.

127. Inoue M, McGurk-Burleson E, Hollis JM, Woo SL: Treatment of medial collateral ligament injury. Part I: the importance of anterior cruciate ligament on varus-valgus knee laxity. Am J Sports Med 15:15–21, 1987.

128. Insall J, Hood R: Bone block transfer of medial head of gastrocnemius for posterior cruciate ligament insufficiency. J Bone Joint Surg 64A:691–699, 1982.

129. Ireland J, Trickey EL, Stoker D: Arthroscopy and arthrography of the knee: a critical review. J Bone Joint Surg 62B:3–6, 1980.

129a. Irrang JL, Dearwater S, Fu FH, Sawhney R: Comparison of continuous passive motion to standard physical therapy in rehabilitation of patients following anterior cruciate ligament reconstruction. *Presented at* the annual meeting of the American Academy of Orthopaedic Surgeons, Washington, DC, February 1992.

130. Iversen BF, Sturup J, Jacobsen K, Anderson J: Implications of muscular defense in testing for the anterior drawer sign in the knee: a stress radiographic investigation. Am J Sports Med 17:409–413, 1989.

131. Jackson D, Jennings L, Maywood R, Berger P: Magnetic resonance imaging of the knee. Am J Sports Med 16:29–38, 1988.

132. Jakob R: Observations on rotatory instability of the lateral compartment of the knee. Acta Orthop Scand 52(191):1–32, 1981.

133. James SL: Biomechanics of knee ligament reconstruction. Clin Orthop 146:90–101, 1980.

134. James S: Knee ligament reconstruction. *In* Evarts CM (ed): Surgery of the Musculoskeletal System, vol 7, pp. 31–110. New York: Churchill-Livingstone, 1983.

135. Jensen J, Slocum D, Larson R, et al: Reconstructive procedures for anterior cruciate ligament insufficiency: a computer analysis of clinical results. Am J Sports Med 11:240–248, 1983.

136. Johnson J, Bach B: Current concepts: Review of posterior cruciate ligament. J Knee Surg 3:143–153, 1990.

137. Johnson L: Lateral capsular complex: anatomical and surgical procedures. Am J Sports Med 7:156–160, 1979.

138. Johnson RJ: The anterior cruciate ligament problem. Clin Orthop 172:14–18, 1983.

139. Johnson RJ, Eriksson E, Haggmark T, Pope M: Five- to ten-year followup evaluation after reconstruction of the anterior cruciate ligament. Clin Orthop 183:122–140, 1984.

140. Johnson RJ, Kettelkamp D, Clark W, Leaverton P: Factors affecting the late results after meniscectomy. J Bone Joint Surg 56A:719–729, 1974.

141. Jokl P, Kaplan N, Stovell P, Keggi K: Non-operative treatment of severe injuries to the medial and anterior cruciate ligaments of the knee. J Bone Joint Surg 66A:741–744, 1984.

142. Jones KC: Reconstruction of the anterior cruciate ligament. J Bone Joint Surg 45A:925–932, 1963.

143. Jones RE, Henley MB, Francis P: Nonoperative management of isolated grade III collateral ligament injury in high school football players. Clin Orthop 213:137–140, 1986.

144. Jonsson T, Althoff B, Peterson L, Renström P: Clinical diagnosis of ruptures of the anterior cruciate ligament: a comparative study of the Lachman test and the anterior drawer sign. Am J Sports Med 10:100–102, 1982.

145. Jonsson T, Peterson L, Renström P, et al: Augmentation with the longitudinal patellar retinaculum in the repair of an anterior cruciate ligament rupture. Am J Sports Med 17:401–408, 1989.

146. Kaeding C, Bergfeld J: Clinical review of PCL laxity. Postgraduate course sponsored by the American Academy of Orthopaedic Surgeons, Rancho Mirage, CA, December 1990.

147. Kannus P: Long-term results of conservatively treated medial collateral ligament injuries of the knee. Clin Orthop 226:103–112, 1988.

148. Kannus P: Knee ligament injuries in adolescents: eight-year followup of conservative management. J Bone Joint Surg 70B:772–776, 1988.

149. Kannus P: Nonoperative treatment of grade II and III sprains of the lateral ligament compartment of the knee. Am J Sports Med 17:83–88, 1989.

150. Kannus P, Järvinen M: Conservatively treated tears of the anterior cruciate ligament: long-term results. J Bone Joint Surg 69A:1007–1012, 1987.
151. Kannus P, Järvinen M: Osteoarthrosis in the knee joint due to chronic posttraumatic insufficiency of the medial collateral ligament: nine-year follow-up. Clin Rheumatol 7:200–207, 1988.
152. Kaplan E: The iliotibial tract: clinical and morphological significance. J Bone Joint Surg 40A:817–832, 1958.
153. Kaplan E: Some aspects of functional anatomy of the human knee joint. Clin Orthop 23:18–29, 1962.
154. Kaplan N, Wickiewicz T, Warren R: Primary surgical treatment of anterior cruciate ligament ruptures. Am J Sports Med 18:354–358, 1990.
155. Kelly M, Flock T, Kinnel J, et al: MR imaging of the knee: clarification of its role. J Arthroscopy Res Surg 7:78–85, 1991.
156. Kennedy J, Alexander I, Hayes K: Nerve supply to the human knee and its functional importance. Am J Sports Med 10:329–335, 1982.
157. Kennedy JC, Fowler PJ: Medial and anterior instability of the knee: an anatomical and clinical study using stress machines. J Bone Joint Surg 53A:1257–1270, 1971.
158. Kennedy J, Galpin R: The use of the medial head of the gastrocnemius muscle in the posterior cruciate deficient knee: indications, technique, and results. Am J Sports Med 10:63–74, 1982.
159. Kennedy JC, Hawkins RJ, Willis RB, et al: Tension studies of human knee ligaments: yield point, ultimate failure, and disruption of the cruciate and tibial collateral ligaments. J Bone Joint Surg 58A:350–355, 1976.
160. Kennedy J, Weinberg H, Wilson A: The anatomy and function of the anterior cruciate ligament: as determined by clinical and morphological studies. J Bone Joint Surg 56A:223–235, 1974.
161. Korn MW, Spitzer R, Robinson K: Is there still a role for knee arthrograph? J Arthroscopy Rel Res 1:40–43, 1985.
162. Krause WR, Pope MH, Johnson RJ, et al: Mechanical changes in the knee after meniscectomy. J Bone Joint Surg 58A:599–604, 1976.
163. Kurosaka M, Yoshiya S, Andrew J, Drish J: A biomechanical comparison of different surgical techniques of graft fixation in an anterior cruciate ligament reconstruction. Am J Sports Med 15:225–229, 1987.
164. Lambert K: Vascularized patellar tendon graft with rigid internal fixation for anterior cruciate ligament insufficiency. Clin Orthop 172:85–89, 1983.
164a. Lane JG, Daniel DD, Stone ML: Prospective evaluation of effect of postoperative immobilization upon complications following anterior cruciate ligament reconstruction. *Presented at* the annual meeting of the American Academy of Orthopaedic Surgeons, Washington, DC, February 1992.
165. Larson RL: Physical examination in the diagnosis of rotatory instability. Clin Orthop 172:38–44, 1983.
166. Larson RL: Chronic medial instability. *In* Evarts CM (ed): Surgery of the Musculoskeletal System, vol 7, pp. 34–56. New York: Churchill-Livingstone, 1983.
167. Larson RL: Augmentation of acute rupture of the anterior cruciate ligament. Orthop Clin North Am 16:135–142, 1985.
168. Larson R, Jones D: Fracture and dislocations of the knee. Part 2: Dislocations and ligamentous injuries of the knee. *In* Rockwood CA, Green DP (eds): Fractures in Adults, 2nd ed, vol 2, pp. 1480–1591. Philadelphia: JB Lippincott, 1984.
169. Last R: The popliteus muscle and the lateral meniscus. J Bone Joint Surg 32B:93–99, 1950.
170. Laws G, Walton M: Fibroblastic healing of grade II ligament injuries: histological and mechanical studies in the sheep. J Bone Joint Surg 70B:390–396, 1988.
171. Lee JK, Yao L, Phelps CT, et al: Anterior cruciate ligament tears: MR imaging compared with arthroscopy and clinical tests. Radiology 166:861–864, 1988.
172. Levinsohn E, Baker B: Pre-arthrotomy diagnostic evaluation of the knee: review of 100 cases diagnosed by arthrography and arthroscopy. Am J Radiol 134:107–111, 1980.
173. Levy I, Torzilli P, Warren R: Effective medial meniscectomy in AP motion of the knee. J Bone Joint Surg 64A:883–888, 1982.
174. Liljedahl SO, Lindvall N, Wetterfars J: Early diagnosis and treatment of acute ruptures of the anterior cruciate ligament: a clinical and arthrographic study of forty-eight cases. J Bone Joint Surg 47A:1503–1513, 1965.
175. Lipke JM, Janecki CJ, Nelson CL, et al: The role of incompetence of the anterior cruciate and lateral ligaments in anterolateral and anteromedial instability: a biomechanical study of cadaver knees. J Bone Joint Surg 63A:954–960, 1981.
176. Lipscomb A, Johnston R, Snyder R, et al: Secondary reconstruction of the anterior cruciate ligament in athletes by using the semitendinosus tendon. Am J Sports Med 7:81–84, 1979.
177. Lipscomb B, Anderson A: Tears of the anterior cruciate ligament in adolescents. J Bone Joint Surg 68A:19–28, 1986.

178. Loos WC, Fox JM, Blazina ME, et al: Acute posterior cruciate ligament injuries. Am J Sports Med 9:86–92, 1981.
179. Losee RE, Jonsson TR, Southwick W: Anterior subluxation of the lateral tibial plateau with diagnostic tests and operative repair. J Bone Joint Surg 60A:1015–1030, 1978.
180. Lucie R, Wiedel J, Messner D: The acute pivot shift—Galway and MacIntosh clinical correlation. Am J Sports Med 12:189–191, 1984.
181. Lynch MA, Henning CE, Glick KR Jr: Knee joint surface changes: long-term follow-up meniscus tear treatment in stable anterior cruciate ligament reconstructions. Clin Orthop 172:148–153, 1983.
182. Lysholm J, Gilquist J: Arthroscopic examination of the posterior cruciate ligament. J Bone Joint Surg 63A:363–366, 1981.
183. MacIntosh D: MacIntosh (over-the-top reconstruction). *In* Crenshaw (ed): Campbell's Operative Orthopaedics, 7th ed, p. 2361. St. Louis: CV Mosby, 1987.
184. Mandelbaum BR, Finerman GA, Reicher MA, et al: Magnetic resonance imaging as a tool for evaluation of traumatic knee injuries: anatomical and pathoanatomical correlations. Am J Sports Med 14:361–370, 1986.
185. Marder R, Raskind J, Carroll M: Prospective evaluation of arthroscopically assisted ACL reconstruction: patella tendon versus semitendinosus and gracilis tendons. Am J Sports Med 19:478–484, 1991.
186. Markolf K, Mensch J, Amstutz H: Stiffness and laxity of the knee—the contributions of the supporting structures: a quantitative in vitro study. J Bone Joint Surg 58A:583–594, 1976.
187. Marshall J: Periarticular osteophyte: initiation and formation in the knee of the dog. Clin Orthop 62:37–47, 1969.
188. Marshall J, Girgis F, Zelko R: The biceps femoris tendon and its functional significance. J Bone Joint Surg 54A:1444–1450, 1972.
189. Marshall JL, Wang JB, Furman W, et al: The anterior drawer sign: what is it? Am J Sports Med 3:152–158, 1975.
190. Marshall J, Warren R, Wickiewicz T: Primary surgical treatment of anterior cruciate lesions. Am J Sports Med 10:103–107, 1982.
191. Marshall J, Warren R, Wickiewicz T, Reider B: The anterior cruciate ligament: a technique of repair and reconstruction. Clin Orthop 143:97–106, 1979.
192. McCarroll J, Rettig A, Shelbourne KD: Anterior cruciate ligament injuries in the young athlete with open physes. Am J Sports Med 16:44–47, 1988.
193. McCormick W, Bagg R, Kennedy C, Leukens C: Reconstruction of the posterior cruciate ligament: preliminary report of a new procedure. Clin Orthop 118:30–34, 1976.
194. McDaniel WJ: Isolated partial tear of the anterior cruciate ligament. Clin Orthop 115:209–212, 1976.
195. McDaniel WJ, Dameron T: Untreated ruptures of the anterior cruciate ligament: a followup study. J Bone Joint Surg 62A:696–705, 1980.
196. McDaniel WJ, Dameron T: The untreated anterior cruciate ligament rupture. Clin Orthop 172:158–163, 1983.
197. McDevitt C, Gilbertson E, Muir A: An experimental model of osteoarthritis: early morphological and biochemical changes. J Bone Joint Surg 59B:24–35, 1977.
198. McMaster W: Isolated posterior cruciate ligament injury: literature review and case report. J Trauma 15:1025–1029, 1975.
199. Meyers MH: Isolated avulsion of the tibial attachment of the posterior cruciate ligament of the knee. J Bone Joint Surg 57A:669–672, 1975.
200. Meyers M, McKeever F: Fracture of the intracondylar eminence of the tibia. J Bone Joint Surg 41A:209–222, 1959.
201. Meyers M, McKeever F: Fracture of the intracondylar eminence of the tibia. J Bone Joint Surg 52A:1677–1684, 1970.
202. Mink JH, Levy T, Crues JV III: MR imaging of the knee: technical factors, diagnostic accuracy, and further pitfalls. Radiology 165:175, 1987.
203. Mink JH, Levy T, Crues JV III: Tears of the anterior cruciate ligament and menisci of the knee: MR imaging evaluation. Radiology 167:769–774, 1988.
204. Mohtadi NG, Webster-Bogaert S, Fowler P: Limitation of motion following ACL reconstruction. Am J Sports Med 19:620–625, 1991.
205. Mok DW, Good C: Non-operative management of acute grade III medial collateral ligament injury of the knee: a prospective study. Injury 20:277–280, 1989.
206. Moore H, Larson R: Posterior cruciate ligament injuries: results of early surgical repair. Am J Sports Med 8:68–78, 1982.
207. Morgan CD, Wojtys E, Cascells CD, Cascells W: Arthroscopic meniscal repair evaluated by second look arthroscopy. Am J Sports Med 19:632–638, 1991.
208. Müller W: The Knee: Form, Function, and Ligament Reconstruction, p. 253. New York: Springer-Verlag, 1983.
209. Nicholas JA: The five-one reconstruction for anteromedial instability of the knee. J Bone Joint Surg 55A:899–922, 1973.

210. Nicholas JA, Freiberger RH, Killoran PJ: Double-contrast arthrography of the knee. J Bone Joint Surg 52A:203–220, 1970.

211. Norwood L, Cross M: Anterior cruciate ligament: functional anatomy of its bundles and rotatory instabilities. Am J Sports Med 7:23–26, 1979.

212. Noyes FR: Functional properties of knee ligaments and alterations induced by immobilization: a correlated biomechanical and histological study in primates. Clin Orthop 123:210, 1977.

213. Noyes FR, Bassett RW, Grood ES, Butler DL: Arthroscopy in acute traumatic hemarthrosis of the knee: incidence of anterior cruciate tears and other injuries. J Bone Joint Surg 62A:687–696, 1980.

214. Noyes FR, Butler DL, Grood ES, et al: Clinical paradoxes of ACL instability and a new test to detect its instability. Orthop Trans 2:36, 1978.

215. Noyes F, Butler D, Grood E, et al: Biomechanical analysis of human ligament grafts used in knee ligament repairs and reconstructions. J Bone Joint Surg 66A:344–352, 1984.

216. Noyes FR, DeLucas JC, Torvik PG: Biomechanics of ACL failure: an analysis of strain rate sensitivity and mechanisms of failure in primates. J Bone Joint Surg 56A:236–253, 1974.

217. Noyes F, Grood E: The strength of the anterior cruciate ligament in humans and rhesus monkeys: age-related and species-related changes. J Bone Joint Surg 58A:1074–1082, 1976.

218. Noyes FR, Grood ES: Diagnosis of knee ligament injuries: clinical concepts. *In* Feagin JA (ed): The Crucial Ligaments, pp. 261–286. New York: Churchill-Livingstone, 1988.

219. Noyes FR, Grood ES, Butler DL, et al: Clinical laxity tests and functional stability of the knee: biomechanical concepts. Clin Orthop 146:84, 1980.

220. Noyes FR, Mangine RE, Barber S: Early knee motion after open and arthroscopic ACL reconstruction. Am J Sports Med 15:149–160, 1987.

221. Noyes FR, Matthews DS, Mooar LA, Grood ES: Symptomatic anterior cruciate deficient knee. Part II: the success of rehabilitation activity modification and counselling of functional disability. J Bone Joint Surg 65A:163–174, 1983.

222. Noyes FR, Mooar PA, Matthews DS, Butler DL: The symptomatic anterior cruciate deficient knee. Part I: the long-term functional disability in the athletically active individual. J Bone Joint Surg 65A:154–162, 1983.

223. Noyes FR, Mooar LA, Moorman CT, McGinnis GH: Partial tears of the ACL—progression to complete ligament deficiency. J Bone Joint Surg 71B:825–827, 1989.

224. O'Brien SJ, Warren RF, Wickiewicz TL, et al: The iliotibial band lateral sling procedure and its effect on the results of ACL reconstruction. Am J Sports Med 19:21–25, 1991.

225. O'Connor RL: Arthroscopy, p. 90. Philadelphia: JB Lippincott, 1977.

226. Odensten M, Hamberg P, Nordin M, et al: Surgical or conservative treatment of the acutely torn anterior cruciate ligament: a randomized study with short-term follow-up observations. Clin Orthop 198:87–93, 1985.

227. Odensten M, Lysholm J, Gillquist J: Suture of fresh ruptures of the anterior cruciate ligament: a five-year followup. Acta Orthop Scand 55:270–272, 1984.

228. Odensten M, Lysholm J, Gillquist J: Course of partial ACL ruptures. Am J Sports Med 13:183–186, 1985.

229. O'Donoghue DH: Surgical treatment of fresh injuries to the major ligaments of the knee. J Bone Joint Surg 32A:721, 1950.

230. O'Donoghue DH: An analysis of the end results of the surgical treatment of major injuries to the ligaments of the knee. J Bone Joint Surg 37A:1–13, 129, 1955.

231. O'Donoghue DH: Reconstruction for medial instability of the knee. J Bone Joint Surg 55A:941–954, 1973.

232. Ogata K, Whiteside LA, Andersen D: The intra-articular effect of various postoperative managements following knee ligament repair. Clin Orthop 150:271, 1980.

233. Ogden J: The uniqueness of growing bones. *In* Rockwood CA Jr, Wilkins KE, King RE (eds): Fractures in Children, vol 3, Chapter 7. Philadelphia: JB Lippincott, 1984.

234. Palmer I: On the injuries to the ligaments of the knee. Acta Chir Scand 81(53):3–282, 1938.

235. Parolie JM, Bergfeld JA: Long-term results of nonoperative treatment of isolated PCL injuries in the athlete. Am J Sports Med 14:35–38, 1986.

236. Pattee G, Fox J, Del Pizzo W, Friedman M: Four to ten year follow-up of unreconstructed ACL tears. Am J Sports Med 17:430–435, 1989.

237. Patterson F, Trickey E: Meniscectomy for tears in the meniscus combined with rupture of the ACL. J Bone Joint Surg 65B:388–390, 1983.

238. Paulos L, Rosenberg T, Parker R: The medial knee ligaments: pathomechanics and surgical repair with the emphasis on the external rotation pivot shift test. Tech Orthop 2:37–46, 1987.

239. Pavlov H, Warren RF, Sherman M, Kayea P: The accuracy of double contrast arthrographic evaluation of the ACL: a retrospective review of 163 knees with surgical confirmation. J Bone Joint Surg 65A:175–183, 1983.

240. Penner DA, Daniel DM, Wood P, Mishra D: An in vitro study of ACL graft placement and isometry. Am J Sports Med 16:238–243, 1988.
241. Polly D, Callaghan J, Sykes R, et al: The accuracy of selective magnetic resonance imaging compared with the findings of arthroscopy of the knee. J Bone Joint Surg 70A:192–198, 1988.
242. Reicher MA, Hartzman S, Bassett RW, et al: MRI imaging of the knee joint. Part II: traumatic disorders. Radiology 162:547–551, 1987.
243. Reider B, Clancy W, Langer L: The diagnosis of cruciate ligament injuries using single contrast arthrography. Am J Sports Med 12:451–454, 1984.
244. Ritter MA, McCarroll J, Wilson FD, Carlson SR: Ambulatory care of medial collateral ligament tears. Phys Sports Med 11:47, 1983.
245. Roberts J: Fractures and dislocations of the knee. *In* Rockwood CA Jr, Wilkins KE, King RE (eds): Fractures in Children, vol 3, Chapter 11. Philadelphia: JB Lippincott, 1984.
246. Rosenberg T, Rasmussen G: Function of the ACL during anterior drawer and Lachman testing: an in vivo analysis in normal knees. Am J Sports Med 12:318–323, 1984.
247. Roth J, Bray R, Best T, et al: Posterior cruciate ligament reconstruction by transfer of the medial gastrocnemius. Am J Sports Med 16:21–28, 1988.
248. Salter R: The biological concept of continuous passive motion of synovial joints: the first 18 years of basic research and its clinical application. Clin Orthop 242:12, 1989.
249. Sandberg R, Balkfors B: Partial ruptures of the ACL: natural course. Clin Orthop 220:176–178, 1987.
250. Sandberg R, Balkfors B, Nilsson B, Westlin N: Operative versus nonoperative treatment of recent injuries to the ligaments of the knee: a prospective randomized study. J Bone Joint Surg 69A:1120, 1987.
251. Sanders W, Wilkins K, Neidere A: Acute insufficiency of the PCL in children. J Bone Joint Surg 62A:129–130, 1980.
252. Satku K, Chew C, Siow H: Posterior cruciate ligament injuries. Acta Orthop Scand 55:26–29, 1984.
253. Satku K, Kumar V, Ngoi S: ACL injuries. J Bone Joint Surg 68B:458–461, 1986.
254. Scapinelli R: Studies on the vasculature of the human knee. J Acta Anat 70:305–331, 1968.
255. Schultz R, Miller D, Kerr C, Micheli L: Mechanoreceptors in human cruciate ligaments. J Bone Joint Surg 66A:1072–1076, 1984.
256. Schutzer S, Christen S, Jacob R: Further observations on the isometricity of the anterior cruciate ligament. Clin Orthop 242:247, 1989.
257. Seebacher J, Inglis A, Marshall J, Warren R: The structure of the posterolateral aspect of the knee. J Bone Joint Surg 64A:536–541, 1982.
258. Seedhom B, Hargreaves D: Transmission of the load in the knee joint with special references to the role of the menisci. Part II: experimental results, discussion and conclusions. Engl Med 8:22–28, 1979.
259. Selesnick FH, Noble HB, Bachman DC, Steinberg FL: Internal derangement of the knee: diagnosis by arthrography, arthroscopy, and arthrotomy. Clin Orthop 198:26–30, 1985.
260. Seto JL, Orofino AS, Morrissey MC, et al: Assessment of quadriceps/hamstring strength, knee ligament stability, functional and sports activity levels five years after anterior cruciate ligament reconstruction. Am J Sports Med 16:170–180, 1988.
261. Sgaglione N, Del Pizzo W, et al: Interpretation of ACL surgery data: comparison and evaluation of existing knee ligament rating systems. *Presented at* the tenth annual meeting of the Arthroscopy Association of North America, San Diego, CA, 1991.
262. Sgaglione N, Warren R, Wickiewicz T, et al: Primary repair with semitendinosus tendon augmentation of acute anterior cruciate ligament injuries. Am J Sports Med 18:64–73, 1990.
263. Shelbourne K: ACL injuries in the child and adolescent. Postgraduate course sponsored by the American Academy of Orthopaedic Surgeons, Rancho Mirage, CA, December, 1990.
264. Shelbourne KD, et al: Arthrofibrosis in acute ACL reconstruction: the effect of timing and rehabilitation. Am J Sports Med 19:332–336, 1991.
265. Shelbourne KD, Baele JR: Treatment of combined ACL and MCL injuries. Am J Knee Surg 1:56–58, 1988.
266. Shelbourne KD, Benedict F, McCarrol JR, et al: Dynamic posterior shift test. Am J Sports Med 19:275–277, 1989.
267. Shelbourne K, Nitz P: Accelerated rehabilitation after anterior cruciate ligament reconstruction. Am J Sports Med 18:292, 1990.
268. Shelbourne KD, Nitz PA: The O'Donoghue trial revisited: combined knee injuries involving anterior cruciate and medial collateral ligament tears. Am J Sports Med 19:474–477, 1991.
269. Shelbourne K, Whitaker J, Podesta L, Reitar I: Anterior cruciate ligament injury: evaluation of intra-articular reconstruction of acute tears without repair—two to seven-year followup of 155 athletes. Am J Sports Med 18:484–489, 1990.

270. Sherman M, Lieber L, Bonamo J, et al: The long term follow-up of primary ACL repair: defining a rationale for augmentation. Am J Sports Med 19:243–255, 1991.
271. Sherman M, Warren R, Marshall J, Savatsky J: A clinical and radiographical analysis of 127 anterior cruciate insufficient knees. Clin Orthop 227:229–237, 1988.
272. Shields C, Silva I, Yee L, Brewster C: Evaluation of the residual instability after arthroscopic meniscectomy in the anterior cruciate deficient knees. Am J Sports Med 15:129–131, 1987.
273. Shino K, Horibe S, Orooro K: Voluntary posterolateral drawer sign in the knee with posterolateral instability. Clin Orthop 215:179–186, 1987.
274. Shoemaker S, Markolf K: The role of the meniscus in the anterior-posterior stability of the loaded anterior cruciate deficient knee. J Bone Joint Surg 68A:71–79, 1986.
275. Silva I, Silver D: Tears of the meniscus as revealed by magnetic resonance imaging. J Bone Joint Surg 70A:199–202, 1988.
276. Singer KM, Henry J: Knee problems in children and adolescents. Clin Sports Med 4:385–397, 1985.
277. Slocum DB, James SL, Larson RL, Singer KM: Clinical tests for anterolateral rotatory instability. Clin Orthop 118:63–69, 1976.
278. Slocum DB, Larson RL: Pes anserinus transplant: a simple surgical procedure for control of rotatory instability of the knee. J Bone Joint Surg 30A:226, 1968.
279. Slocum DB, Larson RL: Rotatory instability of the knee: its pathogenesis in a clinical test to demonstrate its presence. J Bone Joint Surg 50A:211–225, 1968.
280. Slocum DB, Larson RL, James SL: Pes anserinus transplant: impressions after a decade of experience. Am J Sports Med 2:123, 1974.
281. Slocum DB, Larson RL, James SL: Late reconstruction of ligamentous injuries of the medial compartment of the knee. Clin Orthop 100:23, 1974.
282. Southmayd W, Rubin B: Reconstruction of the posterior cruciate ligament using the semimembranosus tendon. Clin Orthop 150:196–197, 1980.
283. Steadman J, Forster R, Silferskiold J: Rehabilitation of the knee. Clin Sports Med 8(3):605, 1989.
284. Strand T, Molster A, Aengesaeter L, et al: Primary repair in posterior cruciate ligament injuries. Acta Orthop Scand 55:545–547, 1984.
285. Strum G, Fox J, Ferkel R, et al: Intra-articular versus intra-articular and extra-articular reconstruction for chronic anterior cruciate ligament instability. Clin Orthop 245:188–197, 1989.
286. Tapper E, Hoover N: Late results after meniscectomy. J Bone Joint Surg 51A:517–526, 1969.
287. Terry G, Hughston J, Norwood L: The anatomy of the iliopatellar band and iliotibial tract. Am J Sports Med 14:39–45, 1986.
288. Thijn C: Accuracy of double contrast arthrography and arthroscopy of the knee joint. Skel Radiol 8:187–192, 1982.
289. Tibone J, Antich T, Perry J, Moynes D: Functional analysis of untreated and reconstructed posterior cruciate ligament injuries. Am J Sports Med 16:217–223, 1988.
290. Tipton C, James SL, Mergner K, et al: Influence of exercise on strength of medial collateral knee ligaments of dogs. Am J Physiol 218:894, 1970.
291. Tolo VT: Congenital absence of the menisci and cruciate ligaments. J Bone Joint Surg 63A:1022–1025, 1981.
292. Torg JS, Conrad W, Caylin V: Clinical diagnosis of anterior cruciate ligament instability in the athlete. Am J Sports Med 4:84–93, 1976.
293. Torisu T: Isolated avulsion fractures to the tibial attachment of the posterior cruciate ligament. J Bone Joint Surg 59A:68–72, 1977.
294. Torisu T: Avulsion fractures of the tibial attachment of the posterior cruciate ligament: indications and results of delayed repair. Clin Orthop 143:107–114, 1979.
295. Trent P, Walker P, Wolf B: Ligament length patterns, strength, and rotational positions of the knee joint. Clin Orthop 117:263–270, 1976.
296. Tria A, Geppert M, McBride M, et al: The triad ratio: a roentgenographic ratio for medial knee injuries. Am J Knee Surg 3:126, 1990.
297. Trickey E: Ruptures of the posterior cruciate ligament of the knee. J Bone Joint Surg 50B:334–341, 1968.
298. Trickey E: Injuries to the posterior cruciate ligament: diagnosis and treatment of early injuries and reconstruction of late instability. Clin Orthop 147:76–81, 1980.
299. Tyrrell R, Gluckert K, Pathria M, Modic M: Fast three-dimensional MR imaging of the knee: comparison with arthroscopy. Radiology 166:865–872, 1988.
300. Walla D, Albright JP, McAuley E, et al: Hamstring control and the unstable anterior cruciate ligament–deficient knee. Am J Sports Med 13:34–39, 1985.
301. Wang C, Walker P: Rotatory laxity of the human knee joint. J Bone Joint Surg 56A:161–170, 1974.
302. Warren R, Levy IM: Meniscal lesions associated with ACL injury. Clin Orthop 172:32–37, 1983.

303. Warren RF, Marshall JL: Injuries of the anterior cruciate and medial collateral ligaments of the knee: a long-term follow-up of 86 cases, part II. Clin Orthop 136:198–211, 1978.

304. Warren RF, Marshall JL: The supporting structures in layers of the medial side of the knee: an anatomical analysis. J Bone Joint Surg 61A:56, 1979.

305. Warren RF, Marshall JL, Girgis F: Prime static stabilizer of the medial side of the knee. J Bone Joint Surg 56A:665, 1974.

306. Wilson W, Scranton P: Combined reconstruction of the anterior cruciate ligament in competitive athletes. J Bone Joint Surg 72A:742–748, 1990.

307. Wirth C, Jager M: Dynamic double tendon replacement of the posterior cruciate ligament. Am J Sports Med 12:39–43, 1984.

308. Woo S, Gomez M, Sites T, et al: The biomechanical and morphological changes in the medial collateral ligament of the rabbit after immobilization and mobilization. J Bone Joint Surg 69A:1200, 1987.

309. Woo S, Inoue M, McGurk-Burleson E, Gomez MA: The treatment of the medial collateral ligament injury. Part II: structure and function of canine knees in response to different treatment regimens. Am J Sports Med 15:22, 1987.

310. Woo S, Young E, Ohland K, et al: The effects of transection of the anterior cruciate ligament on healing of the medial collateral ligament: a biomechanical study of the knee in dogs. J Bone Joint Surg 72A:382, 1990.

311. Woods CW, Chapman DR: Repairable posterior meniscocapsular disruption in ACL injuries. Am J Sports Med 12:381–385, 1984.

312. Woods CW, Stanley RF, Tullas HJ: Lateral capsular sign: x-ray clue to a significant knee instability. Am J Sports Med 7:27–33, 1979.

313. Yaru N, Daniel D, Penner D, Farhoumand I: The effect of tibial attachment site on graft impingement in an anterior cruciate ligament reconstruction. Quoted in Daniel D (ed): Knee Ligaments: Structure, Function, Injury, and Repair, Chapter 28, p. 512. New York: Raven Press, 1990.

314. Zaricznyj B: Avulsion fractures of the tibial eminence: treatment by open reduction and pinning. J Bone Joint Surg 59A:1111–1115, 1977.

CHAPTER 21

Chronic Anterior,

Anterolateral,

and

Anteromedial

Instability

ROBERT S. BURGER, M.D.

ROBERT L. LARSON, M.D.

Chronic knee instability accompanied by a functional disability is usually associated with a tear of one or both cruciate ligaments. Patients with such instability often have a history of repeated episodes of knee injury. The decreased functional use of the involved extremity may lead to uncorrected muscle weakness. The instability may be compensated for by a self-imposed reduction in activity level and maintenance of muscle strength. A recurrence of injury may cause a decrease in use of the extremity, muscle weakness, and return of a functional disability. It is important to investigate the patient's history of the original knee injury and episodes of giving way and their consequences.

In reports of patients with chronic symptomatic knee instability, authors have cited a high percentage of meniscal tears and chondral lesions.[1, 3, 19, 27, 39, 44, 52] Such studies represent a biased population with symptoms. The natural progression of an asymptomatic chronic instability group has not yet been fully investigated. Complete meniscectomy has been cited as a precursor to degenerative changes in the knee.[2, 17, 51, 58, 91, 105] The results of partial meniscectomy and its effect on knee degeneration have been based on only an intermediate range of follow-up and have left the ultimate question about the effectiveness of such procedures unanswered.[32, 67, 74, 95] The presence or absence of a meniscus appears to be one of the chief prognostic factors of long-term knee function.

The extent of damage in the acutely injured knee may not be fully detected by physical examination, radiographic examination, or even arthroscopy. Several reports on magnetic resonance imaging (MRI) studies of patients with anterior cruciate ligament (ACL) tears have shown that more than 80 per cent had an associated osseous lesion.[65, 88, 103] What appears to be an isolated ACL injury may be associated with damage to other secondary stabilizers, which in time may stretch as they provide compensatory restraints for the injured primary stabilizer. Patients who place high demands on the ACL-deficient knee become more symptomatic than those with low-demand activities.[77, 78]

A patient with a chronic history of knee instability should be evaluated to determine the following:

1. The primary complaint (pain, recurrent instability, loss of motion).
2. The cause of the complaint (meniscal, chondral, or ligamentous in origin).
3. The effect on the activities of daily living, work, and recreation.
4. The extent of associated degenerative changes.
5. The status of the primary and secondary restraints.

DIAGNOSIS

History

Joint pain is a frequent complaint of patients with chronic anterior instability. A feeling of instability, episodes of actual giving way, stiffness, swelling, patellofemoral pain, and weakness are common symptoms. Mechanical symptoms such as locking, catching, popping, and giving way suggest meniscal or chondral injuries. Localization of pain to one compartment is consistent with unicompartmental degeneration.

The activity and the mechanism that cause the symptoms and the frequency, intensity, and duration of the symptoms are important for determining the treatment that is necessary. Pain during rest is a poor prognostic sign. The activity modification required and its effect on symptoms must be ascertained. Current and future activity levels required and desired, previous total or partial meniscectomy or meniscal repair, and previous ligament surgery also influence the choice of diagnostic and therapeutic modalities.

Physical Examination

The physical examination (see Chapter 4) is usually more accurate for chronic instability than in the acute situation, in which guarding, muscle spasm, hemarthrosis, and pain may limit findings.[54] Secondary restraints may be stretched, increasing the degree of objective laxity that can be determined on clinical examination.[96]

Evaluation should include the testing of the ligamentous support, the extensor mechanism, and the muscle girth and strength. Evidence of muscle wasting or decreased strength, not only of the muscles about the knee but also the hip and ankle, should be assessed. Loss of muscle strength or instability may be evidenced by an abnormal gait or asymmetry of action on such tests as running in place or the leaning-hop test. Instrumented muscle strength testing may not correlate with function but does provide objective muscle strength and endurance base lines.

The alignment of the extremities for varus angulation, valgus angulation, or recurvatum should be checked. An abnormal varus thrust during gait should be looked for because it may influence the surgical treatment.[4, 48, 75, 82, 87]

Imaging Studies

Routine radiographs should include the flexion weight-bearing view and standing anteroposterior, Merchant's, and lateral views. Full-length standing radiographs may be required in patients with abnormal alignment or degenerative changes in order to determine the precise axis of weight bearing through the joint.

Loss of joint space and the presence of articular defects, condylar flattening, osteophytes, spur formation, soft tissue calcification, subchondral sclerosis or cysts, patellofemoral malalignment, and shifts in weight-bearing alignment are findings that may be present in a patient with chronic instability.

MRI is usually not necessary. It may be indicated when (1) mechanical symptoms consistent with a meniscal tear are present and the patient does not want arthroscopy without further diagnostic proof (MRI is not as accurate, sensitive, or specific in chronic cases as in acute cases);[12, 13] (2) the patient has sustained new contact injuries that require evaluation of meniscal or ligamentous damage; and (3) the findings by clinical and radiographic evaluation are unclear and arthroscopy is not indicated or desired by the patient.

Arthroscopy is indicated in patients with mechanical symptoms that are consistent with osteochondral lesions or meniscal tears that are not improving or that worsen with rest, anti-inflammatory medication, rehabilitation, and activity modification.[19]

ANTERIOR AND ANTEROLATERAL INSTABILITY

Treatment

There are several categories of patients with problems related to chronic anterior or anterolateral instability. Some seek medical attention because of mechanical symptoms produced by a torn cartilage or osteochondral lesion. Some have degenerative changes of the knee that produce discomfort with use as well as the instability. The majority are incapacitated by the pivot-shift phenomenon, which limits their desired activity level.[29]

Symptoms such as locking, catching, a sensation of loose bodies, and the pain that they produce may be relieved by arthroscopic surgery. A decision then has to be made as to whether the instability requires surgical resolution. If a reparable meniscal tear is present (see Chapter 16), the chances of a successful result are enhanced by a simultaneous reconstruction of the ACL.[16, 20, 34, 92, 102, 109] This procedure is the choice for the active patient who plans to continue placing high demands on the knee. The less active patient who is willing to modify activities to the point of eliminating jumping and contact sports may be treated by a rehabilitation program for maintaining muscle strength and by the use of a functional knee brace during less strenuous recreational activities.[8, 27, 28]

Patients whose main problem is functional instability need to be counseled with regard to the alternatives of treatment available. Disabling instability may be relieved by a proper rehabilitation program that includes muscle strengthening, proprioceptive exercises, bracing, and activity modification.[11, 28, 33, 68, 69, 90] Patients who fail such a conservative approach or who insist on a more active lifestyle require ACL reconstruction.[8, 11, 27, 84] The types of ACL reconstructions available and their techniques are discussed in Chapter 20.

There are some patients with lesser degrees of anterolateral instability and only a moderate activity level who may yet have a functional disability in their activities of daily living. These patients are often seen in the more mature age group. An extra-articular procedure to restrain the excessive anterior subluxation of the lateral tibial plateau may be indicated in this circumstance.[3, 10, 22, 23, 35, 38, 43, 47, 55, 64] There is some disagreement as to the value of extra-articular procedures for ACL deficiency. Because of a lower percentage of satisfactory results with extra-articular procedures and the high degree of successful results with intra-articular reconstruction with relative low morbidity, some authors strongly believe that there is no place for the use of extra-articular procedures. In a consensual validation conference sponsored by the American Orthopaedic Society for Sports Medicine, it was agreed that there were some limited indications and that 75 per cent satisfactory results could be expected if a proper isometric attachment site that allows a normal coupling of anterior force on the tibia with its rotational force and yet reduces abnormal subluxation of the lateral tibial plateau is achieved.

Techniques of Lateral Extra-Articular Reconstruction

The rationale for using a lateral extra-articular procedure is to produce a restricting ligament to reduce the abnormal anterolateral translation of the lateral tibial plateau with regard to the lateral femoral condyle. Several techniques have been described.

AUTHORS' PREFERRED TECHNIQUE (LEMAIRE'S PROCEDURE).[62] An extra-articular procedure alone requires tissue of adequate tensile strength to withstand the repetitive rotational forces applied to it. This is achieved in Lemaire's technique by taking a 15- to 20-mm–wide strip of the area between the middle and posterior thirds of the iliotibial tract, detaching it approximately 12 to 15 cm proximally, and pleating the band. It is directed beneath the lateral collateral ligament just distal to its superior insertion (Fig. 21–1A). A 1-cm horizontal incision in the periosteum over the lateral femoral condyle just posterior to the lateral collateral ligament insertion is made, and a similar incision is made parallel to and 2 to 3 cm above the first incision. The periosteum is elevated between these two incisions, forming a subperiosteal tunnel.

A vertical bony tunnel on the lateral femoral condyle is made with the orifices above and below the periosteal bridge that was created. The two drill holes are connected by means of a curved rasp (Fig. 21–1E). A small staple tangent to the lower edge of the proximal drill hole is used to reinforce the bone at this area of stress (Fig. 21–1B). A loop of heavy suture is passed from the distal hole to exit out the proximal drill hole, and the loop is directed from the top of the subperiosteal bridge to exit distally. This loop is tied to a heavy suture in the end of the band and directs the band through its passageway. The end of the pleated iliotibial band is then passed beneath the subperiosteal tissue bridge toward the superior drill hole (Fig. 21–1C).

With the knee in 30° flexion and the tibia in external rotation, tension is placed on the iliotibial band, and four nonabsorbable sutures are used to fix the band at this point. The end of the band is then taken through the superior hole and out the inferior hole. The free end is then passed beneath the lateral collateral ligament, which is sutured to itself, and is reattached at Gerdy's tubercle with nonabsorbable suture (Fig. 21–1D). The point of proximal fixation of the pleated band corresponds to the near-isometric point of the lateral side of the knee, as described by Krakow and Brooks[57] and others.[21, 30, 38] The defect created in the iliotibial tract is closed proximally and continued distally with interrupted sutures. If excessive tightness develops as the closure proceeds distally, the posterior edge of the fascia can be released to provide enough slack to allow closure. A drain is used for 24 hours.

Postoperative care consists of a brace to hold the knee in extension in the immediate postoperative period. No immobilization is used. Quadriceps muscle contraction and straight-leg raising is started the day after surgery on an hourly basis for as long as the patient tolerates. Crutch walking with touch-down weight bearing is continued for 2 weeks, after which a full rehabilitation program for restoring normal walking gait, mobility, and muscle strength is initiated. A progressive return to work and sport activities is begun 6 weeks after surgery if adequate progress in the rehabilitation program has been achieved.

In extra-articular procedures combined with intra-articular ACL reconstruction,[14, 15, 56, 104, 110] a tenodesis of a portion of the iliotibial tract can be used as a simple method to provide lateral support to the healing intra-articular ACL reconstruction. Noyes and Barber[76] found improved results in the combined procedure when using allografts as the intra-articular

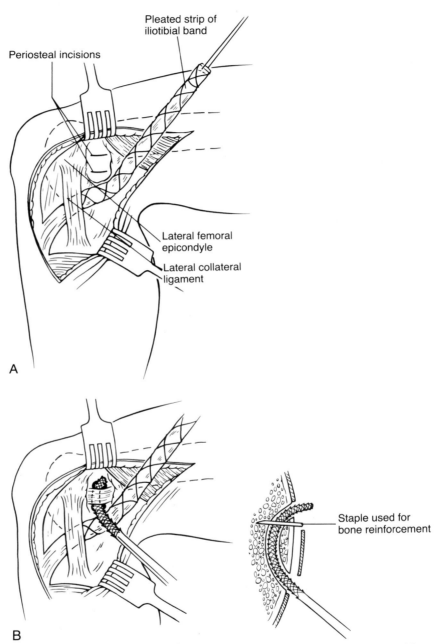

FIGURE 21–1. Lemaire's extra-articular lateral reconstruction. (*A*) A 15- to 20-mm-wide strip of iliotibial band is left attached distally and detached proximally to provide a 12- to 15-cm strip. This strip is pleated with sutures and directed beneath the lateral collateral ligament (LCL). The periosteum is incised just posterior to the femoral attachment of the LCL and a similar incision is made 2 to 3 cm proximal. The periosteum is elevated between these incisions. (*B*) A vertical bony tunnel is created between these two incisions with the use of an awl and a curved rasp.

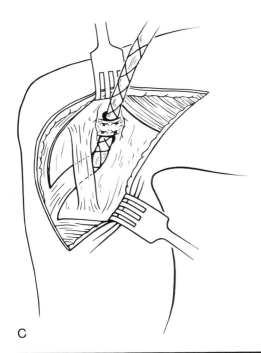

C

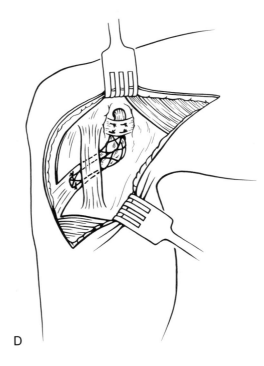

D

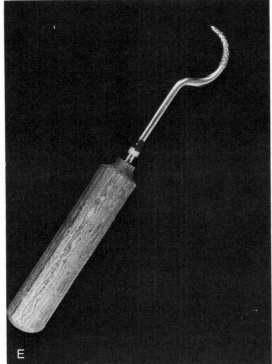

E

FIGURE 21–1 *(continued)* (*C*) The pleated iliotibial strip is passed beneath the periosteal bridge of tissue. (*D*) The strip is then passed through the proximal tunnel opening to exit through the distal tunnel opening and under the LCL, where it is fixed to Gerdy's tubercle. (*E*) The curved rasp used to create the bone tunnel.

graft. The combined procedure was used in patients with above-normal body weight, those with loss of primary and secondary restraints, and those who wished to return to strenuous sports.

MÜLLER'S EXTRA-ARTICULAR PROCEDURE.[72] A skin incision is made 4 cm anterior to the posterior border of the iliotibial tract, starting at the junction of the femoral shaft and lateral condyle. It is extended distally curving toward Gerdy's tubercle and slightly beyond. Two incisions are made in the iliotibial tract. The anterior incision begins between the anterior two thirds and the posterior third and ends just proximal to the joint line. The posterior incision begins 12 to 15 mm posterior to the anterior incision, parallels the anterior incision, and ends at a point just above the joint line (Fig. 21–2A). The strip is left attached proximally and distally and is made 15 to 20 cm in length, but it must extend at least 10 cm above the metaphysis of the femur.

The vastus lateralis is retracted anteriorly to expose the distal shaft of the femur, the lateral condyle, and the intermuscular septum. The superior genicular artery is usually seen in this area and should be ligated. The isometric point for the tenodesis is determined by using a K-wire to temporarily fix the incised band to the femur. This point is usually about 1 cm proximal to the junction of the femoral shaft and the lateral femoral condyle.[21, 30] After the band is impaled at the determined point, the knee is placed through a full range of motion, including internal rotation, which should be full but not excessive, and a determination is made that the sunken strip comes under isometric tension. This should eliminate the pivot shift without overconstraining the tibia.

After the isometric point has been determined, a cannulated drill and

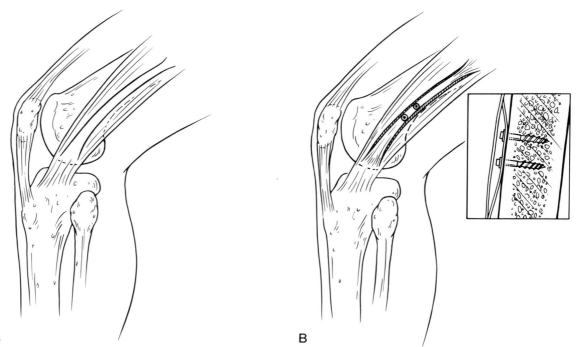

A   B

FIGURE 21–2. Müller's extra-articular reconstruction. (*A*) An incision is made in the iliotibial tract. (*B*) Screw fixation of incised band provides a lateral constraint to forward displacement of tibia.

tap are used, followed by final fixation with a cannulated screw and ligament washer. A second screw and washer are placed 1.5 cm proximal to the first screw to prevent it from turning and loosening postoperatively (Fig. 21–2B). The intra-articular procedure should be completed and laterally fixed before the tenodesis. Interrupted sutures are used to close the tract over the sunken fixed strip.

STEADMAN'S EXTRA-ARTICULAR PROCEDURE.[38] A lateral approach like that just described is used. A strip 2 cm wide by 10 cm in length is isolated from the posterior third of the iliotibial tract. The strip is divided longitudinally into two bands; the posterior band comprises 60 per cent of the total width. A 6.5-mm cancellous screw with a ligament washer is placed on the posterolateral edge of the femoral shaft just proximal to the condylar flare with an anterior-distal orientation (Fig. 21–3A). Each band is reinforced with three sets of heavy nonabsorbable suture. The anterior band is released proximally with enough length to wrap it around the screw (Fig. 21–3B). With tension maintained on the band, the screw is tightened. Because of its position and slight anterior angulation, the screw

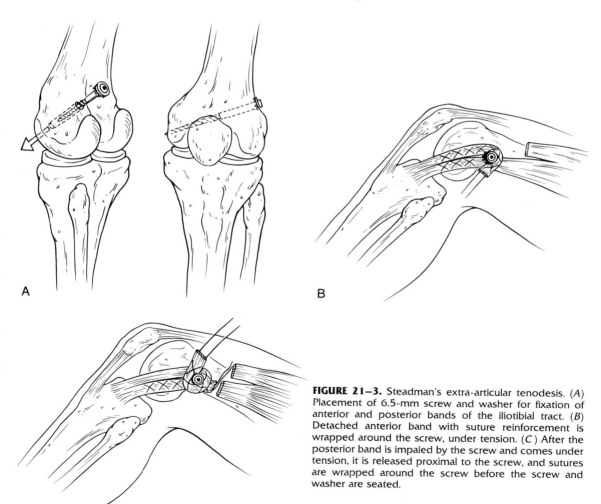

A

B

C

FIGURE 21–3. Steadman's extra-articular tenodesis. (*A*) Placement of 6.5-mm screw and washer for fixation of anterior and posterior bands of the iliotibial tract. (*B*) Detached anterior band with suture reinforcement is wrapped around the screw, under tension. (*C*) After the posterior band is impaled by the screw and comes under tension, it is released proximal to the screw, and sutures are wrapped around the screw before the screw and washer are seated.

impales the posterior band, which tightens with screw advancement. When bone contact by the washer occurs, the posterior band is released proximally, the sutures and band used for reinforcement are wrapped around the screw, and the screw is firmly seated with the knee held in 20° to 30° of flexion (Fig. 21–3C). The knee is then tested for range of motion and to see whether a negative result of Lachman's test has been achieved. The defect in the iliotibial tract is closed.

Chronic Instability Associated With Varus Angulation and Degenerative Changes

Articular cartilage degeneration, an abnormal varus or valgus stance or gait, and loss of motion as a result of degenerative changes associated with a chronic instability require an evaluation; a bony procedure such as a high tibial osteotomy may be necessary. When such late changes have occurred, moderation in activity is required regardless of whether a surgical procedure is indicated.

A varus deformity in a patient with an ACL instability is predisposed to medial meniscal tears, increased compressive forces in the medial joint compartment with resultant medial arthrosis and osteoarthritis, and increased tensile forces on the lateral side that may stretch out the secondary restraints. Medial femoral and notch osteophytes often develop with medial contractures and loss of joint motion. Patellofemoral symptoms may occur. An ACL reconstruction in the presence of genu varum may be doomed to failure.

A high tibial osteotomy to correct alignment and reduce the high adduction forces on the knee is necessary before ACL reconstruction can be considered.[75] Reports of the high tibial osteotomy and ACL reconstructions performed concomitantly have shown good results, although it is a salvage procedure for a significantly disabled knee.[48, 82]

Patients with a varus deformity and moderate to severe degenerative changes should have full-length radiographs and evaluation of the gait in order to determine the extent of the shift of the weight-bearing axis to the medial side and the varus thrust that occurs to the knee during walking.[4, 87] Arthroscopy should be performed in order to debride the knee and to visually evaluate the articular surfaces. The presence of smooth, intact articular cartilage in the lateral and patellofemoral compartments provides a good indication for a high tibial osteotomy.

The technique for high tibial osteotomy[40, 101] is described in Chapter 11. An intra-articular reconstruction with the use of either bone–patellar tendon–bone or semitendinosus tendon as the graft may be used. In some patients, an extra-articular procedure such as that described earlier may be adequate.[48, 82]

Patients with severe degenerative joint changes and loss of motion should first undergo aggressive rehabilitation, activity modification, and bracing. Arthroscopic joint debridement may also provide some temporary relief. The patient's age, the involvement of the joint, and the response and toleration of conservative care are considered in the determination of whether a high tibial osteotomy will provide enough improvement for a significant amount of time or whether more extensive procedures such as total knee replacement or arthrodesis are required.

Results of Treatment

Noyes and associates reported on symptomatic patients with chronic ACL instability treated over a 3-year period with rehabilitation, activity modification, and bracing.[77, 78] One third of the patients improved and compensated to the point of having minimal symptoms with recreational activities; one third remained the same in spite of treatment; and one third did not benefit by the program and required reconstructive surgery or were considering surgery.

Fowler and Regan[27] treated a similar series of patients with diagnostic or surgical arthroscopy and rehabilitation. At 1.5 years after arthroscopy and 5.8 years after injury, two thirds of the patients returned to some level of athletics. Twenty per cent showed evidence of degenerative changes. Other authors have confirmed that a structured and maintained rehabilitation program with arthroscopic procedures such as partial meniscectomy or meniscal repair will allow 30 to 50 per cent of patients with chronic symptomatic ACL insufficiency to return to activities of daily living and low-demand recreational sports without major soft tissue or bony reconstruction.[1, 8, 11, 95] It is emphasized that the knees of these patients were not normal and would continue to have symptoms of some degree with strenuous activities and possible occasional episodes of giving way or reinjury.

Among patients requiring surgical reconstruction of the ACL, the success rate is only slightly below that of those who underwent procedures in the acute phase. Successful results in 70 to 85 per cent of patients have been reported with intra-articular or combined intra- and extra-articular procedures.[7, 15, 36, 49, 50, 56, 70, 94, 104, 110]

ANTEROMEDIAL AND MEDIAL INSTABILITY

Chronic medial or anteromedial instability is the result of previous injury to the medial collateral ligament (MCL), the posterior oblique ligament (POL), the medial capsule, or the semimembranosus complex. These injuries are often associated with ACL injury. Injury to these structures causes excessive abnormal valgus angulation, external rotation, anterior or medial tibial translation, or a combination of instabilities. Rarely does a knee ligament injury produce a one-plane instability; it usually creates a combination of instabilities involving translational as well as rotational components.[29, 41, 60, 85, 96, 97]

Instability involving the medial structures is usually manifested by an uncertainty of support on the inner side of the knee when a valgus thrust is applied to the weight-bearing leg. A change in direction opposite to that of the weight-bearing leg during walking or running produces a sense of insecurity or inward buckling of the knee. This should be differentiated from the sudden pivot shift, in which there is an actual subluxation of the tibia on the femur. An associated ACL insufficiency may produce such giving way, and when present, the associated medial instability may be missed unless specifically looked for. The ACL is the primary restraint to anterior tibial translation and a major secondary restraint to medial joint opening. Knowledge of its status in a patient with anteromedial or medial instability is essential in the planning of appropriate treatment.

The meniscus—medial or lateral—may become injured as a result of excessive stresses and shear forces produced by the rotational instability. Symptoms of mechanical catching or locking that may be present may also confuse the diagnosis.

A complete evaluation of the stabilizing structures of the knee as described in Chapter 4 should be conducted. Special attention is given to the stability on valgus stress at both 0° and 30°, to the results of the Lachman test, and to the results of the anterior drawer test with the leg in external rotation.[97] The latter test as described by Lemaire and colleagues[62, 63] produces a click as the medial tibia is pulled anteriorly, dragging the posterior horn of the medial meniscus underneath the medial femoral condyle when the POL is torn. Differentiation of the types of instabilities present and their severity is important in order to determine the surgical correction required. The surgical results of combined instabilities are less satisfactory than those of reconstruction for a chronic isolated ACL or MCL instability.[5, 25, 26, 41, 60, 80, 108]

Routine radiographs should be evaluated for soft tissue calcifications along the medial side of the knee, osteophytes in the notch, or other bony changes suggestive of degeneration of the joint.

Treatment

The patient's complaints and disability as well as activity levels desired and required should be determined.

Many patients have had a recent injury similar to a previous injury from which they fully recovered. They protect and minimally use the leg and develop muscle atrophy and weakness, of which they might not be aware. A mild medial instability may be present, for which they had previously compensated by muscle strength. The muscle weakness produced by the recent injury produces a chronicity of symptoms. In such a situation, a specific and supervised program of muscle strengthening exercises may be all that is necessary for them to return to their fully compensated level of activity.[6, 24, 26, 28, 37, 45, 53, 71] A rehabilitation program and the possible use of a brace should be the first considerations in the treatment of medial or anteromedial instability.

Failure of nonoperative treatment with a continuation of the functional disability in the desired activities is an indication for a surgical approach to the problem. Most often there is an ACL deficiency in association with the medial instability.[25, 26, 41, 89, 108] This should be the primary structure reconstructed.[26, 93, 108] The medial extra-articular reconstructive procedures may or may not be required, depending on the severity and on whether a global instability is present.[93] If no ACL laxity is present but medial structures are stretched and insufficient, medial reconstruction can be accomplished with the goal of providing medial support to the flexed knee against valgus and rotatory stress.[42]

Surgical Treatment

Techniques for ACL reconstruction are described in Chapter 20. The goals of the surgical approach to the medial side are to preserve the meniscus, establish appropriate tension of the POL, establish continuity and tension of the MCL, and establish the semimembranosus attachments. If tissues of poor quality that are inadequate for providing static support are found, augmentation with autogenous tissue and occasionally dynamic procedures[46, 47, 91, 98–100] to dissipate forces on the reconstructed structures are required. The POL, the MCL, and the posterior horn of the medial meniscus are key structures in establishing medial side stability.[42, 46, 61, 73, 100]

Positioning of the patient and the medial utility incision as described in Chapter 20 are used (see Figs. 20–4, 20–5).

REEFING AND RECONSTRUCTION OF THE POL. Elongation of the POL from previous injury results in excessive external rotation of the tibia and increased stress on the posterior horn of the medial meniscus. Proper tension of this structure must be restored in order for it to regain stabilizing function. If satisfactory tissue with good tensile strength is available, a reefing procedure[46, 61, 100] to take the slack out of the ligament can be used (see Figs. 20–6A, 20–6B). An oblique incision beginning at the medial femoral epicondyle is brought distally and posteriorly to the posterior edge of the tibia; the anteromedial limb of the semimembranosus muscle is its stopping point. The incision is closed by imbricating the posterior edge beneath the anterior portion; mattress sutures are used to take up the amount of slack necessary. The anterior edge is then brought over the closure in a double-breasted manner and sutured with individual mattress sutures. Flexion and extension are checked repeatedly during placement of the sutures to ensure that motion is not compromised and that the sutures do not pull out. The ligament can be advanced by 1 to 2 cm with this method.

If posterior capsular laxity is also present, slack should be taken out of this tissue by detaching its tibial insertion and advancing it distally on the tibia (Fig. 21–4).[61, 100] Reattachment is accomplished with sutures passed through drill holes made from anterior to posterior on the posterior

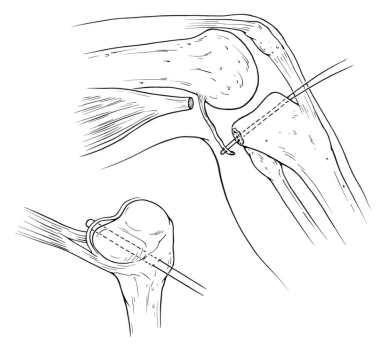

FIGURE 21–4. Distal advancement of the posterior capsule and fixation with suture through drill holes when laxity is present.

tibia. It is necessary to extend the knee to determine the point of attachment that does not interfere with normal motion. Posterior capsular tightening should be completed before tightening of the POL.

AUGMENTATION OF THE POL. Additional support to the POL can be provided by use of the anteromedial limb and the conjoined tendon of the semimembranosus muscle.[46, 61, 72] This can be accomplished in two ways. The anteromedial limb and the conjoined tendon are brought proximally over the imbricated portion of the POL and sutured (see Fig. 20–7B). The anteromedial limb is then detached from its tibial insertion beneath the MCL and reattached superficially to the MCL in line with the portion sewn to the POL. This provides a dynamic pull by the semimembranosus muscle to the POL, augmenting its stabilizing function.

In a technique described by Müller,[72] the posterior half of the anteromedial limb and conjoined tendon (Fig. 21–5) is left attached on the tibia, and the proximal portion is detached and swung proximally in order to attach it superiorly beneath the posterior edge of the MCL. It is sutured both to the tibia and the meniscus to reproduce the natural attachment sites of the POL. Care must be exercised in determining the proximal attachment site that maintains tension with both flexion and extension of the knee.

RECONSTRUCTION OF THE MCL. If the MCL is not too severely attenuated or replaced by inadequate scar tissue, it may be advanced distally on the tibia (Fig. 21–6). It has been found that repositioning distally produces better biomechanical tension of the ligament than does proximal advancement.[9] Although an en bloc advancement of the entire medial capsule and the MCL has been described, this creates abnormal tension to the medial structures and may interfere with normal meniscal function.[66, 81]

Reconstruction of the MCL can be accomplished by using the gracilis tendon (Fig. 21–7).[62, 63] The tendon is detached distally and isolated proximally to above the medial femoral condyle. A vertical incision is

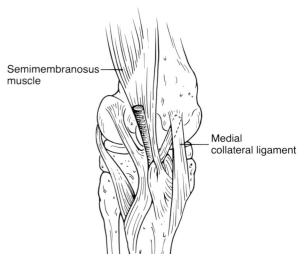

Semimembranosus muscle

Medial collateral ligament

FIGURE 21–5. Müller's procedure for augmenting a deficient posterior oblique ligament. Posterior half of the anteromedial tendon of the semimembranosus muscle is detached proximally and is passed beneath the anterior portion of the tendon and reattached beneath the posterior edge of the superior attachment of the medial collateral ligament (MCL).

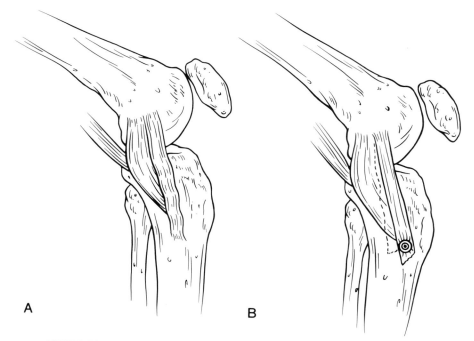

FIGURE 21–6. Distal advancement of the MCL on the tibia for taking out slack.

made along the line of the normal MCL to its distal attachment site (Fig. 21–7A). The distal attachment point is established as the midportion of the distal attachment site. A caliper is used to determine the proximal attachment site near the medial femoral epicondyle in order to make it as isometric as possible. The proximal point of the caliper is firmly fixed with the distal point over the distal attachment site. With the caliper in place over the two attachment sites, the knee is extended. If the distal point goes beyond the point marked, the proximal attachment site is too anterior; if the distal point goes beyond the marked point at 45° and then returns to it, the proximal point is too low. Trial and error will determine the ideal proximal attachment site.

A drill hole is made from the medial femoral epicondyle at this point to exit at the flare posteriorly of the medial femoral condyle. The end of the tendon is passed through this tunnel from posterior to anterior (Fig. 21–7B). It is then laid in the trough of tissue and fixed distally at the predetermined site with a screw and washer or with staples. The two edges of the old MCL are imbricated over the tendon to provide tightening of this tissue with its augmentation (Fig. 21–7C). Full range of motion should be obtained after fixation of the tendon.

The sartorial slide provides a dynamic augmentation to a reefing or repair of the MCL.[46, 61, 100] This is shown in Figures 20–8A and 20–8B.

PES ANSERINUS TRANSFER.[98–100] Proximal transfer of the distal portion of the pes anserinus attachment provides a sling beneath the flare of the medial tibia and a dynamic restraint to excessive external rotation of the tibia.[79, 86] With the improvement of intra-articular reconstruction of the ACL, this procedure is rarely necessary. The procedure can be used in the chronically injured knee as an ancillary back-up to help protect the

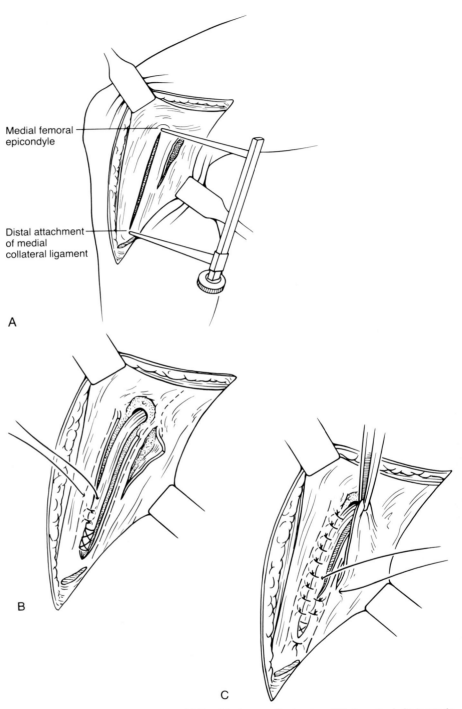

Medial femoral
epicondyle

Distal attachment
of medial
collateral ligament

A

B

C

FIGURE 21–7. Augmentation of the MCL with the gracilis tendon. (*A*) A vertical slit is made in the center of the MCL from its superior to distal attachments. (*B*) The gracilis tendon is detached distally and passed through a drill hole from the posterior medial aspect of the medial femoral condyle to exit at the superior attachment of the MCL. The tendon is placed in the vertical slit and anchored distally. (*C*) The flaps of the deficient MCL are closed over the buried gracilis tendon.

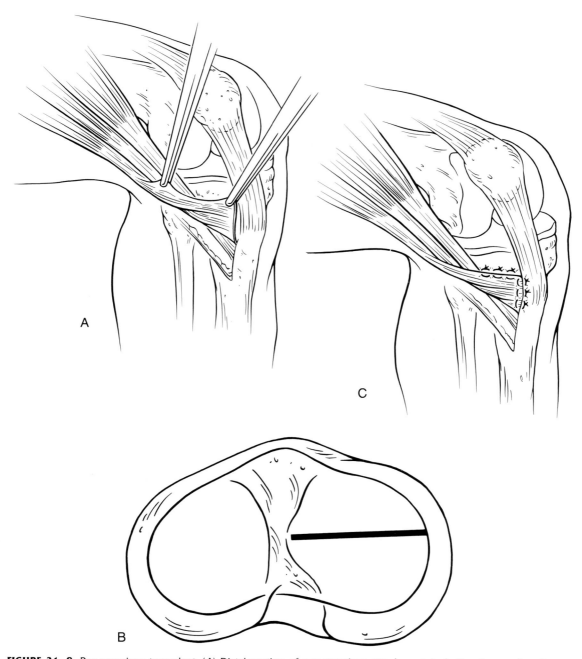

FIGURE 21–8. Pes anserinus transplant. (A) Distal portion of pes anserinus attachment, including the semitendinosus tendon, has been advanced proximally beneath the flare of the medial tibial plateau. (B) This advancement increases the lever arm and makes the semitendinosus muscle a more effective internal rotator of the knee. (C) Depiction of reflected distal attachment of the pes anserinus, showing semitendinosus and gracilis. (D) Reattachment to medial aspect of patellar tendon.

static structures against excessive anteromedial rotation of the tibia. The semitendinosus tendon is the key to the procedure because it must be positioned more proximally at the flare of the proximal tibia to increase its mechanical efficiency as an internal rotator (Figs. 21–8*A*, 21–8*B*). Failure to identify and include the semitendinosus tendon in the transfer was one of the chief causes for inadequacy of the procedure. The pes anserinus transfer does not control anterolateral instability manifested as a pivot-shift phenomenon.

The technique involves identification of the distal portion of the semitendinosus tendon located at the inferior attachment site of the pes anserinus. The distal two thirds of the pes anserinus is detached as far anterior on its tibial attachment site as possible; the detachment must include both the semitendinosus and the gracilis tendons (Fig. 21–8*C*). This tissue is then rotated proximally so the tendons cradle the flare of the medial tibial condyle. It is a mistake to place them too high and lose the sling effect. In mobilizing the inferior portion of the pes anserinus, care is taken to identify and protect the sartorial branch of saphenous nerve, which penetrates the fascia between the sartorius and the gracilis muscles at the musculotendinous junction of the sartorius muscle.[59] Proper tension is required to sustain the muscle power of the pes group. The tendons are sutured to the medial edge of the patellar tendon, beginning distally with an interrupted mattress suture and proceeding proximally (Fig. 21–8*D*). In this region, the inferior branch of the medial genicular artery may be injured, and so hemostasis must be obtained before wound closure.

Range of knee motion must be checked at the conclusion of the surgery. If full motion can be obtained without putting marked stress on the reconstructed tissues, protected mobilization in a hinged brace is used.

Many methods have been described to achieve medial stability. The simplest procedure or procedures that will achieve the goal are most appropriate. The quality of the tissue and the adequacy of remaining intact structures must be assessed. In some cases a simple reefing of the POL is all that is required.

The frequency of surgical reconstruction for chronic anteromedial or medial instability has markedly decreased with the advent of the more precise diagnosis of ACL injury and its treatment. Those cases that do occur are frequently associated with an unrecognized or untreated ACL tear.

Satisfactory results from the surgical treatment for chronic medial instability can be achieved in 70 to 80 per cent of patients.[18, 31, 41, 43, 47, 73, 80, 83, 98, 106, 107] Normalcy in the injured knee in comparison with the contralateral knee is not usually achieved because the repaired and reconstructed tissue does not have the physiologic elasticity, is not as precise in its isometric position, and does not have the tensile strength of an uninjured MCL. Resolution of the functional incapacity is the primary goal to be attained.

REFERENCES

1. Aglietti P, Buzzi R, Basi P: Arthroscopic partial meniscectomy in the anterior cruciate deficient knee. Am J Sports Med 16:597–602, 1983.
2. Allen PR, Denham RA, Swan AV: Late degenerative changes after a meniscectomy: factors affecting the knee after operation. J Bone Joint Surg 66B:666–671, 1984.

3. Andrews JR, Sanders RA, Morin B: Surgical treatment of anterolateral rotatory instability: a followup study. Am J Sports Med 13:112–119, 1985.
4. Andriacchi T: Gait analysis in ACL deficient knees: applications of gait analysis to clinical medicine. *Presented at* the American Academy of Orthopaedic Surgeons, Instructional Course #101, Anaheim, CA, February 1990.
5. Balkfors B: The course of knee ligament injuries. Acta Orthop Scan 53:1, 1982.
6. Ballmer P, Jacob R: The nonoperative treatment of isolated complete tears of the medial collateral ligament of the knee. Arch Orthop Trauma Surg 107:273–276, 1988.
7. Barber F, Small N, Clik J: Anterior cruciate ligament reconstruction by semitendinosus and gracilis tendon autograft. Am J Knee Surg 4:84, 1991.
8. Barrack RL, Bruckner J, Kneisel J, et al: The outcome of non-operatively treated complete tears of the ACL in the active young adults. Clin Orthop 259:192–199, 1990.
9. Bartel DL, Marshall JL, Schieck BS, et al: Surgical repositioning of the medial collateral ligament. J Bone Joint Surg 59A:107–116, 1977.
10. Beyer A, Shields C, Kerlan RK, et al: Extraarticular reconstruction of the anterior cruciate ligament: a long-term followup of 54 cases. Orthop Trans 8:75, 1984.
11. Bonamo J, Fay C, Firestone T: The conservative treatment of the anterior cruciate deficient knee. Am J Sports Med 18:618, 1990.
12. Burger R: Magnetic resonance imaging of the meniscus: how accurate? *Presented at* the 52nd annual meeting of the Western Orthopaedic Association, Honolulu, HI, October 1988.
13. Burger RS, Baciocco E, Conrad S, et al: Magnetic resonance imaging of the meniscus: how accurate? Orthop Trans 13:65, 1989.
14. Clancy W: Anterior cruciate ligament functional instability: a static intraarticular and dynamic extraarticular procedure. Clin Orthop 172:102, 1983.
15. Clancy WG Jr, Nelson DA, Reider B, Narechania RG: Anterior cruciate ligament reconstruction using one-third of the patellar ligament, augmented by extra-articular tendon transfers. J Bone Joint Surg 64A:352–359, 1982.
16. Cooper D, Arnoczky F, Warren R: Arthroscopic meniscal repair. Clin Sports Med 9:589–607, 1990.
17. Cox J, Nye C, Schaffer W, Woodstein I: The degenerative effect of partial and total resection of the medial meniscus in dogs' knees. Clin Orthop 109:178, 1975.
18. D'Arcy J: Pes anserinus transposition for chronic anteromedial rotational instability of the knee. J Bone Joint Surg 60A:66–70, 1978.
19. DeHaven KE: Arthroscopy in the diagnosis and management of the ACL deficient knee. Clin Orthop 172:52–56, 1983.
20. DeHaven K, Sebatianelli W: Open meniscus repairs: indications, technique, and results. Clin Sports Med 9:577–587, 1990.
21. Draganich L, Reider B, Ling M, Samuelson M: An in vitro study of an intraarticular and extraarticular reconstruction in the anterior cruciate ligament deficient knee. Am J Sports Med 18:262–266, 1990.
22. Durken J, Wynne G, Haggerty J: Extraarticular reconstruction of the anterior cruciate ligament insufficient knee: a long-term analysis of the Ellison procedure. Am J Sports Med 17:112, 1989.
23. Ellison A: Distal iliotibial band transfer for anterolateral rotatory instability of the knee. J Bone Joint Surg 61A:330–337, 1979.
24. Ellsasser J: The nonoperative treatment of collateral ligament injuries of the knee in professional football players. J Bone Joint Surg 56A:1185, 1974.
25. Fetto J, Marshall J: Medial collateral ligament injuries of the knee: a rationale for treatment. Clin Orthop 132:206–218, 1978.
26. Fetto J, Marshall J: The natural history and diagnosis of anterior cruciate ligament insufficiency. Clin Orthop 147:29, 1980.
27. Fowler P, Regan W: The patient with a symptomatic chronic anterior cruciate ligament insufficiency: results of minimal arthroscopic surgery and rehabilitation. Am J Sports Med 15:321, 1987.
28. Frieden T, Zätterström R, Lindstrand A, Moritz U: Anterior cruciate insufficient knees treated with physiotherapy: a three-year followup study of patients with late diagnosis. Clin Orthop 263:190–199, 1991.
29. Galway HR, MacIntosh DL: The lateral pivot shift as symptom and sign of anterior cruciate ligament insufficiency. Clin Orthop 147:45–50, 1980.
30. Gibson M, Mikosz R, Reider B, Andriacchi T: Analysis of the Müller anterolateral femoral tibial ligament reconstruction using a computerized knee model. Am J Sports Med 14:371, 1986.
31. Gillespie H: An operation for anteriomedial rotatory instability of the knee. J Bone Joint Surg 62B:457–459, 1980.
32. Gillquist J, Oretor N: Orthoscopic partial meniscectomy: technique and long-term results. Clin Orthop 167:29–33, 1982.
33. Giove TP, Miller SJ 3d, Kent BE, et al: Non-operative treatment of the torn anterior cruciate ligament. J Bone Joint Surg 65A:184–192, 1983.

34. Hanks G, Gause TM, Handel JA, Kalenak A: Meniscus repair in the anterior cruciate deficient knee. Am J Sports Med 18:606–623, 1990.

35. Hanks G, Joyner D, Kalenak A: Anterolateral rotatory instability of the knee: an analysis of the Ellison procedure. Am J Sports Med 9:225–232, 1981.

36. Harter R, Osternig L, Singer K: Instrumented Lachman tests for the evaluation of anterior laxity after reconstruction of the anterior cruciate ligament. J Bone Joint Surg 71A:975–983, 1989.

37. Hastings DE: The nonoperative management of collateral ligament injuries of the knee. Clin Orthop 147:22, 1980.

38. Higgins R, Steadman J: Anterior cruciate ligament repairs in world class skiers. Am J Sports Med 15:439, 1987.

39. Hirschman HP, Daniel DM, Miyasaka K: The fate of unoperated knee ligament injuries. *In* Daniel DM (ed): Knee Ligaments: Structure, Function, Injury and Repair, pp. 481–503. New York: Raven Press, 1980.

40. Holden D, James S, Larson R, Slocum D: Proximal tibial osteotomy in patients who are 50 years old or less: a long-term followup study. J Bone Joint Surg 70A:977, 1988.

41. Hughston J, Andrews J, Cross M, Moshi A: Classification of knee ligament instabilities. Part I: the medial compartment in cruciate ligaments. J Bone Joint Surg 58A:159–172, 1976.

42. Hughston J, Eilers A: The role of the posterior oblique ligament in repairs of acute medial ligament tears of the knee. J Bone Joint Surg 55A:923–940, 1973.

43. Hunter S, Andrews J, McLeod W, et al: Surgical reconstruction of chronic anteromedial rotatory instability of the knee. Am J Sports Med 7:165–168, 1979.

44. Indelicato P: Non-operative treatment of complete tears of the medial collateral ligament of the knee. J Bone Joint Surg 65A:323, 1983.

45. Indelicato P, Bittar E: A perspective of lesions associated with ACL insufficiency of the knee. Clin Orthop 198:77–80, 1985.

46. James SL: Biomechanics of knee ligament reconstruction. Clin Orthop 146:90–101, 1980.

47. James SL: Knee ligament reconstruction. *In* Evarts MC (ed): Surgery of Muskuloskeletal System, vol 3, pp. 31–110. New York: Churchill-Livingstone, 1983.

48. James SL: Alignment abnormalities in ACL deficient knees: Definitions, diagnosis, and treatment. *Presented at* the American Academy of Orthopaedic Surgeons, CME Course: Anterior and posterior cruciate ligament injuries of the knee, Rancho Mirage, CA, December 1990.

49. Jensen JE, Slocum DB, Larson RL, et al: Reconstruction procedures for anterior cruciate ligament insufficiency: a computer analysis of clinical results. Am J Sports Med 11:240–248, 1983.

50. Johnson R, Eriksson E, Haggmark T, Pope MH: Five- to ten-year follow-up evaluation after reconstruction of the anterior cruciate ligament. Clin Orthop 183:122–140, 1984.

51. Johnson RJ, Kettelkamp D, Clark W, Leaverton P: Factors affecting the late results after meniscectomy. J Bone Joint Surg 56A:719–729, 1974.

52. Woods CW, Chapman DR: Repairable posterior meniscocapsular disruption in ACL injuries. Am J Sports Med 12:381–385, 1984.

53. Jokl P, Kaplan N, Stovell P, Keggi K: Non-operative treatment of severe injuries to the medial and anterior cruciate ligament of the knee. J Bone Joint Surg 66A:741–744, 1984.

54. Jonsson T, Althoff B, Peterson L, Renstrom P: Clinical diagnosis of ruptures of the anterior cruciate ligament: a comparative study of the Lachman test and the anterior drawer test. Am J Sports Med 10:100–102, 1982.

55. Kennedy J, Stewart R, Walker D: An early analysis of the Ellison procedure. J Bone Joint Surg 60A:1031, 1978.

56. Kornblatt I, Warren R, Wickiewicz T: Combined intraarticular quadriceps tendon substitution and extraarticular lateral sling procedure for chronic anterior cruciate ligament insufficiency. Am J Knee Surg 4:63, 1991.

57. Krakow D, Brooks R: Optimization of knee ligament position for lateral extraarticular reconstruction. Am J Sports Med 11:293–301, 1983.

58. Krause WR, Pope MH, Johnson RJ: Mechanical changes in the knee after arthroscopic meniscectomy. J Bone Joint Surg 58A:599, 1976.

59. Larson R: Complications of dislocations and ligamentous injuries of the knee. *In* Epps C (ed): Complications in Orthopedic Knee Surgery, vol 2, p. 495. Philadelphia: JB Lippincott, 1978.

60. Larson R: Combined instability of the knee. Clin Orthop 147:68–75, 1980.

61. Larson RL, Burger RS: Medial instability of the knee. *In* Chapman MW (ed): Operative Orthopaedics. Philadelphia: JB Lippincott, in press.

62. Lemaire M, Combelles F: Technique actuelle de platie ligamentaire pour rupture ancienne du ligament croise anterieur. Rev Chir Orthop 66:522–525, 1980.

63. Lemaire M, Miremad C: Les instabilites chroniques anteriieures et internes du genou: traitement. Rev Chir Orthop 69:591–601, 1983.

64. Losee RE, Jonsson TR, Southwick W: Anterior subluxation of the lateral tibial plateau with diagnostic tests and operative repair. J Bone Joint Surg 60A:1015–1030, 1978.

65. Marks P, Fowler PJ, Vellet D: MRI detected bone lesions in anterior cruciate injured

knees. *Presented at* the biannual meeting of the International Arthroscopy Association, Toronto, 1991.

66. Mauck H: A new operative procedure for instability of the knee. J Bone Joint Surg 18:984–990, 1936.
67. Metcalf R, Coward D, Rosenberg T: Arthroscopic partial meniscectomy: a five-year follow-up study. Orthop Trans 7:504, 1983.
68. McDaniel N, Dameron T: Untreated ruptures of the anterior cruciate ligament. J Bone Joint Surg 62A:696, 1980.
69. McDaniel N, Dameron T: The untreated anterior cruciate ligament. Clin Orthop 172:158, 1983.
70. Mitsou A, Vallianatos P, Piskopakis N, Maheras S: Anterior cruciate ligament reconstruction by over-the-top repair combined with popliteus tendon plasty. J Bone Joint Surg 72B:398, 1990.
71. Mok D, Good C: Non-operative management of acute grade III medial collateral ligament injury of the knee: a prospective study. Injury 20:277, 1989.
72. Müller W: The Knee: Form, Function, and Ligament Reconstruction. New York: Springer-Verlag, 1983.
73. Nicholas J: The 5-1 reconstruction for anteromedial instability of the knee: indications, technique, and results in 52 patients. J Bone Joint Surg 55A:899–922, 1973.
74. Northmore-Ball MD, Chir MB, Dandy D: Long-term results of arthroscopic partial meniscectomy. Clin Orthop 167:3335–3342, 1982.
75. Noyes FR: The cruciate ligaments: alignment and associated ligament laxities, ACL and PCL injuries of the knee. *Presented at* the American Academy of Orthopaedic Surgeons, CME Course, Monterey, CA, 1989.
76. Noyes FR, Barber SD: The effect of an extra-articular procedure on allograft reconstruction for chronic ruptures of the anterior cruciate ligament. *Presented at* the Combined Session of International Arthroscopy Association and International Society of the Knee, Toronto, 1991.
77. Noyes F, Matthews D, Mooar P, Butler D: The symptomatic anterior cruciate deficient knee. Part I: the long-term functional disability in athletically active individuals. J Bone Joint Surg 65A:154–162, 1983.
78. Noyes F, Matthews D, Mooar P, Grood E: The symptomatic anterior cruciate deficient knee. Part II: the results of rehabilitation, activity modification, and counselling on functional disability. 65A:163–174, 1983.
79. Noyes F, Sonstegard D: Biomechanical function of the pes anserinus at the knee and the effects of its transplantation. J Bone Joint Surg 55A:1225–1241, 1973.
80. O'Donoghue D: Analysis of the end results of surgical treatment of major injuries to the ligaments of the knee. J Bone Joint Surg 37A:1–13, 1955.
81. O'Donoghue D: Reconstruction for medial instability of the knee: technique and results in 60 cases. J Bone Joint Surg 55A:941–955, 1973.
82. O'Neill D, James SL: Valgus osteotomy with anterior cruciate laxity. *Presented at* the American Academy of Orthopaedic Surgeons, CME Course, Rancho Mirage, CA, December 1990.
83. Oretop N, Gillquist J, Liljedahl S: Long-term results of surgery for non-acute anteromedial rotatory instability of the knee. Acta Orthop Scand 50:329, 1979.
84. Pattee G, Fox JM, Del Pizzo W, Friedman MJ: Four to ten year followup of unreconstructed anterior cruciate ligament tears. Am J Sports Med 17:430–435, 1989.
85. Paulos L, Rosenberg T, Parker R: The medial knee ligaments: pathomechanics and surgical repair with the emphasis on the external rotation pivot shift test. Tech Orthop 2:37–46, 1987.
86. Perry J, Fox JM, Boitano MA, et al: Functional evaluation of the pes anserinus transfer by electomyography and gait analysis. J Bone Joint Surg 62A:973–980, 1980.
87. Prodomous C, Andriacchi T, Galante J: A relationship between gait and clinical changes following a high tibial osteotomy. J Bone Joint Surg 67A:1188, 1985.
88. Rosen MA, Jackson DW, Berger PE: Occult osseous lesions documented by MRI associated with anterior cruciate ruptures. *Presented at* the annual meeting of the Arthroscopy Association of North America, Anaheim, CA, 1991.
89. Sandberg R, Balkfors B, Nilsson B, Westlin N: Operative versus non-operative treatment of recent injuries to the ligaments of the knee: a prospective randomized study. J Bone Joint Surg 69A:1120–1126, 1987.
90. Satku K, Kumar V, Ngoi S: Anterior cruciate ligament injuries—to counsel or to operate? J Bone Joint Surg 68B:458, 1986.
91. Seedhom B, Hargreaves D: Transmission of the load in the knee joint with special references to the role of the menisci. Part II: experimental results, discussion and conclusions. Eng Med 8:22–228, 1979.
92. Shelbourne K: Treatment of meniscal injuries in ACL deficient knees. *Presented at* the American Academy of Orthopaedic Surgeons, CME Course: Anterior and posterior cruciate ligament injuries of the knee, Rancho Mirage, CA, December 1990.
93. Shelbourne KD, Baele JR: Treatment of combined ACL and MCL injuries. Am J Knee Surg 1:56–58, 1988.

94. Shelbourne K, Whitaker J, McCarroll JR, et al: Anterior cruciate ligament injury: evaluation of intraarticular reconstruction of acute tears without repair—two to seven-year followup of 155 athletes. Am J Sports Med 18:484–489, 1990.
95. Shields C, Silva J, Yee L, Brewster C: Evaluation of residual instability after arthroscopic meniscectomy in anterior cruciate deficient knees. Am J Sports Med 15:129–131, 1987.
96. Slocum D, James S, Larson R, Singer K: Clinical tests for anterolateral rotatory instability of the knee. Clin Orthop 118:63–69, 1976.
97. Slocum D, Larson R: Rotatory instability of the knee: its pathogenesis and the clinical test to determine its presence. J Bone Joint Surg 50A:211–225, 1968.
98. Slocum D, Larson R: Pes anserinus transplant: a simple surgical procedure for control of rotatory instability of the knee. J Bone Joint Surg 50A:226–242, 1968.
99. Slocum D, Larson R, James S: Pes anserinus transplant: impressions after a decade of experience. Am J Sports Med 2:123–136, 1974.
100. Slocum D, Larson R, James S: Late reconstruction of ligamentous injuries to the medial compartment of the knee. Clin Orthop 100:23–66, 1974.
101. Slocum D, Larson R, James S, Greenier R: High tibial osteotomy. Cling Orthop 104:239, 1974.
102. Sommerlath K: The prognosis of repaired and intact menisci in unstable knees—a comparative study. J Arthroscopy 4:93–95, 1991.
103. Speer KP, Spritzer CE, Garrett WE, et al: Osseous injury associated with acute tears of the anterior cruciate ligament. *Presented at* the annual meeting of the American Society of Sports Medicine, Anaheim, CA, 1991.
104. Strum G, Fox J, Ferkel R, et al: Intraarticular versus intraarticular and extraarticular reconstruction for chronic anterior cruciate ligament instability. Clin Orthop 245:188, 1989.
105. Tapper E, Hoover N: Late results after meniscectomy. J Bone Joint Surg 51A:517–526, 1969.
106. Umansky A: The milch fasciodesis for the reconstruction of the tibial collateral ligament. J Bone Joint Surg 34A:202–206, 1952.
107. Unverferth LJ, Olix MI, Ketterer WF: A clinical follow-up of pes anserinus transplantation for chronic anteromedial rotatory instability of the knee. Clin Orthop 134:149–152, 1978.
108. Warren R, Marshall J: Injuries of the anterior cruciate and medial collateral ligaments of the knee. Clin Orthop 136:198, 1978.
109. Wickiewicz T: Meniscal injuries in the cruciate deficient knee. Clin Sports Med 9:681, 1990.
110. Wilson W, Scranton P: Combined reconstruction of the anterior cruciate ligament in competitive athletes. J Bone Joint Surg 72A:742, 1990.

CHAPTER 22

Chronic

Posterior and

Posterolateral

Laxity

WILLIAM A. GRANA, M.D.

■

The posterior cruciate ligament (PCL) functions as one of the main guides to motion of the knee and, with the anterior cruciate ligament (ACL), contributes to the "screw home" mechanism of the knee.[1, 5, 13, 18, 19, 26, 42] However, the anatomy, the function, and the pathophysiologic processes surrounding the effects of injury on this ligament, as well as its relationship to the posterolateral structures of the knee, are not as well understood as are those of the ACL. The PCL is injured less frequently; the reported injury occurrence varies from 5 to 10 per cent of all ligament injuries.[5, 7, 13, 23, 24] Loos and associates indicated a 0.7 per cent occurrence of PCL injuries among over 11,000 surgically treated knees.[26] Because of this lesser frequency, there is a lower index of suspicion for injury of the PCL and this diagnosis is often missed; treatment, therefore, is frequently late or delayed. Part of the dilemma in the diagnosis of posterior laxity of the knee is the relationship between the function of the PCL and the ligamentous structure of the posterolateral corner of the knee and the effects of injury to each on overall posterior and posterolateral rotary instability (Fig. 22–1).

Surgical repair of acute bony avulsion of the tibial attachment of the PCL has historically been reported to yield good results, but some authors have expressed concern about interstitial injury to the ligament before bony avulsion.[5, 45] Most authors have recommended acute repair of the PCL after its disruption, although with some degree of pessimism about the success of this procedure.[1, 19, 23, 24, 28, 40] There does not seem to be consensus about the best way to treat the acute injury; some authors prefer nonoperative management, and some prefer surgical repair with or without augmentation.[6, 11–13, 19, 28, 33, 40, 42, 45] Perhaps because of this controversy over both the management and the difficulty in diagnosis of the acute injury and over the resultant differing advice to patients, physicians tend to see patients with chronic rather than acute problems. It may also be that the manifestation of the effects of injury to the posterolateral structures comes later and the development of rotary instability increases the disability of patients.

The majority of PCL injuries are a result of high-velocity trauma, as

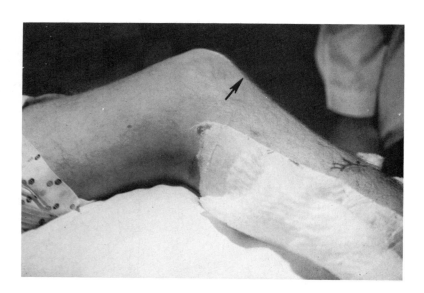

FIGURE 22–1. The appearance of posterior sag (*arrow*) of the tibia is indicative of injury to the posterior cruciate ligament (PCL) and also may be the beginning of a dilemma for the patient in terms of the diagnosis, evaluation, and management of this problem.

occurs in motor vehicle accidents, although some authors have shown that such injuries can also occur during sports activities, especially football and soccer.[7, 13, 23, 32] Therefore, in the athlete, PCL injury is far less common than other ligamentous injuries, and the results of PCL stabilization are less predictable than those of ACL reconstruction. Many authors have recommended nonoperative treatment for the isolated PCL injury.[13, 33, 42] Nonetheless, aggressive treatment, whether nonoperative or operative, for the preservation of the meniscus is important because of the concern about the development of degenerative changes of the patellofemoral and tibiofemoral joints after PCL injury. Other investigators have raised concerns about this potential for articular cartilage damage and therefore believe that even in isolated PCL insufficiency, operative treatment is indicated.[2, 5, 10, 38, 47] There clearly remains controversy about the management of chronic isolated PCL insufficiency. On the contrary, when PCL injuries are associated with injury of the posterolateral corner, instability and disability are much more common, and there are more frequent complaints of pain, giving way, recurrent swelling, and meniscal symptoms.[42] In addition, there is a significant increase in patellofemoral pressure as the knee goes from 15° to 90° of flexion with this combination of PCL and posterolateral insufficiency.[14] Therefore, the chronic combined posterior laxity is best managed operatively.

The purpose of this chapter is to discuss the management of chronic laxity of the PCL and the arcuate ligament complex.

ANATOMY OF THE POSTERIOR CRUCIATE LIGAMENT

Although the anatomy of the PCL has been discussed in Chapter 3, a brief review is worthwhile. The PCL is extra-articular and has a synovial covering of its medial, lateral, and anterior aspects. Distally on the tibia, the PCL blends with the posterior capsule and periosteum. It is vertically angled forward 30° to 45° depending on the degree of knee flexion (Fig. 22–2). It is more vertical in extension and more horizontal in flexion. There are an anterior portion and a posterior portion of the ligament; the posterior component is thinner. The anterior fibers are taut in flexion and lax in extension (Figs. 22–3, 22–4). The PCL is about 3.25 to 4.00 cm in length and between 10 and 15 mm wide. The ligament fans out at the femoral attachment in the shape of a semicircle, 32 mm in its greatest width. The tibial attachment is a depression in the posterior tibia between the two plateaus about 1 cm below the tibial surface.[14, 19, 46] Of importance is that the tibial attachment is not at the level of joint but significantly below it. This point is particularly important when a reconstruction of the PCL is accomplished (Fig. 22–5). The meniscofemoral ligaments of Wrisberg and Humphrey are posterior and anterior, respectively, to the PCL, and they arise from the lateral meniscus or the tibia near the insertion of the PCL and run obliquely to the origin of the PCL on the femur. The ligament of Wrisberg can have a significant role as a restraint to straight posterior laxity in isolated injury of the PCL.[17]

The lateral compartment of the knee extends from the lateral border of the patellar tendon to the PCL posteriorly. The anatomically important structures of the lateral side are the lateral capsular ligaments, the arcuate ligament complex, the iliotibial band, the biceps femoris muscle and

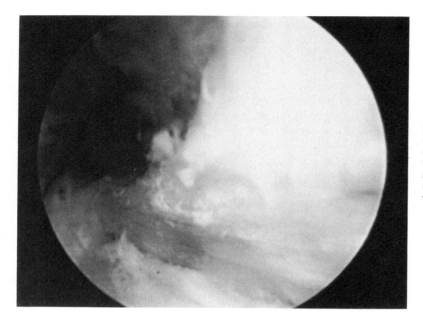

FIGURE 22–2. The PCL is vertically angled forward 30° to 45° depending on the degree of knee flexion. This arthroscopic perspective shows the forward inclination of the PCL, as well as the winding course of its fibers.

tendon, and the peroneal nerve. The capsular portion of the posterolateral corner of the knee has been termed the arcuate ligament complex by several authors.[14, 18, 29] The posterolateral aspect of the knee is divided into three distinct layers. The deep layer is the lateral part of the capsule, which divides into two layers just posterior to the iliotibial tract. These layers encompass three ligaments: the lateral collateral ligament, the fabellofibular ligament, and the arcuate ligament. The popliteus tendon is also in the deep layer and functions with the posterolateral corner ligaments to prevent posterolateral laxity.[18, 35]

The arcuate ligament complex consists of the posterolateral ligaments

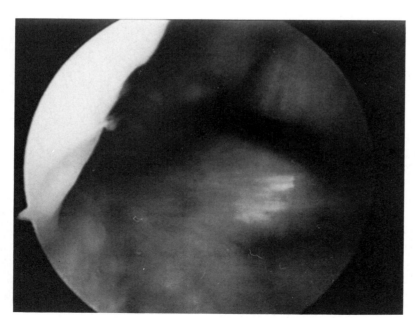

FIGURE 22–3. The posterior fibers of the PCL are taut in extension, whereas the anterior fibers are lax in extension.

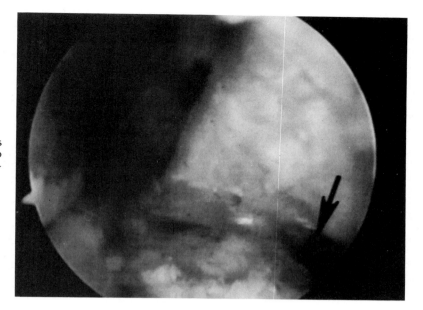

FIGURE 22–4. The anterior fibers of the PCL are taut in flexion to 90° (*arrow*), and the posterior fibers are lax.

(the arcuate ligament, the fabellofibular ligament, and the lateral collateral ligament) and the aponeurotic and tendinous portions of the popliteal tendon and the popliteus muscle; this muscle works in concert with the lateral head of the gastrocnemius muscle to restrain posterolateral laxity of the tibia.[15, 18, 35]

The posterior third of the capsular ligament, consisting of the meniscofemoral and meniscotibial portions, is reinforced by the popliteus muscle-tendon unit. This muscle-tendon unit consists of medial fibers that attach to the lateral meniscus and lateral fibers, which form the tendon of insertion of the popliteus muscle into the lateral femoral condyle. These components of the popliteus muscle, together with the condensation of

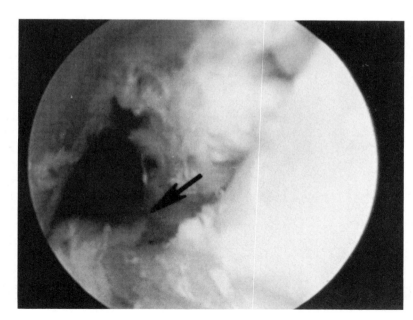

FIGURE 22–5. The tibial attachment (*arrow*) is a depression in the posterior tibia between the two plateaus about 1 cm below the tibial surface. This point is particularly salient when a reconstruction of the PCL is accomplished.

fasciae over the posterior surface of the muscle, form the so-called arcuate ligament. The arcuate ligament is the most important stabilizer of the posterolateral corner of the knee. The arcuate ligament, the lateral collateral ligament, and the fabellofibular ligament together form the arcuate ligament complex. With the PCL, the arcuate ligament complex protects against excessive posterior and posterolateral excursion of the tibia on the femur.[15, 35]

BIOMECHANICS OF POSTERIOR CRUCIATE AND POSTEROLATERAL LIGAMENT FUNCTION

The PCL has been called the primary stabilizer of the knee by some authors and provides up to 95 per cent of the total restraint to posterior displacement of the tibia on the femur. The PCL contributes to the screw home mechanism of the knee by providing a guide for the motion of the tibia on the femur.[14–16, 18]

If the PCL is sectioned, there is no increase in rotational laxity in the knee. After sectioning, there is a small amount of posterior translation of the tibia on the femur in extension, but in flexion there is much more translation. Therefore, the posterior capsule blocks laxity in extension, and the posterior drawer test is more sensitive in flexion. Furthermore, immobilization in extension and neutral rotation protects a reconstructed PCL if the posterior capsule is intact. The removal of only the PCL produces no change in the limits for tibial rotation or for varus and valgus angulation. The removal of the posterolateral extra-articular restraints increases the amount of external rotation and varus angulation. This increase in external rotation is highest at 30° of flexion and lowest at 90° of flexion with an intact PCL. With removal of the PCL, this external rotation increases significantly.[16]

Varus angulation is normal as long as the lateral collateral ligament is intact. When this ligament is cut, there is a notable increase in varus angulation with the knee flexed at 15°. Further sectioning of the arcuate ligament complex and the popliteal tendon adds significantly to the varus angulation. Removal of the PCL also produces additional increases in varus angulation, which further increases with more flexion. When the PCL is sectioned after the lateral collateral ligament and the posterolateral capsular structures have been cut, a large increase in posterior translation and varus rotation occurs. In all angles of flexion, the arcuate ligament complex functions as the principal structure that enables varus angulation and external rotation of the tibia, whereas the PCL is the principal structure that enables posterior translation. However, at angles of flexion at 30° or less, the amount of posterior translation after sectioning of only the lateral collateral ligament in the deep structures is similar to that noted after isolated sectioning of the PCL.[14, 15]

These results, as well as those described earlier in this chapter, demonstrate the importance of the combined action of the PCL and the arcuate ligament complex in the prevention of posterior translation, varus angulation, and external rotation of the tibia. In general, an isolated injury to the PCL does not produce posterolateral laxity. In addition, these results may help explain the wide variability of function of the knees of patients who have sustained PCL injuries. Patients who have an isolated

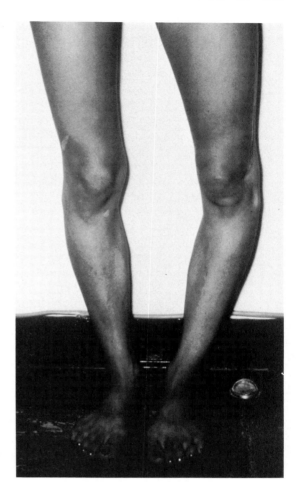

FIGURE 22–6. A combined injury of the arcuate ligament complex and the PCL produces instability in flexion from 0° to 30° in the most severe instances, there is varus posterolateral thrust such as that seen here.

injury of the PCL may maintain good function of the knee in positions that are close to extension. On the other hand, those patients who have a combined injury of the posterolateral capsule and the PCL have instability in flexion of 0° to 30°, and therefore function is impaired in these positions (Fig. 22–6).

During stance phase of normal gait, knee motion is predominantly from 0° to 40°. The PCL is stressed maximally in terminal stance. Strain in the PCL decreases from full extension to 20° of flexion; when the knee flexes beyond 20°, the strain markedly increases in the PCL. With an incompetent PCL, the stress is transferred to the secondary restraints (the posteromedial and posterolateral capsules), and there is increased posterior shear force on the articular cartilage. Therefore, a patient with posterolateral laxity as well as PCL insufficiency is much more likely to experience functional problems and articular cartilage damage because of loss of this secondary restraint.[14–16, 41]

NATURAL HISTORY OF CHRONIC POSTERIOR AND POSTEROLATERAL LAXITY

Patients who have PCL insufficiency usually have a history of significant injury of the knee. Football, basketball, soccer, and skiing are sports commonly associated with the occurrence of PCL injury. In addition, vehicular trauma (car and motorcycle) is another common mechanism of injury as the knee strikes the dashboard in a car or the surface of the road after a motorcycle accident. In the majority of patients, the mechanism of injury is an anterior force to a flexed knee or a shear or twist injury as a valgus or varus force is applied to the knee. In a smaller group of patients, hyperextension of the knee is the mechanism of injury.[7, 13, 23, 24, 26, 28, 32, 39, 42]

In patients who have chronic posterior insufficiency, the end result is affected by a history of meniscectomy, the presence of chondromalacia of the patella, or the presence of quadriceps weakness. Patients who have multidirectional instability are more likely to develop all of these complications. It is common for such a patient's initial injury problem to be missed, and therefore the patient does not come to the orthopaedist for care until one of the complications develops or unless the patient has instability of the knee. The outcome for an individual patient appears to depend on the presence of rotational instability. A more aggressive approach is recommended for such a patient.[42]

The PCL, being in a central location in the knee near the longitudinal axis of rotation, undergoes the least strain of all the knee stabilizers with any applied stress. Because of its central location, high tensile strength, and protected environment, it is the primary stabilizer of the knee. It is thus doubtful that any external applied force could disrupt this ligament without first tearing other major structures. Therefore, in repair of ligamentous disruptions that involve the PCL, careful attention to repair and to augmentation of the secondary restraints may determine the prognosis for long-term function.[18, 19, 29]

DIAGNOSIS OF POSTERIOR LAXITY

The purpose of a test for posterior laxity is to detect abnormal translation or rotation of the tibial plateau on the femur. The posterior drawer test and the posterior sag test are performed with the knee in 90° of flexion with the foot fixed on the examining table, and the profile of the affected anterior proximal tibia is compared with that of the opposite (unaffected) side (Fig. 22–7). The tibia may be stressed posteriorly while the examiner palpates the patient's femoral condyles and the anterior edge of the tibial plateau in order to determine their relationship. The amount of posterior translation of the tibia determines the amount of posterolateral laxity (Fig. 22–8).[6, 20, 23, 24, 31]

A modification of this procedure is the quadriceps active test, which is performed with the knee in 90° of flexion with the foot fixed on the table. The patient is asked to actively contract the quadriceps muscle or to attempt to slide the foot forward on the table. This results in anterior translation of the tibia in the patient who has a disruption of the PCL as a result of the anterior pull of the quadriceps muscle. The affected knee is compared with the contralateral (normal) knee (Fig. 22–9).[8, 25, 37]

Posterolateral laxity is best detected by the reverse pivot shift, defined by Jakob and collaborators.[22] The test is performed with the knee flexed as the examiner palpates the tibial tubercle (Fig. 22–10). The knee is extended, and as the tibia moves from the flexed, subluxated, externally rotated position to the extended reduced position, there is a "clunk" near

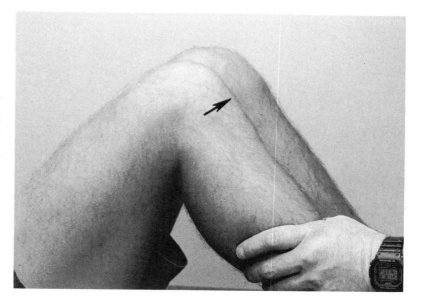

FIGURE 22–7. The posterior drawer test and the posterior sag test are performed with the knee in 90° of flexion with the foot fixed on the examining table, and the profile of the affected anterior proximal tibia (*arrow*) is compared with that of the opposite (unaffected) side.

full extension (Fig. 22–11). When the test is carried out with the tibia externally rotated, the palpable "clunk" is maximized. In a modification of the reverse pivot shift described by Shelbourne and colleagues, the hip and knee are flexed to 90°, and then the knee is slowly extended passively. In the knee with posterior instability, the tibia suddenly reduces as the knee joint nears full extension, and a jerk or "clunk" is felt by both the patient and the examiner. The test is performed with the patient's hamstrings tight in order to produce a dynamic rather than a passive type test.[36]

Another method of evaluating posterolateral instability is with the patient lying supine and the hips and knees of both extremities flexed

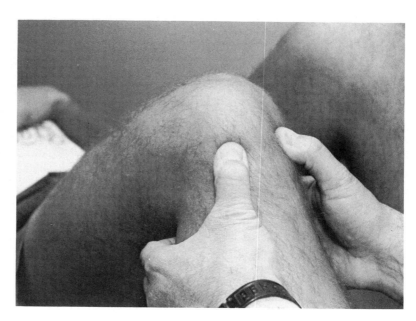

FIGURE 22–8. The examiner palpates the femoral condyles and the anterior edge of the tibial plateau in order to determine their relationship. The amount of posterior translation of the tibia determines the amount of posterior laxity.

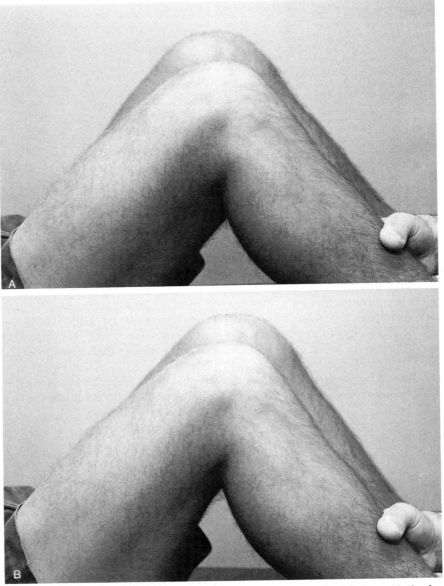

FIGURE 22–9. Quadriceps active test is done with the knee in 90° of flexion with the foot fixed on the table. The patient is asked to actively contract the quadriceps muscle or to attempt to slide the foot forward on the table (*B*). This results in the anterior translation of the tibia in the patient who has a disruption of the PCL. When the patient relaxes (*A*), the anterior tibial crest sags posteriorly again.

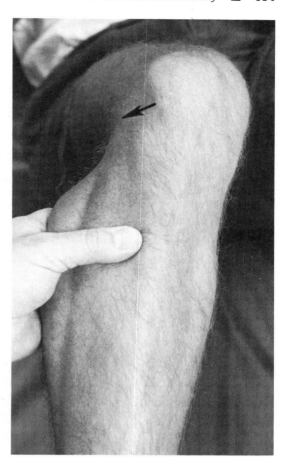

FIGURE 22–10. Posterolateral laxity is best detected by the reverse pivot shift. The test is performed with the knee flexed as the examiner palpates the tibial tubercle with the tibia externally rotated. In this position, the tibial plateau (*arrow*) is subluxated posterolaterally.

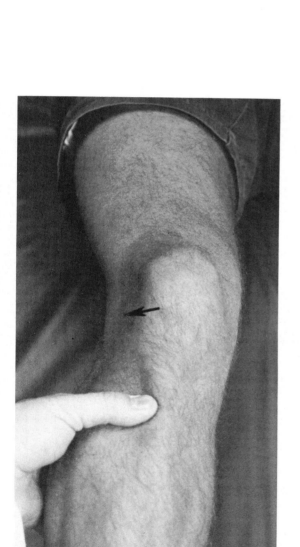

FIGURE 22–11. In the reverse pivot shift, as the knee is extended and the tibia goes from the flexed, subluxated position to the extended reduced position (*arrow*), there is a "clunk" near full extension.

90°. The examiner grasps both of the patient's feet and externally rotates them. A positive result is excessive external rotation of the affected tibia, as recognized from the position of the foot and also by a slight posterior sag at the affected lateral tibial tubercle (Fig. 22–12).[1, 20, 21]

Hughston and colleagues pointed out the frequent association of lateral ligament injury with PCL injury. They demonstrated the frequency of the association between injury to the arcuate ligament complex and injury to the posterolateral capsular structures and the association of these injuries with posterolateral rotary instability, as diagnosed by the posterolateral drawer test and the external rotation recurvatum test. In addition, these patients often have increased varus or valgus stress laxity in extension. The presence of such laxity should heighten the index of suspicion that a PCL injury is present.[1, 19, 21]

Because most PCL injuries result from major violence, there should be a high index of suspicion of PCL damage when such violence is associated with a significant knee injury. The presence of varus or valgus instability at 0° of extension and a posterior drawer sign are the most reliable physical findings in a patient with posterior laxity.

The problem in straight posterior instability is to define the neutral point for the knee—that is, to distinguish posterior laxity from anterior laxity. This can be very difficult in a chronically injured patient, particularly when a PCL injury is combined with an ACL injury as well. Anteroposterior lateral stress radiographs are useful in the evaluation of such complex laxity and therefore play an important role in the evaluation of a patient with combined PCL-ACL laxity. The amount of translation is measured from comparably obtained stress films of the injured and uninjured knees.[33]

Objective laxity testing with a laxity-testing device is useful for documenting the amount of straight posterior laxity. However, the accuracy of such testing may be diminished by the presence of posterolateral laxity.[32] Extreme care must be taken in evaluating a patient with a posterior injury. Differences between the injured and uninjured knees of 5 mm or

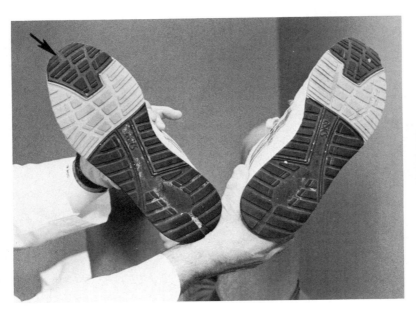

FIGURE 22–12. In posterolateral laxity, excessive external rotation of the affected tibia, as shown on the left (*arrow*), is recognized by the position of the foot.

more usually indicate significant or complete injury to the PCL. The normal right-left difference should be in the range of 1 to 2 mm. In ACL insufficiency, there is a distinct correlation between the amount of increased laxity and the function of the knee; however, in PCL insufficiency, this correlation has not been found.[32, 42] Nevertheless, patients with functional problems usually have a significant decrease in quadriceps strength in the affected knee in comparison with the uninjured knee, and therefore isokinetic testing offers predictive value for the PCL-injured patient.

When there are a high index of suspicion and inconclusive physical findings, arthroscopy is useful in the evaluation of this injury. In addition, examination with the patient under anesthesia along with the arthroscopy can help prevent misdiagnosis or clarify a suspected isolated tear. Good results are associated with correct, complete acute diagnosis, with younger patients with athletic rather than motor vehicle injuries, and with tears that are not midsubstance.

NONOPERATIVE MANAGEMENT OF THE CHRONIC PCL INJURY

In order to treat posterior instability, the assessment of the patient must include a careful evaluation for rotary instability and for the presence of degenerative change in the tibiofemoral or patellofemoral joint. If there are associated ligamentous injuries with manifested multidirectional instability—whether ACL, arcuate ligament complex, or medial injury—acute repair and reconstruction should be accomplished. However, in a patient who manifests only straight posterior instability, as determined by physical examination, radiographic studies, examination with the patient under anesthesia, and arthroscopy, nonoperative management may be undertaken.[42]

Nonoperative management of the isolated PCL injury focuses on protection with the knee in full extension and on early passive motion progressing to active motion, within the limits of pain. Quadriceps strengthening progresses from straight-leg raises to short-arc and long-arc resistive exercises with hamstring stretching and eccentric hamstring curls.[13, 32]

The steps are as follows: For the first 1 to 3 weeks, the patient is managed in a knee immobilizer for weight bearing as tolerated, initially with crutches and then without crutches. The patient begins active range-of-motion exercises as quickly as pain and swelling permit. Nonsteroidal anti-inflammatory medication is useful for reducing the swelling, as is local application of ice three to four times a day for 20 to 30 minutes. As the range of motion permits, active exercise is begun, initially with straight-leg raising without weights and progressing to the use of weights, with a maximum of 15 pounds for three to four sets of 10 twice a day. When these exercises are performed without pain, short-arc quadriceps exercises begin and continue until the patient is able to use 20 pounds for three to four sets of 10 twice a day. As gait improves and the patient is able to walk without a limp and without crutches, long-arc quadriceps exercises and hamstring curls with weight are begun; the weight is gradually increased until the patient achieves maximal strength. The goal is to have hamstring strength that is 70 per cent of the quadriceps strength.

As the patient approaches full strength, somewhere between the third and sixth weeks, proprioceptive activity begins. Muscle control is facilitated in all planes by the use of a balance or wobble board and by plyometric exercises with a minitrampoline or a jump rope. Such activity aids in the return of proprioception and coordination. Sports-specific drills are implemented, first with jogging and then with figure 8 running, and sports-specific skills such as catching or throwing a ball are incorporated. A brace is worn throughout this period of functional activity once strength allows such a return.

Results of Nonoperative Management

The results of nonoperative management, primarily in an athletic population, have been presented by several authors. These results indicate that patients who return to sports are more satisfied if the strength of the quadriceps is greater in the injured knee than in the uninjured knee. There is little relationship between the amount of posttranslation and the ability to return to a sport. If patients can decrease the posterior drawer by internal rotation of the tibia during activity, success is more likely.[9, 10, 13, 32, 42] In addition, Parolie and Bergfeld noted that if there is more than 15 mm of posterior laxity that does not decrease with internal rotation or if there is 5 to 15 mm of posterior laxity that is associated with other major ligamentous injury, surgical treatment should be accomplished.[32]

The success of nonoperative treatment results from the patient's ability to "set the knee in full extension," as defined by Cain and Schwab in their study of a professional football player. Electromyographic recordings revealed that the quadriceps muscle of the PCL-deficient knee contracted before heel strike, as opposed to the uninvolved knee, in which it contracted after heel strike.[4] In addition, Tibone and co-workers noted that the gastrocnemius muscle group plays a significant role in this extension mechanism as well.[41] This probably accounts for Parolie and Bergfeld's finding that 2 to 3 per cent of college football seniors examined in a predraft physical for the National Football League are found to have chronic PCL-deficient knees but are successful in the sport at an elite level.[32]

Parolie and Bergfeld, in their study of nonoperative management, reported that 80 per cent of patients were satisfied with the results of management and 84 per cent returned to their previous sport, 68 per cent at the same level of performance and 16 per cent at a decreased level of performance. The difference in results of ligament laxity testing in injured and uninjured knees was not related to the patients' return to sports or to satisfaction with the results of management.[32]

Fowler and Messieh noted that although a significant number of patients have laxity according to objective criteria, acceptable functional stability in these patients occurs without absolute static stability. Fowler and Messieh found that in a group of 13 patients, all were able to return to their previous activities and experienced no limitations with regard to their injured knees. Fowler and Messieh concluded that nonoperative treatment of isolated PCL injury in athletes is a viable alternative to repair and reconstruction.[13]

Dejour and associates outlined three potential phases of adaptation.[10] The first phase is a period of functional adaptation lasting for 3 to 18 months after injury. Re-education of the quadriceps significantly helps in this adaptation. The second phase is that of functional tolerance, which enables the patient to return to sports. This phase lasts about 15 years, but if there is multidirectional instability, slow and progressive deterioration of the patellofemoral and tibiofemoral articular surfaces may occur, resulting in the third phase of osteoarthritis, which appears 15 to 20 years after injury. An important point to remember is that a number of studies have documented that a nonoperative treatment program for isolated PCL injuries seems be as beneficial to patients as is surgical repair or reconstruction of the isolated injury.

With these results in mind and the finding of an isolated PCL injury, a nonoperative program, including a brace, can be recommended with confidence and with a basis in scientific fact as PCL laxity is now understood.

OPERATIVE MANAGEMENT OF THE CHRONIC PCL INJURY

Avulsion of the Tibial Attachment of the PCL

The operative methods for management of a patient with PCL insufficiency or with combined posterolateral instability have been described in a variety of ways. Trickey[45] described reattachment of the avulsed tibial attachment of the PCL as a treatment for posterior instability.[45] More recently, Meyers described his experience with this method of management in 14 isolated avulsion fractures of the posterior tibial attachment of the PCL.[27] Two of these injuries were treated late by advancement of the tibia, and union was obtained with good function. An isolated tibial attachment by avulsion of bone can be fixed with a 6.5-mm cancellous screw or a 4.5-mm malleolar screw with or without a small metal washer. As an alternative, if the fragments are comminuted, sutures can be placed through the ligament and brought out through drill holes in the bone. Torisu reported good results with a similar approach to chronic injury.[43, 44]

The approach for this type of injury and reconstruction is generally posteriorly with the patient prone. Burks and Schaffer described a simplified approach with the patient prone.[3] The skin incision is a gentle curve with the horizontal portion near the flexion crease of the knee and with the vertical limb overlying the medial aspect of the belly of the medial gastrocnemius muscle. The incision is carried down through the fascial layer and vertically over the medial head of the gastrocnemius muscle. The medial sural cutaneous nerve is usually distal to the horizontal limit of the incision. The medial border of the gastrocnemius muscle is identified, and the interval is developed between it and the semimembranosus tendon by blunt dissection. The posterior joint capsule is reached by lateral retraction of the medial head of the gastrocnemius muscle. No tension is applied to the neurovascular structures that are protected by this muscle belly. The posterior aspect of the proximal tibia and the posterior portion of the femoral condyles are palpable. A portion of the tendon of the medial head of the gastrocnemius muscle may be released from the distal femur if additional exposure laterally is needed. Slight knee flexion aids in the exposure. A vertical incision is made through the posterior capsule, and the contents of the posterior intercondylar notch and the tibial attachment of the PCL are then accessible. The screw can be directed perpendicular to the posterior aspect of the proximal tibia when the avulsion fracture is reduced.

Meyers reported good results in a series of 14 patients treated in this manner. However, no instrumented laxity testing or clinical classification system was used for evaluation.[27]

Intra-Articular Reconstruction of the PCL

Müller reported the use of the quadriceps tendon, patellar expansion, and the patellar tendon as a method of reconstruction for the PCL. Although he provided no results, he did indicate that as a result of his experience, "we have become hesitant to perform true reconstruction of the PCL and are conducting further cases with a modified technique in order to evaluate the long term results."[29]

Both Hughston and Degenhardt[20] and Roth and collaborators[34] described the use of the medial head of the gastrocnemius muscle for reconstruction of the PCL with differing results. Hughston and Degenhardt followed 29 patients for a mean period of 45 months after reconstruction and found that 86 per cent had subjectively improved and 77 per cent were functionally good. Forty per cent had a moderately positive posterior drawer test. In Roth and collaborators' group, 31 patients were reviewed an average of 53 months after surgery. Sixty-nine per cent of the patients had subjectively improved; however, 91 per cent continued to have pain, and 59 per cent continued to experience giving way. Patients in whom an associated collateral ligament procedure was accomplished experienced significantly better results than did those who underwent only PCL surgery. Roth and collaborators' conclusion was that "we do not recommend this procedure as a primary PCL reconstruction." It appears that most authors have discarded this procedure because of the recurrence of laxity.

Clancy recommended the use of the bone–patellar tendon–bone graft for the posterior cruciate ligament and reported the results of this procedure.[5] He managed 33 patients with chronic instability in this manner and evaluated 23 patients who returned for evaluation after a minimal follow-up interval of 2 years. Of these, 13 had undergone treatment for a chronic problem. The overall static and functional result was graded as good or excellent in 11. However, no objective laxity testing was conducted with these patients. Feagin also used this method for the management of PCL insufficiency and reported the technique in his book *The Crucial Ligaments*.[12]

Wirth and Jager described the use of semitendinosus and gracilis tendons in 12 patients with an average follow-up interval of 32 months. All patients were subjectively satisfied, but most still had a positive posterior drawer test. Wirth and Jager believed that the reconstruction was an excellent alternative treatment for PCL instability.[48]

The author's preferred treatment is to use a central third of the patellar tendon or a patellar tendon allograft for substitution of the PCL. This substitution is accomplished through an arthroscopically assisted technique with interference screw fixation of the bone–patellar tendon–bone graft.

Technique of PCL Reconstruction

The patient is appropriately anesthetized with a general anesthetic or with epidural anesthesia. The tourniquet is used as needed because it is necessary to make incisions during the procedure, but a fluid pump is used for the arthroscopic portion of the procedure and may enable the patient to undergo the procedure without any anesthesia. The patient is supine on the operating table, and the knee is flexed at 90°, prepared, and draped appropriately. An image intensifier is useful to verify tibial pin placement. Routine arthroscopy is performed, injury to the PCL is identified, appropriate articular cartilage and meniscal procedures are performed, and the arthroscopically assisted intra-articular reconstruction of the PCL is accomplished. It is preferable to have a 70°-angled arthroscope available, although it is not mandatory.

The anterior portals are the usual inferolateral and inferomedial portals placed adjacent to the patellar tendon at its medial and lateral margins in the anteromedial and anterolateral sulcus. With the arthroscope through the notch viewing from the medial side and with operating instruments from the lateral side, the old PCL stump and scar are cleared from the notch in order to facilitate exposure of the posterior aspect of the joint. Then, under direct vision with the arthroscope through the notch, a posteromedial portal is created. Through this portal, with the use of a full radius shaver and a burr, the PCL fossa on the tibia is exposed and freshened to a raw, bony surface. The point for the PCL drill guide is identified 1 cm below the articular surface of the tibia. The PCL tibial guide is used for placing the guide pin, and its position is verified with the image intensifier (Fig. 22–13).

Minimal abrasion of the medial femoral condylar attachment of the ACL is accomplished. For the placement of the drill hole for the graft, the femoral drill guide is positioned with the knee in 90° of flexion, and the drill is guided at the midpoint of the notch on the medial femoral condyle and then moved posteriorly from the edge of the articular surface 3 to 4 mm.

When the preparation of the notch is completed, a patellar tendon graft is obtained. If an allograft is to be used, the allograft is prepared while the notch preparation is ongoing. In the case of the patellar tendon graft, the central third is used. In the case of an allograft, a 12- to 14-mm graft is used. Appropriate small incisions are made on the tibia and the femur for the cannulated reamers and for fixation of the grafts. Appropriate drill holes are made with the use of cannulated reamers over the guide pins that have been placed with the drill guides.

The graft is then passed anteriorly with the use of a ligature passer and the arthroscope, and the posterior medial portal is used for grasping forceps to help the bone block turn the corner. A plastic ligament passing tube is useful for this purpose. The graft is fixed with 6.5-mm cancellous screws by an interference fit technique.

Usually, this technique is accomplished in tandem with posterolateral reconstruction and at the completion of the passage of the graft, but

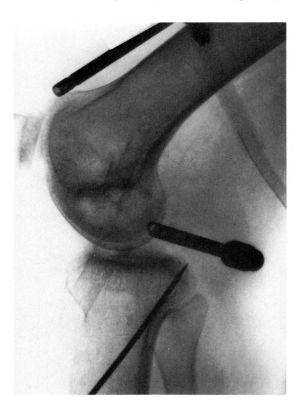

FIGURE 22–13. An image intensifier or permanent plain radiograph is needed for verifying the position of the tibial pin placement. The tibial pin should be placed about 1 cm below the articular surface of the tibia.

before fixation, the posterolateral reconstruction is accomplished. The author's preferred technique of reconstruction is elaborated later in this chapter.

Postoperative care includes a splint in full extension that is removed for passive range-of-motion exercise. A continuous passive motion (CPM) device, if preferred, may be used intermittently when the patient is awake for 30 to 60 minutes at a time, three or four times a day. However, most patients do just as well without the CPM device. The patient is hospitalized, usually for 1 to 2 nights. During the hospitalization, the patient begins an exercise program that includes multiangle isometric exercises, three sets of 10, twice a day at 0°, 20°, and 40° for the quadriceps muscle. Heel slides to 30° are accomplished, and patellar mobilization is performed annually in order to facilitate the motion. Three sets of 10 ankle pumps and straight-leg raising in the brace in 0° of extension are accomplished twice a day. Finally, hip adduction and abduction strengthening exercises, three sets of 10, twice a day in the brace, are performed. Weight bearing, initially touchdown and then partial weight bearing, is allowed over the first 10 days after surgery.

During the first week after discharge, all of these exercises are continued, and toe raises with the splint in place are added. These are done bilaterally in three to four sets of 10. A portable, battery-operated muscle stimulator is used for the quadriceps muscle. Over the ensuing 5 weeks, the immobilizer is continued until the third week, and then the patient uses a hinged knee immobilizer that allows motion to 60° and weight bearing is increased to full. Heel slides are increased to 60°, and closed-chain kinetic exercise for strengthening the quadriceps and the hamstring muscles is begun. The crutches are discontinued at the time of full weight bearing.

In 6 weeks the patient should be able to perform full weight bearing. Use of the immobilizer is continued, the heel slides are increased to 90°, and lying extension is increased from 45° to 0°. If a swimming pool is available, walking in water can begin, as can standing hamstring curls without weight.

After the sixth week and up through the 12th week a full range of motion is gradually allowed; swimming and bicycling are permitted, and full range of motion is obtained. Resistance for the closed-chain kinetic exercise is increased, and at week 12 use of the hinge brace is discontinued, and the patient begins an activity program that progresses to a running program during the fourth to sixth months. After the sixth month, cutting, pivoting, and pliometric exercise are begun and isokinetic testing is allowed. Between the ninth and 12th months, return to full sports activity is allowed, depending on return of skills and full strength.

A form-fitted brace is used for the PCL-deficient patient after surgery and during return to impact-loading activity. The author's patients use such a brace for approximately 18 months postoperatively or indefinitely, depending on the individual patient's preference. The primary purpose is to protect the graft from the forces that tend to produce posterior sag after surgery. Quadriceps rehabilitation is of the utmost importance for these patients, as noted earlier. A specifically designed, shell type, dynamic orthosis helps reestablish the relationship of the femur and the tibia in the PCL-reconstructed knee.

Posterolateral Corner Reconstruction

The literature contains few descriptions of reconstruction for posterolateral instability.[11, 21] Hughston and Jacobson wrote about the treatment of chronic posterolateral rotary instability, in which their operative approach was to advance the arcuate ligament complex and its osseous attachment anteriorly and distally on the femur. They reported a series of 141 knees in 140 patients who were followed 2 to 13 years after surgery. Of the reconstructions, 85 per cent were rated as good, 14 per cent as fair, and 1 per cent as poor. Subjectively, 78 per cent of the patients considered the result good and 22 per cent fair; no one rated the result as poor. Functionally, these results were rated as good by 80 per cent of the patients, fair by 16 per cent, and poor by 4 per cent.[21]

Müller described tightening of the arcuate ligament complex on the tibia as well as the reinforcement of the posterolateral corner with a portion of the biceps tendon or iliotibial band. He called this procedure the popliteus bypass. No results of this procedure were reported; however, he noted that the popliteus corner is seldom repaired alone, but it is generally repaired as part of an operation for combined instability or as a step in the correction of a global posterior instability in which the PCL is reconstructed as well.[30]

The author's procedure for posterolateral laxity is a combination of Hughston's advancement of the arcuate ligament complex and Müller's popliteus bypass. It is virtually always performed as a second step in intra-articular reconstruction of the PCL, as outlined earlier, or of the

ACL. Therefore, the patient is supine on the operating table with knees flexed to 90°. An incision is made along the posterior edge of the iliotibial band, beginning about 5 cm above the patella, extending distally to Gerdy's tubercle (Fig. 22–14). The iliotibial band is dissected anteriorly just enough to expose the posterior corner. The arcuate ligament complex, including the lateral collateral ligament, the fabellofibular and arcuate ligaments, and the popliteus muscle, are dissected free as a single flap. They are taken up with a 1-cm² bone block, outlined with an osteotome (Fig. 22–15). A burr is then used to create a cancellous bed on the lateral side of the femoral condyle in order to allow the flap to be advanced anteriorly 0.5 to 1.0 cm. The knee is taken through a range of motion in order to make certain that the point is an isometric point when the flap is fixed. The bone block is recessed slightly and fixed down with a cancellous screw and a flat metal washer. Before fixation, the second portion of the procedure is performed.

The popliteus bypass can be accomplished with a strip of the biceps tendon that is approximately half of the tendon, but the author prefers using a semitendinosus free graft when available. Alternatively, the surgery can also be accomplished with a portion of the bone–patellar tendon–bone allograft used for the intra-articular PCL reconstruction. When the semitendinosus or bone–patellar tendon–bone allograft is used, it is passed through a drill hole from anterior to posterior to the posterolateral corner of the tibia. It is then brought proximally along the course of the popliteal tendon and fixed with the cancellous screw and a washer

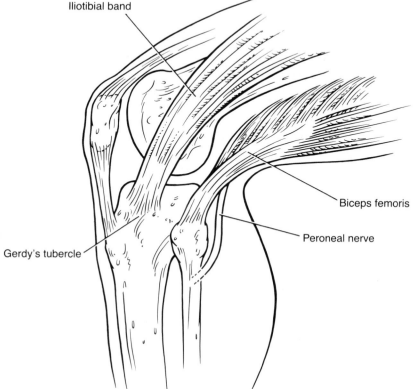

Iliotibial band

Biceps femoris

Peroneal nerve

Gerdy's tubercle

FIGURE 22–14. An incision for posterolateral reconstruction is made along the posterior edge of the iliotibial band, beginning about 5 cm above the patella and extending distally to Gerdy's tubercle.

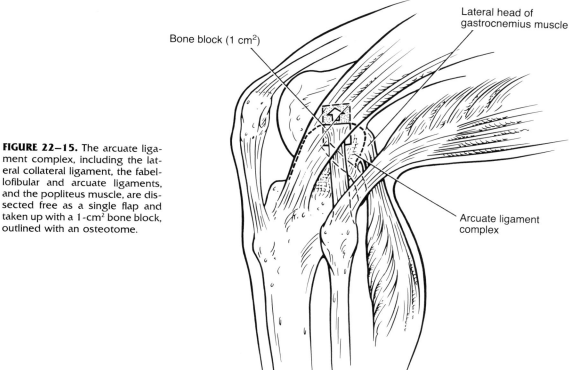

Bone block (1 cm²)

Lateral head of
gastrocnemius muscle

Arcuate ligament
complex

FIGURE 22–15. The arcuate ligament complex, including the lateral collateral ligament, the fabellofibular and arcuate ligaments, and the popliteus muscle, are dissected free as a single flap and taken up with a 1-cm² bone block, outlined with an osteotome.

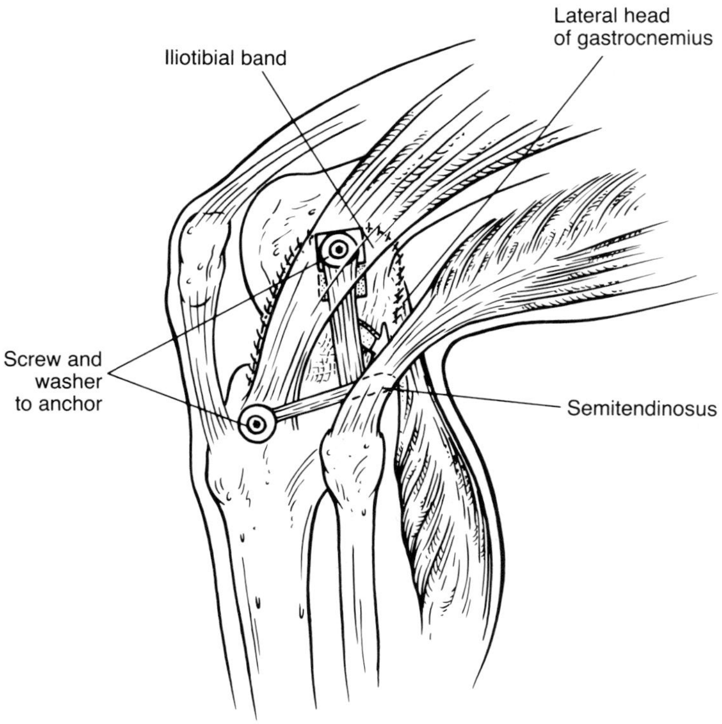

Iliotibial band

Lateral head
of gastrocnemius

Screw and
washer
to anchor

Semitendinosus

FIGURE 22–16. Semitendinosus muscle is passed through a drill hole anterior to posterior at the posterolateral corner of the tibia. It is then brought proximally along the course of the popliteal tendon and fixed with a cancellous screw and a washer along with the flap of the arcuate ligament complex.

on the femoral side and with a cancellous screw and a ligament washer on the tibial side (Fig. 22–16). If a bone–patellar tendon–bone block is used, it is brought through the tunnel as usual, and a hole is made in the femoral condyle in order to bury the bone block on the other end of the patellar tendon graft. In this case, a second screw is used for an interference fit. If the biceps tendon is used, it is taken down and brought along the course of the popliteal tendon, but sutures are passed from front to back in order to fix it down at the posterolateral corner of the tibia as well. It is also fixed on the femur with the cancellous screw and a ligament washer.

The final step in the procedure is to bring the lateral gastrocnemius muscle around for suturing over the posterior edge of the advanced arcuate ligament complex. After the grafts are fixed, the stability of the knee is rechecked; the posterolateral subluxation should be eliminated. The rehabilitation follows, stepwise, the PCL protocol that was outlined earlier in this chapter.

SUMMARY

In summary, the management of posterolateral laxity of the knee depends on the specific ligamentous injury and the functional problems that result from any anatomic disruption. There is no doubt that the management of PCL insufficiency is not well understood because of its infrequent occurrence. Nonoperative treatment is recommended for isolated PCL injuries without evidence of multidirectional instability. However, in patients who have meniscal disorder and appear to have developed patellofemoral or tibiofemoral articular complaints, reconstruction is probably indicated. Operative management is recommended for multidirectional or complex posterolateral instability by an intra-articular reconstruction of the PCL and an extra-articular soft tissue reconstruction of the posterolateral corner. These procedures should involve tightening of the arcuate ligament complex and enforcement of it with some local graft or allograft material. The patients should be treated postoperatively in extension in order to prevent posterolateral sag as long as the posterior capsule is intact, and patients treated nonoperatively or operatively should have the use of an individually fitted brace.

REFERENCES

1. Baker CL, Norwood LA, Hughston JC: Acute combined posterior cruciate and posterolateral instability of the knee. Am J Sports Med 12:204–208, 1984.
2. Bray RC, Dandy DJ: Meniscal lesions and chronic anterior cruciate ligament deficiency: meniscal tears occurring before and after reconstruction. J Bone Joint Surg 71B:128–130, 1989.
3. Burks RT, Schaffer JJ: A simplified approach to the tibial attachment of the posterior cruciate ligament. Clin Orthop 254:216–219, 1990.
4. Cain TE, Schwab GH: Performance of an athlete with straight posterior knee instability. Am J Sports Med 9:203–208, 1981.
5. Clancy WG: Knee ligamentous injury in sports: the past, present, and future. Med Sci Sports 15:9–14, 1983.
6. Clancy WG, Shelbourne KD, Zoellner GB, et al: Treatment of knee joint instability secondary to rupture of the posterior cruciate ligament: report of a new procedure. J Bone Joint Surg 65A:310–322, 1983.

7. Cross MJ, Powell JF: Long-term followup of posterior cruciate ligament rupture: a study of 116 cases. Am J Sports Med 12:292–297, 1984.
8. Daniel DM, Stone ML, Barnett P, Sachs R: Use of the quadriceps active test to diagnose posterior cruciate ligament disruption and measure posterior laxity of the knee. J Bone Joint Surg 70A:386–391, 1988.
9. Degenhardt TC: Chronic posterior cruciate ligament instability: nonoperative management. Orthop Trans 5:486–487, 1981.
10. Dejour H, Walch G, Peyrot J, Eberhard PH: The natural history of rupture of the posterior cruciate ligament. Fr J Orthop Surg 2:112–120, 1988.
11. DeLee JC, Riley MB, Rockwood CA: Acute posterolateral rotatory instability of the knee. Am J Sports Med 11:199–207, 1983.
12. Feagin JA: The Crucial Ligaments. New York: Churchill Livingstone, 1988.
13. Fowler PJ, Messieh SS: Isolated posterior cruciate ligament injuries in athletes. Am J Sports Med 15:553–557, 1987.
14. Girgis FG, Marshall JL, Monajem ARS: The cruciate ligaments of the knee joint: anatomical, functional and experimental analysis. Clin Orthop 106:216–231, 1975.
15. Gollehon DL, Torzilli PA, Warren RF: The role of the posterolateral and cruciate ligaments in the stability of the human knee. J Bone Joint Surg 69A:233–242, 1987.
16. Grood ES, Stowers SF, Noyes FR: Limits of movement in the human knee. J Bone Joint Surg 70A:88–97, 1988.
17. Heller L, Langman J: The menisco-femoral ligaments of the human knee. J Bone Joint Surg 46B:307–313, 1964.
18. Hughston JC, Andrews JR, Cross MJ, et al: Classification of knee ligament instabilities: parts I and II. J Bone Joint Surg 58A:159–179, 1976.
19. Hughston JC, Bowden JA, Andrews JR, et al: Acute tears of the posterior cruciate ligament: results of operative treatment. J Bone Joint Surg 62A:438–450, 1980.
20. Hughston JC, Degenhardt TC: Reconstruction of the posterior cruciate ligament. Clin Orthop 164:59–77, 1982.
21. Hughston JC, Jacobson KE: Chronic posterolateral rotatory instability of the knee. J Bone Joint Surg 67A:351–359, 1985.
22. Jakob RP, Hassler H, Staeubli HU: Observations on rotatory instability of the lateral compartment of the knee. Acta Orthop Scand 191:6–27, 1981.
23. Kennedy JC, Grainger RW: The posterior cruciate ligament. J Trauma 7:367–376, 1967.
24. Kennedy JC, Roth JH, Walker DM: Posterior cruciate ligament injuries. Orthop Dig 7:19–31, 1979.
25. Loomer RL: A test for knee posterolateral rotatory instability. Clin Orthop 264:235–238, 1991.
26. Loos WC, Fox JM, Blazina ME, et al: Acute posterior cruciate ligament injuries. Am J Sports Med 9:86–92, 1981.
27. Meyers MH: Isolated avulsion of the tibial attachment of the posterior cruciate ligament of the knee. J Bone Joint Surg 57A:669–672, 1975.
28. Moore HA, Larson RL: Posterior cruciate ligament injuries: results of early surgical repair. Am J Sports Med 8:68–78, 1980.
29. Müller W: The Knee: Form, Function, and Ligament Reconstruction, pp. 214–220. Berlin: Springer-Verlag, 1983.
30. Müller W: The Knee: Form, Function, and Ligament Reconstruction, pp. 234–240. Berlin: Springer-Verlag, 1983.
31. Ogata K, McCarthy JA, Dunlap J, Manske PR: Pathomechanics of posterior sag of the tibia in posterior cruciate deficient knees: an experimental study. Am J Sports Med 16:630–636, 1988.
32. Parolie JM, Bergfeld JA: Long-term results of nonoperative treatment of isolated posterior cruciate ligament injuries in the athlete. Am J Sports Med 14:35–38, 1986.
33. Rijke AM, Tegtmeyer CJ, Weiland DJ, McCue FC: Stress examination of the cruciate ligaments: a radiologic Lachman test. Radiology 165:867–869, 1987.
34. Roth JH, Bray RC, Best TM, et al: Posterior cruciate ligament reconstruction by transfer of the medial gastrocnemius tendon. Am J Sports Med 16:21–28, 1988.
35. Seebacher JR, Inglis AE, Marshall JL, Warren RF: The structure of the posterolateral aspect of the knee. J Bone Joint Surg 64A:536–541, 1982.
36. Shelbourne KD, Benedict F, McCarroll JR, Rettig AC: Dynamic posterior shift test: an adjuvant in evaluation of posterior tibial subluxation. Am J Sports Med 17:275–277, 1989.
37. Shino K, Horibe S, Ono K: The voluntarily evoked posterolateral drawer sign in the knee with posterolateral instability. Clin Orthop 215:179–186, 1987.
38. Sommerlatch C, Gillquist J: Knee function after meniscus repair and total meniscectomy: a seven year follow up study. J Arthroscop Rel Surg 3:166–169, 1987.
39. Starr DE: Repair of old ligamentous injuries of the knee. Clin Orthop 23:162–170, 1962.
40. Strand T, Molster AO, Engesaeter LB, et al: Primary repair in posterior cruciate ligament injuries. Acta Orthop Scand 55:545–547, 1984.
41. Tibone JE, Antich TJ, Perry J, Moynes D: Functional analysis of untreated and reconstructed posterior cruciate ligament injuries. Am J Sports Med 16:217–223, 1988.

42. Torg JS, Barton TM, Pavlov H, Stine R: Natural history of the posterior cruciate ligament-deficient knee. Clin Orthop 246:208–216, 1989.
43. Torisu T: Avulsion fracture of the tibial attachment of the posterior cruciate ligament: indications and results of delayed repair. Clin Orthop 143:107–114, 1979.
44. Torisu T: Isolated avulsion fracture of the tibial attachment of the posterior cruciate ligament. J Bone Joint Surg 59A:68–72, 1977.
45. Trickey EL: Rupture of the posterior cruciate ligament of the knee. J Bone Joint Surg 50B:334–341, 1968.
46. Van Dommelen BA, Fowler PJ: Anatomy of the posterior cruciate ligament: a review. Am J Sports Med 17:24–29, 1989.
47. Wickiewicz TL: Meniscal injuries in the cruciate-deficient knee. Clin Sports Med 9:681–694, 1991.
48. Wirth CJ, Jager M: Dynamic double tendon replacement of the posterior cruciate ligament. Am J Sports Med 12:39–43, 1984.

CHAPTER 23

Allograft and Synthetic Reconstruction of the Ligaments of the Knee

WILLIAM A. GRANA, M.D.

■

For more than 15 years, the author has had an interest in the use of synthetic materials for the reconstruction of ligaments of the knee because of the potential benefits to the patient. The concept of atraumatic arthroscopic placement of a synthetic material to produce immediate stability without lengthy rehabilitation makes this procedure an extremely desirable option. However, there are many potential problems. The natural cruciate ligament has unique mechanical properties that make it strong enough to resist sudden large loads but still return to its original configuration without plastic deformation. Moreover, in the normal working range of load, it must withstand unlimited cycles of smaller force without plastic change. No current synthetic material can reproduce these qualities.

Another concept that is very attractive is for the synthetic material to serve as a lattice for the regrowth of a ligament.[35][40] Some of the author's original investigation was with this concept in mind, but as yet there is no material adequate for this purpose. Moreover, the fibrous tissue that grows into such porous materials is not the same as normal ligament.[2]

Finally, the option that seems to have worked best is use of the synthetic material as an augmentation of autogenous or allograft tissue in order to provide immediate stability until the biologic graft has completed its process of maturation. Then it will not matter if the synthetic fails.[44]

The purpose of this chapter is to present the current status of synthetic materials and allograft tissue in reconstructive surgery for instability of the knee. With regard to the synthetics, the focus is on the anterior cruciate ligament (ACL), inasmuch as the materials available in the United States are for this purpose and because the most frequent clinical problems are those affecting the ACL. The challenge in the design of an artificial ligament is to develop a substitute whose characteristics duplicate those of the original ligament. Materials of adequate strength have been developed, but reproducing the viscoelastic properties of the human ACL has not been accomplished. The history of synthetic ligaments is an interesting account of the development and marketing of implant materials for human use.

SYNTHETIC LIGAMENT RECONSTRUCTION

Historical Review

The Richards Company developed the Polyflex ligament, made of ultra-high-weight polyethylene, which was shaped into a solid rod. At the end of the ligament was a threaded metal fixture that allowed the polyethylene to be fixed through femoral and tibial drill holes. This material was extremely strong but stiff and brittle.[9] This ligament was sold for human use with little experimental research to document its efficacy. Virtually all of these ligaments failed in human use. The material was ultimately withdrawn from the market, and the experience left a tainted association about the term "synthetic ligament."

The Proplast ligament was a stent made of polyaramide fibers embedded in fluorinated ethylene propylene copolymer. It was coated with a carbon fiber and a polytetrine composite in order to facilitate collagen ingrowth. The graft was fixed through tibial and femoral drill holes with a staple at each end. The ultimate fixation was to the bone of the femoral and tibial drill holes by ingrowth.[9] This ligament was designed to be used with an extra-articular reconstruction. At the time, the Proplast was also used as a leader for autogenous grafts if additional length was required to anchor to bone.[25] When it was used as a prosthesis, there were multiple problems related to the stiffness of the material. The majority of these grafts failed, and clinical use was discontinued early in the trials.[9]

Carbon fiber was used as a ligament substitute in several different ways during the development of synthetic ligaments in the United States.[2] In addition, carbon fiber was in widespread use in Europe and other parts of the world.[26, 45] Initially, the prosthesis was made of pure carbon fiber with the concept that it would serve as a lattice for soft tissue ingrowth. Carbon fiber was ultimately used as a composite in which the carbon was coated with polycaprolactone and polylactic acid. The coating was resorbable, and as ingrowth occurred, the coating would disappear.[52] A variety of preclinical studies with this material demonstrated that fibrous tissue would grow into the carbon fiber graft. Fibroblasts would extrude collagen parallel to the carbon fibers. However, this material was found to be 60 per cent type I and 40 per cent type III collagen, thereby resembling a scar type of tissue rather than a ligament, which is normally 85 per cent type I and 15 per cent type III.[2] Moreover, the strength properties of carbon fiber were not adequate for the ACL, having a strength of approximately 425 newtons. However, it was believed that such rapid ingrowth of collagen obviated the need for a stronger material. However, the formation of a scar rather than a ligament, as well as the weakness of the material, resulted in breakage and failure. The problems associated with carbon fiber abrasion and breakage resulted in synovitis and chronic effusion.[19, 41, 45] The material was eliminated for synthetic replacement because of these problems.

The Xenograft was a bovine tendon chemically treated to prevent immunogenic response, according to the concept that it produced a lattice of collagen for fibrous tissue ingrowth.[30–32] The Xenograft is no longer available for implantation because it did not pass the U.S. Food and Drug Administration (FDA) approval process. In clinical trials, there was evidence that the graft did not provide biologic compatibility in the joint, and as a result, there was a significant problem with infection.[49]

Finally, a Dexon absorbable graft made of braided polyglycolic acid was used by Cabaud and co-workers, but only for implantation in animals.[13, 43] This animal experimentation revealed the graft was not durable whether used alone or in combination with a permanent synthetic material such as polyester (Dacron). Again, the concept was of a lattice that would fill in with fibrous tissue, and eventually the synthetic would be absorbed, leaving only the autologous tissue or a very small amount of foreign material. Unfortunately, the material failed early in implantation and was abandoned.[43]

Most of these grafts were heralded by much fanfare and hope but failed to stand the test of even short-term animal and clinical experimentation. To date, three materials have passed the FDA approval process and are currently on the market, primarily for salvage procedures. Each material is reviewed in the following sections with a description of its design and physical properties, the concept of its use, and the results from clinical trials. It is unclear what the future for synthetics is in the United States, but at this time, caution is to be used. Only with longer follow-up intervals and better design of materials will it be known whether any synthetic will stand the test of time and achieve the goals that have been set for the ideal device. The future is exciting, but this enthusiasm must be balanced with common sense about what is best for the patient on the basis of the specific clinical situation.[18]

FDA Regulation of Ligament Devices[16]

The Bureau of Chemistry of the U.S. Department of Agriculture enforced the Food and Drug Act of 1926 until 1927 when this agency was reformed. It was renamed the Food and Drug Administration (FDA) in 1931. In 1940, the FDA was transferred from the Department of Agriculture to the Federal Security Agency, which today is called the Department of Health and Human Services. In 1938, a new Food and Drug Cosmetic Act, signed by President Franklin D. Roosevelt, authorized inspection of pharmaceutical companies and established regulations for drug manufacturers that required scientific proof that products could be used safely. It also allowed therapeutic devices to be regulated for the first time and made it unlawful to sell devices that were dangerous or marketed with false claims.

In 1976, the medical device amendment of the federal Food and Drug Cosmetic Act was amended. These amendments identified three classes of devices according to the degree of regulatory control required. The amendments defined the legal role of panels of non-FDA experts to review evidence of device safety and effectiveness. In 1982, the Center for Devices and Radiologic Health was created. This center became responsible for review of applications of the marketing of prosthetic ligament devices. The Orthopaedic and Rehabilitation Devices panel reviews applications for prosthetic ligament devices and consists of seven voting members and two nonvoting members, all of whom represent consumer and industry interests, and a variety of expert clinical and scientific consultants. This group is responsible for the approval process for prosthetic ligament devices.

A device manufacturer may apply for an investigational device exemption on the basis of data obtained through literature, laboratory, or animal studies that demonstrate that the device is reasonably safe and effective for use on human subjects during carefully controlled trials. The application must also contain the design for clinical trials and an analysis of risk to the patient. The manufacturer must identify clinical investigators and the investigational review boards that will monitor the investigation. If an investigational device exemption is completed, then a manufacturer may provide data of the scientific proof and effectiveness of the new device. A manufacturer submits a pre–market approval (PMA) application in order to obtain FDA approval to market the device. PMA is recommended by the Orthopaedic and Rehabilitation Devices panel on the basis of their knowledge of the field and their review of the PMA application. The FDA makes a final decision of whether to grant or withhold PMA. In the United States, only three materials have received the PMA from the FDA. This includes the 3M polypropylene ligament augmentation device (LAD), the Stryker Meadox Dacron prosthesis, and the Gore-Tex polytetrafluoroethylene prosthesis. These devices are the focus of the remainder of this discussion on synthetic ligaments.

Design and Biomechanics

The ideal synthetic ligament is a material whose physical properties duplicate those of the ACL, especially with regard to its ability to withstand repetitive load without plastic deformation. The material must be strong but not brittle, and there remains the question "How much is enough?" There is always the risk of capturing the joint with a strong but stiff graft. In Chapter 3 it was noted that the physical properties of the ACL have not been duplicated in any synthetic material currently in use.

A second requirement is that the material be biocompatible. There must be no reactivity of the joint to the material even in the event of abrasion of small particles from the material as a result of impingement or chronic wear. There must be no immunologic phenomena and no systemic effects. There must be both short- and long-term tolerance, as demonstrated in both short- and long-term clinical trials.

Third, the material must be easily inserted, preferably by arthroscopic technique. At the same time, it must be easily explanted if it fails. Explantation must be accomplished without destruction of autologous tissue, which would thereby produce further laxity or functional problems.

Finally, the material must be priced within reason and therefore available to as many patients as possible. The material must be adequately tested through both animal and clinical trials, as noted in the FDA approval process. There should be no promotion of the device until this testing is complete or, preferably, before a 5-year clinical trial in humans.

The biomechanical terms that define mechanical properties in these ligaments are listed as follows:

Ultimate tensile strength (breaking point) is the point at which all components of a material fail. The ultimate tensile strength of the ACL is approximately 1700 newtons.

Elastic deformation occurs when an object is loaded from its original resting state to a new resting state and then returns to that original resting state upon removal of the load.

Plastic deformation occurs when an object does not return to the original resting state when the load is removed, thereby becoming permanent deformed.

Yield point is the point at which the material begins plastic deformation.

Fatigue strength is the ultimate tensile strength after cyclic loading. Three common methods of fatigue testing are tension, flexion, and twisting. The knee has been estimated to undergo approximately 4 million cycles per year with an averaged daily load in walking of 210 newtons, and so when fatigue testing is conducted, researchers must consider how the material is cycled, how many times it is cycled, and what loads were applied.

Abrasion is the wear produced through the rubbing of two surfaces. In the case of synthetic ligaments, wear particles can be produced and can in turn produce foreign body synovitis.

Stiffness is an object's resistance to deformation as a result of change in force.

Biological degradation occurs as a result of the body's environment, inasmuch as the material may be affected by ongoing changes within this environment. Many synthetics undergo loss of strength in a synovial fluid environment.[9]

Specific Materials

Information on a number of these products is provided in Table 23–1.

TABLE 23–1. Competing Anterior Cruciate Ligament Replacement Products

Characteristics	Normal Human Anterior Cruciate Ligament (16 to 26 Years)	Patellar Tendon	Semitendinosus	Gore-Tex	Gore-Tex II	3M Kennedy LAD	Stryker 130-20/25
Type of substitute		Alone	Doubled	Permanent prosthesis	Permanent prosthesis	Augmentation graft	Permanent prosthesis
Material		Autologous allograft	Autologous allograft	PTFE (Teflon)	PTFE with sheath	Braided polypropylene	Polyester (Dacron)
Fixation		Biologic/steel sutures/internal screw	Sutures/staples/biologic	Screws	Screws	Staple-femur/biologic-tibia	Staples
Ultimate tensile load (newtons)	1703 to 2000	2800	2700	5300	5300	1500, 1730	3631
Ultimate strain (percentage)	25 to 30	—	21	8 to 10	8 to 10	22	18.7
Stiffness (newton/mm)	200 to 300	675	430	365	400	61	365
Drill hole diameter (mm)		8 to 10	7 to 9	6.5	7.9	6.0	5.0
Functional placement		Either	Either	Over the top	Over the top	Over the top	Either

LAD, ligament augmentation device; PTFE, polytetrafluoroethylene.

THE 3M POLYPROPYLENE LIGAMENT AUGMENTATION DEVICE (LAD)

ACL reconstruction is generally performed with an autogenous tissue such as the hamstring tendons or the patellar tendon. These graft tissues are initially strong but become weak during the first few weeks after surgery. During this time, the graft is susceptible to stretch or injury from repetitive loading in the rehabilitation period.[3, 4, 14] The LAD (Fig. 23–1) is a permanent, nonabsorbable implant for augmenting an autogenous or allograft tissue in ACL reconstruction. The LAD is implanted in parallel with the biologic graft for the purpose of enhancing graft strength and sharing load with the graft. The concept is that the LAD protects the graft during the postoperative period of weakness while still providing early stability to the joint.[44]

In theory, load distribution between the LAD and the biologic graft depends on the stiffness of the LAD, the graft tissue used, and the suture connection between the two materials. As the stiffness of the graft decreases, the contribution of the biologic graft to load sharing decreases, and as the stiffness of the graft increases, the contribution increases. The LAD protects the biologic graft from excessive stress when the graft tissue is weak. As the graft tissue heals and regains stiffness, the proportion of the load carried by the biologic graft increases, thereby producing a stimulus for remodeling and avoiding stress shielding when the graft is strong. A variety of studies have demonstrated that the LAD initially provides graft strength and fixation during the early postoperative period and shares load with the biologic graft.[21, 50]

The LAD is a flat braid constructed from bundles or "tows" of polypropylene filament. Each filament is 43 microns in diameter, and its breaking strength is more than 135,000 psi. Each "tow" contains 180 filaments. The device is fabricated in two widths, 6 mm and 8 mm. The device is approximately 1.5 mm thick and is supplied in lengths ranging from 6 to 25 mm in 1-cm increments in order to allow sizing to the particular autologous tissue used.[44]

The physical properties are equivalent to those of the normal ACL: a tensile strength of 1730 newtons; elongation of 22 per cent, and stiffness

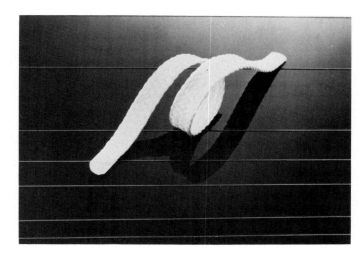

FIGURE 23–1. 3M ligament augmentation device (LAD).

of 280 newtons/mm (3-cm length). Cyclic fatigue studies showed a 9 per cent strength loss and a 4 per cent creep after 1 million tensile load cycles between 50 and 500 newtons. Bending fatigue studies showed a 23 per cent strength loss and 4.5 per cent creep after 10 million tensile load cycles between 150 and 300 newtons with flexion between 15° and 40°. Fatigue failure did not occur during any of the cyclic testing.[44]

Clinical studies have been conducted with this device. Initially, these studies were conducted by Kennedy[44] and subsequently by a number of other investigators. The clinical results can best be summarized by a long-term study presented at the American Orthopaedic Society for Sports Medicine Specialty Day Meeting in February 1990. Results of Kennedy's original work were presented by Fowler and associates.[17] One hundred forty-three procedures were reviewed retrospectively by telephone interview and chart review. A total of 100 patients were available for follow-up after an average of 7.5 years (range was 5.5 to 9.0 years). Ninety per cent of the patients' results were rated good to excellent in terms of activity level, function, limitation, pain, swelling, and giving way. Eighty-nine per cent of the patients participated in activities on the same level as they had before injury. Seventy-eight per cent had no giving way, and 87 per cent were functioning with no or minor limitations with regard to the knee. Seventy-four per cent required no further surgery, and there was documentation in one patient of a traumatic tear of a reconstruction 8 years postoperatively during a rugby match. Six per cent of the patients required subsequent meniscal surgery. Ninety-six per cent of the patients stated that they would be willing to repeat the procedure if necessary. These results appear promising with regard to the safety of the device and the functional result.[17]

However, another study by Daniels and colleagues indicates that there is little difference between the use of an augmented autogenous reconstruction and the use of an autogenous reconstruction by itself. Results with regard to function, swelling, and stability appear to be approximately the same; however, Daniels and colleagues noted the low risk involved with using the polypropylene braid, including a lower incidence of joint effusion. They were able to perform biopsies in several of the patients and noted very minimal amounts of particulate debris in the sampled tissue. They emphasized the importance of surgical techniques to reduce the chances of impingement or abrasion of the graft. Their conclusions were that patients with augmented grafts and those with nonaugmented grafts showed good clinical results.[15]

The concept of load sharing of a synthetic material with a biologic graft seems theoretically feasible and appears to have scientific support. Whether there is a significant improvement in the results awaits a prospective study of augmented and nonaugmented grafts.

THE STRYKER DACRON LIGAMENT PROSTHESIS

Dacron has been studied extensively in animal models as a replacement for the ACL and has shown promise because of its ability to support and enhance fibrous tissue ingrowth.[35, 40] Pull strength from bone has been shown to be superior to that of other synthetics.[5] Dacron has been used both as an augmentation and as a prosthesis (Fig. 23–2), and the work in animal models indicates that it functions primarily as a prosthesis.[28]

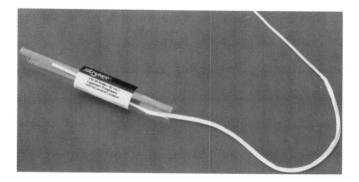

FIGURE 23-2. Stryker Meadox Dacron prosthesis.

The ligament is designed as a graft 8 mm in diameter with a knitted velour outer sheath and an inner core of four woven Dacron tapes. Mechanical properties of the graft are an ultimate tensile strength of 3600 newtons with a mean ultimate elongation of 18.7 per cent and plastic deformation of less than 1 per cent after 10 million tensile load cycles. Fatigue life is 324 million cycles with a tensile load level of 210 newtons. The graft has been used as an augmentation of the iliotibial band taken through a tibial drill hole and over the top of the femur. The graft has also been used as a pure prosthesis and taken through a drill hole on both the tibia and the femur. The comparison of the augmented and nonaugmented reconstructions shows that there is no difference in the results of the two procedures. The graft therefore acts as a pure prosthesis rather than a scaffold or a stint. The graft is surgically inserted by either an open technique or an arthroscopic technique with special attention to notchplasty. Fixation is with a specially designed staple.[6, 7]

The published results of this surgery with a group of patients, considered a salvage group with one to two previous surgeries per patient for ACL insufficiency, showed that the functional rating improved from 40 to 81 points and the activity level from 2 to 4. Seventy-five per cent of the patients had a negative Lachman sign, a negative drawer test, and a negative pivot shift test at follow-up. The mean follow-up time was 21 months. The overall failure rate was 21.5 per cent; in this group of patients, 2 per cent experienced synovitis, 2 per cent experienced septic arthritis, and 1 per cent experienced extra-articular infection. Graft failure occurred at a rate of 4 per cent. As with the LAD, this graft seems safe to use, but there are higher complication and failure rates than with an autologous procedure.[28]

The most recent information on this graft is from Wilk and Richmond, who presented a 5-year follow-up of a multicenter study in which this prosthesis was used. It reveals an overall failure rate of 35.7 per cent in a group of 84 patients. This was demonstrated by a Lachman sign or an anterior drawer of more than grade 2+, a positive pivot shift, test, or instrumented laxity testing showing a difference of more than 3 mm. Therefore, this study demonstrates a significant deterioration of results over the previous 2 years of follow-up. The conclusion of this work was that although the Dacron ligament achieved the short-term goal of restoration stability and improvement of function, it did not provide long-term stability for the ACL-deficient knee.[53]

THE GORE-TEX PROSTHESIS

The Gore-Tex graft (Fig. 23–3) is made of braided bundles of a single fiber of expanded polytetrafluoroethylene. There is an eyelet at each end of the graft for fixation to bone with a cortical screw. The braid is said to allow more even load distribution through the prosthesis, and the eyelets are for mechanical fixation by standard bicortical screws. The graft is designed to be used as a prosthesis. Because of its strength and stiffness, preconditioning of the graft and placement are important aspects of the technique of the procedure.[8]

Physical and physiologic properties of the ligament include an ultimate tensile strength of 4448 newtons, a stiffness of 322 newtons/mm, maximal elongation of 8.9 per cent, and a fatigue strength of 100 per cent after 3.7×10^7 load cycles at a load of 111 newtons. The mode of cyclic testing was bending, and the ultimate strength of these samples was not impaired by the cyclic loading when tested to failure. As with the Dacron graft, there is significant ingrowth of fibrous tissue, but pull-out strength in animal experiments was slightly less than for the Dacron.[8, 10, 48]

The surgical technique is to place the implant in bone tunnels in the tibia and the femur by use of an over-the-top routing on the femoral condyle. The eyelets of the graft are fixed to the bone with screws in order to provide the initial fixation by bicortical screws. Ultimate fixation is achieved through osseous and fibrous tissue ingrowth into and through the device in the bone tunnels. A wide notchplasty is accomplished to prevent abrasion, and no extra-articular back-up procedure is performed.[1] The graft must be preconditioned by applying at least 200 newtons (45 pounds) of tension to the tibial eyelet with the knee in full extension and with the femoral end of the graft fixed. If the knee is overtightened by placement of the tibial eyelet too far distally, high ligament forces are generated with extension. This problem has been studied and reported on previously in a detailed description in the work of More and Markolf.[36]

Early experience with the Gore-Tex prosthesis, as with other synthetics, was promising. In evaluations of both primary and salvage procedures, 87 per cent of all patients had satisfactory results. However, even in these early studies, problems with the use of the prosthesis included partial or

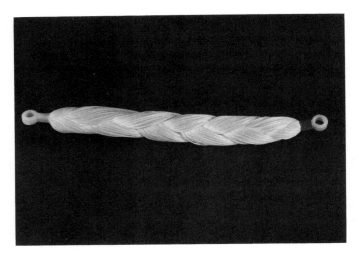

FIGURE 23–3. Gore-Tex ligament prosthesis.

complete tear, sterile effusions, and synovial irritation. Placement of the graft and avoidance of abrasion are crucial. The results for the salvage were less promising than those for the primary procedure. Again, 87 per cent of the patients had an improvement in anterior instability, but 70 per cent had pain. In these early results, 18 per cent of patients had a sensation of or actual giving way; 59 per cent had some degree of pivot shift, 54 per cent had a complication; and 20 per cent had recurrent instability. Four of the patients with recurrent instability were documented to have graft failure.[22] In a 3-year period, there was indication of deterioration of results.[54] There was an increase in instability symptoms, swelling, and laxity. Three predictors of later failure at 2 years were identified as subjective symptoms of swelling, subjective symptoms of giving way, and an increased anterior drawer. The 5-year follow-up, as presented by Gore-Tex, revealed that 25 per cent of the patients experienced giving way and 48 per cent had a pivot shift. Fourteen to 15 per cent of patients had some degree of swelling. By 5 years, approximately 10 per cent of the devices were removed because of failure or recurrent instability.[1, 20] Furthermore, there was documentation of synovial irritation and effusion from particulate polytetrafluoroethylene in the joint.[19] Gore-Tex now has a Generation II graft that provides better protection from the abrasion problem.[18] What the future is for the Gore-Tex graft is uncertain at this time.

The Future for Synthetics

The future for synthetics is uncertain. Currently, the best concept seems to be the use of a synthetic as an augmentation device with load sharing of biologic tissue, whether allograft or autograft. On the other hand, there is some evidence that the augmentation device does not serve any useful role, inasmuch as in some studies the results are not affected by the use of the augmentation device. The initial enthusiasm of the early 1980s for the use of a synthetic has abated. Many surgeons have substituted the use of an allograft for a synthetic. There is a need for better materials designed with the viscoelastic properties of the cruciate ligament in mind as well as for biologic compatibility with the joint. To date, such a material is not available. The author does not find any current reasonable use for a prosthetic material except in a patient who declines the use of an allograft. However, Robert L. Larson believes that synthetics are a reasonable alternative to the use of an allograft when reconstruction of a "salvage" knee is performed.

ALLOGRAFT RECONSTRUCTION OF THE LIGAMENTS OF THE KNEE

Use of an allograft to reconstruct one or both of the cruciate ligaments of the knee offers the potential advantages of not having to sacrifice functional tissue from another site, acting as a biologic graft, duplicating the anatomic properties of the ACL graft, and availability of various sizes and shapes of grafts, which can be fashioned by the surgeon and can be amenable to long-term storage. All of these potential advantages are tempered by concerns regarding immunogenicity and transmission of chronic infectious diseases. These concerns have resulted in techniques for processing and preserving allografts. Deep-frozen tissue, freeze-dried tissue, and tissue sterilized by means of gamma radiation or gas such as ethylene oxide have been used. The concerns about the effects of these preparation methods have led to a variety of studies of allograft properties before insertion.[33]

Allografts have been used for repair of rotator cuff tendon defects as well as in other tendon and reconstructive surgery in the past.[37] A variety of studies have shown that fascia lata femoris, bone–patellar tendon–bone, and ACL allografts can be used to reconstruct the ACL.[38, 39] The allografts undergo necrosis, revascularization, and remodeling. However, the mechanical properties of the allografts become weaker with poorer elongation and lower maximal load at ultimate failure.

A second concern about allografts is the inflammatory response that they may provoke. It appears that deep freezing, freeze drying, and gamma irradiation all significantly reduce this problem. However, freeze drying with ethylene oxide has been shown to produce a consistent articular reaction after allograft implantation. There are collagen debris, lymphocytic response, and destruction of the graft. Synovial biopsy shows a chronic inflammatory process, and the allograft demonstrates areas of focal necrosis and inflammation. For these reasons, ethylene oxide sterilization has been discarded as a method of preparation of allografts.[23, 24, 42] Gamma irradiation also changes the mechanical properties of the graft by altering the collagenous structure. Therefore, all of the preservation methods result in some degree of weakening of the graft.[29, 33] Even fresh-frozen allograft tissue may have diminished physical properties in comparison with the same autogenous tissue.[46]

Disease Transmission in Allograft Surgery[11, 12, 27]

The causes of infections associated with tissue transplants include bacterial, viral, microbacterial, fungal, and other rare pathogens. Both local and systemic infections have been recognized. All infections can result in severe morbidity for the patient as well as the loss of therapeutic efficiency of the graft. The removal of the graft may become necessary if conservative medical therapy is not successful. Local infection may lead to systemic dissemination. In some reports of orthopaedic transplantation, bone transplantation has resulted in bacterial infection, hepatitis, and acquired immunodeficiency syndrome in the recipient. At the time of this writing, there are no reported cases of infectious complications from the use of allograft tendon materials for the reconstruction of the cruciate ligament. However, the potential still exists. Prevention of disease transmission depends on an effective screening process. There are rigid standards for donor screening and for microbiologic and serologic testing, and if these guidelines are followed, the estimated risk of disease transmission is less than 1 per 1 million.

Current Utilization

Current recommendations are to use fresh-frozen allograft material, which is prepared by being slowly frozen to minus 80°C at a rate of approximately

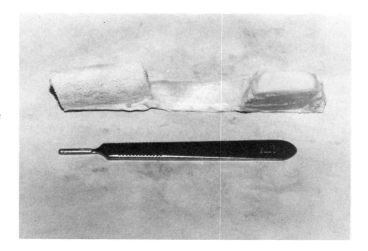

FIGURE 23–4. Bone–patellar tendon–bone allograft.

1°C per minute. This procedure seems to have the least effect on the mechanical properties of the collagen, and biologic compatibility and decreased reactivity are maintained when the graft is implanted in the joint.

The author has used allograft material for failed autograft reconstructions or for complex instability problems, but not as a primary procedure in routine ACL reconstruction. The indications for its use have been in a patient whose knee has been multiply reconstructed or in failed repair of ACL insufficiency in which both patellar tendon and hamstring tendons have been used. The author has also used allografts primarily for posterior cruciate ligament (PCL) insufficiency or for complex cruciate insufficiency by which both the ACL and the PCL must be reconstructed. Surgical technique includes arthroscopic methods of insertion and follows the same rehabilitation guidelines as in autograft reconstruction. The advantages of allograft over autograft reconstruction are that a larger graft can be obtained and can be shaped appropriately with a bone plug for interference screw fixation (Fig. 23–4).

There are few results reported of allograft reconstruction. The published results in the literature are difficult to compare because different tissues and different rehabilitation protocols are used.[34, 47, 51] There are no consistent follow-up protocols. In the published studies, there were no reports of rejection or chronic disease transmission. However, the ultimate role of the allograft remains undefined at this point. The author believes that its use should be confined to the salvage procedure or the complex instability problem.

REFERENCES

1. Ahlfeld SK, Larson RL, Collins HR: Anterior cruciate reconstruction in the chronically unstable knee using an expanded polytetrafluoroethylene (PTFE) prosthetic ligament. Am J Sports Med 15:326–330, 1987.
2. Alexander H, Parsons JR, Weiss AB: Preclinical evaluation of ligament reconstruction with an absorbable polymer-coated carbon-fiber stent (Integraft*). *In* Friedman MJ, Ferkel RD (eds): Prosthetic Ligament Reconstruction of the Knee, pp. 41–51. Philadelphia: WB Saunders, 1988.
3. Alm A, Stromberg B: Vascular anatomy of the patellar and cruciate ligaments: a microangiographic and histologic investigation in the dog. Acta Chir Scand (Suppl) 445:25–35, 1974.

4. Alm A, Stromberg B: Transposed medial third of patellar ligament in reconstruction of the anterior cruciate ligament: a surgical and morphologic study in dogs. Acta Chir Scand (Suppl) 445:37–49, 1974.

5. Arnoczky SP, Torzilli PA, Warren RF, Allen AA: Biologic fixation of ligament prostheses and augmentations: an evaluation of bone ingrowth in the dog. Am J Sports Med 16(2):106–112, 1988.

6. Bhate AP, Lemons JE, Devrnja R, Rigney ED: Durability Characterization of Stryker Dacron Prosthetic Ligaments. Oakland, NJ: Meadox Medicals, Inc., 1978.

7. Bhate AP, Lemons JE, Moseley J: Viscoelastic Characterization of Stryker Dacron Ligament Prostheses. Birmingham: Department of Engineering, University of Alabama; and Oakland, NJ: Meadox Medicals, Inc., 1978.

8. Bolton CW, Bruchman WC: The Gore-Tex expanded polytetrafluoroethylene prosthetic ligament. Clin Orthop 196:202–213, 1985.

9. Bonnarens FO, Drez D: Biomechanics of artificial ligaments and associated problems. *In* Jackson DW, Drez D (eds): The Anterior Cruciate Deficient Knee, pp. 239–253. St. Louis: CV Mosby, 1987.

10. Bruchman WC, Bain JR, Bolton CW: Prosthetic replacement of the cruciate ligaments with expanded polytetrafluoroethylene. *In* Feagin JA (ed): The Crucial Ligaments. New York: Churchill Livingstone, 1988.

11. Buck BE, Malinin TI, Brown MD: Bone transplantation and human immunodeficiency virus: an estimate risk of acquired immunodeficiency syndrome (AIDS). Clin Orthop 240:129–136, 1989.

12. Buck BE, Resnick L, Shah SM, et al: Human immunodeficiency virus cultured from bone: implications for transplantation. Clin Orthop 251:249–253, 1990.

13. Cabaud HE, Feagin JA, Rodkey WG: Acute anterior cruciate ligament injury and repair reinforced with a biodegradable material device for repair and reconstruction of injured tendons. Am J Sports Med 13:242–247, 1985.

14. Clancy WC, Narenchiania RG, Rosenberg TD, et al: Anterior and posterior cruciate ligament reconstruction in rhesus monkeys: a histological, micrographic, and biomechanical analysis. J Bone Joint Surg 63A:1270–1284, 1981.

15. Daniel DM, Woodward EP, Losse GM, Stone ML: The Marshall/MacIntosh anterior cruciate ligament reconstruction with the Kennedy ligament augmentation device: report of the United States clinical trials. *In* Friedman MJ, Ferkel RD (eds): Prosthetic Ligament Reconstruction of the Knee, pp. 71–78. Philadelphia: WB Saunders, 1988.

16. Ferl JG, Goldenthal KL, Mishra NK: FDA regulation of prosthetic ligament devices. *In* Friedman MJ, Ferkel RD (eds): Prosthetic Ligament Reconstruction of the Knee, pp. 202–208. Philadelphia: WB Saunders, 1988.

17. Fowler PJ, Roth JH, MacKinlay D: Long Term Follow-Up of Intra-Articular ACL Reconstructions Augmented With Braided Polypropylene (Kennedy LAD). *Presented at* the American Orthopaedic Society for Sports Medicine Specialty Day Meeting, New Orleans, February 1990.

18. Friedman MJ, Ferkel RD: Prosthetic Ligament Reconstruction of the Knee. Philadelphia: WB Saunders, 1988.

19. Fu FH: Evaluation of Prosthetic Debris. *Presented at* the Seventh International Symposium on Advances in Cruciate Ligament Reconstruction of the Knee: Autogenous vs. Prosthetic. University of California, Los Angeles, Palm Desert, CA, March 1990.

20. Gore WL & Associates: The Gore-Tex Cruciate Ligament Prosthesis: Five-Year Clinical Results. Flagstaff, AZ: WL Gore & Associates, Inc., 1989.

21. Hanley P, Lew WD, Lewis JL, et al: Load sharing and graft forces in anterior cruciate ligament reconstructions with the ligament augmentation device. Am J Sports Med 17:414–422, 1989.

22. Indelicato PA, Pascale MS, Huegel MO: Early experience with the Gore-Tex polytetrafluoroethylene anterior cruciate ligament prosthesis. Am J Sports Med 17:55–62, 1989.

23. Jackson DW, Grood ES, Arnoczky SP, et al: Freeze-dried anterior cruciate ligament allografts: preliminary studies in a goat model. Am J Sports Med 15:295–303, 1987.

24. Jackson DW, Windler GE, Simon TM: Intraarticular reaction associated with the use of freeze-dried, ethylene oxide–sterilized bone–patella tendon–bone allografts in the reconstruction of the anterior cruciate ligament. Am J Sports Med 18:1–11, 1990.

25. James SL, Woods GW, Homsy CA, et al: Cruciate ligament stents in reconstruction of the unstable knee. Clin Orthop 143:90–96, 1979.

26. Jenkins DHR: The repair of cruciate ligaments with flexible carbon fibre. J Bone Joint Surg 60B:520–522, 1978.

27. Kakaiya R, Miller WV, Gudino MD: Tissue transplant–transmitted infections. Transfusion 31:277–284, 1991.

28. Lukianov AV, Richmond JC, Barrett GR, Gillquist J: A multicenter study on the results of anterior cruciate ligament reconstruction using a Dacron ligament prosthesis in "salvage" cases. Am J Sports Med 17:380–386, 1989.

29. McCarthy J, Blomstrom G, Steadman J, et al: ACL Reconstruction Using Cryopreserved Patellar Tendon Allografts: A Biomechanical and Histological Evaluation. Marietta, GA: Cryolife, Inc.

30. McMaster WC: A histologic assessment of canine anterior cruciate substitution with bovine xenograft. Clin Orthop 196:196–201, 1985.
31. McMaster WC: Biomechanics profile of the ProCol cruciate bioprosthesis. *In* Friedman MJ, Ferkel RD (eds): Prosthetic Ligament Reconstruction of the Knee, pp. 89–94. Philadelphia: WB Saunders, 1988.
32. McMaster WC: Open anterior cruciate ligament reconstruction with ProCol Bioprosthesis: results at 24 months—U.S. series. *In* Friedman MJ, Ferkel RD (eds): Prosthetic Ligament Reconstruction of the Knee, pp. 95–100. Philadelphia: WB Saunders, 1988.
33. Meyers JF: Allograft reconstruction of the anterior cruciate ligament. Clin Sports Med 10:487, 1991.
34. Meyers JF, Caspari RB, Cash JD, et al: Arthroscopic Evaluation of Allograft Anterior Cruciate Ligament Reconstruction. *Presented at* the Arthroscopy Association of North America Annual Meeting, Orlando, FL, April 1990.
35. Meyers JF, Grana WA, Lesker PA: Reconstruction of the anterior cruciate ligament in the dog: Comparison of results obtained with three different porous synthetic materials. Am J Sports Med 7:85–90, 1979.
36. More RC, Markolf KL: Measurement of stability of the knee and ligament force after implantation of a synthetic anterior cruciate ligament. J Bone Joint Surg 70A:1020–1031, 1988.
37. Neviaser SJ, Neviaser RJ, Neviaser TJ: The repair of chronic massive ruptures of the rotator cuff of the shoulder by use of a freeze-dried rotator cuff. J Bone Joint Surg 60A:681–684, 1978.
38. Nikolaou PK, Seaber AV, Glisson RR, et al: Anterior cruciate ligament allograft transplantation: long-term function, histology, revascularization, and operative technique. Am J Sports Med 14:348–360, 1986.
39. Noyes FR, Barber SD, Mangine RE: Bone–patellar ligament–bone and fascia lata allografts for reconstruction of the anterior cruciate ligament. J Bone Joint Surg 72A:1125–1136, 1990.
40. Park JP, Grana WA, Chitwood JS: A high-strength Dacron augmentation for cruciate ligament reconstruction: a two-year canine study. Clin Orthop 196:175–185, 1985.
41. Parson JR, Bhayani S, Alexander H, Weiss AB: Carbon fiber debris within the synovial joint: A time-dependent mechanical and histologic study. Clin Orthop 196: 69–76, 1985.
42. Roberts TS, Drez D, McCarthy W, Pain R: Anterior cruciate ligament reconstruction using freeze-dried, ethylene oxide-sterilized, bone–patellar tendon–bone allografts: Two year results in thirty-six patients. Am J Sports Med 19:35–40, 1991.
43. Rodkey WG, Cabaud HE, Feagin JA, Perlik PC: A partially biodegradable material device for repair and reconstruction of injured tendons: Experimental studies. Am J Sports Med 13:242–247, 1985.
44. Roth JH, Kennedy JC: Polypropylene-braid–augmented anterior cruciate ligament reconstruction. *In* Friedman MJ, Ferkel RD (eds): Prosthetic Ligament Reconstruction of the Knee, pp. 79–88. Philadelphia: WB Saunders, 1988.
45. Rushton N, Dandy DJ, Naylor CPE: The clinical arthroscopic and histological finding after replacement of the anterior cruciate ligament with carbon fibre. J Bone Joint Surg 65B:308–309, 1983.
46. Schmidt F, Biles J, Egle DM, et al: Study of Mechanical Properties of Allograft Materials for ACL Reconstruction. Unpublished work, June 1988.
47. Shino K, Kawasaki T, Hirose H, et al: Replacement of the anterior cruciate ligament by an allogenic tendon graft: an operation for chronic ligamentous insufficiency. J Bone Joint Surg 68B:739–746, 1986.
48. Stonebrook SN, Berman AB, Bruchman WC, Bain JR: Functional biomechanics of the Gore-Tex cruciate-ligament prosthesis: effects of implant tensioning. *In* Friedman MJ, Ferkel RD (eds): Prosthetic Ligament Reconstruction of the Knee, pp. 140–148. Philadelphia: WB Saunders, 1988.
49. Teitge RA: Anterior Cruciate Ligament Reconstruction Using Bovine Xenograft Prosthesis. *Presented at* the American Orthopaedic Society for Sports Medicine Annual Meeting, Nashville, 1985.
50. Van Kampen CL: Biomechanics of the 3M Kennedy LAD. St. Paul, MN: 3M Orthopedic Products Division.
51. Wainer RA, Clarke TJ, Poehling GG: Arthroscopic reconstruction of the anterior cruciate ligament using allograft tendon. Arthroscopy 4:199–205, 1988.
52. Weiss AB, Blazina ME, Goldstein AR, Alexander H: Ligament replacement with an absorbable copolymer carbon fiber scaffold—early clinical experience. Clin Orthop 196:77–85, 1985.
53. Wilk RM, Richmond JC: Dacron Ligament Reconstruction for Chronic ACL Insufficiency: 5 Year Follow-Up. *Presented at* the American Orthopaedic Society for Sports Medicine Annual Meeting, Orlando FL, July 1991.
54. Woods GA, Indelicato PA, Prevot TJ: The Gore-Tex anterior cruciate ligament prosthesis: two versus three year results. Am J Sports Med 19:48–55, 1991.

CHAPTER 24

Complications in

Arthroscopic and

Ligamentous

Knee Surgery

JONATHAN GREENLEAF, M.D.

ROBERT L. LARSON, M.D.

■

Knee surgery has evolved into a plethora of newer techniques since 1970. Modalities such as arthroscopy, computed tomography, and magnetic resonance imaging have opened up new diagnostic opportunities. Modernization of surgical techniques for anterior cruciate ligament (ACL) reconstruction and accelerated rehabilitation programs have helped to decrease morbidity. The frequency of complications such as limited motion after knee surgery has been reduced. Arthroscopic surgical techniques have allowed ACL replacement with only limited surgical exposure. In spite of these refinements, complications are a source of continued concern. Complications should be recognized, evaluated, and given thoughtful consideration.

COMPLICATIONS IN ARTHROSCOPIC SURGERY

Jackson and Dandy,[35] in 1976, described arthroscopic complications. At that time, most complications were caused by breakage of arthroscopic instruments in the joint. Researchers have conducted several retrospective and prospective large-scale surveys of complications ranging from common problems such as hemarthrosis to very uncommon problems such as gas gangrene and false aneurysms of the popliteal artery.

Several studies have been conducted in order to determine the incidence of complications relating to arthroscopic procedures.[11, 59, 68, 71, 72] The Arthroscopy Association of North America (AANA), in a national survey (1986) of 395,566 arthroscopies, reported that 375,069 were of the knee.[71] The complication rate for arthroscopic surgery of all joints was 0.56 per cent. The survey was a retrospective poll that relied solely on the memory of the surgeons. A more accurate prospective survey was taken during a 19-month period (1986 to 1988) with monthly reporting by 21 experienced arthroscopists.[72] In the 10,282 procedures reported, there were 173 complications—a complication rate of 1.7 per cent (Table 24–1).

The types and percentages of complications seen in this study are given in Table 24–2. No vascular injuries were reported. The remaining 6.9 per cent were miscellaneous complications.

TABLE 24–1. Incidence of Complications for Specific Procedures: Arthroscopic

Procedure	Complication Percentage
Lateral release	8.0
ACL reconstruction: synthetic	5.2
ACL: allograft	3.7
ACL: autogenous	2.2
Abrasion arthroplasty	2.1
Outside-inside meniscus repair	2.1
Synovectomy	2.0
Medial meniscus repair	1.8
Medial meniscectomy	1.8
Lateral meniscectomy	1.6
Shaving chondroplasty	1.6
Plica excision	1.4
Lateral meniscus repair	0.0

Modified from Small NC: Complications in arthroscopic surgery performed by experienced arthroscopists. Arthroscopy 4:215–221, 1988.
ACL, anterior cruciate ligament.

TABLE 24–2. General Arthroscopic Complications

Complication	Percentage of Total Number of Arthroscopic Procedures	Percentage of Complications
Hemarthrosis	1.00	60.0
Infection	0.20	12.1
Thromboembolic	0.12	6.9
Anesthesia	0.10	6.4
Instrument failure	0.05	2.9
Reflex sympathetic dystrophy	0.04	2.3
Ligament injury	0.02	1.2
Neurologic injury	0.01	0.06
Vascular injury	0.00	0.00

Modified from Small NC: Complications in arthroscopic surgery performed by experienced arthroscopists. Arthroscopy 4:215–221, 1988.
For a total of 10,282 procedures.

A large orthopaedic group described complications in one series of 2640 cases and in a second series of the next 2739 cases.[59, 68] The first series had a complication rate of 8.2 per cent; the second series had a complication rate of 6.1 per cent. Age (over 50 years) and tourniquet time (more than 60 minutes) were the factors found to most predictably increase the risk of a complication.

Anesthesia

Anesthesia risks for arthroscopic surgery are similar to those of any other type of orthopaedic knee surgery. The most important consideration concerning arthroscopic complications is the type of anesthetic, be it general, epidural, spinal, or local. The rate of anesthesia-related mortality is approximately 0.01 per cent in surgical cases.[16, 21, 44] Among patients aged 10 to 40 years who undergo elective surgery, the mortality rates are close to zero.[44]

General anesthesia used for arthroscopy produced 63 complications in the 1986 survey by AANA.[71] Cardiac arrhythmia, pneumonia, and aspiration pneumonitis were the most frequent complications. Spinal anesthesia produced cases of urinary retention and single cases each of cardiac arrest, temporary ascending paralysis, and respiratory arrest. Local anesthetics, particularly with epinephrine, caused blistering, superficial infections, skin slough, and grand mal seizure. Anesthetic complications accounted for 3.7 per cent of all complications in the first AANA study.

The rate of arthroscopic complications not caused by anesthesia ranges from 1.68 to 8.2 per cent.[68, 71, 72] Sherman and associates' study[68] of 2640 arthroscopies revealed 126 major complications, which included infections, hemarthrosis, adhesions, effusions, neurologic problems, RSD, and instrument breakage. Minor complications were difficulties with wound healing and ecchymosis.

Hemarthrosis

Hemarthrosis is reported to occur in 1 to 5 per cent of all knee arthroscopies.[11, 59, 68, 72, 73] There were 104 incidents of hemarthrosis (60 per cent) of the 173 complications reported by Small.[72] Hemarthrosis was associated most frequently with partial medial meniscectomy and arthroscopic lateral release.

Infection

Deep infections occur in 0.04 to 0.08 per cent of knee arthroscopies.[11, 59] Problems with portal healing and superficial drainage are seen in a significantly larger percentage, perhaps up to 3 per cent of all arthroscopies. *Staphylococcus aureus* was the most common bacterial agent; *Staphylococcus epidermidis* and *Streptococcus* species were present in a small number of patients. The average interval between the procedure and discovery of the infection was 11.7 days in the 1988 AANA report. Prophylactic antibiotics were used in four of the 19 patients who developed an infection.

Aritomi and Yamamoto[2] reported two cases of *Pseudomonas aeruginosa* infection in 58 knee arthroscopies. There have also been case reports of some unusual infections such as meningococcal septicemia, toxic shock syndrome, gas gangrene, and *Clostridium* pyoarthrosis.[5, 9, 39]

Intra-articular steroid injection at the time of arthroscopy has been reported to increase the risk of postoperative septic arthritis. Its use may also mask the early stages of infection.[50]

D'Angelo and Ogilvie-Harris[9] performed a retrospective review of 4000 arthroscopic procedures with an overall deep infection rate of 0.23 per cent. Conclusions from their review were that there were no statistical risk factors for the development of septic arthritis after arthroscopic surgery. Pain, redness, and swelling in the first 2 weeks after operative arthroscopy are suggestive of infection. Prompt diagnosis and treatment with appropriate antibiotics, repeated arthroscopy, and placement of suction irrigation systems are successful. Antibiotic prophylaxis was believed to be cost beneficial in reducing the morbidity rate in arthroscopic surgery.

Thromboembolic Complications

Thromboembolic disease has been found to be a significant complication in arthroscopic surgery.[80] The 1986 AANA study[71] and the 1988 prospective study by Small[72] revealed that thromboembolic disease was the first (34 per cent) and third (7 per cent) most frequently reported complication in the two studies. Thrombosis was seen to occur in 0.1 to 3.2 per cent of arthroscopy patients. A tourniquet was used in eight of 12 cases. The average tourniquet time was 50 minutes with an average pressure of 350 mm Hg. Four pulmonary emboli were documented; none was fatal. In Sherman and associates' study,[68] no pulmonary emboli were noted. There is no conclusive evidence that the use of a tourniquet or various tourniquet pressures affect the incidence of thrombophlebitis during arthroscopic surgery.

Instrument Failures

With modern arthroscopic techniques and instruments, the incidence of instrument failure has been noted to range between 0.05 and 0.1 per cent.[59, 68, 71, 72] Instrument breakage was related to long operative procedures and occurred most often in arthroscopic partial lateral meniscectomy and meniscal repair.

Neurologic Injury

Complications such as RSD and injuries to the neurovascular structures around the knee have been relatively uncommon.[62, 68, 73] RSD occurred in 0.04 per cent of 10,282 patients.[71] One neurologic injury was to the saphenous nerve after medial meniscal repair. The reported incidence of neurologic injury is 0.4 to 1.6 per cent.[71, 72] All the neurologic problems in Sherman and associates' series[68] related to postoperative hyperesthesias or paresthesias in the distribution of the sartorial or infrapatellar branch of the saphenous nerve.

Complications in Arthroscopic Surgery by Procedure

From all data on arthroscopic procedures, it appears that diagnostic arthroscopy had the lowest overall complication rate: between 0.7 and 2.1 per cent.[11, 69, 71, 72] Arthroscopic surgical procedures had complication rates of 1.2 to 10 per cent. Lateral retinacular release (7 to 10 per cent), chondroplasty (5 to 10 per cent), and partial lateral meniscectomy (3 to 8 per cent) had the highest incidences of complications. A complication rate of 1.6 per cent was reported in 3874 meniscal procedures.[72, 73] The incidence of complications in arthroscopic meniscal repairs was surprisingly less (1.2 per cent). These complications included one case each of hemarthrosis, saphenous nerve injury, and instrument failure.

Unusual Complications

A case of resection of the patellar ligament during arthroscopic synovectomy was reported.[4] It was not recognized at the time of surgery but was detected 10 days later when the patient complained of anterior knee pain and inability to extend the knee. A patellar ligament reconstruction was required.

A report of gas gangrene after arthroscopic ACL repair revealed another severe complication that can occur.[39] Extensive fasciotomy, debridement, antibiotic therapy, and five sessions of hyperbaric oxygen in a pressure chamber resulted in a functionally intact extremity.

Extra-articular fluid dissections and pneumoscrotum have also been reported.[27, 51] The pneumoscrotum was thought to be caused by a loose connection of the collapsible plastic bags of saline on the inflow tubing. The air injected to the knee leaked into the subcutaneous tissue through multiple puncture sites. The pain produced by the condition was completely resolved in 7 days with no treatment.

Extra-articular fluid extravasation has a potential for decreasing the blood supply to the leg. Lack of joint distention, an increasing amount of fluid that produces distention of the joint, or increased thigh tension during arthroscopy indicates extravasation of fluid. Methods of preventing this complication include palpation of the thigh during the procedure, avoiding knee flexion past 30° to 45° with the knee fully distended, and an adequate outflow system. Excessive joint distention and increased fluid pressure can cause rupture of the suprapatellar pouch.[51]

Extravasation of fluid can also occur during arthroscopy in the presence of a capsular defect that allows fluid to escape into the calf.[19, 57] Precautions should be in effect in performing arthroscopy after acute trauma to the knee. Continuous monitoring both of the volume of irrigation fluid and of calf tension is necessary.

Prepatellar bursitis resulted from loss of an excised meniscal fragment into the subcutaneous tissue during an attempt at fragment extraction.[36] The fragment could be palpated 4 weeks later in the prepatellar bursa. Surgical removal with local anesthetic was required.

A fistula between the knee joint and the prepatellar bursa developed after an arthroscopic lateral release.[25] Recurrent effusion in the knee and prepatellar bursa had been present for 4 months after the arthroscopic surgery. A surgical closure of the edges of the bursa resolved the problem.

Vascular complications associated with arthroscopic procedures are rare, accounting for less than 1 per cent of all complications. Popliteal artery injury and venous aneurysm have been reported.[37, 76] Genicular artery injuries rarely occur. Two cases have been reported: one with a false aneurysm of the lateral inferior genicular artery, and one with a false aneurysm of the descending genicular artery.[79] The proximity of the genicular arteries to the joint line—particularly the lateral genicular artery—makes them vulnerable to injury during establishment of the portals of entry. Prompt resection of the false aneurysms produced excellent results.

Conclusions

According to the current literature, total complication rates in arthroscopic surgery range between 1.7 and 8 per cent. Hemarthrosis was the most frequent complication. Lateral retinacular release and partial medial meniscectomy (excluding arthroscopically assisted ligament procedures) had the highest complication rate. Statistical data have shown a higher incidence of complications in cases involving industrial injury. One study showed a lower risk of complications in patients less than 30 years old with tourniquet time of less than 40 minutes.[68] The use of a tourniquet by itself has no effect on the complication rate, but a tourniquet time of longer than 60 minutes places a patient statistically at a higher risk for development of complications.

One study suggested that surgical experience did not affect the complication rate.[68] In a study in 1986, Small[71] compared complications reported in a retrospective survey by the AANA with a prospective study reported in 1988.[72] Meniscal repair complications were reduced from 2.5 per cent in the 1986 study to 1.2 per cent in the 1988 report. This reduction was thought to be attributable to better educational efforts in describing the neurovascular structures around the knee and how to avoid injury to them.

COMPLICATIONS IN LIGAMENTOUS KNEE SURGERY

Complications of knee ligament surgery can be classified into general and intraoperative categories. The general group includes anesthetic complications, wound problems, deep venous thrombosis, RSD, and compartmental syndrome and neurovascular injuries. The intraoperative category relates to specific ligament reconstruction. Graft donor site complications, postoperative graft impingement, patellofemoral pain, quadriceps weakness, and growth plate injuries are involved.

Anesthetic Morbidity and Mortality

Rates of anesthesia-related mortality from ligament surgery of the knee are similar in arthroscopic and other open knee surgery in matched age and patient health groups. The literature indicates an anesthesia-related mortality rate of approximately 0.01 per cent.[16, 21, 44]

Hematoma and Hemarthrosis

A tourniquet is routinely used in knee ligament reconstruction procedures around the knee. The vascular anastomosis around the knee makes these structures vulnerable to injury from trauma or surgical exposure (Fig. 24–1). The lateral superior and inferior genicular arteries, the medial superior and inferior genicular arteries, and their communicating branches may be torn or cut during a necessary dissection for ligamentous repair and reconstruction. DeLee[11] and Patterson and Trickey[54] reported hemarthrosis

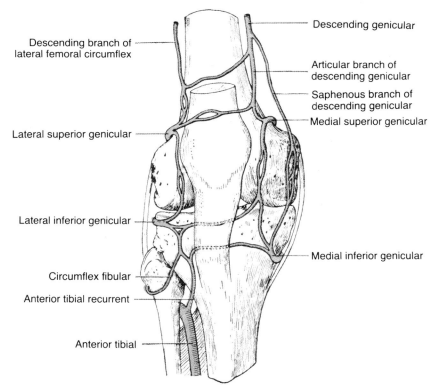

FIGURE 24–1. Anterior view of the knee showing the genicular arteries and their anastomoses. Note the position of the lateral inferior genicular artery at the joint line level. (From Gross CM [ed]: Gray's Anatomy of the Human Body, 29th ed. Philadelphia: Lea and Febiger, 1973.)

rates of 2 to 5 per cent in ACL reconstruction. For this reason, it is wise to use closed suction drainage in the immediate postoperative period in order to minimize the accumulation of blood in the knee joint or deep tissues. Suction drainage should be continued for no more than 48 hours after surgery.

Vascular Injuries

The incidence of vascular injuries in surgical reconstruction has been reported to be between 0 and 0.01 per cent.[11, 66, 72] If such injuries are recognized and repaired immediately, minimal residual disability will result. When both the popliteal vein and the popliteal artery have been injured, repair of the artery is the primary concern. The vein is frequently left unrepaired in the expectation that collateral return circulation will develop. This development may be a slow process, with a problem of recurrent edema of the leg when patients are on their feet for long periods.

Knee dislocation is the most frequent cause of vascular injuries about the knee; the incidence of popliteal artery injury is 32 per cent.[24, 42] Vascular lesions occur in 40 per cent of straight anterior or posterior dislocations. For vascular repairs performed within 8 hours of the injury, there is an 80 to 90 per cent rate of limb salvage. Irreversible changes occur after 6 to 8 hours of ischemia. Acute attention to vascular status and aggressive use of arteriography are recommended in order to prevent long-term vascular sequelae.[49]

An unusual vascular complication was reported after a synthetic ACL was placed in the over-the-top position.[63] The popliteal artery was found trapped between the ligamentous graft and the bone during exploration. A satisfactory result was obtained with bypass of the entrapped segment.

Tourniquet Complications

Complications from pneumatic tourniquet use during ligamentous knee surgery are tourniquet ischemia, paresthesias, and paralysis.[14, 62, 66] Delay in recovery of peripheral nerves after knee surgery may be attributable to a resolving compression syndrome caused by the pneumatic tourniquet.[62, 66] Studies have shown reduced conduction velocity at the site of the tourniquet with normal conduction velocities distal to the tourniquet. Histologic studies have shown demyelinization under the tourniquet areas. A study by Dobner and Nitz[14] showed electromyographic evidence of denervation and slight functional loss of the extremity during testing 6 weeks after medial or lateral meniscectomy. It is probable that long tourniquet times of more than 60 minutes caused some postoperative tourniquet nerve injury, although most such injuries have been transient in nature.

Wound Infections

The incidence of wound infections in open ACL reconstructions ranges from 0.3 to 12.5 per cent.[22, 29, 69] In one study,[66] six infections were reported among 390 cases; of these, three were deep infections. None occurred within the first 8 weeks after surgery. The organisms most often noted after ACL reconstruction surgery were *Staphylococcus aureus* and *Staphylococcus epidermidis*. After open wound debridement and intravenous administration of antibiotics, the infections resolved in all patients. Graf and Uhr[22] reported one superficial infection with no occurrences of postoperative septic arthritis in more than 100 ACL reconstructions. Data from two series of knee reconstructions show a decreased incidence of infection with perioperative antibiotic coverage.[9, 15] Prophylactic intravenous antibiotic therapy is recommended before knee ligament surgery.

Deep Venous Thrombosis

Deep venous thrombosis occurs in 0.75 to 3.5 per cent of all knee ligament reconstruction cases.[66] The incidence of thromboembolic disease that follows knee ligament surgery is less than that in total knee arthroplasty surgery. This is probably because the patients who undergo ligament surgery are generally younger and more active. Cases of pulmonary embolism after ACL reconstruction have been reported.[54] In view of the low rate of thrombophlebitis, prophylactic measures have not routinely been taken, and risk/benefit ratios may not warrant prophylaxis in the young patient before ligamentous surgery.

Reflex Sympathetic Dystrophy

RSD encompasses a large number of symptoms, including limb atrophy, osteoporosis, hypervascularity, and hypersensitivity to painful stimuli. A definition given by Schutzer and Gossling[67] is a "departure from the orderly and predictable response of an extremity to some form of internal or external trauma." It is manifested by four characteristics: (1) intense or unduly prolonged pain; (2) vasomotor disturbances; (3) delayed functional recovery; and (4) trophic changes that may include edema, atrophy, or fibrosis. Poehling and colleagues[58] suggested that the presence of two or more of these characteristics implies the presence of this clinical syndrome. RSD is usually associated with injuries involving soft tissues, with fractures, with long periods of immobilization, and with nerve injury. No definitive estimate of the incidence is available. A study of 3000 knee injuries by Tietjen[78] revealed that 27 patients had persistent complaints for which a diagnosis could not be established. Fourteen of the 27 had clinical and radiologic findings that were consistent with RSD of the knee.

Sensitivity to light touch, skin redness or mottling, atrophy around the knee joint, and increased temperatures (sometimes coolness) are important clinical findings. Thermography, bone scan, and a trial with sympathetic block can be useful for making the diagnosis. Osteoporosis is a radiographic characteristic of the disorder.[78]

Standard treatment of RSD consists of prolonged sympathetic blocks via epidural catheter, continuous passive motion, gentle physical therapy, and analgesics.[17, 41, 67, 78] Other treatments that have been suggested include corticosteroids, propranolol, electroacupuncture, and deep-friction massage.

The diagnosis of RSD requires a high index of suspicion. Studies have shown that patients with pain syndromes treated with vasoactive therapy (amitriptyline, reserpine, guanethidine, nifedipine, sympathetic block, and sympathectomy) within 1 year of onset have better results than those whose treatment begins after 1 year.[38, 58] RSD should be considered in any patient in whom the course of rehabilitation departs from an orderly and predictable pattern after injury or surgery.[58]

Nerve Injuries

Sensory branches around the knee may be injured by traction, compression from other structures, or cutting during the surgical exposure. Two sensory nerves on the medial side of the knee are particularly vulnerable: the infrapatellar and the sartorial branches of the saphenous nerve. The saphenous nerve lies beneath the sartorius muscle. As it passes between the sartorius muscle and the gracilis tendon, it gives off the infrapatellar branch, which travels anteriorly toward the tibial tubercle, and the sartorial branch, which travels distally to supply sensation to the medial aspect of the calf.

The infrapatellar branch may be cut by the surgical incision necessary to expose the structures on the medial aspect, or it may be traumatized so that a neuroma develops. Cutting the nerve results in loss of sensation to the anteromedial proximal aspect of the knee. Although this loss of sensation may be annoying to the patient, it produces no functional deficit and in time may be tolerated. If a neuroma develops, it becomes a source of persistent discomfort. An injection of a local anesthetic into the localized tender area helps in diagnosing the problem if relief is immediately produced. If a steroid injection does not resolve the pain, a surgical en bloc excision is required.

Poehling and colleagues[58] reported 35 cases of RSD, all of which had evidence of insult to the infrapatellar branch. They suggested that care be taken during arthroscopy to avoid injuring the nerve. Transillumination of the lateral joint line often shows the vein that runs parallel to the joint line. The nerve runs with this vein, and injury can be prevented by directing portals of entry away from the vein.

The sartorial branch is most often injured when exposure of the pes anserinus tendon is required. When the nerve is cut, numbness on the anteromedial aspect of the calf is produced. If the nerve becomes compressed by a pes anserinus transfer or by fibrous tissue, a localized painful area may develop. A surgical procedure to eliminate the nerve compression is required in order to alleviate the symptoms.

Other small sensory nerves may be injured by arthroscopic or surgical procedures about the knee. Symptoms vary from areas of exquisite tenderness (neuropraxia) to areas of loss of sensation. Localized injection of a mixture of steroid and local anesthetic may resolve the symptoms.

The peroneal nerve lies directly behind the fibular head in close proximity to the biceps tendon on the lateral side of the knee. During surgical procedures around this area, care should be taken to identify and protect the nerve from injury or traction. Excessive varus stress to the knee may cause injury that is often associated with rupture of the lateral collateral ligaments. Peroneal nerve injury is sometimes associated with fractures of the fibular head. Neuropraxic lesions begin to show recovery by 3 months. Exploration is not usually indicated before 3 months unless the associated injury requires a surgical correction. Resection of bruised nerve tissue and anastomosis of a cut nerve have a relatively poor prognosis. If the nerve is intact, neurolysis should be performed only if surgical exploration is required.

When a medial meniscal repair is performed at the same time as ACL reconstruction, the saphenous nerve is also at risk. In a survey of complications sponsored by the AANA, there were 73 complications in 3034 meniscal repairs, a complication rate of 2.5 per cent. There were 30 saphenous nerve injuries (1 per cent) in this series.[73]

Skin Necrosis

Postoperative hematoma and infection are the chief causes of wound dehiscence. Adequate hemostasis before wound closure and the use of a suction drain for the first 24 to 48 hours after surgery are the most helpful procedures in preventing a hematoma. Prophylactic antibiotic given intravenously at the beginning of surgery, irrigation with an antibiotic solution during surgery, and the use of intravenous antibiotics for 24 hours after surgery help to saturate any developing hematoma with the drugs.

Skin incisions from previous surgery need to be evaluated in subsequent surgical procedures. Blood flow to the skin may be diminished between close incisions. Incorporating the previous incision into the current incision or planning incisions that will provide skin flaps with adequate blood supply are the techniques necessary for preventing necrosis.

COMPLICATIONS RELATING TO ACL SURGERY

Limitation of knee motion, patellofemoral pain, and quadriceps weakness have been designated as the most frequent complications that occur after ACL surgery. Sachs and collaborators[65] showed a strong interrelationship among the three. They surmised that flexion contracture caused patellofemoral irritability and that either or both in combination resulted in quadriceps weakness.

Limitation of Knee Motion

Limited knee motion is the single most frequent cause of postoperative problems with knee ligament reconstruction. It may be caused by any one or a combination of prolonged immobilization, technical problems relating to graft placement or tensioning, development of arthrofibrosis, infection, or RSD.

Arthrofibrosis and the infrapatellar contracture syndrome have been described by Paulos and co-workers[56] and others.[20, 22, 26, 29, 66, 74] Arthrofibrosis can occur in the intercondylar notch, the suprapatellar pouch, or the intracondylar and supracondylar region. Various authors who have described this problem have shown that it occurs in open and arthroscopic ACL reconstructions.

The incidence of limited knee motion is 7 to 32 per cent of the cases reported in the literature.[13, 22, 26, 29, 69] Flexion contracture is defined as a lack of full extension to within 10° or limitation of flexion to less than

130°. Open surgery and surgery performed within the first week after injury increase the risk of postoperative limitation of motion, according to Graf and associates.[23]

Among patients who underwent ACL reconstructions and were immobilized first for 3 weeks in 30° of flexion and then for 3 to 5 weeks in a hinged cast or brace with a 30° extension stop, there was a 29 per cent incidence of flexion contracture of more than 5° one year after surgery. This incidence was decreased from 32 to 11 per cent by immobilization in full extension for 10 to 14 days after surgery in patients for whom the patellar tendon was the graft source. Among patients with hamstring tendon grafts, the incidence was reduced from 24 to 0 per cent with this treatment.[66]

The use of continuous passive motion has provided varying degrees of success in preventing limited motion. Graf and Uhr[22] believed that its use provided a decrease in the number of patients requiring manipulation or surgery after ACL reconstruction. Sachs and collaborators[66] believed that its use does not play much of a role in postoperative rehabilitation.

Harner and colleagues[26] reported an 11.1 per cent incidence of limited knee motion after ACL reconstruction. The suggested risk factors included being male, undergoing ACL reconstruction less than 1 month after injury, and undergoing a concurrent extra-articular procedure.

Ligamentous surgery performed within 1 to 4 weeks after initial injury has been implicated by other authors as a risk factor in producing limited motion.[23, 75] The inflammatory response after an acute injury, coupled with the healing response to the surgical procedure, was incriminated as the reason for the increase.

Early recognition and appropriate treatment are the key factors in preventing long-term effects of limited motion. There is a trend toward initial immobilization in full extension if immobilization is used at all. Preferably, early protected motion is instituted in all patients with ACL reconstructions. If a surgical procedure is required, the timing is critical. It may be necessary to provide treatment for reducing inflammation and increasing quadriceps strength before surgical release and debridement of fibrotic tissue can be considered. For a 15° flexion contracture 6 weeks after surgery, either arthroscopic or open lysis of adhesions should be considered if the qualifications just described have been met and the patient is not responding to knee and patellar mobilization techniques or other nonoperative stretching methods such as the drop-out cast (Fig. 24–2), desubluxation hinged casts (Fig. 24–3), or dynamic extension brace (Fig. 24–4).

Patellofemoral Pain

The incidence of patellofemoral pain and patellar tendinitis after ACL reconstruction with the central third of the patellar tendon has been high in the postoperative period.[29, 65, 66] A review by Sachs and collaborators[66] of 126 patients revealed a 19 per cent incidence of patellofemoral pain 1 year after surgery. Of 36 patients who had a normal patellofemoral joint at surgery, only one third had a normal patellofemoral finding on clinical examination 1 year later. Patellar tendinitis can also occur during the rehabilitation period. These symptoms can correlate with aggressive pro-

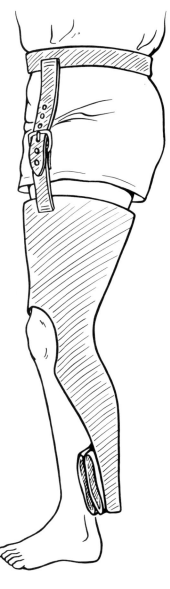

FIGURE 24–2. Drop-out cast (MacIntosh): With control of the upper thigh, the tibia can be wedged into extension by placing pads between the distal tibia and posterior shell of the cast. Gradually increasing the thickness of the felt wedges provides low forces over a long period of time. The patient is able to walk with this cast. (Modified from Paulos LE, Rosenberg TD, Drawbert J, et al: Infrapatellar contracture syndrome: an unrecognized cause of knee stiffness with patella entrapment and patella infera. Am J Sports Med 15:331–341, 1987.)

gressive resistance exercises. Graf and Uhr[22] found that 6 per cent of patients complained of parapatellar pain. These symptoms generally resolve with rest, anti-inflammatory agents, and eccentric quadriceps exercise programs. A common complaint is pain in kneeling on the donor graft site for prolonged periods of time.

Other long-term patellofemoral problems such as patellar fracture[47] (see Fig. 24–5) and patellar tendon rupture[6] have been reported in the literature, although they are unusual.

Quadriceps Weakness

Weakness of the quadriceps muscle, defined as strength of less than 80 per cent of that of the opposite leg, was present 1 year after surgery in 65

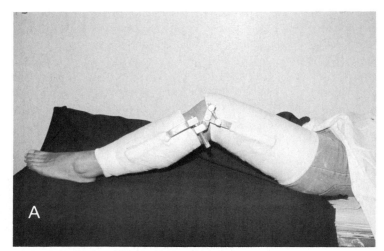

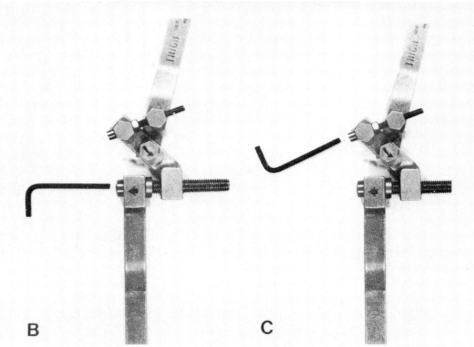

FIGURE 24–3. *(A)* An extension-desubluxation hinge. This is incorporated into a plaster thigh cuff and a lower leg cylinder. *(B)* Tightening of the distal threads pulls the proximal tibia forward. *(C)* Tightening of the proximal threads extends the knee. (From Larson RL: Complications of dislocations and ligamentous injuries. *In* Epps CH [ed]: Complications in Orthopaedic Surgery, 2nd ed, p. 562. Philadelphia: JB Lippincott, 1986.)

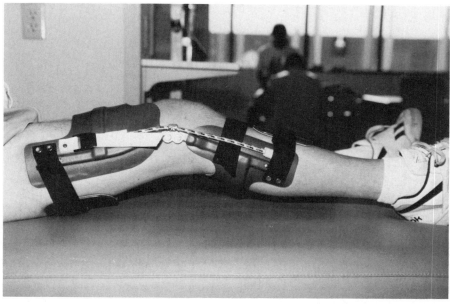

FIGURE 24–4. Dynamic extension brace used to provide an anterior pull on the proximal tibia for flexion contracture. The elastic strap can be adjusted to provide more anterior tibial force as required by degree of flexion contracture. (Courtesy of B. Lantz. Brace is MKSII PCL orthosis manufactured by Vixie Enterprises, Eugene, Oregon.)

per cent of 126 patients who had undergone ACL reconstructive surgery, according to the study by Sachs and collaborators.[66] This weakness was shown to be more pronounced in patients whose donor site was the patellar tendon than in patients who had hamstring grafts. In a comparison of allografts as the donor tissue with autografts,[28] 68 per cent of patients in the allograft group were asymptomatic and had 80 per cent or more of quadriceps strength. Of the autograft group, only 20 per cent had attained 80 per cent quadriceps strength. Of this group, 60 per cent also had discomfort at the donor site or patellofemoral discomfort.

COMPLICATIONS RELATED TO GRAFT SELECTION

Synthetic

The most frequent complications encountered with synthetic grafts are acute and chronic effusions associated with certain grafts. These effusions tend to subside after several months' duration.[30] Breakage can occur and is often related to impingement of the graft upon the bony tunnels and intercondylar notch areas of the femur. Four-year results have shown an average failure rate of the Gore-Tex graft of approximately 34 per cent.[18, 30, 55] Other synthetic grafts such as the Leeds-Keio graft and the Stryker Medox polyester (Dacron) ligament have shown similar rates of breakage. Particulate deposition in the synovium of the knee joint has been associated with wear and breakage of synthetic grafts.[30, 52, 64] This has been of particular concern in the use of the carbon fiber–augmented prosthesis.[52, 53]

Allograft

Different types of allograft tissues have been used for ligament reconstruction about the knee, including freeze-dried fascia lata, the Achilles tendon, and patellar tendon with bone. Freeze drying and ethylene oxide sterilization have insignificant effects on the initial mechanical properties of ligament-bone allografts. Reduced pull-out load has been recorded after ethylene oxide sterilization.[33] There may be reduced or delayed osteogenesis associated with ethylene oxide sterilized bone.[33, 46] Residual ethylene oxide in tendon allografts has also caused a reactive synovitis, as reported by Roberts and co-workers[60] and Jackson and associates.[34]

One of the main theoretical detriments to the use of allografts is the possible transmission of viral diseases such as hepatitis and the human immunodeficiency virus (HIV).[7, 33, 34, 45] The risk of transmitting HIV with bone and soft tissue allografts is extremely low with the use of fresh-frozen or freeze-dried allografts.[7] Safeguards regarding donor selection, HIV screening, and hepatitis screening have reduced the risks. Risk of transmission of HIV infection with an allograft has been calculated to be less than one in 1 million if all current laboratory techniques are used to exclude potentially infected persons from the donor pool.[7] A single case of transmission of HIV has been reported by the Centers for Disease Control through bone transplantation. The allograft was obtained from a living donor who had acquired immunodeficiency syndrome (AIDS) at the time of transplantation. This procedure was performed before 1985, when current standards of screening were not in effect.[46] The virus is not killed by freeze-drying, washing, or freezing. Sterilization with ionizing radiation in low doses may not be effective because many retroviruses are radioresistant.[33, 34, 45]

A weak immune response has been shown to occur in a small percentage of allograft patients. Some theoretical data have suggested that hypervascularization and weakening of soft tissue allografts could potentially occur after a period of several months in vivo.[31]

Graft Harvest

PATELLAR TENDON, BONE–TENDON–BONE. Patellar fractures, both acute and chronic stress fractures,[47] have been mentioned in several case reports (Fig. 24–5). Avoidance of making bone plugs too deep and beveling edges of the patella may help to decrease the incidence of this problem.

SEMITENDINOSUS HARVESTING. The harvest of hamstring tendons for ligament reconstruction may cause injury to the infrapatellar or sartorial branch of the saphenous nerve. This can be avoided through awareness of where the nerve is in relation to the tendon of the semitendinosus muscle.[40]

TECHNICAL COMPLICATIONS

Graft Impingement

Impingement is a complication of ligament reconstruction that can cause limitation of motion or abrasion of the graft, resulting in weakness and

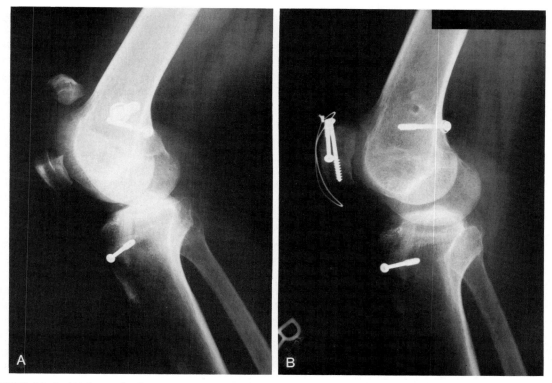

FIGURE 24–5. *(A)* A patellar fracture occurred in a 20-year-old white male 1 year after anterior cruciate ligament reconstruction with the central third of the patellar tendon. While fishing, he fell directly onto his knee, sustaining this midportion transverse patellar fracture. *(B)* This fracture was treated by tension band fixation technique. The patient achieved full recovery without pain.

disruption.[13, 20, 22, 29] Graft impingement may be caused by inappropriate placement of the tibial or femoral tunnel. Care must be taken not to place the tibial tunnel too far laterally. Notchplasty should be performed when required, but overaggressive notchplasty should be avoided. Removal of the normal weight-bearing articular surface of the lateral femoral condyle or aggressive superior notchplasties may cause scarring, crepitus, and early degenerative changes in the patellofemoral joint.

Femoral tunnel placement affects the tension and isometry of the graft. Care must be taken to avoid an angle in the femoral tunnel that does not leave bone stock adequate for holding fixation of the femoral portion of the graft. Anterior placement of a femoral graft results in increased tension of the graft in flexion. Posterior placement of the graft results in nonisometric placement of the reconstruction, causing excessive tightening in extension.[70] Nonisometric placement of the graft may result in plastic deformation, loss of motion, and increased intra-articular joint pressures during motion.

Abrasion at Tunnel Sites

Abrasion at tibial and femoral tunnel sites can cause wear and rupture of the graft. This is a well-described entity with synthetic type grafts.[18, 55] Care should be taken to align tibial and femoral bone tunnels in as much a linear fashion as possible. Chamfering of the posterior portion of the tibial tunnel and anterior portion of the femoral tunnel or smoothing the posterolateral groove when an over-the-top technique is used is necessary for minimizing abrasion of the graft. When interference type screws are used, care should be taken to place the screws so that they do not advance beyond the bony portion of the graft material. The screw should be placed so that the tips do not impinge upon the graft when the knee is flexed.

Graft Fixation

The adequacy of fixation of the graft should be evaluated in the operating room before the incision is closed. Several fixation techniques have been used and include sutures tied over buttons, sutures tied around screw posts, Kurosaka screws with interference fit, and staples.[10, 61] Published studies concerning pull-out strengths of all of these devices show that the double-back staple method, as discussed by Robertson and colleagues,[61] and Kurosaka interference screws provide the most rigid fixation.[3, 13] Large, nonabsorbable sutures tied around screw posts or ligament washers have also been shown to be effective. The most important factor is that secure rigid fixation is accomplished intraoperatively. Loss of fixation of the graft has been described with the use of an interference screw that was placed in divergence from the bone plug. The use of guide wires with cannulated screws may alleviate this problem. Breakage of the metal fixation with migration of metal fragments has also been reported.[77]

COMPLICATIONS IN TREATING LIGAMENT INJURIES IN THE ADOLESCENT WITH OPEN PHYSES

Adolescent athletes have shown that they are capable of sustaining significant ligamentous injuries to the knee.[1, 8, 12, 43, 48] The most common are midsubstance and tibial avulsion to the ACL.[1, 8, 12, 43] These younger patients experience a significant number of meniscal tears, the majority of which are reparable.[48] Complication rates for meniscal repair in adolescent patients are usually lower and healing rates are higher than in older patients. As with any meniscal repair, care must be taken to isolate and avoid injuring neurovascular structures around the knee.

Reconstruction of the ACL in adolescents has been investigated. McCarroll and associates' series[48] of 24 reconstructions showed no growth disturbances after a follow-up interval of more than 2 years, even with femoral and tibial drill holes. Lipscomb and Anderson[43] also drilled across both the femoral and tibial epiphyses and reported only one growth disturbance, which they attributed to a technical error of stapling both tibial and femoral epiphyses. They no longer use staples. Henning (quoted by McCarroll and associates[48]) reported a series of 33 ACL reconstructions in patients with open growth plates; there was one growth abnormality in the distal lateral femoral physis that caused significant genu valgum. Henning changed his approach to one of using an over-the-top procedure, taking precautions when using a notchplasty and drilling across the epiphysis. A growth disturbance rate of 1 to 3 per cent occurs when both tibial and femoral drill holes are used. In most of these series, no intra-articular reconstructions were used until the growth plates had begun to blur and started to close. On the basis of the possible consequences of a significant leg length discrepancy or angular deformity in the younger adolescent or child, intra-articular reconstruction with tibial and femoral drill holes should be delayed when possible until growth plates begin to close.

SUMMARY

Major complications that cause significant morbidity or even death do occur with ligament reconstruction procedures. Anesthetic complications and postoperative complications such as thromboembolism and pulmonary embolus are significant medical problems that must be addressed both pre- and postoperatively. Deep infection with any type of knee surgery may have disastrous complications. These complications are infrequent. With careful preoperative screening and continued intra- and postoperative planning, the incidence of these severe complications will decrease.

Minor complications and persistent problems after significant knee surgery, such as lack of appropriate joint position sense, poor range of motion, and persistent pain, continue to occur. Arthroscopic knee surgery, although seemingly innocuous, has been shown to have significant consequences even when performed by experienced arthroscopists. With complication rates ranging from 2 to 8 per cent, arthroscopy is a procedure that requires careful attention to detail. Technical considerations with cruciate ligament reconstruction and improvements in education continue to bring complication rates in this type of surgery down. The advent of rigid fixation and of early motion in all types of knee surgery has helped decrease morbidity and lessen the frequency of some complications.

REFERENCES

1. Angel KR, Hall DJ: Anterior cruciate ligament injury in children and adolescents. Arthroscopy 5:192–196, 1989.
2. Aritomi H, Yamamoto M: A method of arthroscopic surgery: clinical evaluation of synovectomy with electric resectoscope and removal of loose bodies in the knee joint. Orthop Clin North Am 10:565–584, 1979.
3. Bach BR Jr: Potential pitfalls of Kurosaka screw interference fixation for ACL surgery. Am J Knee Surg 2:76–82, 1989.
4. Bachner E, Parker R, Zaas R: Resection of the patellar ligament: a complication of arthroscopic synovectomy. Arthroscopy 5:76–78, 1989.
5. Berhang AM: Clostridium pyoarthrosis following arthroscopic surgery. Arthroscopy 3:56–58, 1987.
6. Bonamo J, Krinick RM, Sporn AA: Rupture of the patellar ligament after use of its central third for anterior cruciate reconstruction. J Bone Joint Surg 66A:1294–1297, 1984.
7. Buck BE, Malinin TI, Brown MD: Bone transplantation and human immunodeficiency virus: an estimate of risk of acquired immunodeficiency syndrome (AIDS). Clin Orthop 240:129–136, 1989.
8. Clanton TO, DeLee JC, Sanders B, et al: Knee ligament injuries in children. J Bone Joint Surg 61A:1195–1201, 1979.
9. D'Angelo GL, Ogilvie-Harris DJ: Septic arthritis following arthroscopy with cost/benefit analysis of antibiotic prophylaxis. J Arthroscopic Rel Surg 4:10–14, 1988.
10. Daniel DM: Principles of knee ligament surgery. *In* Daniel DM, Akeson WA, O'Connor JJ (eds): Knee Ligaments: Structure, Function, Injury, and Repair, pp. 11–29. New York: Raven Press, 1990.
11. DeLee JC: Complications of arthroscopy and arthroscopic surgery: results of a national survey. Arthroscopy 1:214–220, 1985.

12. DeLee JC, Curtis R: Anterior cruciate ligament insufficiency in children. Clin Orthop 172:112–118, 1983.

13. Diefendorf DR, Friedman MJ: Arthroscopic anterior cruciate ligament reconstruction: an overview. *In* Sherman OH, Minkoff J (eds): Arthroscopic Surgery. Baltimore: Williams & Wilkins, 1990.

14. Dobner JJ, Nitz AJ: Post-meniscectomy tourniquet palsy and functional sequelae. Am J Sports Med 10:211–214, 1982.

15. Eltham RD: Clean air operating environment and superficial infection. *In* Utoff H (ed): Current Concepts of Infection in Orthopaedics, pp. 33–37. Berlin: Springer-Verlag, 1985.

16. Epstein RM: Morbidity and mortality from anesthesia: a continuing problem. Anesthesiology 4:388–389, 1978.

17. Ficat R, Hungerford D: Disorders of the Patello-Femoral Joint, pp. 149–169. Baltimore: William & Wilkins, 1977.

18. Fox JM, Karzel RP, Diefendorf DR, et al: Four year experience with Gore-Tex prosthetic ligament in ACL deficient knees. *Presented at* the 57th annual meeting of the American Association of Orthopaedic Surgeons, New Orleans, February 1990.

19. Fruengaard S, Holm A: Compartment syndrome complications in arthroscopy surgery: brief report. J Bone Joint Surg 70B:146–147, 1988.

20. Fullerton LR Jr, Andrews JR: Mechanical block to extension following augmentation of the anterior cruciate ligament: case report. Am J Sports Med 12:166–169, 1984.

21. Goldstein A Jr, Keats AS: The risk of anesthesia. Anesthesiology 33:130–141, 1970.

22. Graf B, Uhr F: Complications of intra-articular anterior cruciate reconstruction. Clin Sports Med 7:835–848, 1988.

23. Graf BK, Ott JW, Lange RH, et al: Risk Factors for Restricted Motion After Anterior Cruciate Reconstruction: A Retrospective Study of 323 Patients. *Presented at* the 58th annual meeting of the American Association of Orthopaedic Surgeons, Anaheim, CA, March 1991.

24. Green NE, Allen BL: Vascular injuries associated with dislocation of the knee. J Bone Joint Surg 59A:236–239, 1977.

25. Hadied A: An unusual complication of arthroscopy: a fistula between the knee and prepatellar bursa. Case report. J Bone Joint Surg 66A:624, 1984.

26. Harner CD, Fu JH, Irrgang JJ, et al: Loss of Knee Motion Following Arthroscopic Anterior Cruciate Ligament Reconstruction. *Presented at* the 58th annual meeting of the American Association of Orthopaedic Surgeons, Anaheim, CA, March 1991.

27. Henderson C, Hopson C: Pneumoscrotum as a complication of arthroscopy. J Bone Joint Surg 64A:1238–1240, 1982.

28. Huegel M, Indelicato PA: Trends in rehabilitation following anterior cruciate reconstruction. Clin Sports Med 7:801–811, 1988.

29. Hughston J: Complications of anterior cruciate ligament surgery. Orthop Clin North Am 16:237–240, 1985.

30. Indelicato P, Woods GA, Prevot TJ, et al: The Gore-Tex Anterior Cruciate Ligament Prosthesis: Two Versus Three Year Results. *Presented at* the 57th annual meeting of the American Association of Orthopaedic Surgeons, New Orleans, February 1990.

31. Jackson D: The Future of Ligament Reconstruction. AAOS Continuing Education Course, ACL-PCL, Rancho Mirage, CA, December 1990.

32. Jackson DW, Grood ES, Arnoczky SP, et al: Freeze dried anterior cruciate ligament allografts: preliminary studies in a goat model. Am J Sports Med 15:295–303, 1987.

33. Jackson DW, Grood ES, Wilcox P, et al: The effects of processing techniques on the mechanical properties of bone–anterior cruciate ligament–bone allografts: an experimental study in goats. Am J Sports Med 16:101–105, 1988.

34. Jackson DW, Windler GE, Simon TM: Intra-articular reaction associated with the use of freeze-dried, ethylene oxide sterilized bone–patellar tendon–bone allografts in the reconstruction of the anterior cruciate ligament. Am J Sports Med 18:1–11, 1989.

35. Jackson RW, Dandy DJ: Arthroscopy of the Knee. New York: Grune and Stratton, 1976.

36. Janecki C, Hechtman K: Prepatellar bursitis: a complication of arthroscopic surgery of the knee due to a lost meniscal fragment. Arthroscopy 5:342–343, 1989.

37. Jimenez F, Utrilla A, Cuesta C, et al: Popliteal artery and venous aneurysm as a complication of arthroscopic meniscectomy. J Trauma 28:1404–1405, 1988.

38. Katz MM, Hungerford DS: Reflex sympathetic dystrophy affecting the knee. J Bone Joint Surg 69B:797–803, 1987.

39. Ketterle R, Beckurts T, Kovacs J, et al: Gas-gangrene following arthroscopic surgery: arthroscopy. J Arthroscop Rel Surg 5:79–83, 1989.

40. Kummell BM, Zazaris GA: Preservation of infrapatellar branch of saphenous nerve during knee surgery. Orthop Rev 43:45, 1974.

41. Lankford LL, Thompson JE: Reflex sympathetic dystrophy, upper and lower extremity: diagnosis and management. Instructional Course Lectures AAOS 26:163–178, 1977.

42. Larson RL: Complications of dislocations and ligamentous injuries. *In* Epps CH Jr (ed): Complications in Orthopaedic Surgery, 2nd ed, pp. 557–584. Philadelphia: JB Lippincott, 1986.

43. Lipscomb B, Anderson A: Tears of the anterior cruciate ligament in adolescents. J Bone Joint Surg 68A:19–28, 1986.
44. Lunn JN, Hunter AR, Scott DB: Anaesthesia related surgical mortality. Anaesthesia 38:1090–1096, 1983.
45. Malinin T: Preparation and banking of bone and tendon allografts. *In* Sherman OH, Minkoff J (eds): Arthroscopic Surgery. Baltimore: Williams & Wilkins, 1990.
46. Manning JB, Meyers JF: Allograft anterior cruciate ligament reconstruction: technique and pitfalls. *In* Sherman OH, Minkoff J (eds): Arthroscopic Surgery. Baltimore: Williams & Wilkins, 1990.
47. McCarroll JR: Fracture of the patella during a golf swing following reconstruction of the anterior cruciate ligament: a case report. Am J Sports Med 11:26–27, 1983.
48. McCarroll JR, Rettig AC, Shelbourne KD: Anterior cruciate ligament injuries in the young athlete with open physes. Am J Sports Med 16:44–47, 1988.
49. McCoy GF, Hannon DG, Barr RJ, Templeton J: Vascular injury associated with low velocity dislocations of the knee. J Bone Joint Surg 69B:285–287, 1987.
50. Montgomery SC, Campbell J: Septic arthritis following arthroscopy and intra-articular steroids. J Bone Joint Surg 71B:540, 1989.
51. Noyes FR, Spievack ES: Extraarticular fluid dissection in tissues during arthroscopy: a report of clinical cases and a study of intraarticular and thigh pressures in cadavers. Am J Sports Med 10:346–351, 1982.
52. Olson EJ, Kang JD, Fu FH, et al: The biochemical and histological effects of artificial ligament wear particles: *in vitro* and *in vivo* studies. Am J Sports Med 16:558–570, 1988.
53. Parsons JR, Byani S, Alexander H, et al: Carbon fiber debris within the synovial joint: time dependent mechanical and histological studies. Orthop Transac 7:246, 1983.
54. Patterson FWN, Trickey EL: Anterior cruciate reconstruction using part of the patellar tendon as a free graft. J Bone Joint Surg 68B:453–457, 1986.
55. Paulos LE, Rosenberg TD, Tearse DS, Grewe SR: Gore-Tex Prosthetic ACL Reconstruction: A Long-Term Follow-Up. *Presented at* the 57th annual meeting of the American Association of Orthopaedic Surgeons, New Orleans, February 1990.
56. Paulos LE, Rosenberg TD, Drawbert J, et al: Infrapatellar contracture syndrome: an unrecognized cause of knee stiffness with patella entrapment and patella infera. Am J Sports Med 15:331–341, 1987.
57. Peek RD, Haynes PW: Compartment syndrome as a complication of arthroscopy: a case report and a study of interstitial pressures. Am J Sports Med 12:464–468, 1984.
58. Poehling GG, Pollock FE Jr, Korman LA: Reflex sympathetic dystrophy of the knee after sensory nerve injury. Arthroscopy 4:31–35, 1988.
59. Rames R, Fox J, Del Pizzo W: Arthroscopy—"No Problem Surgery": A Follow-Up Analysis of Complications of the Next 2739 cases. *Presented at* Specialty Day Arthroscopic Association of North America, 58th annual meeting of the American Association of Orthopaedic Surgeons, Anaheim, CA, March 1991.
60. Roberts TS, Drez D, McCarthy W, et al: Anterior cruciate ligament reconstruction using freeze-dried, ethylene oxide sterilized bone–patellar tendon–bone allografts: two year results in 36 patients. Am J Sports Med 19:35–41, 1991.
61. Robertson D, Daniel D, Biden E: Soft tissue fixation to bone. Am J Sports Med 14:398–403, 1986.
62. Rorabeck CH, Kennedy JC: Tourniquet-induced nerve ischemia complicating knee ligament surgery. Am J Sports Med 8:98–102, 1980.
63. Roth JH, Bray RC: Popliteal artery injury during anterior cruciate ligament reconstruction: brief report. J Bone Joint Surg 70B:840, 1988.
64. Roth JH, Shkrum MJ, Bray RC: Synovial reaction associated with disruption of polypropylene braid-augmented intra-articular anterior cruciate ligament reconstruction: a case report. Am J Sports Med 16:301–305, 1988.
65. Sachs RA, Daniel DM, Stone ML, Garfein RF: Patello-femoral problems after ACL reconstruction. Am J Sports Med 17:760–766, 1989.
66. Sachs RA, Reznik A, Daniel DM, Stone ML: Complications of knee ligament surgery. *In* Daniel DM (ed): Knee Ligaments: Structure, Function, Injury, and Repair, pp. 505–520. New York: Raven Press, 1990.
67. Schutzer S, Gossling H: The treatment of reflex sympathetic dystrophy syndrome. J Bone Joint Surg 66A:625–629, 1984.
68. Sherman OH, Fox JM, Snyder SJ, et al: Arthroscopy—"no problem surgery." J Bone Joint Surg 68A:256–265, 1986.
69. Sherman OH, Minkoff J: Complications of arthroscopic anterior cruciate ligament technique. *In* Sherman OH, Minkoff J (eds): Arthroscopic Surgery. Baltimore: Williams & Wilkins, 1990.
70. Siegel MG, Grood E, Hefzy S, et al: Analysis and placement of the anterior cruciate ligament substitute. Orthop Transac 8:69, 1984.
71. Small NC: Complications in arthroscopy: the knee and other joints. Arthroscopy 2:253–258, 1986.

72. Small NC: Complications in arthroscopic surgery performed by experienced arthroscopists. Arthroscopy 4:215–221, 1988.
73. Small NC: Complications in arthroscopic meniscal surgery. Clin Sports Med 9:609–617, 1990.
74. Sprague N, O'Connor R, Fox J: Arthroscopic treatment of post-operative knee arthrofibrosis. Clin Orthop 166:165–172, 1982.
75. Strum GM, Friedman MJ, Fox JM, et al: Acute anterior cruciate ligament reconstruction: analysis of complications. Clin Orthop 253:184–189, 1990.
76. Tawes RL, Etheredge SN, Webb RL, et al: Popliteal artery injury complicating arthroscopic meniscectomy. Am J Surg 156:136–138, 1988.
77. Thomson JD, Talbert CJ, Jackson IP: Late breakage of orthopaedic stapling causing peroneal nerve palsy. Am J Sports Med 18:109–111, 1990.
78. Tietjen R: Reflex sympathetic dystrophy of the knee. Clin Orthop 209:234–243, 1986.
79. Vincent GM, Stanish WD: False aneurysm after arthroscopic meniscectomy. J Bone Joint Surg 72A:770, 1990.
80. Walker RH, Dellingham M: Thrombophlebitis following arthroscopic surgery of the knee. Contemp Orthop 6:29–33, 1983.

Index